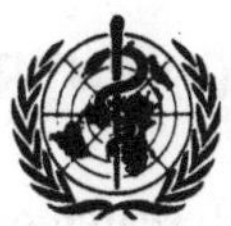

WORLD HEALTH ORGANIZATION

INTERNATIONAL AGENCY FOR RESEARCH ON CANCER

IARC MONOGRAPHS

ON THE

EVALUATION OF CARCINOGENIC RISKS TO HUMANS

Some Chemicals that Cause Tumours of the Kidney or Urinary Bladder in Rodents and Some Other Substances

VOLUME 73

This publication represents the views and expert opinions
of an IARC Working Group on the
Evaluation of Carcinogenic Risks to Humans,
which met in Lyon,

13–20 October 1998

1999

IARC MONOGRAPHS

In 1969, the International Agency for Research on Cancer (IARC) initiated a programme on the evaluation of the carcinogenic risk of chemicals to humans involving the production of critically evaluated monographs on individual chemicals. The programme was subsequently expanded to include evaluations of carcinogenic risks associated with exposures to complex mixtures, life-style factors and biological agents, as well as those in specific occupations.

The objective of the programme is to elaborate and publish in the form of monographs critical reviews of data on carcinogenicity for agents to which humans are known to be exposed and on specific exposure situations; to evaluate these data in terms of human risk with the help of international working groups of experts in chemical carcinogenesis and related fields; and to indicate where additional research efforts are needed.

The lists of IARC evaluations are regularly updated and are available on Internet: http://www.iarc.fr/.

This project was supported by Cooperative Agreement 5 UO1 CA33193 awarded by the United States National Cancer Institute, Department of Health and Human Services. Additional support has been provided since 1986 by the European Commission, since 1993 by the United States National Institute of Environmental Health Sciences and since 1995 by the United States Environmental Protection Agency through Cooperative Agreement Assistance CR 824264.

©International Agency for Research on Cancer, 1999

Distributed by IARC*Press* (Fax: +33 4 72 73 83 02; E-mail: press@iarc.fr)
and by the World Health Organization Distribution and Sales, CH-1211 Geneva 27.
(Fax: +41 22 791 4857)

Publications of the World Health Organization enjoy copyright protection in accordance with the provisions of Protocol 2 of the Universal Copyright Convention.
All rights reserved. Application for rights of reproduction or translation, in part or *in toto*, should be made to the International Agency for Research on Cancer.

IARC Library Cataloguing in Publication Data

Some chemicals that cause tumours of the kidney or urinary bladder in rodents and some other substances /
IARC Working Group on the Evaluation of Carcinogenic Risks to Humans (1999 : Lyon, France).

(IARC monographs on the evaluation of carcinogenic risks to humans ; 73)

1. Urologic neoplasms – congresses 2. Kidney neoplasms – congresses
I. IARC Working Group on the Evaluation of Carcinogenic Risks to Humans
II. Series

ISBN 92 832 1273 8 (NLM Classification: W1)
ISSN 1017-1606

PRINTED IN FRANCE

CONTENTS

NOTE TO THE READER

The term 'carcinogenic risk' in the *IARC Monographs* series is taken to mean the probability that exposure to an agent will lead to cancer in humans.

Inclusion of an agent in the *Monographs* does not imply that it is a carcinogen, only that the published data have been examined. Equally, the fact that an agent has not yet been evaluated in a monograph does not mean that it is not carcinogenic.

The evaluations of carcinogenic risk are made by international working groups of independent scientists and are qualitative in nature. No recommendation is given for regulation or legislation.

Anyone who is aware of published data that may alter the evaluation of the carcinogenic risk of an agent to humans is encouraged to make this information available to the Unit of Carcinogen Identification and Evaluation, International Agency for Research on Cancer, 150 cours Albert Thomas, 69372 Lyon Cedex 08, France, in order that the agent may be considered for re-evaluation by a future Working Group.

Although every effort is made to prepare the monographs as accurately as possible, mistakes may occur. Readers are requested to communicate any errors to the Unit of Carcinogen Identification and Evaluation, so that corrections can be reported in future volumes.

IARC WORKING GROUP ON THE EVALUATION OF CARCINOGENIC RISKS TO HUMANS: SOME CHEMICALS THAT CAUSE TUMOURS OF THE KIDNEY OR URINARY BLADDER IN RODENTS AND SOME OTHER SUBSTANCES

Lyon, 13–20 October 1998

LIST OF PARTICIPANTS

Members[1]

S.J. Borghoff, Chemical Industry Institute of Toxicology, PO Box 12137, Research Triangle Park, NC 27709, United States

G. Brambilla, Department of Internal Medicine, University of Genoa, viale Benedetto XV, 2, 16132 Genoa, Italy

T.E. Bunton, Division of Comparative Medicine, School of Medicine, Johns Hopkins University, 456 Ross Research Building, 720 Rutland Avenue, Baltimore, MD 21205, United States

C.C. Capen, The Ohio State University, Department of Veterinary Biosciences, 1925 Coffey Road Columbus, OH 43210, United States (*Chairman*)

S.M. Cohen, University of Nebraska Medical Center, Department of Pathology and Microbiology, 98135 Nebraska Medical Center, Omaha, NE 68198-3135, United States

L. Fishbein, 4320 Ashford Lane, Fairfax, VA 22032, United States

S. Fukushima, Department of Pathology, Osaka City University Medical School, 1-4-3 Asahi-machi, Abeno-ku, Osaka 545 8585, Japan

M. Gérin, University of Montréal, Department of Occupational and Environmental Health, Faculty of Medicine, CP 6128—Station A, Montreal, Québec H3C 3J7, Canada

G.C. Hard, American Health Foundation, 1 Dana Road, Valhalla, NY 10595, United States

M. Hayashi, Division of Genetics and Mutagenesis, National Institute of Hygienic Sciences, 1-18-1 Kami Yoga Setagaya-ku, Tokyo 158-8501, Japan

---

[1] Unable to attend: J.K. Haseman, Biostatistics Branch, National Institute of Environmental Health Sciences, PO Box 12233 – Mail op A3-03, Research Triangle Park, NC 27709, United States; S. Vamvakas, Institut für Toxikologie, Universität Würzburg, Versbacher Strasse 9, 97078 Würzburg, Germany

R.J. Kavlock, Reproductive Toxicology Division, National Health and Environmental Health Effects Research Laboratory, US Environmental Protection Agency, MD-71, Research Triangle Park, NC 27711, United States

B.G. Lake, BIBRA International, Woodmansterne Road, Carshalton, Surrey SM5 4DS, United Kingdom

L.D. Lehman-McKeeman, Procter & Gamble Co., Miami Valley Laboratories, PO Box 538707, Cincinnati, OH 45239-8707, United States

S. Olin, International Life Sciences Institute, Risk Science Institute, 1126 Sixteenth Street NW, Washington DC 20036, United States

J.H. Olsen, Danish Cancer Society, Institute of Cancer Epidemiology, Box 839, 2100 Copenhagen Ø, Denmark

T. Partanen, Finnish Institute of Occupational Health, Topeliuksenkatu 41 a A, 00250 Helsinki, Finland

T. Sanner, Department for Environmental and Occupational Cancer, The Norwegian Radium Hospital, Montebello, 0310 Oslo, Norway

R. Schulte-Hermann, Institut für Tumorbiologie-Krebsforschung der Universität Wien, Borschkegasse 8a, 1090 Vienna, Austria

B. Terracini, Centro per la Prevenzione Oncologica, Università di Torino, via Santena 7, 10126 Turin, Italy (*Vice-Chairman*)

J.M. Ward, National Cancer Institute, NCI-FCC, FVC-201, PO Box B, Frederick, MD 21702-1201, United States

M.D. Waters, National Health and Environmental Effects Research Laboratory, US Environmental Protection Agency, MD-51A, Research Triangle Park, NC 27711, United States

J. Whysner, Toxicology & Risk Assessment Program, American Health Foundation, 1 Dana Road, Valhalla, NY 10595-1599, United States

Representatives/Observers

American Industrial Health Council

R.H. Adamson, National Soft Drink Association, 1101—16th Street, NW, Washington DC 20036-4877, United States

R.M. David, Health and Environment Laboratories, Eastman Kodak Company, Rochester, NY 14652-6272, United States

European Centre for Ecotoxicology and Toxicology of Chemicals

J. Foster, Zeneca, Pathology and Toxicology Support Section, Zeneca Central Toxicology Laboratory, Alderley Park, Macclesfield, Cheshire SK10 4TJ, United Kingdom

Food Directorate, Health Protection Branch

E. Vavasour, Chemical Health Hazard Assessment Division, Bureau of Chemical Safety, Food Directorate, Health Protection Branch, Postal Locator: 2204D1, Ottawa, Ontario K1A OL2, Canada

Secretariat

E. Heseltine (*Editor*), Lajarthe, 24290 St Léon-sur-Vézère, France
E. Smith, International Programme on Chemical Safety, WHO, Geneva, Switzerland

IARC

R. Baan, Unit of Carcinogen Identification and Evaluation
M. Blettner[1], Unit of Carcinogen Identification and Evaluation
M. Friesen, Unit of Gene–Environment Interactions
C. Genevois-Charmeau, Unit of Carcinogen Identification and Evaluation
Y. Grosse, Unit of Carcinogen Identification and Evaluation
V. Krutovskikh, Unit of Multistage Carcinogenesis
C. Malaveille, Unit of Endogenous Cancer Risk Factors
D. McGregor, Unit of Carcinogen Identification and Evaluation
C. Partensky, Unit of Carcinogen Identification and Evaluation
J. Rice, Unit of Carcinogen Identification and Evaluation (*Head of Programme*)
E. Ward[2], Environmental Cancer Epidemiology
J. Wilbourn, Unit of Carcinogen Identification and Evaluation (*Responsible Officer)*

Technical assistance

M. Lézère
A. Meneghel
D. Mietton
J. Mitchell
S. Reynaud
S. Ruiz

Present addresses:
[1] Department of Epidemiology and Medical Statistics, School of Public Health, Postfach 100131, 33501 Bielefeld, Germany
[2] National Institute for Occupational Safety and Health (NIOSH), 4676 Columbia Parkway, Cincinnati, OH 45226, United States

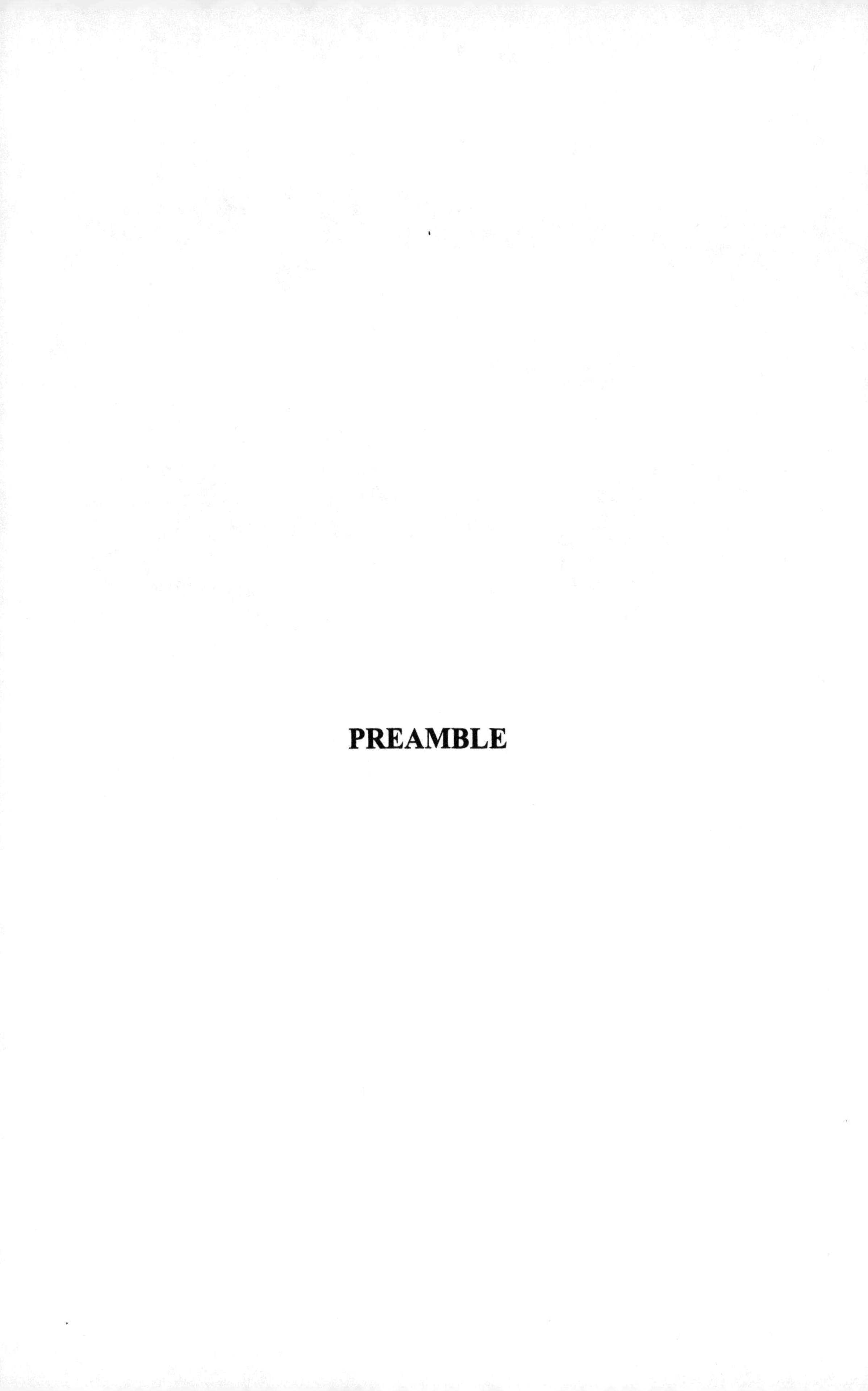

PREAMBLE

IARC MONOGRAPHS PROGRAMME ON THE EVALUATION OF CARCINOGENIC RISKS TO HUMANS

PREAMBLE

1. BACKGROUND

In 1969, the International Agency for Research on Cancer (IARC) initiated a programme to evaluate the carcinogenic risk of chemicals to humans and to produce monographs on individual chemicals. The Monographs programme has since been expanded to include consideration of exposures to complex mixtures of chemicals (which occur, for example, in some occupations and as a result of human habits) and of exposures to other agents, such as radiation and viruses. With Supplement 6 (IARC, 1987a), the title of the series was modified from *IARC Monographs on the Evaluation of the Carcinogenic Risk of Chemicals to Humans* to *IARC Monographs on the Evaluation of Carcinogenic Risks to Humans*, in order to reflect the widened scope of the programme.

The criteria established in 1971 to evaluate carcinogenic risk to humans were adopted by the working groups whose deliberations resulted in the first 16 volumes of the *IARC Monographs series*. Those criteria were subsequently updated by further ad-hoc working groups (IARC, 1977, 1978, 1979, 1982, 1983, 1987b, 1988, 1991a; Vainio *et al.*, 1992).

2. OBJECTIVE AND SCOPE

The objective of the programme is to prepare, with the help of international working groups of experts, and to publish in the form of monographs, critical reviews and evaluations of evidence on the carcinogenicity of a wide range of human exposures. The *Monographs* may also indicate where additional research efforts are needed.

The *Monographs* represent the first step in carcinogenic risk assessment, which involves examination of all relevant information in order to assess the strength of the available evidence that certain exposures could alter the incidence of cancer in humans. The second step is quantitative risk estimation. Detailed, quantitative evaluations of epidemiological data may be made in the *Monographs*, but without extrapolation beyond the range of the data available. Quantitative extrapolation from experimental data to the human situation is not undertaken.

The term 'carcinogen' is used in these monographs to denote an exposure that is capable of increasing the incidence of malignant neoplasms; the induction of benign neoplasms may in some circumstances (see p. 19) contribute to the judgement that the exposure is carcinogenic. The terms 'neoplasm' and 'tumour' are used interchangeably.

Some epidemiological and experimental studies indicate that different agents may act at different stages in the carcinogenic process, and several mechanisms may be involved. The aim of the *Monographs* has been, from their inception, to evaluate evidence of carcinogenicity at any stage in the carcinogenesis process, independently of the underlying mechanisms. Information on mechanisms may, however, be used in making the overall evaluation (IARC, 1991a; Vainio *et al.*, 1992; see also pp. 25–27).

The *Monographs* may assist national and international authorities in making risk assessments and in formulating decisions concerning any necessary preventive measures. The evaluations of IARC working groups are scientific, qualitative judgements about the evidence for or against carcinogenicity provided by the available data. These evaluations represent only one part of the body of information on which regulatory measures may be based. Other components of regulatory decisions vary from one situation to another and from country to country, responding to different socioeconomic and national priorities. **Therefore, no recommendation is given with regard to regulation or legislation, which are the responsibility of individual governments and/or other international organizations.**

The *IARC Monographs* are recognized as an authoritative source of information on the carcinogenicity of a wide range of human exposures. A survey of users in 1988 indicated that the *Monographs* are consulted by various agencies in 57 countries. About 3000 copies of each volume are printed, for distribution to governments, regulatory bodies and interested scientists. The Monographs are also available from IARC*Press* in Lyon and via the Distribution and Sales Service of the World Health Organization in Geneva.

3. SELECTION OF TOPICS FOR MONOGRAPHS

Topics are selected on the basis of two main criteria: (a) there is evidence of human exposure, and (b) there is some evidence or suspicion of carcinogenicity. The term 'agent' is used to include individual chemical compounds, groups of related chemical compounds, physical agents (such as radiation) and biological factors (such as viruses). Exposures to mixtures of agents may occur in occupational exposures and as a result of personal and cultural habits (like smoking and dietary practices). Chemical analogues and compounds with biological or physical characteristics similar to those of suspected carcinogens may also be considered, even in the absence of data on a possible carcinogenic effect in humans or experimental animals.

The scientific literature is surveyed for published data relevant to an assessment of carcinogenicity. The IARC information bulletins on agents being tested for carcinogenicity (IARC, 1973–1996) and directories of on-going research in cancer epidemiology (IARC, 1976–1996) often indicate exposures that may be scheduled for future meetings. Ad-hoc working groups convened by IARC in 1984, 1989, 1991, 1993 and 1998 gave recommendations as to which agents should be evaluated in the IARC Monographs series (IARC, 1984, 1989, 1991b, 1993, 1998a,b).

As significant new data on subjects on which monographs have already been prepared become available, re-evaluations are made at subsequent meetings, and revised monographs are published.

4. DATA FOR MONOGRAPHS

The *Monographs* do not necessarily cite all the literature concerning the subject of an evaluation. Only those data considered by the Working Group to be relevant to making the evaluation are included.

With regard to biological and epidemiological data, only reports that have been published or accepted for publication in the openly available scientific literature are reviewed by the working groups. In certain instances, government agency reports that have undergone peer review and are widely available are considered. Exceptions may be made on an ad-hoc basis to include unpublished reports that are in their final form and publicly available, if their inclusion is considered pertinent to making a final evaluation (see pp. 25–27). In the sections on chemical and physical properties, on analysis, on production and use and on occurrence, unpublished sources of information may be used.

5. THE WORKING GROUP

Reviews and evaluations are formulated by a working group of experts. The tasks of the group are: (i) to ascertain that all appropriate data have been collected; (ii) to select the data relevant for the evaluation on the basis of scientific merit; (iii) to prepare accurate summaries of the data to enable the reader to follow the reasoning of the Working Group; (iv) to evaluate the results of epidemiological and experimental studies on cancer; (v) to evaluate data relevant to the understanding of mechanism of action; and (vi) to make an overall evaluation of the carcinogenicity of the exposure to humans.

Working Group participants who contributed to the considerations and evaluations within a particular volume are listed, with their addresses, at the beginning of each publication. Each participant who is a member of a working group serves as an individual scientist and not as a representative of any organization, government or industry. In addition, nominees of national and international agencies and industrial associations may be invited as observers.

6. WORKING PROCEDURES

Approximately one year in advance of a meeting of a working group, the topics of the monographs are announced and participants are selected by IARC staff in consultation with other experts. Subsequently, relevant biological and epidemiological data are collected by the Carcinogen Identification and Evaluation Unit of IARC from recognized sources of information on carcinogenesis, including data storage and retrieval systems such as MEDLINE and TOXLINE.

For chemicals and some complex mixtures, the major collection of data and the preparation of first drafts of the sections on chemical and physical properties, on analysis, on production and use and on occurrence are carried out under a separate contract funded by the United States National Cancer Institute. Representatives from industrial associations may assist in the preparation of sections on production and use. Information on production and trade is obtained from governmental and trade publications and, in some cases, by direct contact with industries. Separate production data on some agents may not be available because their publication could disclose confidential information. Information on uses may be obtained from published sources but is often complemented by direct contact with manufacturers. Efforts are made to supplement this information with data from other national and international sources.

Six months before the meeting, the material obtained is sent to meeting participants, or is used by IARC staff, to prepare sections for the first drafts of monographs. The first drafts are compiled by IARC staff and sent before the meeting to all participants of the Working Group for review.

The Working Group meets in Lyon for seven to eight days to discuss and finalize the texts of the monographs and to formulate the evaluations. After the meeting, the master copy of each monograph is verified by consulting the original literature, edited and prepared for publication. The aim is to publish monographs within six months of the Working Group meeting.

The available studies are summarized by the Working Group, with particular regard to the qualitative aspects discussed below. In general, numerical findings are indicated as they appear in the original report; units are converted when necessary for easier comparison. The Working Group may conduct additional analyses of the published data and use them in their assessment of the evidence; the results of such supplementary analyses are given in square brackets. When an important aspect of a study, directly impinging on its interpretation, should be brought to the attention of the reader, a comment is given in square brackets.

7. EXPOSURE DATA

Sections that indicate the extent of past and present human exposure, the sources of exposure, the people most likely to be exposed and the factors that contribute to the exposure are included at the beginning of each monograph.

Most monographs on individual chemicals, groups of chemicals or complex mixtures include sections on chemical and physical data, on analysis, on production and use and on occurrence. In monographs on, for example, physical agents, occupational exposures and cultural habits, other sections may be included, such as: historical perspectives, description of an industry or habit, chemistry of the complex mixture or taxonomy. Monographs on biological agents have sections on structure and biology, methods of detection, epidemiology of infection and clinical disease other than cancer.

For chemical exposures, the Chemical Abstracts Services Registry Number, the latest Chemical Abstracts Primary Name and the IUPAC Systematic Name are recorded; other synonyms are given, but the list is not necessarily comprehensive. For biological agents, taxonomy and structure are described, and the degree of variability is given, when applicable.

Information on chemical and physical properties and, in particular, data relevant to identification, occurrence and biological activity are included. For biological agents, mode of replication, life cycle, target cells, persistence and latency and host response are given. A description of technical products of chemicals includes trade names, relevant specifications and available information on composition and impurities. Some of the trade names given may be those of mixtures in which the agent being evaluated is only one of the ingredients.

The purpose of the section on analysis or detection is to give the reader an overview of current methods, with emphasis on those widely used for regulatory purposes. Methods for monitoring human exposure are also given, when available. No critical evaluation or recommendation of any of the methods is meant or implied. The IARC published a series of volumes, *Environmental Carcinogens: Methods of Analysis and Exposure Measurement* (IARC, 1978–93), that describe validated methods for analysing a wide variety of chemicals and mixtures. For biological agents, methods of detection and exposure assessment are described, including their sensitivity, specificity and reproducibility.

The dates of first synthesis and of first commercial production of a chemical or mixture are provided; for agents which do not occur naturally, this information may allow a reasonable estimate to be made of the date before which no human exposure to the agent could have occurred. The dates of first reported occurrence of an exposure are also provided. In addition, methods of synthesis used in past and present commercial production and different methods of production which may give rise to different impurities are described.

Data on production, international trade and uses are obtained for representative regions, which usually include Europe, Japan and the United States of America. It should not, however, be inferred that those areas or nations are necessarily the sole or major sources or users of the agent. Some identified uses may not be current or major applications, and the coverage is not necessarily comprehensive. In the case of drugs, mention of their therapeutic uses does not necessarily represent current practice, nor does it imply judgement as to their therapeutic efficacy.

Information on the occurrence of an agent or mixture in the environment is obtained from data derived from the monitoring and surveillance of levels in occupational environments, air, water, soil, foods and animal and human tissues. When available, data on the generation, persistence and bioaccumulation of the agent are also included. In the case of mixtures, industries, occupations or processes, information is given about all agents present. For processes, industries and occupations, a historical description is also given, noting variations in chemical composition, physical properties and levels of occupational exposure with time and place. For biological agents, the epidemiology of infection is described.

Statements concerning regulations and guidelines (e.g., pesticide registrations, maximal levels permitted in foods, occupational exposure limits) are included for some countries as indications of potential exposures, but they may not reflect the most recent situation, since such limits are continuously reviewed and modified. The absence of information on regulatory status for a country should not be taken to imply that that country does not have regulations with regard to the exposure. For biological agents, legislation and control, including vaccines and therapy, are described.

8. STUDIES OF CANCER IN HUMANS

(*a*) *Types of studies considered*

Three types of epidemiological studies of cancer contribute to the assessment of carcinogenicity in humans—cohort studies, case–control studies and correlation (or ecological) studies. Rarely, results from randomized trials may be available. Case series and case reports of cancer in humans may also be reviewed.

Cohort and case–control studies relate the exposures under study to the occurrence of cancer in individuals and provide an estimate of relative risk (ratio of incidence or mortality in those exposed to incidence or mortality in those not exposed) as the main measure of association.

In correlation studies, the units of investigation are usually whole populations (e.g. in particular geographical areas or at particular times), and cancer frequency is related to a summary measure of the exposure of the population to the agent, mixture or exposure circumstance under study. Because individual exposure is not documented, however, a causal relationship is less easy to infer from correlation studies than from cohort and case–control studies. Case reports generally arise from a suspicion, based on clinical experience, that the concurrence of two events—that is, a particular exposure and occurrence of a cancer—has happened rather more frequently than would be expected by chance. Case reports usually lack complete ascertainment of cases in any population, definition or enumeration of the population at risk and estimation of the expected number of cases in the absence of exposure. The uncertainties surrounding interpretation of case reports and correlation studies make them inadequate, except in rare instances, to form the sole basis for inferring a causal relationship. When taken together with case–control and cohort studies, however, relevant case reports or correlation studies may add materially to the judgement that a causal relationship is present.

Epidemiological studies of benign neoplasms, presumed preneoplastic lesions and other end-points thought to be relevant to cancer are also reviewed by working groups. They may, in some instances, strengthen inferences drawn from studies of cancer itself.

(*b*) *Quality of studies considered*

The Monographs are not intended to summarize all published studies. Those that are judged to be inadequate or irrelevant to the evaluation are generally omitted. They may be mentioned briefly, particularly when the information is considered to be a useful supplement to that in other reports or when they provide the only data available. Their inclusion does not imply acceptance of the adequacy of the study design or of the analysis and interpretation of the results, and limitations are clearly outlined in square brackets at the end of the study description.

It is necessary to take into account the possible roles of bias, confounding and chance in the interpretation of epidemiological studies. By 'bias' is meant the operation of factors in study design or execution that lead erroneously to a stronger or weaker association than in fact exists between disease and an agent, mixture or exposure circumstance. By 'confounding' is meant a situation in which the relationship with disease is made to appear stronger or weaker than it truly is as a result of an association between the apparent causal factor and another factor that is associated with either an increase or decrease in the incidence of the disease. In evaluating the extent to which these factors have been minimized in an individual study, working groups consider a number of aspects of design and analysis as described in the report of the study. Most of these considerations apply equally to case–control, cohort and correlation studies. Lack of clarity of any of these aspects in the reporting of a study can decrease its credibility and the weight given to it in the final evaluation of the exposure.

Firstly, the study population, disease (or diseases) and exposure should have been well defined by the authors. Cases of disease in the study population should have been identified in a way that was independent of the exposure of interest, and exposure should have been assessed in a way that was not related to disease status.

Secondly, the authors should have taken account in the study design and analysis of other variables that can influence the risk of disease and may have been related to the exposure of interest. Potential confounding by such variables should have been dealt with either in the design of the study, such as by matching, or in the analysis, by statistical adjustment. In cohort studies, comparisons with local rates of disease may be more appropriate than those with national rates. Internal comparisons of disease frequency among individuals at different levels of exposure should also have been made in the study.

Thirdly, the authors should have reported the basic data on which the conclusions are founded, even if sophisticated statistical analyses were employed. At the very least, they should have given the numbers of exposed and unexposed cases and controls in a case–control study and the numbers of cases observed and expected in a cohort study. Further tabulations by time since exposure began and other temporal factors are also important. In a cohort study, data on all cancer sites and all causes of death should have been given, to reveal the possibility of reporting bias. In a case–control study, the effects of investigated factors other than the exposure of interest should have been reported.

Finally, the statistical methods used to obtain estimates of relative risk, absolute rates of cancer, confidence intervals and significance tests, and to adjust for confounding should have been clearly stated by the authors. The methods used should preferably have been the generally accepted techniques that have been refined since the mid-1970s. These methods have been reviewed for case–control studies (Breslow & Day, 1980) and for cohort studies (Breslow & Day, 1987).

(*c*) *Inferences about mechanism of action*

Detailed analyses of both relative and absolute risks in relation to temporal variables, such as age at first exposure, time since first exposure, duration of exposure, cumulative exposure and time since exposure ceased, are reviewed and summarized when available. The analysis of temporal relationships can be useful in formulating models of carcinogenesis. In particular, such analyses may suggest whether a carcinogen acts early or late in the process of carcinogenesis, although at best they allow only indirect inferences about the mechanism of action. Special attention is given to measurements of biological markers of carcinogen exposure or action, such as DNA or protein adducts, as well as markers of early steps in the carcinogenic process, such as proto-oncogene mutation, when these are incorporated into epidemiological studies focused on cancer incidence or mortality. Such measurements may allow inferences to be made about putative mechanisms of action (IARC, 1991a; Vainio *et al.*, 1992).

(*d*) *Criteria for causality*

After the individual epidemiological studies of cancer have been summarized and the quality assessed, a judgement is made concerning the strength of evidence that the agent, mixture or exposure circumstance in question is carcinogenic for humans. In making its judgement, the Working Group considers several criteria for causality. A strong association (a large relative risk) is more likely to indicate causality than a weak association, although it is recognized that relative risks of small magnitude do not imply lack of causality and may be important if the disease is common. Associations that are replicated in several studies of the same design or using different epidemiological approaches or under different circumstances of exposure are more likely to represent a causal relationship than isolated observations from single studies. If there are inconsistent results among investigations, possible reasons are sought (such as differences in amount of exposure), and results of studies judged to be of high quality are given more weight than those of studies judged to be methodologically less sound. When suspicion of carcinogenicity arises largely from a single study, these data are not combined with those from later studies in any subsequent reassessment of the strength of the evidence.

If the risk of the disease in question increases with the amount of exposure, this is considered to be a strong indication of causality, although absence of a graded response is not necessarily evidence against a causal relationship. Demonstration of a decline in risk after cessation of or reduction in exposure in individuals or in whole populations also supports a causal interpretation of the findings.

Although a carcinogen may act upon more than one target, the specificity of an association (an increased occurrence of cancer at one anatomical site or of one morphological type) adds plausibility to a causal relationship, particularly when excess cancer occurrence is limited to one morphological type within the same organ.

Although rarely available, results from randomized trials showing different rates among exposed and unexposed individuals provide particularly strong evidence for causality.

When several epidemiological studies show little or no indication of an association between an exposure and cancer, the judgement may be made that, in the aggregate, they show evidence of lack of carcinogenicity. Such a judgement requires first of all that the studies giving rise to it meet, to a sufficient degree, the standards of design and analysis described above. Specifically, the possibility that bias, confounding or misclassification of exposure or outcome could explain the observed results should be considered and excluded with reasonable certainty. In addition, all studies that are judged to be methodologically sound should be consistent with a relative risk of unity for any observed level of exposure and, when considered together, should provide a pooled estimate of relative risk which is at or near unity and has a narrow confidence interval, due to sufficient population size. Moreover, no individual study nor the pooled results of all the studies should show any consistent tendency for the relative risk of cancer to increase with increasing level of exposure. It is important to note that evidence of lack of carcinogenicity obtained in this way from several epidemiological studies can apply only to the type(s) of cancer studied and to dose levels and intervals between first exposure and observation of disease that are the same as or less than those observed in all the studies. Experience with human cancer indicates that, in some cases, the period from first exposure to the development of clinical cancer is seldom less than 20 years; latent periods substantially shorter than 30 years cannot provide evidence for lack of carcinogenicity.

9. STUDIES OF CANCER IN EXPERIMENTAL ANIMALS

All known human carcinogens that have been studied adequately in experimental animals have produced positive results in one or more animal species (Wilbourn *et al.*, 1986; Tomatis *et al.*, 1989). For several agents (aflatoxins, 4-aminobiphenyl, azathioprine, betel quid with tobacco, bischloromethyl ether and chloromethyl methyl ether (technical grade), chlorambucil, chlornaphazine, ciclosporin, coal-tar pitches, coal-tars, combined oral contraceptives, cyclophosphamide, diethylstilboestrol, melphalan, 8-methoxypsoralen plus ultraviolet A radiation, mustard gas, myleran, 2-naphthylamine, nonsteroidal oestrogens, oestrogen replacement therapy/steroidal oestrogens, solar radiation, thiotepa and vinyl chloride), carcinogenicity in experimental animals was established or highly suspected before epidemiological studies confirmed their carcinogenicity in humans (Vainio *et al.*, 1995). Although this association cannot establish that all agents and mixtures that cause cancer in experimental animals also cause cancer in humans, nevertheless, **in the absence of adequate data on humans, it is biologically plausible and prudent to regard agents and mixtures for which there is *sufficient evidence* (see p. 24) of carcinogenicity in experimental animals as if they presented a carcinogenic risk to humans**. The possibility that a given agent may cause cancer through a species-specific mechanism which does not operate in humans (see p. 27) should also be taken into consideration.

The nature and extent of impurities or contaminants present in the chemical or mixture being evaluated are given when available. Animal strain, sex, numbers per group, age at start of treatment and survival are reported.

Other types of studies summarized include: experiments in which the agent or mixture was administered in conjunction with known carcinogens or factors that modify carcinogenic effects; studies in which the end-point was not cancer but a defined precancerous lesion; and experiments on the carcinogenicity of known metabolites and derivatives.

For experimental studies of mixtures, consideration is given to the possibility of changes in the physicochemical properties of the test substance during collection, storage, extraction, concentration and delivery. Chemical and toxicological interactions of the components of mixtures may result in nonlinear dose–response relationships.

An assessment is made as to the relevance to human exposure of samples tested in experimental animals, which may involve consideration of: (i) physical and chemical characteristics, (ii) constituent substances that indicate the presence of a class of substances, (iii) the results of tests for genetic and related effects, including studies on DNA adduct formation, proto-oncogene mutation and expression and suppressor gene inactivation. The relevance of results obtained, for example, with animal viruses analogous to the virus being evaluated in the monograph must also be considered. They may provide biological and mechanistic information relevant to the understanding of the process of carcinogenesis in humans and may strengthen the plausibility of a conclusion that the biological agent under evaluation is carcinogenic in humans.

(*a*) *Qualitative aspects*

An assessment of carcinogenicity involves several considerations of qualitative importance, including (i) the experimental conditions under which the test was performed, including route and schedule of exposure, species, strain, sex, age, duration of follow-up; (ii) the consistency of the results, for example, across species and target organ(s); (iii) the spectrum of neoplastic response, from preneoplastic lesions and benign tumours to malignant neoplasms; and (iv) the possible role of modifying factors.

As mentioned earlier (p. 11), the *Monographs* are not intended to summarize all published studies. Those studies in experimental animals that are inadequate (e.g., too short a duration, too few animals, poor survival; see below) or are judged irrelevant to the evaluation are generally omitted. Guidelines for conducting adequate long-term carcinogenicity experiments have been outlined (e.g. Montesano *et al.*, 1986).

Considerations of importance to the Working Group in the interpretation and evaluation of a particular study include: (i) how clearly the agent was defined and, in the case of mixtures, how adequately the sample characterization was reported; (ii) whether the dose was adequately monitored, particularly in inhalation experiments; (iii) whether the doses and duration of treatment were appropriate and whether the survival of treated animals was similar to that of controls; (iv) whether there were adequate numbers of animals per group; (v) whether animals of each sex were used; (vi) whether animals were allocated randomly to groups; (vii) whether the duration of observation was adequate; and (viii) whether the data were adequately reported. If available, recent data on the incidence of specific tumours in historical controls, as well as in concurrent controls, should be taken into account in the evaluation of tumour response.

When benign tumours occur together with and originate from the same cell type in an organ or tissue as malignant tumours in a particular study and appear to represent a stage in the progression to malignancy, it may be valid to combine them in assessing tumour incidence (Huff *et al.*, 1989). The occurrence of lesions presumed to be pre-neoplastic may in certain instances aid in assessing the biological plausibility of any neoplastic response observed. If an agent or mixture induces only benign neoplasms that appear to be end-points that do not readily progress to malignancy, it should nevertheless be suspected of being a carcinogen and requires further investigation.

(*b*) *Quantitative aspects*

The probability that tumours will occur may depend on the species, sex, strain and age of the animal, the dose of the carcinogen and the route and length of exposure. Evidence of an increased incidence of neoplasms with increased level of exposure strengthens the inference of a causal association between the exposure and the development of neoplasms.

The form of the dose–response relationship can vary widely, depending on the particular agent under study and the target organ. Both DNA damage and increased cell division are important aspects of carcinogenesis, and cell proliferation is a strong determinant of dose–response relationships for some carcinogens (Cohen & Ellwein, 1990). Since many chemicals require metabolic activation before being converted into their reactive intermediates, both metabolic and pharmacokinetic aspects are important in determining the dose–response pattern. Saturation of steps such as absorption, activation, inactivation and elimination may produce nonlinearity in the dose–response relationship, as could saturation of processes such as DNA repair (Hoel *et al.*, 1983; Gart *et al.*, 1986).

(*c*) *Statistical analysis of long-term experiments in animals*

Factors considered by the Working Group include the adequacy of the information given for each treatment group: (i) the number of animals studied and the number examined histologically, (ii) the number of animals with a given tumour type and (iii) length of survival. The statistical methods used should be clearly stated and should be the generally accepted techniques refined for this purpose (Peto *et al.*, 1980; Gart *et al.*, 1986). When there is no difference in survival between control and treatment groups, the Working Group usually compares the proportions of animals developing each tumour type in each of the groups. Otherwise, consideration is given as to whether or not appropriate adjustments have been made for differences in survival. These adjustments can include: comparisons of the proportions of tumour-bearing animals among the effective number of animals (alive at the time the first tumour is discovered), in the case where most differences in survival occur before tumours appear; life-table methods, when tumours are visible or when they may be considered 'fatal' because mortality rapidly follows tumour development; and the Mantel-Haenszel test or logistic regression, when occult tumours do not affect the animals' risk of dying but are 'incidental' findings at autopsy.

In practice, classifying tumours as fatal or incidental may be difficult. Several survival-adjusted methods have been developed that do not require this distinction (Gart *et al.*, 1986), although they have not been fully evaluated.

10. OTHER DATA RELEVANT TO AN EVALUATION OF CARCINOGENICITY AND ITS MECHANISMS

In coming to an overall evaluation of carcinogenicity in humans (see pp. 25–27), the Working Group also considers related data. The nature of the information selected for the summary depends on the agent being considered.

For chemicals and complex mixtures of chemicals such as those in some occupational situations or involving cultural habits (e.g. tobacco smoking), the other data considered to be relevant are divided into those on absorption, distribution, metabolism and excretion; toxic effects; reproductive and developmental effects; and genetic and related effects.

Concise information is given on absorption, distribution (including placental transfer) and excretion in both humans and experimental animals. Kinetic factors that may affect the dose–response relationship, such as saturation of uptake, protein binding, metabolic activation, detoxification and DNA repair processes, are mentioned. Studies that indicate the metabolic fate of the agent in humans and in experimental animals are summarized briefly, and comparisons of data on humans and on animals are made when possible. Comparative information on the relationship between exposure and the dose that reaches the target site may be of particular importance for extrapolation between species. Data are given on acute and chronic toxic effects (other than cancer), such as organ toxicity, increased cell proliferation, immunotoxicity and endocrine effects. The presence and toxicological significance of cellular receptors is described. Effects on reproduction, teratogenicity, fetotoxicity and embryotoxicity are also summarized briefly.

Tests of genetic and related effects are described in view of the relevance of gene mutation and chromosomal damage to carcinogenesis (Vainio *et al.*, 1992; McGregor *et al.*, 1999). The adequacy of the reporting of sample characterization is considered and, where necessary, commented upon; with regard to complex mixtures, such comments are similar to those described for animal carcinogenicity tests on p. 18. The available data are interpreted critically by phylogenetic group according to the end-points detected, which may include DNA damage, gene mutation, sister chromatid exchange, micronucleus formation, chromosomal aberrations, aneuploidy and cell transformation. The concentrations employed are given, and mention is made of whether use of an exogenous metabolic system *in vitro* affected the test result. These data are given as listings of test systems, data and references. The Genetic and Related Effects data presented in the *Monographs* are also available in the form of Graphic Activity Profiles (GAP) prepared in collaboration with the United States Environmental Protection Agency (EPA) (see also

Waters *et al.*, 1987) using software for personal computers that are Microsoft Windows® compatible. The EPA/IARC GAP software and database may be downloaded free of charge from *www.epa.gov/gapdb*.

Positive results in tests using prokaryotes, lower eukaryotes, plants, insects and cultured mammalian cells suggest that genetic and related effects could occur in mammals. Results from such tests may also give information about the types of genetic effect produced and about the involvement of metabolic activation. Some end-points described are clearly genetic in nature (e.g., gene mutations and chromosomal aberrations), while others are to a greater or lesser degree associated with genetic effects (e.g. unscheduled DNA synthesis). In-vitro tests for tumour-promoting activity and for cell transformation may be sensitive to changes that are not necessarily the result of genetic alterations but that may have specific relevance to the process of carcinogenesis. A critical appraisal of these tests has been published (Montesano *et al.*, 1986).

Genetic or other activity manifest in experimental mammals and humans is regarded as being of greater relevance than that in other organisms. The demonstration that an agent or mixture can induce gene and chromosomal mutations in whole mammals indicates that it may have carcinogenic activity, although this activity may not be detectably expressed in any or all species. Relative potency in tests for mutagenicity and related effects is not a reliable indicator of carcinogenic potency. Negative results in tests for mutagenicity in selected tissues from animals treated *in vivo* provide less weight, partly because they do not exclude the possibility of an effect in tissues other than those examined. Moreover, negative results in short-term tests with genetic end-points cannot be considered to provide evidence to rule out carcinogenicity of agents or mixtures that act through other mechanisms (e.g. receptor-mediated effects, cellular toxicity with regenerative proliferation, peroxisome proliferation) (Vainio *et al.*, 1992). Factors that may lead to misleading results in short-term tests have been discussed in detail elsewhere (Montesano *et al.*, 1986).

When available, data relevant to mechanisms of carcinogenesis that do not involve structural changes at the level of the gene are also described.

The adequacy of epidemiological studies of reproductive outcome and genetic and related effects in humans is evaluated by the same criteria as are applied to epidemiological studies of cancer.

Structure–activity relationships that may be relevant to an evaluation of the carcinogenicity of an agent are also described.

For biological agents—viruses, bacteria and parasites—other data relevant to carcinogenicity include descriptions of the pathology of infection, molecular biology (integration and expression of viruses, and any genetic alterations seen in human tumours) and other observations, which might include cellular and tissue responses to infection, immune response and the presence of tumour markers.

11. SUMMARY OF DATA REPORTED

In this section, the relevant epidemiological and experimental data are summarized. Only reports, other than in abstract form, that meet the criteria outlined on p. 11 are considered for evaluating carcinogenicity. Inadequate studies are generally not summarized: such studies are usually identified by a square-bracketed comment in the preceding text.

(*a*) *Exposure*

Human exposure to chemicals and complex mixtures is summarized on the basis of elements such as production, use, occurrence in the environment and determinations in human tissues and body fluids. Quantitative data are given when available. Exposure to biological agents is described in terms of transmission and prevalence of infection.

(*b*) *Carcinogenicity in humans*

Results of epidemiological studies that are considered to be pertinent to an assessment of human carcinogenicity are summarized. When relevant, case reports and correlation studies are also summarized.

(*c*) *Carcinogenicity in experimental animals*

Data relevant to an evaluation of carcinogenicity in animals are summarized. For each animal species and route of administration, it is stated whether an increased incidence of neoplasms or preneoplastic lesions was observed, and the tumour sites are indicated. If the agent or mixture produced tumours after prenatal exposure or in single-dose experiments, this is also indicated. Negative findings are also summarized. Dose–response and other quantitative data may be given when available.

(*d*) *Other data relevant to an evaluation of carcinogenicity and its mechanisms*

Data on biological effects in humans that are of particular relevance are summarized. These may include toxicological, kinetic and metabolic considerations and evidence of DNA binding, persistence of DNA lesions or genetic damage in exposed humans. Toxicological information, such as that on cytotoxicity and regeneration, receptor binding and hormonal and immunological effects, and data on kinetics and metabolism in experimental animals are given when considered relevant to the possible mechanism of the carcinogenic action of the agent. The results of tests for genetic and related effects are summarized for whole mammals, cultured mammalian cells and nonmammalian systems.

When available, comparisons of such data for humans and for animals, and particularly animals that have developed cancer, are described.

Structure–activity relationships are mentioned when relevant.

For the agent, mixture or exposure circumstance being evaluated, the available data on end-points or other phenomena relevant to mechanisms of carcinogenesis from studies in humans, experimental animals and tissue and cell test systems are summarized within one or more of the following descriptive dimensions:

(i) Evidence of genotoxicity (structural changes at the level of the gene): for example, structure–activity considerations, adduct formation, mutagenicity (effect on specific genes), chromosomal mutation/aneuploidy

(ii) Evidence of effects on the expression of relevant genes (functional changes at the intracellular level): for example, alterations to the structure or quantity of the product of a proto-oncogene or tumour-suppressor gene, alterations to metabolic activation/inactivation/DNA repair

(iii) Evidence of relevant effects on cell behaviour (morphological or behavioural changes at the cellular or tissue level): for example, induction of mitogenesis, compensatory cell proliferation, preneoplasia and hyperplasia, survival of premalignant or malignant cells (immortalization, immunosuppression), effects on metastatic potential

(iv) Evidence from dose and time relationships of carcinogenic effects and interactions between agents: for example, early/late stage, as inferred from epidemiological studies; initiation/promotion/progression/malignant conversion, as defined in animal carcinogenicity experiments; toxicokinetics

These dimensions are not mutually exclusive, and an agent may fall within more than one of them. Thus, for example, the action of an agent on the expression of relevant genes could be summarized under both the first and second dimensions, even if it were known with reasonable certainty that those effects resulted from genotoxicity.

12. EVALUATION

Evaluations of the strength of the evidence for carcinogenicity arising from human and experimental animal data are made, using standard terms.

It is recognized that the criteria for these evaluations, described below, cannot encompass all of the factors that may be relevant to an evaluation of carcinogenicity. In considering all of the relevant scientific data, the Working Group may assign the agent, mixture or exposure circumstance to a higher or lower category than a strict interpretation of these criteria would indicate.

(*a*) *Degrees of evidence for carcinogenicity in humans and in experimental animals and supporting evidence*

These categories refer only to the strength of the evidence that an exposure is carcinogenic and not to the extent of its carcinogenic activity (potency) nor to the mechanisms involved. A classification may change as new information becomes available.

An evaluation of degree of evidence, whether for a single agent or a mixture, is limited to the materials tested, as defined physically, chemically or biologically. When the agents evaluated are considered by the Working Group to be sufficiently closely related, they may be grouped together for the purpose of a single evaluation of degree of evidence.

(i) *Carcinogenicity in humans*

The applicability of an evaluation of the carcinogenicity of a mixture, process, occupation or industry on the basis of evidence from epidemiological studies depends on the variability over time and place of the mixtures, processes, occupations and industries. The Working Group seeks to identify the specific exposure, process or activity which is considered most likely to be responsible for any excess risk. The evaluation is focused as narrowly as the available data on exposure and other aspects permit.

The evidence relevant to carcinogenicity from studies in humans is classified into one of the following categories:

Sufficient evidence of carcinogenicity: The Working Group considers that a causal relationship has been established between exposure to the agent, mixture or exposure circumstance and human cancer. That is, a positive relationship has been observed between the exposure and cancer in studies in which chance, bias and confounding could be ruled out with reasonable confidence.

Limited evidence of carcinogenicity: A positive association has been observed between exposure to the agent, mixture or exposure circumstance and cancer for which a causal interpretation is considered by the Working Group to be credible, but chance, bias or confounding could not be ruled out with reasonable confidence.

Inadequate evidence of carcinogenicity: The available studies are of insufficient quality, consistency or statistical power to permit a conclusion regarding the presence or absence of a causal association between exposure and cancer, or no data on cancer in humans are available.

Evidence suggesting lack of carcinogenicity: There are several adequate studies covering the full range of levels of exposure that human beings are known to encounter, which are mutually consistent in not showing a positive association between exposure to the agent, mixture or exposure circumstance and any studied cancer at any observed level of exposure. A conclusion of 'evidence suggesting lack of carcinogenicity' is inevitably limited to the cancer sites, conditions and levels of exposure and length of observation covered by the available studies. In addition, the possibility of a very small risk at the levels of exposure studied can never be excluded.

In some instances, the above categories may be used to classify the degree of evidence related to carcinogenicity in specific organs or tissues.

(ii) *Carcinogenicity in experimental animals*

The evidence relevant to carcinogenicity in experimental animals is classified into one of the following categories:

Sufficient evidence of carcinogenicity: The Working Group considers that a causal relationship has been established between the agent or mixture and an increased incidence of malignant neoplasms or of an appropriate combination of benign and malignant neoplasms in (a) two or more species of animals or (b) in two or more independent studies in one species carried out at different times or in different laboratories or under different protocols.

Exceptionally, a single study in one species might be considered to provide sufficient evidence of carcinogenicity when malignant neoplasms occur to an unusual degree with regard to incidence, site, type of tumour or age at onset.

Limited evidence of carcinogenicity: The data suggest a carcinogenic effect but are limited for making a definitive evaluation because, e.g. (a) the evidence of carcinogenicity is restricted to a single experiment; or (b) there are unresolved questions regarding the adequacy of the design, conduct or interpretation of the study; or (c) the agent or mixture increases the incidence only of benign neoplasms or lesions of uncertain neoplastic potential, or of certain neoplasms which may occur spontaneously in high incidences in certain strains.

Inadequate evidence of carcinogenicity: The studies cannot be interpreted as showing either the presence or absence of a carcinogenic effect because of major qualitative or quantitative limitations, or no data on cancer in experimental animals are available.

Evidence suggesting lack of carcinogenicity: Adequate studies involving at least two species are available which show that, within the limits of the tests used, the agent or mixture is not carcinogenic. A conclusion of evidence suggesting lack of carcinogenicity is inevitably limited to the species, tumour sites and levels of exposure studied.

(*b*) *Other data relevant to the evaluation of carcinogenicity and its mechanisms*

Other evidence judged to be relevant to an evaluation of carcinogenicity and of sufficient importance to affect the overall evaluation is then described. This may include data on preneoplastic lesions, tumour pathology, genetic and related effects, structure–activity relationships, metabolism and pharmacokinetics, physicochemical parameters and analogous biological agents.

Data relevant to mechanisms of the carcinogenic action are also evaluated. The strength of the evidence that any carcinogenic effect observed is due to a particular mechanism is assessed, using terms such as weak, moderate or strong. Then, the Working Group assesses if that particular mechanism is likely to be operative in humans. The strongest indications that a particular mechanism operates in humans come from data on humans or biological specimens obtained from exposed humans. The data may be considered to be especially relevant if they show that the agent in question has caused changes in exposed humans that are on the causal pathway to carcinogenesis. Such data may, however, never become available, because it is at least conceivable that certain compounds may be kept from human use solely on the basis of evidence of their toxicity and/or carcinogenicity in experimental systems.

For complex exposures, including occupational and industrial exposures, the chemical composition and the potential contribution of carcinogens known to be present are considered by the Working Group in its overall evaluation of human carcinogenicity. The Working Group also determines the extent to which the materials tested in experimental systems are related to those to which humans are exposed.

(*c*) *Overall evaluation*

Finally, the body of evidence is considered as a whole, in order to reach an overall evaluation of the carcinogenicity to humans of an agent, mixture or circumstance of exposure.

An evaluation may be made for a group of chemical compounds that have been evaluated by the Working Group. In addition, when supporting data indicate that other, related compounds for which there is no direct evidence of capacity to induce cancer in humans or in animals may also be carcinogenic, a statement describing the rationale for this conclusion is added to the evaluation narrative; an additional evaluation may be made for this broader group of compounds if the strength of the evidence warrants it.

The agent, mixture or exposure circumstance is described according to the wording of one of the following categories, and the designated group is given. The categorization of an agent, mixture or exposure circumstance is a matter of scientific judgement, reflecting the strength of the evidence derived from studies in humans and in experimental animals and from other relevant data.

Group 1 —The agent (mixture) is carcinogenic to humans.
The exposure circumstance entails exposures that are carcinogenic to humans.

This category is used when there is *sufficient evidence* of carcinogenicity in humans. Exceptionally, an agent (mixture) may be placed in this category when evidence of carcinogenicity in humans is less than sufficient but there is *sufficient evidence* of carcinogenicity in experimental animals and strong evidence in exposed humans that the agent (mixture) acts through a relevant mechanism of carcinogenicity.

Group 2

This category includes agents, mixtures and exposure circumstances for which, at one extreme, the degree of evidence of carcinogenicity in humans is almost sufficient, as well as those for which, at the other extreme, there are no human data but for which there is evidence of carcinogenicity in experimental animals. Agents, mixtures and exposure circumstances are assigned to either group 2A (probably carcinogenic to humans) or group 2B (possibly carcinogenic to humans) on the basis of epidemiological and experimental evidence of carcinogenicity and other relevant data.

Group 2A—The agent (mixture) is probably carcinogenic to humans.
The exposure circumstance entails exposures that are probably carcinogenic to humans.

This category is used when there is *limited evidence* of carcinogenicity in humans and *sufficient evidence* of carcinogenicity in experimental animals. In some cases, an agent (mixture) may be classified in this category when there is *inadequate evidence* of carcinogenicity in humans, *sufficient evidence* of carcinogenicity in experimental animals and strong evidence that the carcinogenesis is mediated by a mechanism that also operates in humans. Exceptionally, an agent, mixture or exposure circumstance may be classified in this category solely on the basis of *limited evidence* of carcinogenicity in humans.

Group 2B—The agent (mixture) is possibly carcinogenic to humans.
The exposure circumstance entails exposures that are possibly carcinogenic to humans.

This category is used for agents, mixtures and exposure circumstances for which there is *limited evidence* of carcinogenicity in humans and less than *sufficient evidence* of carcinogenicity in experimental animals. It may also be used when there is *inadequate evidence* of carcinogenicity in humans but there is *sufficient evidence* of carcinogenicity in experimental animals. In some instances, an agent, mixture or exposure circumstance for which there is *inadequate evidence* of carcinogenicity in humans but *limited evidence* of carcinogenicity in experimental animals together with supporting evidence from other relevant data may be placed in this group.

Group 3—The agent (mixture or exposure circumstance) is not classifiable as to its carcinogenicity to humans.

This category is used most commonly for agents, mixtures and exposure circumstances for which the *evidence of carcinogenicity* is *inadequate* in humans and *inadequate* or *limited* in experimental animals.

Exceptionally, agents (mixtures) for which the *evidence of carcinogenicity* is *inadequate* in humans but *sufficient* in experimental animals may be placed in this category when there is strong evidence that the mechanism of carcinogenicity in experimental animals does not operate in humans.

Agents, mixtures and exposure circumstances that do not fall into any other group are also placed in this category.

Group 4—The agent (mixture) is probably not carcinogenic to humans.

This category is used for agents or mixtures for which there is *evidence suggesting lack of carcinogenicity* in humans and in experimental animals. In some instances, agents or mixtures for which there is *inadequate evidence* of carcinogenicity in humans but *evidence suggesting lack of carcinogenicity* in experimental animals, consistently and strongly supported by a broad range of other relevant data, may be classified in this group.

References

Breslow, N.E. & Day, N.E. (1980) *Statistical Methods in Cancer Research*, Vol. 1, *The Analysis of Case–Control Studies* (IARC Scientific Publications No. 32), Lyon, IARC

Breslow, N.E. & Day, N.E. (1987) *Statistical Methods in Cancer Research*, Vol. 2, *The Design and Analysis of Cohort Studies* (IARC Scientific Publications No. 82), Lyon, IARC

Cohen, S.M. & Ellwein, L.B. (1990) Cell proliferation in carcinogenesis. *Science*, **249**, 1007–1011

Gart, J.J., Krewski, D., Lee, P.N., Tarone, R.E. & Wahrendorf, J. (1986) *Statistical Methods in Cancer Research*, Vol. 3, *The Design and Analysis of Long-term Animal Experiments* (IARC Scientific Publications No. 79), Lyon, IARC

Hoel, D.G., Kaplan, N.L. & Anderson, M.W. (1983) Implication of nonlinear kinetics on risk estimation in carcinogenesis. *Science*, **219**, 1032–1037

Huff, J.E., Eustis, S.L. & Haseman, J.K. (1989) Occurrence and relevance of chemically induced benign neoplasms in long-term carcinogenicity studies. *Cancer Metastasis Rev.*, **8**, 1–21

IARC (1973–1996) *Information Bulletin on the Survey of Chemicals Being Tested for Carcinogenicity/Directory of Agents Being Tested for Carcinogenicity*, Numbers 1–17, Lyon

IARC (1976–1996)

Directory of On-going Research in Cancer Epidemiology 1976. Edited by C.S. Muir & G. Wagner, Lyon

Directory of On-going Research in Cancer Epidemiology 1977 (IARC Scientific Publications No. 17). Edited by C.S. Muir & G. Wagner, Lyon

Directory of On-going Research in Cancer Epidemiology 1978 (IARC Scientific Publications No. 26). Edited by C.S. Muir & G. Wagner, Lyon

Directory of On-going Research in Cancer Epidemiology 1979 (IARC Scientific Publications No. 28). Edited by C.S. Muir & G. Wagner, Lyon

Directory of On-going Research in Cancer Epidemiology 1980 (IARC Scientific Publications No. 35). Edited by C.S. Muir & G. Wagner, Lyon

Directory of On-going Research in Cancer Epidemiology 1981 (IARC Scientific Publications No. 38). Edited by C.S. Muir & G. Wagner, Lyon

Directory of On-going Research in Cancer Epidemiology 1982 (IARC Scientific Publications No. 46). Edited by C.S. Muir & G. Wagner, Lyon

Directory of On-going Research in Cancer Epidemiology 1983 (IARC Scientific Publications No. 50). Edited by C.S. Muir & G. Wagner, Lyon

Directory of On-going Research in Cancer Epidemiology 1984 (IARC Scientific Publications No. 62). Edited by C.S. Muir & G. Wagner, Lyon

Directory of On-going Research in Cancer Epidemiology 1985 (IARC Scientific Publications No. 69). Edited by C.S. Muir & G. Wagner, Lyon

Directory of On-going Research in Cancer Epidemiology 1986 (IARC Scientific Publications No. 80). Edited by C.S. Muir & G. Wagner, Lyon

Directory of On-going Research in Cancer Epidemiology 1987 (IARC Scientific Publications No. 86). Edited by D.M. Parkin & J. Wahrendorf, Lyon

Directory of On-going Research in Cancer Epidemiology 1988 (IARC Scientific Publications No. 93). Edited by M. Coleman & J. Wahrendorf, Lyon

Directory of On-going Research in Cancer Epidemiology 1989/90 (IARC Scientific Publications No. 101). Edited by M. Coleman & J. Wahrendorf, Lyon

Directory of On-going Research in Cancer Epidemiology 1991 (IARC Scientific Publications No.110). Edited by M. Coleman & J. Wahrendorf, Lyon

Directory of On-going Research in Cancer Epidemiology 1992 (IARC Scientific Publications No. 117). Edited by M. Coleman, J. Wahrendorf & E. Démaret, Lyon

Directory of On-going Research in Cancer Epidemiology 1994 (IARC Scientific Publications No. 130). Edited by R. Sankaranarayanan, J. Wahrendorf & E. Démaret, Lyon

Directory of On-going Research in Cancer Epidemiology 1996 (IARC Scientific Publications No. 137). Edited by R. Sankaranarayanan, J. Wahrendorf & E. Démaret, Lyon

IARC (1977) *IARC Monographs Programme on the Evaluation of the Carcinogenic Risk of Chemicals to Humans*. Preamble (IARC intern. tech. Rep. No. 77/002), Lyon

IARC (1978) *Chemicals with* Sufficient Evidence *of Carcinogenicity in Experimental Animals*—IARC Monographs *Volumes 1–17* (IARC intern. tech. Rep. No. 78/003), Lyon

IARC (1978–1993) *Environmental Carcinogens. Methods of Analysis and Exposure Measurement*:

Vol. 1. Analysis of Volatile Nitrosamines in Food (IARC Scientific Publications No. 18). Edited by R. Preussmann, M. Castegnaro, E.A. Walker & A.E. Wasserman (1978)

Vol. 2. Methods for the Measurement of Vinyl Chloride in Poly(vinyl chloride), Air, Water and Foodstuffs (IARC Scientific Publications No. 22). Edited by D.C.M. Squirrell & W. Thain (1978)

Vol. 3. Analysis of Polycyclic Aromatic Hydrocarbons in Environmental Samples (IARC Scientific Publications No. 29). Edited by M. Castegnaro, P. Bogovski, H. Kunte & E.A. Walker (1979)

Vol. 4. Some Aromatic Amines and Azo Dyes in the General and Industrial Environment (IARC Scientific Publications No. 40). Edited by L. Fishbein, M. Castegnaro, I.K. O'Neill & H. Bartsch (1981)

Vol. 5. Some Mycotoxins (IARC Scientific Publications No. 44). Edited by L. Stoloff, M. Castegnaro, P. Scott, I.K. O'Neill & H. Bartsch (1983)

Vol. 6. N-Nitroso Compounds (IARC Scientific Publications No. 45). Edited by R. Preussmann, I.K. O'Neill, G. Eisenbrand, B. Spiegelhalder & H. Bartsch (1983)

Vol. 7. Some Volatile Halogenated Hydrocarbons (IARC Scientific Publications No. 68). Edited by L. Fishbein & I.K. O'Neill (1985)

Vol. 8. Some Metals: As, Be, Cd, Cr, Ni, Pb, Se, Zn (IARC Scientific Publications No. 71). Edited by I.K. O'Neill, P. Schuller & L. Fishbein (1986)

Vol. 9. Passive Smoking (IARC Scientific Publications No. 81). Edited by I.K. O'Neill, K.D. Brunnemann, B. Dodet & D. Hoffmann (1987)

*Vol. 10. Benzene and Alkylated Benzenes (*IARC Scientific Publications No. 85). Edited by L. Fishbein & I.K. O'Neill (1988)

Vol. 11. Polychlorinated Dioxins and Dibenzofurans (IARC Scientific Publications No. 108). Edited by C. Rappe, H.R. Buser, B. Dodet & I.K. O'Neill (1991)

Vol. 12. Indoor Air (IARC Scientific Publications No. 109). Edited by B. Seifert, H. van de Wiel, B. Dodet & I.K. O'Neill (1993)

IARC (1979) *Criteria to Select Chemicals for* IARC Monographs (IARC intern. tech. Rep. No. 79/003), Lyon

IARC (1982) *IARC Monographs on the Evaluation of the Carcinogenic Risk of Chemicals to Humans*, Supplement 4, *Chemicals, Industrial Processes and Industries Associated with Cancer in Humans* (IARC Monographs, Volumes 1 to 29), Lyon

IARC (1983) *Approaches to Classifying Chemical Carcinogens According to Mechanism of Action* (IARC intern. tech. Rep. No. 83/001), Lyon

IARC (1984) *Chemicals and Exposures to Complex Mixtures Recommended for Evaluation in IARC Monographs and Chemicals and Complex Mixtures Recommended for Long-term Carcinogenicity Testing* (IARC intern. tech. Rep. No. 84/002), Lyon

IARC (1987a) *IARC Monographs on the Evaluation of Carcinogenic Risks to Humans*, Supplement 6, *Genetic and Related Effects: An Updating of Selected* IARC Monographs *from Volumes 1 to 42*, Lyon

IARC (1987b) *IARC Monographs on the Evaluation of Carcinogenic Risks to Humans*, Supplement 7, *Overall Evaluations of Carcinogenicity: An Updating of* IARC Monographs *Volumes 1 to 42*, Lyon

IARC (1988) *Report of an IARC Working Group to Review the Approaches and Processes Used to Evaluate the Carcinogenicity of Mixtures and Groups of Chemicals* (IARC intern. tech. Rep. No. 88/002), Lyon

IARC (1989) *Chemicals, Groups of Chemicals, Mixtures and Exposure Circumstances to be Evaluated in Future IARC Monographs, Report of an ad hoc Working Group* (IARC intern. tech. Rep. No. 89/004), Lyon

IARC (1991a) *A Consensus Report of an IARC Monographs Working Group on the Use of Mechanisms of Carcinogenesis in Risk Identification* (IARC intern. tech. Rep. No. 91/002), Lyon

IARC (1991b) *Report of an ad-hoc* IARC Monographs *Advisory Group on Viruses and Other Biological Agents Such as Parasites* (IARC intern. tech. Rep. No. 91/001), Lyon

IARC (1993) *Chemicals, Groups of Chemicals, Complex Mixtures, Physical and Biological Agents and Exposure Circumstances to be Evaluated in Future* IARC Monographs, *Report of an ad-hoc Working Group* (IARC intern. Rep. No. 93/005), Lyon

IARC (1998a) *Report of an ad-hoc* IARC Monographs *Advisory Group on Physical Agents* (IARC Internal Report No. 98/002), Lyon

IARC (1998b) *Report of an ad-hoc* IARC Monographs *Advisory Group on Priorities for Future Evaluations* (IARC Internal Report No. 98/004), Lyon

McGregor, D.B., Rice, J.M. & Venitt, S., eds (1999) *The Use of Short and Medium-term Tests for Carcinogens and Data on Genetic Effects in Carcinogenic Hazard Evaluation* (IARC Scientific Publications No. 146), Lyon, IARC

Montesano, R., Bartsch, H., Vainio, H., Wilbourn, J. & Yamasaki, H., eds (1986) *Long-term and Short-term Assays for Carcinogenesis—A Critical Appraisal* (IARC Scientific Publications No. 83), Lyon, IARC

Peto, R., Pike, M.C., Day, N.E., Gray, R.G., Lee, P.N., Parish, S., Peto, J., Richards, S. & Wahrendorf, J. (1980) Guidelines for simple, sensitive significance tests for carcinogenic effects in long-term animal experiments. In: *IARC Monographs on the Evaluation of the Carcinogenic Risk of Chemicals to Humans*, Supplement 2, *Long-term and Short-term Screening Assays for Carcinogens: A Critical Appraisal*, Lyon, pp. 311–426

Tomatis, L., Aitio, A., Wilbourn, J. & Shuker, L. (1989) Human carcinogens so far identified. *Jpn. J. Cancer Res.*, **80**, 795–807

Vainio, H., Magee, P.N., McGregor, D.B. & McMichael, A.J., eds (1992) *Mechanisms of Carcinogenesis in Risk Identification* (IARC Scientific Publications No. 116), Lyon, IARC

Vainio, H., Wilbourn, J.D., Sasco, A.J., Partensky, C., Gaudin, N., Heseltine, E. & Eragne, I. (1995) *Identification of human carcinogenic risk in* IARC Monographs. *Bull. Cancer,* **82**, 339–348 (in French)

Waters, M.D., Stack, H.F., Brady, A.L., Lohman, P.H.M., Haroun, L. & Vainio, H. (1987) Appendix 1. Activity profiles for genetic and related tests. In: *IARC Monographs on the Evaluation of Carcinogenic Risks to Humans*, Suppl. 6, *Genetic and Related Effects: An Updating of Selected IARC Monographs from Volumes 1 to 42*, Lyon, IARC, pp. 687–696

Wilbourn, J., Haroun, L., Heseltine, E., Kaldor, J., Partensky, C. & Vainio, H. (1986) Response of experimental animals to human carcinogens: an analysis based upon the IARC Monographs Programme. *Carcinogenesis*, **7**, 1853–1863

GENERAL REMARKS ON THE SUBSTANCES CONSIDERED

This seventy-third volume of *IARC Monographs* covers 20 individual compounds and three groups of compounds (cyclamates, saccharin and its salts, and nitrilotriacetic acid and its salts). All but two of these, *meta*-dichlorobenzene and methyl *tert*-butyl ether, were evaluated by previous IARC working groups (Table 1).

Since the previous evaluations, new data have become available, and the Preamble to the *IARC Monographs* has been modified to permit more explicit inclusion of mechanistic considerations and of data on aspects other than cancer in the evaluation process (Vainio *et al.*, 1992). In particular, evidence has accumulated concerning certain pathological processes that lead to tumour development in the kidney and urinary bladder of rats exposed to some chemicals. These include specifically the role of alpha-2 urinary (α_{2u}) globulin-associated nephropathy in the development of epithelial neoplasms of the renal cortex in male rats, and the roles of bladder stones and certain amorphous urinary precipitates in carcinogenesis in the urinary bladder of rats. Specific guidelines have been developed on the use of information on the mechanisms of induction of tumours of the kidney, urinary bladder and thyroid gland in rodents in evaluating the carcinogenicity of certain chemicals (Capen *et al.*, 1999), and these guidelines were used where appropriate in making the current evaluations.

References

Capen, C.C., Dybing, E., Rice, J.M. & Wilbourn, J.D., eds (1999) *Species Differences in Thyroid, Kidney and Urinary Bladder Carcinogenesis* (IARC Scientific Publications No. 147), Lyon, IARC

Vainio, H., Magee, P., McGregor, D. & McMichael, A.J., eds (1992) *Mechanisms of Carcinogenesis in Risk Identification* (IARC Scientific Publications No. 116), Lyon, IARC

Table 1. Previous evaluations of agents considered in this volume

Agent	*IARC Monographs* volume		Degree of carcinogenicity		Overall evaluation of carcinogenicity to humans
	Number	Year	Human	Animal	
Allyl isothiocyanate	36, Suppl. 7	1987	I (ND)	L	3
ortho-Anisidine	27, Suppl. 7	1987	I (ND)	S	2B
Atrazine	53	1991	I	L	2B[a]
Butyl benzyl phthalate	29, Suppl. 7	1987	I (ND)	I	3
Chloroform	20, Suppl. 7	1987	I	S	2B
Chlorothalonil	30, Suppl. 7	1987	I (ND)	L	3
Cyclamates	22, Suppl. 7	1987	I	L	3
ortho-Dichlorobenzene	29, Suppl. 7	1987	I (ND)	I	3
para-Dichlorobenzene	29, Suppl. 7	1987	I (ND)	S	2B
Hexachlorobutadiene	20, Suppl. 7	1987	I (ND)	L	3
Hexachloroethane	20, Suppl. 7	1987	I (ND)	L	3
d-Limonene	56	1993	I (ND)	L	3
Melamine	39, Suppl. 7	1987	I (ND)	I	3
Nitrilotriacetic acid and its salts	48	1990	I (ND)	S	2B
Paracetamol (Acetaminophen)	50	1990	I	L	3
ortho-Phenylphenol	30, Suppl. 7	1987	I (ND)	I	3
Potassium bromate	40, Suppl. 7	1987	I (ND)	S	2B
Quercetin	31, Suppl. 7	1987	I (ND)	L	3
Saccharin	22, Suppl. 7	1987	I	S	2B
Simazine	53	1991	I	I	3
Sodium *ortho*-phenylphenate	30, Suppl. 7	1987	I (ND)	S	2B

I, inadequate evidence; ND, no data; L, limited evidence; S, sufficient evidence; 2B, possibly carcinogenic to humans; 3, not classifiable as to its carcinogenicity to humans (see also Preamble, pp. 23–27)

[a] Mechanistic data were taken into account in making the overall evaluation.

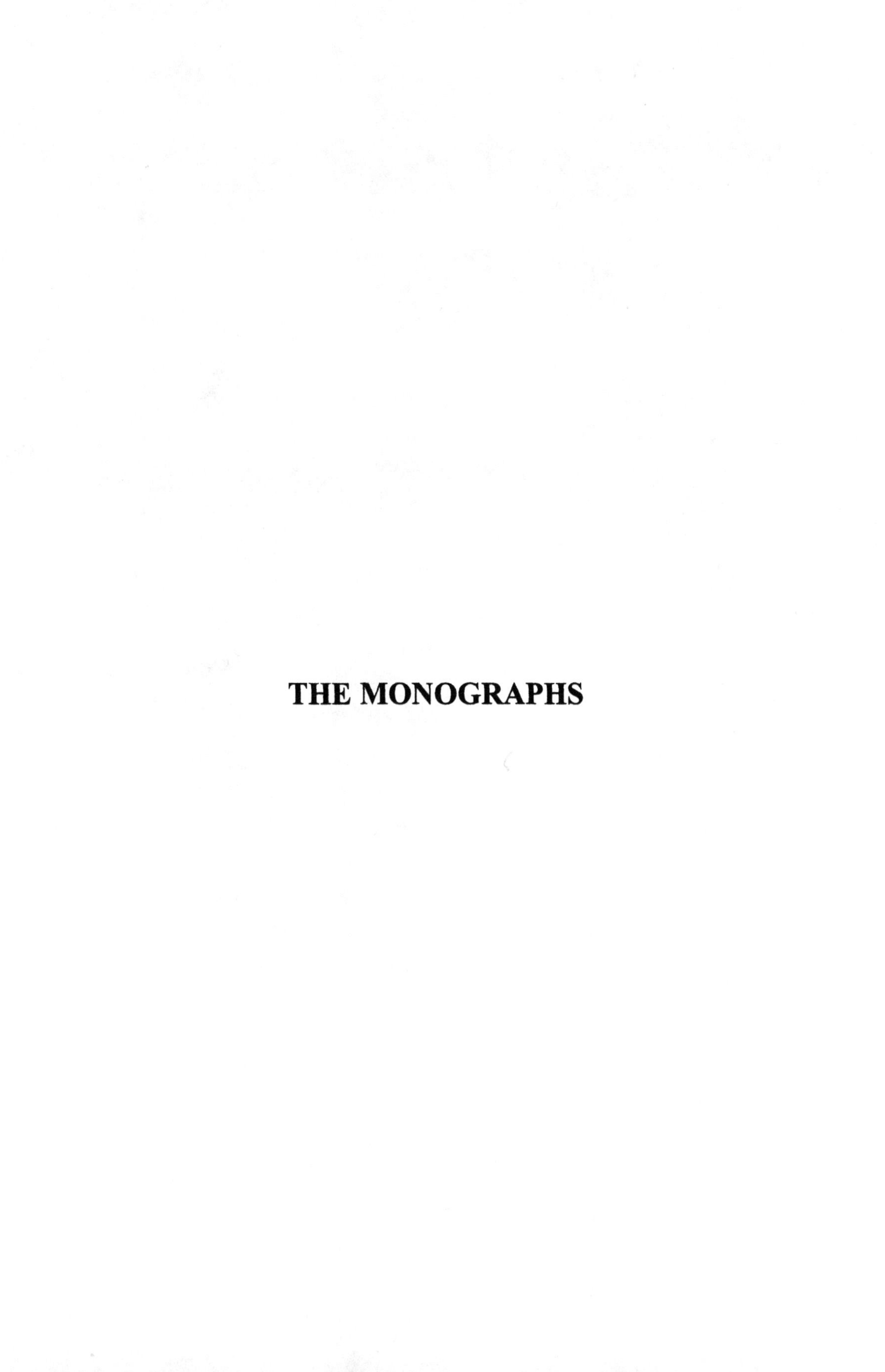

THE MONOGRAPHS

ALLYL ISOTHIOCYANATE

This substance was considered by previous working groups, in 1984 (IARC, 1985) and 1987 (IARC, 1987). Since that time, new data have become available, and these have been incorporated into the monograph and taken into consideration in the present evaluation.

1. Exposure Data

1.1 Chemical and physical data

1.1.1 *Nomenclature*

Chem. Abstr. Serv. Reg. No.: 57-06-7
Deleted CAS Reg. No.: 50888-64-7; 50978-48-8; 58391-87-0; 107231-30-1
Chem. Abstr. Name: 3-Isothiocyanato-1-propene
IUPAC Systematic Name: Allyl isothiocyanate
Synonyms: AITC; allyl mustard oil; allyl senevolum; allyl thioisocyanate; 3-isothiocyanato-1-propene; isothiocyanic acid, allyl ester; mustard oil; oleum sinapis; 2-propenyl isothiocyanate; volatile mustard oil; volatile oil of mustard

1.1.2 *Structural and molecular formulae and relative molecular mass*

$$H_2C{=}CH{-}CH_2N{=}C{=}S$$

C_4H_5NS Relative molecular mass: 99.16

1.1.3 *Chemical and physical properties of the pure substance*

(*a*) *Description*: Colourless or pale-yellow, very refractive liquid with a very pungent, irritating odour and acrid taste (Budavari, 1996)
(*b*) *Boiling-point*: 152°C (Lide, 1997)
(*c*) *Melting-point*: –80°C (Lide, 1997)
(*d*) *Density*: 1.0126 g/cm³ at 20°C (Lide, 1997)
(*e*) *Solubility*: Sparingly soluble in water; very soluble in benzene, ethyl ether and ethanol; miscible with most organic solvents (Budavari, 1996; Lide, 1997)
(*f*) *Vapour pressure*: 1.33 kPa at 38.3°C (Verschueren, 1996)
(*g*) *Octanol/water partition coefficient (P)*: log P, 2.11 (Verschueren, 1996)
(*h*) *Conversion factor*: mg/m³ = 4.06 × ppm

1.2 Production and use

Information available in 1995 indicated that allyl isothiocyanate was produced in Germany, Japan, Mexico and the United States (Chemical Information Services, 1995).

Allyl isothiocyanate is used as a flavouring agent, in medicine as a rubefacient (counterirritant), as a fumigant, in ointments, in mustard plasters, as an adjuvant, as a fungicide, as a repellent for cats and dogs and as a preservative in animal feed (National Toxicology Program, 1991).

1.3 Occurrence

1.3.1 *Natural occurrence*

Allyl isothiocyanate is the chief constituent of natural mustard oil. It is also found in cooked cabbage, horseradish and black mustard seed (National Toxicology Program, 1991).

1.3.2 *Occupational exposure*

No information on occupational exposure to allyl isothiocyanate was available to the Working Group.

1.3.3 *Dietary intake*

The average daily intake of individuals in the United States was estimated to be less than 6 mg/day on the basis of annual usage in 1970 and estimated exposure to allyl isothiocyanate in foods (Food & Drug Administration, 1975).

1.4 Regulations and guidelines

In the former Czechoslovakia, the 8-h time-weighted average exposure limit for allyl isothiocyanate in workplace air was 0.3 mg/m^3 (International Labor Office, 1991).

No international guidelines for allyl isothiocyanate in drinking-water have been established (WHO, 1993).

2. Studies of Cancer in Humans

No data were available to the Working Group.

3. Studies of Cancer in Experimental Animals

Previous evaluation

Allyl isothiocyanate was tested for carcinogenicity by gastric intubation in mice of one strain and in rats of one strain. In mice, no increase in the incidence of tumours was observed. An increased incidence of epithelial hyperplasia and transitional-cell papillomas of the urinary bladder was observed in male rats only, and some subcutaneous fibrosarcomas occurred in female rats given the high dose (IARC, 1985).

New studies

Groups of 20 female A/J mice were given 1 or 5 μmol of allyl isothiocyanate per mouse by gavage in saline or corn oil and then 10 μmol of 4-(methylnitrosamino)-1-(3-pyridyl)butanone (NNK) in 0.1 ml saline or saline alone. Sixteen weeks after these treatments, the animals were killed and pulmonary adenomas were counted. The tumour incidence was 100% in all groups receiving NNK. No statistically significant difference in tumour multiplicity was seen, with 11.1, 11.6 and 9.5 tumour per animal in the controls and in the groups receiving 1 and 5 μmol allyl isothiocyanate, respectively. The incidences of lung adenomas in mice receiving saline were 20 and 10% for those given corn oil and allyl isothiocyanate with multiplicities of 0.3 and 0.2, respectively (Jiao *et al.*, 1994a).

4. Other Data Relevant to an Evaluation of Carcinogenicity and its Mechanisms

4.1 Absorption, distribution, metabolism and excretion

4.1.1 *Humans*

Four adult volunteers (two men, two women, aged 20–45) ingested 10 g brown mustard with bread, and a control group of four participants ate bread without mustard. In a second experiment, 20 g of brown mustard were eaten in turkey or chicken sandwiches. In both experiments, urine samples were collected at various intervals up to 48 h following the meal. The major urinary metabolite was *N*-acetyl-*S*-(*N*-allylthiocarbamoyl)-L-cysteine, the *N*-acetylcysteine conjugate of allyl isothiocyanate, but none was found after 12 h. Excretion of this metabolite was dose-dependent (Jiao *et al.*, 1994b).

4.1.2 *Experimental systems*

Male and female Fischer 344 rats (8–10 weeks old) and male and female B6C3F$_1$ mice (6–8 weeks old) were given [^{14}C]allyl isothiocyanate in a solution of ethanol: Emulphor EL-620:water (1:1:8) at doses of 25.2 or 252 μmol/kg [2.5 or 25 mg/kg bw] by gavage, 25 mg/kg bw by injection into a tail vein for studies of distribution or injection into an exposed femoral vein for studies of biliary excretion. The radiolabel was cleared primarily in urine (70–80%) and exhaled air (13–15%), with lesser amounts in faeces (3–5%) in both species. The major metabolite detected in rat and mouse urine was the mercapturic acid, *N*-acetyl-*S*-(*N*-allylthiocarbamoyl)-L-cysteine, while mouse urine also contained three other major and two minor metabolites. The metabolism of allyl isothiocyanate by male and female rats was similar, but the females excreted more than twice as much urine as the males. Major sex- and species-related differences in the tissue distribution of allyl isothiocyanate were restricted to the urinary bladder. Thus, the urinary bladder of male rats contained five times higher concentrations of allyl isothiocyanate-derived radiolabel that that of male mice at early time points, but all of the allyl isothiocyanate-derived radiolabel was cleared from male rat bladder by 24 h (Ioannou *et al.*, 1984). Similar results were obtained by Bollard *et al.* (1997) after oral administration of allyl isothiocyanate (2.5 or 25 mg/kg bw) to male and female Fischer 344 rats and B6C3F$_1$ mice.

The urinary excretion of allyl isothiocyanate in male Fischer 344 rats did not change with age, but 27-month-old rats showed increased excretion of volatile metabolites and decreased $^{14}CO_2$ production and faecal excretion (Borghoff & Birnbaum, 1986).

Allyl isothiocyanate is a highly reactive compound, which has been shown *in vitro* to form adducts with proteins (Kawakishi & Kaneko, 1987) and glutathione (Kawakishi & Kaneko, 1985).

Oral administration of allyl isothiocyanate, benzyl isothiocyanate or phenethyl isothiocyanate to male Fischer 344 rats inhibited the formation of the α-hydroxylation products of *N*-nitrosopyrrolidine and NNK in liver microsomes (Chung *et al.*, 1984).

All of a series of isothiocyanates (including allyl isothiocyanate, benzyl isothiocyanate, phenethyl isothiocyanate, and 1-hexylisothiocyanate) inhibited dealkylation of pentoxyresorufin more readily than that of ethoxyresorufin in liver microsomes prepared from male Fischer 344 rats treated with phenobarbital or 3-methylcholanthrene. Allyl isothiocyanate and its glutathione conjugate were the weakest inhibitors in the series (Conaway *et al.*, 1996). The chemopreventive activity of isothiocyanates has been correlated to inhibition of this microsomal enzyme (Yang *et al.*, 1994).

Allyl isothiocyanate altered the expression of xenobiotic-metabolizing enzymes such as monooxygenases, amino transferases and glutathione transferases in the liver, small intestine and serum of rats (Lewerenz *et al.*, 1988a; Bogaards *et al.*, 1990). *N*-Nitrosodimethylamine demethylase activity in rat and human liver microsomes was significantly inhibited by arylalkyl isothiocyanates such as benzyl isothiocyanate and phenethyl isothiocyanate at micromolar concentrations, but very weakly inhibited by allyl isothiocyanate and other alkyl isothiocyanates (Jiao *et al.*, 1996).

4.2 Toxic effects

4.2.1 *Humans*

Allyl isothiocyanate irritates the mucous membranes and induces eczematous or vesicular skin reactions (Gaul, 1964). Contact dermatitis was reported in a waitress who handled salad plants, and patch tests with radishes and with allyl isothiocyanate produced positive reactions (Mitchell & Jordan, 1974).

Allyl isothiocyanate was cytostatic and cytotoxic towards a human colon carcinoma cell line, HT29; this activity was reduced when the cells were treated with sodium butyrate or dimethylformamide (Musk & Johnson, 1993a). The authors speculated that allyl isothiocyanate protects against the development of colorectal cancer by selectively inhibiting the growth of transformed cell clones within the gastrointestinal mucosa.

4.2.2 *Experimental systems*

The oral LD_{50} of allyl isothiocyanate dissolved in corn oil was reported to be 339 mg/kg bw in rats (Jenner *et al.*, 1964); in mice, the subcutaneous LD_{50} of a 10%

solution of allyl isothiocyanate in corn oil was 80 mg/kg bw (Klesse & Lukoschek, 1955). The compound strongly irritates skin and mucous membranes (Gosselin *et al.*, 1982).

A single administration of the compound in corn oil by gavage caused growth retardation and dose-related, non-specific signs of toxicity at doses of 200 and 400 mg/kg bw in rats and 100–800 mg/kg bw in mice. In a 14-day experiment in which mice and rats received doses of 3–50 and 25–400 mg/kg bw, respectively, dose-dependent thickening of the stomach mucosa was seen. Rats also showed adhesion of the stomach wall to the peritoneum, and mice given the highest dose developed thickening of the urinary bladder wall. Doses of ≥ 200 mg/kg bw in rats and of ≥ 50 mg/kg bw in mice were lethal. In a study lasting 103 weeks, daily doses of 12 or 25 mg/kg bw caused a slight, dose-related decrease in body-weight gain and mean survival time, and an increased incidence of cytoplasmic vacuolization was noted in the livers of male mice (National Toxicology Program, 1982).

Administration to rats of 0.5 mg allyl isothiocyanate by intraperitoneal injection of 0.1% in the diet for 30 days resulted in reduced blood clotting and prothrombin times, an increase in total plasma phospholipids, increased concentrations of total lipids and cholesterol in the liver and decreased activity of D-amino acid oxidase (Muztar *et al.*, 1979a,b) and xanthine oxidase (Huque & Ahmad, 1975). Feeding allyl isothiocyanate increased the urine volume and increased the uric acid, creatinine and glucose concentrations in the urine of Sprague-Dawley rats (Muztar *et al.*, 1979b).

Allyl isothiocyanate exerts slight goitrogenic activity. Rats weighing 150–320 g given 2–4 mg as a single dose by gavage in water showed inhibited uptake of iodine into the thyroid gland (Langer & Štolc, 1963). Studies *in vitro* indicated that this effect may be due to inhibition of inorganic iodide storage and of organic binding of iodine (Langer & Greer, 1968).

Male outbred rats (Shoe; WIST) (70–90 g) were given allyl isothiocyanate in paraffin oil by gavage at doses of 0, 10, 20 or 40 mg/kg bw on five days per week for up to six weeks (Lewerenz *et al.*, 1988b). The highest dose decreased body weight and thymus weight, reduced the blood glucose and serum globulin concentrations, increased the percentage of neutrophils and decreased the percentage of lymphocytes after two weeks; changes in urinary specific gravity, a slight but significant increase in aspartate aminotransferase activity and histological changes in the kidneys, indicative of renal dysfunction, were also seen at this dose. This investigation did not show that allyl isothiocyanate had a goitrogenic effect, as reported by Langer and Štolc (1963). There were no significant changes in thyroid weight in rats treated for up to four weeks.

Both glutathione and L-cysteine conjugates of allyl isothiocyanate were cytotoxic to RL-4 rat hepatocytes. Since glutathione conjugates cannot enter the cell, their toxicity was suggested to be due to release of free isothiocyanates (Bruggeman *et al.*, 1986).

4.3 Reproductive and developmental effects

4.3.1 *Humans*

No data were available to the Working Group.

4.3.2 *Experimental systems*

Allyl isothiocyanate has been tested for developmental toxicity by exposing CD-1 mice to doses of up to 28 mg/kg bw per day, Wistar rats to 18.5 mg/kg bw per day, Syrian hamsters to 23.8 mg/kg bw per day and Dutch-belted rabbits to 12.3 mg/kg bw per day throughout their respective major organogenesis periods. No evidence of maternal toxicity and no treatment-related malformations were observed in any species. There was some increase in the incidence of resorbed fetuses in mice, the average number of live pups per litter being 9.9 at the highest dose and 11 in the controls, while the percentage of dead implants was 14 at this dose and 5.7 in the controls. No adverse developmental effects were seen when limited numbers of Wistar rats received up to 120 mg/kg bw by oral intubation on day 12 or 13 gestation. When Holtzman rats received up to 100 mg/kg bw by subcutaneous injection on days 8 and 9 of gestation, the incidence of resorptions was increased at the high dose (IARC, 1985).

4.4 Genetic and related effects

4.4.1 *Humans*

No data were available to the Working Group.

4.4.2 *Experimental systems* (see Table 1 for references)

Inconsistent results for gene mutation in *Salmonella typhimurium* TA100 and TA98 were found with and without exogenous metabolic activation. Allyl isothiocyanate did not induce gene mutation in *Salmonella* strains TA1535, TA1537 or TA1538 in the absence of exogenous metabolic activation, but it induced mutation in *Escherichia coli* with exogenous metabolic activation. Allyl isothiocyanate at a very high dose induced chromosomal aberrations in *Allium cepa*. Sex-linked recessive lethal mutations were induced in *Drosophila melanogaster*. The compound induced gene mutation in mouse lymphoma L5178Y cells in the absence of exogenous metabolic activation. It did not induce sister chromatid exchange in Chinese hamster ovary cells in the absence of exogenous metabolic activation, but inconsistent results were obtained in assays for chromosomal aberration in mammalian cells *in vitro*. In single studies, allyl isothiocyanate was reported to induce aneuploidy and cell transformation in a Chinese hamster cell line at the extremely low concentration of 5 pg/mL and chromosomal aberrations in human cells *in vitro*, but it did not induce aneuploidy or cell transformation in human fibroblasts *in vitro*. It did not induce dominant lethal mutations in mice and did not give rise to unscheduled DNA synthesis in the liver of rats exposed *in vivo*.

Mustard oil, which is reported to contain more than 90% allyl isothiocyanate, induced sex-linked recessive lethal mutations in *Drosophila melanogaster* but did not induce aneuploidy. It did not induce chromosomal aberrations in human embryonic lung cells *in vitro* and did not induce any 'genetic effect' in *Saccharomyces cerevisiae* in a host-mediated assay. It did not induce chromosomal aberrations in bone marrow or dominant lethal mutations in rats treated *in vivo*.

Table 1. Genetic and related effects of allyl isothiocyanate

Test system	Results[a]		Dose[b] (LED or HID)	Reference
	Without exogenous metabolic system	With exogenous metabolic system		
Salmonella typhimurium TA100, TA98, reverse mutation	+	NT	25	Yamaguchi (1980)
Salmonella typhimurium TA100, TA98, reverse mutation	–	–	500 μg/plate	Kasamaki *et al.* (1982)
Salmonella typhimurium TA100, TA1535, TA98 reverse mutation	–	–	0.1 μL/plate	Eder *et al.* (1980)
Salmonella typhimurium TA1535, TA1537, TA1538, reverse mutation	–	–	100 μg/plate	Yamaguchi (1980)
Salmonella typhimurium TA100, reverse mutation	–	+	0.25 μL/plate	Neudecker & Henschler (1985)
Escherichia coli WP67, reverse mutation	–	+	99	Rihová (1982)
Allium cepa, chromosomal aberrations	+	NT	20 000	Sharma & Sharma (1962)
Drosophila melanogaster, sex-linked recessive lethal mutations	+		NR	Auerbach & Robson (1944)
Gene mutation, mouse lymphoma L5178Y cells, *tk* locus *in vitro*	+	NT	0.4	McGregor *et al.* (1988)
Sister chromatid exchange, Chinese hamster ovary cells *in vitro*	–	NT	3.0	Musk *et al.* (1995)
Chromosomal aberrations, Chinese hamster B241 cells *in vitro*	+	NT	0.0001	Kasamaki *et al.* (1982)
Chromosomal aberrations, Chinese hamster ovary cells *in vitro*	–	NT	3.0	Musk *et al.* (1995)
Chromosomal aberrations, Chinese hamster B241 cells *in vitro*	+	NT	0.0005	Kasamaki *et al.* (1987)
Chromosomal aberrations, transformed Indian muntjac cells *in vitro*	–	NT	0.8	Musk & Johnson (1993b)
Aneuploidy, Chinese hamster B241 cells *in vitro*	+	NT	0.0005	Kasamaki *et al.* (1987)
Cell transformation, Chinese hamster B241 cells with confirmation *in vivo*	+	NT	0.0005	Kasamaki *et al.* (1987)
Chromosomal aberrations, human HAIN-55 fibroblasts *in vitro*	+	NT	0.002	Kasamaki *et al.* (1987)
Aneuploidy, human HAIN-55 cells *in vitro*	–	NT	0.002	Kasamaki *et al.* (1987)
Cell transformation, human HAIN-55 cells *in vitro*	–	NT	0.002	Kasamaki *et al.* (1987)
Dominant lethal mutation, mice *in vivo*	–		19 ip × 1	Epstein *et al.* (1972)

Table 1 (contd)

Test system	Results[a]		Dose[b] (LED or HID)	Reference
	Without exogenous metabolic system	With exogenous metabolic system		
Unscheduled DNA synthesis, rat hepatocytes *in vivo*	–		125 po × 1	Bechtel *et al.* (1998)
Mustard oil reported to contain > 90% allyl isothiocyanate				
Drosophila melanogaster, sex-linked recessive lethal mutations	+		NR, spray	Auerbach & Robson (1947)
Drosophila melanogaster, aneuploidy	–		NR, spray	Auerbach & Robson (1947)
Chromosomal aberrations, human embryonic lung cells *in vitro*	–	NT	10	Food & Drug Administration (1975)
Host-mediated assay, *Saccharomyces cerevisiae* in mouse peritoneal cavity	–		130 po × 1	Food & Drug Administration (1975)
Chromosomal aberrations, rat bone-marrow cells *in vivo*	–		100 po × 1	Food & Drug Administration (1975)
Dominant lethal mutation, rats *in vivo*	–		100 po × 1	Food & Drug Administration (1975)

[a] +, positive; –, negative; NT, not tested
[b] LED, lowest effective dose; HID, highest ineffective dose; unless otherwise stated, in-vitro test, μg/mL; in-vivo test, mg/kg bw per day; ip, intraperitoneal; NR, not reported; po, oral

5. Summary of Data Reported and Evaluation

5.1 Exposure data

Exposure to allyl isothiocyanate occurs as a result of its presence in foods as the chief constituent of mustard oil and as a flavouring agent.

5.2 Human carcinogenicity data

No data were available to the Working Group.

5.3 Animal carcinogenicity data

Allyl isothiocyanate was tested for carcinogenicity in one experiment in mice and one experiment in rats by oral administration. No increase in tumour incidence was observed in mice. An increased but low incidence of transitional-cell hyperplasia and papillomas of the urinary bladder was observed in male rats, and there was a low incidence of subcutaneous fibrosarcomas in female rats given the high dose.

5.4 Other relevant data

Major sex- and species-related differences in the tissue distribution of allyl isothiocyanate were restricted to the urinary bladder, where higher concentrations of allyl isothiocyanate-derived radiolabel were found in the bladders of male rats than in mice or female rats. Rodents and humans both metabolize allyl isothiocyanate to *N*-acetyl-*S*-(*N*-allyl thiocarbamoyl)-L-cysteine. Allyl isothiocyanate appears to be an irritant in both rodents and humans.

Allyl isothiocyanate was not teratogenic to mice, rats, hamsters or rabbits, but resorptions were seen in mice and rats.

No data were available on the genetic and related effects of allyl isothiocyanate in humans. The available data do not allow a conclusion about the genotoxicity of allyl isothiocyanate in expertimental systems *in vivo*. There is evidence for genotoxic effects in mammalian cells *in vitro*. It was not mutagenic to bacteria.

5.5 Evaluation

There is *inadequate evidence* in humans for the carcinogenicity of allyl isothiocyanate.

There is *limited evidence* in experimental animals for the carcinogenicity of allyl isothiocyanate.

Overall evaluation

Allyl isothiocyanate is *not classifiable as to its carcinogenicity to humans (Group 3)*.

6. References

Auerbach, C. & Robson, J.M. (1944) Production of mutations by allyl isothiocyanate. *Nature*, **54**, 81

Auerbach, C. & Robson, J.M. (1947) Tests of chemical substances for mutagenic action. *Proc. R. Soc. Edinburgh*, **62B**, 284–291

Bechtel, D., Henderson, L. & Proudlock, R. (1998) Lack of UDS activity in the livers of rats exposed to allylisothiocyanate. *Teratog. Carcinog. Mutag.*, **18**, 209–217

Bogaards, J.J.P., van Ommen, B., Falke, H.E., Williams, M.I. & van Bladeren, P.J. (1990) Glutathione *S*-transferase subunit induction patterns of brussels sprouts, allyl isothiocyanate and goitrin in rat liver and small intestinal mucosa: A new approach for the identification of inducing xenobiotics. *Food chem. Toxicol.*, **28**, 81–88

Bollard, M., Stribbling, S., Mitchell, S. & Caldwell, J. (1997) The disposition of allyl isothiocyanate in the rat and mouse. *Food chem. Toxicol.*, **35**, 933–943

Borghoff, S.J. & Birnbaum, L.S. (1986) Age-related changes in the metabolism and excretion of allyl isothiocyanate. A model compound for glutathione conjugation. *Drug Metab. Disposition*, **14**, 417–422

Bruggeman, I.M., Temmink, J.H.M. & van Bladeren, P.J. (1986) Glutathione- and cysteine-mediated cytotoxicity of allyl and benzyl isothiocyanate. *Toxicol. appl. Pharmacol.*, **83**, 349–359

Budavari, S., ed. (1996) *The Merck Index*, 12th Ed., Whitehouse Station, NJ, Merck & Co., Inc., p. 54

Chemical Information Services (1995) *Directory of World Chemical Producers 1995/96 Standard Edition*, Dallas, TX, p. 442

Chung, F.-L., Juchatz, A., Vitarius, J. & Hecht, S.S. (1984) Effects of dietary compounds on α-hydroxylation of *N*-nitrosopyrrolidine and *N′*-nitrosonornicotine in rat target tissues. *Cancer Res.*, **44**, 2924–2928

Conaway, C.C., Jiao, D. & Chung, F.-L. (1996) Inhibition of rat liver cytochrome P450 isozymes by isothiocyanates and their conjugates: A structure–activity relationship study. *Carcinogenesis*, **17**, 2423–2427

Eder, E., Neudecker, T., Lutz, D. & Henschler, D. (1980) Mutagenic potential of allyl and allylic compounds. *Biochem. Pharmacol.*, **29**, 993–998

Epstein, S.S., Arnold, E., Andrea, J., Bass, W. & Bishop, Y. (1972) Detection of chemical mutagens by the dominant lethal assay in the mouse. *Toxicol. appl. Pharmacol*, **23**, 288–325

Food & Drug Administration (1975) *Evaluation of Health Aspects of Mustard and Oil of Mustard and Food Ingredients* (PB-254 528), Springfield, VA, Federtion of American Societies for Experimental Biology, National Technical Information Service

Gaul, L.E. (1964) Contact dermatitis from synthetic oil of mustard. *Arch. Dermatol.*, **90**, 158–159

Gosselin, R.E., Hodge, H.C., Smith, R.P. & Gleason, M.N., eds (1982) *Clinical Toxicology of Commercial Products. Acute Poisoning*, 4th Ed., Baltimore, MD, Williams & Wilkins, p. II-216

Huque, T. & Ahmad, P. (1975) Effect of allyl isothiocyanate on blood and urine levels of uric acid and glucose in rats. *Bangladesh J. Biol. Agric.*, **4**, 12–13

IARC (1985) *IARC Monographs on the Evaluation of Carcinogenic Risk of Chemicals to Humans*, Vol. 36, *Allyl Compounds, Aldehydes, Epoxides and Peroxides*, Lyon, pp. 55–68

IARC (1987) *IARC Monographs on the Evaluation of Carcinogenic Risks to Humans*, Suppl. 7, *Overall Evaluations of Carcinogenicity: An Updating of* IARC Monographs *Volumes 1 to 42*, Lyon, p. 56

International Labour Office (1991) *Occupational Exposure Limits for Airborne Toxic Substances*, 3rd. Ed. (Occupational Safety and Health Series No. 37), Geneva, p. 12

Ioannou, Y.M., Burka, L.T. & Matthews, H.B. (1984) Allyl isothiocyanate: Comparative disposition in rats and mice. *Toxicol. appl. Pharmacol.*, **75**, 173–181

Jenner, P.M., Hagan, E.C., Taylor, J.M., Cook, E.L. & Fitzhugh, O.G. (1964) Food flavourings and compounds of related structure. I. Acute oral toxicity. *Food Cosmet. Toxicol.*, **2**, 327–343

Jiao, D., Eklind, K.I., Choi, C.-I., Desai, D.H., Amin, S.G. & Chung, F.-L. (1994a) Structure–activity relationships of isothiocyanates as mechanism-based inhibition of 4-(methylnitrosamino)-1-(3-pyridyl)butanone-induced lung tumorigenesis in A/J mice. *Cancer Res.*, **54**, 4327–4333

Jiao, D., Ho, C.-T., Foiles, P. & Chung, F.-L. (1994b) Identification and quantification of the *N*-acetylcysteine conjugate of allyl isothiocyanate in human urine after ingestion of mustard. *Cancer Epidemiol. Biomarkers Prev.*, **3**, 487–492

Jiao, D., Conaway, C.C., Wang, M.-H., Yang, C.S., Koehl, W. & Chung, F.-L. (1996) Inhibition of *N*-nitrosodimethylamine demethylase in rat and human liver microsomes by isothiocyanates and their glutathione, L-cysteine and *N*-acetyl-L-cysteine conjugates. *Chem. Res. Toxicol.*, **9**, 932–938

Kasamaki, A., Takahashi, H., Tsumura, N., Niwa, J., Fujita, T. & Urasawa, S. (1982) Genotoxicity of flavoring agents. *Mutat. Res.*, **105**, 387–392

Kasamaki, A., Yasuhara, T. & Urasawa, S. (1987) Neoplastic transformation of Chinese hamster cells *in vitro* after treatment with flavoring agents. *J. toxicol. Sci.*, **12**, 383–396

Kawakishi, S. & Kaneko, T. (1985) Interaction of oxidized glutathione with allyl isothiocyanate. *Phytochemistry*, **24**, 715–718

Kawakishi, S. & Kaneko, T. (1987) Interaction of proteins with allyl isothiocyanate. *J. agric. Food Chem.*, **35**, 85–88

Klesse, P. & Lukoschek, P. (1955) [Investigations of the bacteriostatic action of some mustard oils.] *Arzneimittelforsch.*, **5**, 505–507 (in German)

Langer, P. & Greer, M.A. (1968) Antithyroid activity of some naturally occurring isothiocyanates in vitro. *Metabolism*, **17**, 596–605

Langer, P. & Štolc, V. (1963) Goitrogenic activity of allylisothiocyanate—a widespread natural mustard oil. *Endocrinology*, **76**, 151–155

Lewerenz, H.-J., Plass, R. & Macholz, R. (1988a) Effect of allyl isothiocyanate on hepatic monooxygenases and serum transferases in rats. *Toxicol. Lett.*, **45**, 65–70

Lewerenz, H.-J., Plass, R., Bleyl, D.W.R. & Macholz, R. (1988b) Short-term toxicity study of allyl isothiocyanate in rats. *Die Nahrung*, **32**, 723–728

Lide, D.R., ed. (1997) *CRC Handbook of Chemistry and Physics*, 78th Ed., Boca Raton, FL, CRC Press, p. 3-289

McGregor, D.B., Brown, A., Cattanach, P., Edwards, I., McBride, D., Riach, C. & Caspary, W.J. (1988) Responses of the L5178Y *tk*+/*tk*- mouse lymphoma cell forward mutation assay: III. 72 coded chemicals. *Environ. mol. Mutag.*, **12**, 85–154

Mitchell, J.C. & Jordan, W.P. (1974) Allergic contact dermatitis from the radish, *Raphanus sativus*. *Br. J. Dermatol.*, **91**, 183–189

Musk, S.R.R. & Johnson, I.T. (1993a) Allyl isothiocyanate is selectively toxic to transformed cells of the human colorectal tumor line HT29. *Carcinogenesis*, **14**, 2079–2083

Musk, S.R.R. & Johnson, I.T. (1993b) The clastogenic effects of isothiocyanates. *Mutat. Res.*, **300**, 111–117

Musk, S.R.R., Smith, T.K. & Johnson, I.T. (1995) On the cytotoxicity and genotoxicity of allyl and phenethyl isothiocyanates and their parent glucosinolates sinigrin and gluconasturtiin. *Mutat. Res.*, **348**, 19–23

Muztar, A.J., Ahmad, P., Huque, T. & Slinger, S.J. (1979a) A study of the chemical binding of allyl isothiocyanate with thyroxine and of the effect of allyl isothiocyanate on lipid metabolism in the rat. *Can. J. Physiol. Pharmacol.*, **57**, 385–389

Muztar, A.J., Huque, T., Ahmad, P. & Slinger, S.J. (1979b) Effect of allyl isothiocyanate on plasma and urinary concentrations of some biochemical entities in the rat. *Can. J. Physiol. Pharmacol.*, **57**, 504–509

National Toxicology Program (1982) *Carcinogenesis Bioassay of Allyl Isothiocyanate (CAS No. 57-06-7) in F344/N Rats and B6C3F$_1$ Mice (Gavage Study)* (NTP No. 81-36; NIH Publication No. 83-1790), Washington DC, US Department of Health and Human Services

National Toxicology Program (1991) *NTP Chemical Repository Data Sheet: Allyl Isothiocyanate*, Research Triangle Park, NC

Neudecker, T. & Henschler, D. (1985) Allyl isothiocyanate is mutagenic in *Salmonella typhimurium*. *Mutat. Res.*, **156**, 33–37

Rihová, E. (1982) Mutagenic effects of allyl isothiocyanate in *Escherichia coli* WP 67. *Folia microbiol.*, **27**, 25–31

Sharma, A.K. & Sharma, A. (1962) A study of the importance of nucleic acids in controlling chromosome breaks induced by different compounds. *Nucleus*, **5**, 127–136

Verschueren, K. (1996) *Handbook of Environmental Data on Organic Chemicals*, 3rd Ed., New York, Van Nostrand Reinhold Co., pp. 163–164

WHO (1993) *Guidelines for Drinking Water Quality*, 2nd Ed., Vol. 1, *Recommendations*, Geneva

Yamaguchi, T. (1980) Mutagenicity of isothiocyanates, isocyanates and thioureas on *Salmonella typhimurium*. *Agric. Biol. Chem.*, **44**, 3017–3018

Yang, C.S., Smith, T.J. & Hong, J.Y. (1994) Cytochrome P-450 enzymes as targets for chemoprevention against chemical carcinogenesis and toxicity: Opportunities and limitations. *Cancer Res.*, **54** (Suppl. 7), 1982s–1986s

ortho-ANISIDINE

This substance was considered by previous working groups, in 1981 (IARC, 1982) and 1987 (IARC, 1987). Since that time, new data have become available, and these have been incorporated into the monograph and taken into consideration in the present evaluation.

1. Exposure Data

1.1 Chemical and physical data

1.1.1 *Nomenclature*

Chem. Abstr. Serv. Reg. No.: 90-04-0

Chem. Abstr. Name: 2-Methoxybenzenamine

IUPAC Systematic Name: *o*-Anisidine

Synonyms: *ortho*-Aminoanisole; 2-aminoanisole; *ortho*-aminomethoxybenzene; 2-aminomethoxybenzene; 1-amino-2-methoxybenzene; 2-methoxy-1-aminobenzene; *ortho*-methoxyaniline; 2-methoxyaniline; 2-methoxybenzenamine; *ortho*-methoxyphenylamine; 2-methoxyphenylamine

1.1.2 *Structural and molecular formulae and relative molecular mass*

NH_2

OCH_3

C_7H_9NO Relative molecular mass: 123.15

1.1.3 *Chemical and physical properties of the pure substance*

(*a*) *Description*: Yellowish liquid; becomes brownish on exposure to air (Budavari, 1996)

(*b*) *Boiling-point*: 224°C (Lide, 1997)

(*c*) *Melting-point*: 6.2°C (Lide, 1997)

(*d*) *Density*: 1.096 g/cm^3 at 20°C (Lide, 1997)

(*e*) *Solubility*: Slightly soluble in water; soluble in ethanol, diethyl ether and acetone (Lide, 1997)

(*f*) *Stability*: Susceptible to oxidation in air (National Toxicology Program, 1991) (*g*) *Octanol/water partition coefficient (P)*: log P, 0.95 (calculated), 1.18 (measured) (Verschueren, 1996).

(*h*) *Conversion factor*: mg/m³ = 5.04 × ppm

1.2 Production and use

Information available in 1995 indicated that *ortho*-anisidine was produced in Armenia, China, France, Germany, India, Japan, the Ukraine and the United Kingdom (Chemical Information Services, 1995).

ortho-Anisidine is used as a chemical intermediate (e.g. in the manufacture of azo or triphenylmethane dyes and pharmaceuticals), as a corrosion inhibitor for steel storage and as an antioxidant for some polymercaptan resins (National Toxicology Program, 1991).

1.3 Occurrence

1.3.1 *Natural occurrence*

ortho-Anisidine is not known to occur naturally.

1.3.2 *Occupational exposure*

According to the 1981–83 National Occupational Exposure Survey (National Institute for Occupational Safety and Health, 1998), approximately 700 workers in the United States were potentially exposed to *ortho*-anisidine. Occupational exposure to *ortho*-anisidine may occur during its production and during its use as a chemical intermediate, corrosion inhibitor or antioxidant.

1.3.3 *Environmental occurrence*

ortho-Anisidine has been identified in wastewater from chemical plants and from oil refineries, and in cigarette smoke (National Library of Medicine, 1998a).

According to the United States Environmental Protection Agency Toxic Chemical Release Inventory for 1987, 1600 kg of *ortho*-anisidine were released into the air, 280 kg were discharged into water, and 110 kg were released onto the land from manufacturing and processing facilities in the United States. By 1996, 690 kg were released into the air and 13 kg discharged into water (National Library of Medicine, 1998b).

1.4 Regulations and guidelines

The American Conference of Governmental Industrial Hygienists (1997) has recommended an 8-h time-weighted average threshold limit value of 0.5 mg/m³, with a notation for potential dermal absorption, for occupational exposure to *ortho*-anisidine in workplace air. Similar values have been used as standards or guidelines in many other countries (International Labour Office, 1991).

No international guidelines for *ortho*-anisidine in drinking-water have been established (WHO, 1993).

2. Studies of Cancer in Humans

No data were available to the Working Group.

3. Studies of Cancer in Experimental Animals

Previous evaluation

ortho-Anisidine hydrochloride was tested for carcinogenicity in one study in mice and one study in rats by oral administration in the diet. It produced transitional-cell carcinomas of the urinary bladder in animals of each species and sex (IARC, 1982).

New studies

In a model of urinary bladder carcinogenesis, groups of 15 male Fischer 344 rats, six weeks of age, were given 0.05% *N*-nitroso-*N*,4-hydroxybutylamine (NHBA) in the drinking-water for four weeks. They were then fed diets with or without a supplement of 1700 mg/kg diet (ppm) *ortho*-anisidine for the first two weeks and 425 ppm thereafter for an additional 30 weeks. Ten animals received *ortho*-anisidine without prior NHBA administration. The incidence of papillary or nodular hyperplasia in the urinary bladder, derived by assessing the number of lesions per unit length of mucosa, was significantly higher ($p < 0.01$) in the group receiving *ortho*-anisidine plus NHBA (13/16) than in the group given NHBA alone (2/13). No lesions were observed in animals receiving *ortho*-anisidine alone (Ono *et al.*, 1992).

4. Other Data Relevant to an Evaluation of Carcinogenicity and its Mechanisms

4.1 Absorption, distribution, metabolism and excretion

4.1.1 *Humans*

No data were available to the Working Group.

4.1.2 *Experimental systems*

Horseradish peroxidase oxidized *ortho*-anisidine via a nitrogen-centred cation radical to the diimine, quinone imine and an azo dimer *in vitro*. The metabolism led to covalent binding to calf thymus DNA. Metabolites of *ortho*-anisidine were consistently more reactive with protein and glutathione than metabolites of *para*-anisidine (Thompson & Eling, 1991). [The Working Group noted that studies with mammalian enzymes have not been carried out.]

4.2 Toxic effects

4.2.1 *Humans*

No data were available to the Working Group.

4.2.2 *Experimental systems*

The oral LD_{50} of *ortho*-anisidine has been reported to be 2000 mg/kg bw in rats, 870 mg/kg bw in rabbits and 1400 mg/kg bw in mice. Its subacute effects include haematological changes, anaemia and nephrotoxicity (Prosolenko, 1975).

ortho-Anisidine induced methaemoglobinaemia in CBA mice and Alpk:APfSD rats after oral administration (Ashby *et al.*, 1991). The authors suggested that their results indicate that *ortho*-anisidine is distributed and *N*-oxidized in rodents.

Male and female B6C3F_1 mice were fed diets containing up to 30 000 mg/kg of diet (ppm) *ortho*-anisidine hydrochloride for seven weeks. A dose-dependent depression in mean body-weight gain of up to 40% was observed. The spleens of mice given doses > 10 000 mg/kg of diet were black and enlarged. Female mice that received doses of 2500 or 5000 mg/kg of diet for up to 103 weeks developed more cystic hyperplasia of the uterus and endometrium than did control animals. Mice of each sex at 30 000 mg/kg of diet had an increased incidence of hyperplasia of the bladder (National Cancer Institute, 1978).

Feeding of diets containing up to 30 000 mg/kg (ppm) *ortho*-anisidine hydrochloride to Fischer 344 rats for seven weeks led to reductions in weight gain of up to 52% in males and 27% in females. Feeding of diets containing 1000 or 3000 mg/kg resulted in granular spleens in males but not in females; the spleens of rats of each sex given diets containing *ortho*-anisidine at > 10 000 mg/kg were dark and granular. A dose of 10 000 mg/kg of diet for up to 103 weeks resulted in depressions of body-weight gain of 21% in males and 11% in females. Male and female rats fed diets containing 5000 or 10 000 mg/kg *ortho*-anisidine hydrochloride developed non-neoplastic lesions of the thyroid gland and kidney more frequently than did control animals (National Cancer Institute, 1978).

4.3 Reproductive and developmental effects

No data were available to the Working Group.

4.4 Genetic and related effects

4.4.1 *Humans*

No data were available to the Working Group.

4.4.2 *Experimental systems* (see Table 1 for references)

ortho-Anisidine did not induce reverse mutation in *Escherichia coli* or in *Salmonella typhimurium* strains TA100, TA1535, TA1537, TA1538, TA98 or YG1012. In the presence of exogenous metabolic activation, it induced mutations in strain YG1029, both YG strains having elevated levels of *N*-acetyltransferase. *ortho*-Anisidine did not induce sex-linked recessive lethal mutations in *Drosophila*. It gave rise to gene mutations in

Table 1. Genetic and related effects of *ortho*-anisidine

Test system	Results[a]		Dose[b] (LED or HID)	Reference
	Without exogenous metabolic system	With exogenous metabolic system		
Salmonella typhimurium TA100, TA98, TA1535, TA1537, reverse mutation	–	–	10 800 µg/plate	Haworth *et al.* (1983)
Salmonella typhimurium TA100, TA98, TA1535, TA1537, TA1538, reverse mutation	–	–	10 000 µg/plate	Dunkel *et al.* (1985)
Salmonella typhimurium YG1012 (TA1538 with *N*-acetyltransferase gene), reverse mutation	–	–	Not reported	Thompson *et al.* (1992)
Salmonella typhimurium YG1029 (TA100 with *N*-acetyltransferase gene), reverse mutation	–	+	62 µg/plate	Thompson *et al.* (1992)
Escherichia coli WP2*uvrA*, reverse mutation	–	–	10 000 µg/plate	Dunkel *et al.* (1985)
Drosophila melanogaster, sex-linked recessive lethal mutations	–		2000 ppm inj	Yoon *et al.* (1985)
DNA strand breaks/cross-links, mouse lymphoma L5178Y cells *in vitro*	–	+	150	Garberg *et al.* (1988)
Gene mutation, mouse lymphoma L5178Y cells, *tk* locus *in vitro*	+	+	123	Wangenheim & Bolcsfoldi (1988)
Sister chromatid exchange, Chinese hamster ovary cells *in vitro*	+	+	38	Galloway *et al.* (1987)
Chromosomal aberrations, Chinese hamster ovary cells *in vitro*	+	+	1200	Galloway *et al.* (1987)
Cell transformation, Syrian hamster embryo cells, clonal assay	+	NT	500	Kerkaert *et al.* (1998)
Host-mediated assay, *Escherichia coli* in blood of mouse, DNA repair *in vivo*	–		1300 po × 1	Hellmer & Bolcsfoldi (1992)
Host-mediated assay, *Escherichia coli* in blood of mouse, DNA repair *in vivo*	+		310 ip × 1	Hellmer & Bolcsfoldi (1992)
DNA single-strand break, liver, thymus and testis of Sprague-Dawley rats *in vivo*	–		700 po × 1	Ashby *et al.* (1991)
DNA single-strand break, liver, kidney, spleen and bladder of Wistar rats *in vivo*	–		500 po × 1	Ashby *et al.* (1991)
DNA single-strand break, liver and bladder of Wistar rats *in vivo*	–		750 ip × 1	Ashby *et al.* (1991)
DNA breaks, bladder and colon of CD-1 mice *in vivo*	+		690 po × 1	Sasaki *et al.* (1998)

Table 1 (contd)

Test system	Results[a]		Dose[b] (LED or HID)	Reference
	Without exogenous metabolic system	With exogenous metabolic system		
Unscheduled DNA synthesis, rat hepatocytes *in vivo*	–		1104 po × 1	Ashby *et al.* (1991)
Unscheduled DNA synthesis, rat kidney cells *in vivo*	–		500 ip × 1	Tyson & Mirsalis (1985)
Gene mutation, mouse bladder cells *in vivo*, *lacI* transgenic model	(+)		750 po × 3	Ashby *et al.* (1994)
Gene mutation, mouse liver cells *in vivo*, *lacI* transgenic model	-		750 po × 10	Ashby *et al.* (1994)
Micronucleus formation, CBA mouse bone-marrow cells *in vivo*	–		690 po × 1–3	Ashby *et al.* (1991)
Micronucleus formation, $B6C3F_1$ mouse bone-marrow cells *in vivo*	–		500 ip × 3	Ashby *et al.* (1991)
Micronucleus formation, mouse bone-marrow cells *in vivo*	?		800 ip × 1	Morita *et al.* (1997)
Micronucleus formation, AP and Fischer 344 rat bone-marrow cells *in vivo*	–		1380 po × 1	Ashby *et al.* (1991)
Micronucleus formation, rats liver cells *in vivo*	–		1104 po × 1	Ashby *et al.* (1991)
Binding (covalent) to DNA, $B6C3F_1$ mouse bladder and liver *in vivo*	–		750 po × 1	Ashby *et al.* (1994)
Inhibition of gap-junctional intercellular communication, 3PC mouse keratinocytes *in vitro*	+	NT	1232	Jansen & Jongen (1996)

[a] +, positive; (+), weakly positive; –, negative; NT, not tested; ?, inconclusive
[b] LED, lowest effective dose; HID, highest ineffective dose; unless otherwise stated, in-vitro test, µg/mL; in-vivo test, mg/kg bw per day; inj, injection; po, oral; ip, intraperitoneal

mouse lymphoma L5178Y cells *in vitro* both in the presence and absence of exogenous metabolic activation, while DNA breaks and cross-links were observed only in the presence of an exogenous metabolic system. Sister chromatid exchange and chromosomal aberrations were induced in Chinese hamster ovary cells *in vitro*, both in the presence and absence of exogenous metabolic activation. In the absence of exogenous metabolic activation, *ortho*-anisidine induced cell transformation in Syrian hamster embryo cells *in vitro*. *ortho*-Anisidine did not bind covalently to DNA in mouse bladder or liver cells *in vivo*; it did not induce single-strand breaks in liver, thymus, testis, kidney, spleen or bladder DNA of rats treated *in vivo*, nor did it induce unscheduled DNA synthesis in rat hepatocytes or kidney cells *in vivo*. In mice treated *in vivo*, *ortho*-anisidine gave rise to breaks in bladder and colon DNA but not in DNA of stomach, kidney, liver, lung, brain or bone marrow. *ortho*-Anisidine induced DNA repair in *E. coli* in a host-mediated assay in male mice when the animals were treated intraperitoneally but not when they were treated by oral gavage. *ortho*-Anisidine weakly induced gene mutation in the *lacI* transgene in mouse bladder but not in liver. It did not induce micronuclei in bone marrow of mice or in bone-marrow or liver cells of rats treated *in vivo*.

ortho-Anisidine inhibited gap-junctional intercellular communication in mouse hepatocytes in the absence of an exogenous metabolic system *in vitro*.

5. Summary of Data Reported and Evaluation

5.1 Exposure data

Exposure to *ortho*-anisidine may occur during its production and its use as a chemical intermediate, a corrosion inhibitor and an industrial antioxidant.

5.2 Human carcinogenicity data

No data were available to the Working Group.

5.3 Animal carcinogenicity data

ortho-Anisidine hydrochloride was tested for carcinogenicity in one study in mice and one study in rats by oral administration in the diet. It produced transitional-cell carcinomas of the urinary bladder in animals of each species and sex.

5.4 Other relevant data

Limited information was available to the Working Group on the metabolism of *ortho*-anisidine. It was shown to be *O*-dealkylated in rat liver microsomes.

ortho-Anisidine at a high dose increased the incidence of hyperplasia of the bladder in male and female mice.

No data were available on the developmental and reproductive effects of *ortho*-anisidine.

No data were available on the genetic and related effects of *ortho*-anisidine in humans. No conclusion can be drawn about its genotoxicity in experimental animals *in vivo*; however, *ortho*-anisidine induced gene mutation in bladder cells in an assay in transgenic mice. There is no evidence that it has genotoxic effects in mammalian cells *in vitro*. *ortho*-Anisidine was not mutagenic to bacteria.

5.5 Evaluation

There is *inadequate evidence* in humans for the carcinogenicity of *ortho*-anisidine.

There is *sufficient evidence* in experimental animals for the carcinogenicity of *ortho*-anisidine.

Overall evaluation

ortho-Anisidine is *possibly carcinogenic to humans (Group 2B)*.

6. References

American Conference of Governmental Industrial Hygienists (1997) *1997 TLVs® and BEIs®*, Cincinnati, OH, p. 16

Ashby, J., Lefevre, P.A., Tinwell, H., Brunborg, G., Schmezer, P., Pool-Zobel, B., Shanu-Wilson, R., Holme, J.A., Soderlund, E.J., Gulati, D. & Wojciechowski, J.P. (1991) The non-genotoxicity to rodents of the potent rodent bladder carcinogens *o*-anisidine and *p*-cresidine. *Mutat. Res.*, **250**, 115–133

Ashby, J., Short, J.M., Jones, N.J., Lefevre, P.A., Provost, G.S., Rogers, B.J., Martin, E.A., Parry, J.M., Burnette, K., Glickman, B.W. & H. Tinwell (1994) Mutagenicity of o-anisidine to the bladder of *lacI*-transgenic B6C3F1 mice: Absence of ^{14}C or ^{32}P bladder DNA adduction. *Carcinogenesis*, **15**, 2291–2296

Budavari, S., ed. (1996) *The Merck Index*, 12th Ed., Whitehouse Station, NJ, Merck & Co., Inc., p. 113

Chemical Information Services (1995) *Directory of World Chemical Producers 1995/96 Edition*, Dallas, TX, p. 66

Dunkel, V.C., Zeiger, E., Brusick, D., McCoy, E., McGregor, D., Mortelmans, K., Rosenkranz, H.S. & Simmon, V.F. (1985) Reproducibility of microbial mutagenicity assays: II. Testing of carcinogens and noncarcinogens in *Salmonella typhimurium* and *Escherichia coli*. *Environ. Mutag.*, **7** (Suppl. 5), 1–248

Galloway, S.M., Armstrong, M.J., Reuben, C., Colman, S., Brown, B., Cannon, C., Bloom, A.D., Nakamura, F., Ahmed, M., Duk, S., Rimpo, J., Margolin, B.H., Resnick, M.A., Anderson, B. & Zeiger, E. (1987) Chromosome aberrations and sister chromatid exchanges in Chinese hamster ovary cells: Evaluations of 108 chemicals. *Environ. mol. Mutag.*, **10** (Suppl. 10), 1–175

Garberg, P., Akerblom, E.L. & Bolcsfoldi, G. (1988) Evaluation of a genotoxicity test measuring DNA-strand breaks in mouse lymphoma cells by alkaline unwinding and hydroxyapatite elution. *Mutat. Res.*, **203**, 155–176

Haworth, S., Lawlor, T., Mortelmans, K., Speck, W. & Zeiger, E. (1983) Salmonella mutagenicity test results for 250 chemicals. *Environ. Mutag.*, **5** (Suppl. 1), 1–142

Hellmer, L. & Bolcsfoldi, G. (1992) An evaluation of the *E. coli K-12 uvrB/recA* DNA repair host-mediated assay. II. *In vivo* results for 36 compounds tested in the mouse. *Mutat. Res.*, **272**, 161–173

IARC (1982) *IARC Monographs on the Evaluation of the Carcinogenic Risk of Chemicals to Humans*, Vol. 27, *Some Aromatic Amines, Anthraquinones and Nitroso Compounds, and Inorganic Fluorides used in Drinking-water and Dental Preparations*, Lyon, pp. 63–80

IARC (1987) *IARC Monographs on the Evaluation of Carcinogenic Risks to Humans*, Suppl. 7, *Overall Evaluations of Carcinogenicity: An Updating of* IARC Monographs *Volumes 1 to 42*, Lyon, p. 57

International Labour Office (1991) *Occupational Exposure Limits for Airborne Toxic Substances*, 3rd. Ed. (Occupational Safety and Health Series No. 37), Geneva, pp. 26–27

Jansen, L.A.M. & Jongen, W.M.F. (1996) The use of initiated cells as a test system for the detection of gap junctional intracellular communication. *Carcinogenesis*, **17**, 33–339

Kerckaert, G.A., LeBoeuf, R.A. & Isfort, R.J. (1998) Assessing the predictiveness of the Syrian hamster embryo cell transformation assay for determining the rodent carcinogenic potential of single ring aromatic/nitroaromatic amine compounds. *Toxicol. Sci.*, **41**, 189–197

Lide, D.R., ed. (1997) *CRC Handbook of Chemistry and Physics*, 78th Ed., Boca Raton, FL, CRC Press, p. 3-23

Morita, T., Asano, N., Awogi, T., Sasaki, Y.F., Sato, S., Shimada, H., Sutou, S., Suzuki, T., Wakata, A., Sofuni, T. & Hayashi, M. (1997) Evaluation of the rodent micronucleus assay in the screening of IARC carcinogens (Groups 1, 2A and 2B). The summary report of the 6th collaborative study by CSGMT/JEMS.MMS. *Mutat. Res.*, **389**, 3–122

National Cancer Institute (1978) *Bioassay of o-Anisidine Hydrochloride for Possible Carcinogenicity* (Tech. Rep. Ser. No. 89; DHEW Publ. No (NIH) 78-1339), Washington DC, US Government Printing Office

National Institute for Occupational Safety and Health (1998) *National Occupational Exposure Survey 1981–83*, Cincinnati, OH

National Library of Medicine (1998a) *Hazardous Substances Data Bank (HSDB)*, Bethesda, MD [Record No. 2073]

National Library of Medicine (1998b) *Toxic Chemical Release Inventory 1987 & 1996* (TRI87 & TRI96), Bethesda, MD

National Toxicology Program (1991) *NTP Chemical Repository Data Sheet: ortho-Anisidine*, Research Triangle Park, NC

Ono, S., Kurata, Y, Shichino, Y., Sano, M. & Fukushima, S. (1992) Synergism of environmental carcinogens and promoters on bladder cancer development initiated by *N*-butyl-*N*-(4-hydroxybutyl)nitrosamine in F344 rats. *Jpn. J. Cancer Res.*, **83**, 955–963

Prosolenko, N.V. (1975) [Comparative toxicological evaluation of methoxyanilines (*o*- and *p*-anisidines)]. *Tr. Khar'k. Gos. med. Inst.*, **124,** 11–14 (in Russian)

Sasaki, Y.F., Nishidate, E., Su, Y. Q., Matsusaka, N., Tsuda, S., Susa, N., Furukawa, Y. & Ueno, S. (1998) Organ-specific genotoxicity of the potent rodent bladder carcinogens *o*-anisidine and *p*-cresidine. *Mutat. Res.*, **412**, 155-160

Thompson, D.C. & Eling, T.E. (1991) Reactive intermediates formed during peroxidative oxidation of anisidine isomers. *Chem. Res. Toxicol.*, **4**, 474–481

Thompson, D.C., Josephy, P.D., Chu, J.W.K. & Eling, T.E. (1992) Enhanced mutagenicity of anisidine isomers in bacterial strains containing elevated *N*-acetyltransferase activity. *Mutat. Res.*, **279**, 83–89

Tyson, C.K. & Mirsalis, J.C. (1985) Measurement of unscheduled DNA synthesis in rat kidney cells following in vivo treatment with genotoxic agents. *Environ. Mutag.*, **7**, 889–899

Verschueren, K. (1996) *Handbook of Environmental Data on Organic Chemicals*, 3rd Ed., New York, Van Nostrand Reinhold Co., pp. 205–206

Wangenheim, J. & Bolcsfoldi, G. (1988) Mouse lymphoma L5178Y thymidine kinase locus assay of 50 compounds. *Mutagenesis*, **3**, 193–205

WHO (1993) *Guidelines for Drinking Water Quality*, 2nd Ed., Vol. 1, *Recommendations*, Geneva

Yoon, J.S., Mason, J.M., Valencia, R., Woodruff, R.C. & Zimmering, S. (1985) Chemical mutagenesis testing in Drosophila. IV. Results of 45 coded compounds tested for the National Toxicology Program. *Environ. Mutag.*, **7**, 349–367

ATRAZINE

This substance was considered by a previous working group, in 1990 (IARC, 1991). Since that time, new data have become available, and these have been incorporated into the monograph and taken into consideration in the present evaluation.

1. Exposure Data

1.1 Chemical and physical data

1.1.1 *Nomenclature*

Chem. Abstr. Serv. Reg. No.: 1912-24-9

Deleted CAS Reg. Nos: 11121-31-6; 12040-45-8; 12797-72-7; 39400-72-1; 69771-31-9; 93616-39-8

Chem. Abstr. Name: 6-Chloro-*N*-ethyl-*N*′-(1-methylethyl)-1,3,5-triazine-2,4-diamine

IUPAC Systematic Name: 6-Chloro-N^2-ethyl-N^4-isopropyl-1,3,5-triazine-2,4-diamine

Synonyms: 2-Chloro-4-(ethylamino)-6-(isopropylamino)triazine; 2-chloro-4-(ethylamino)-6-(isopropylamino)-*s*-triazine; 2-chloro-4-ethylamino-6-isopropylamino-1,3,5-triazine

1.1.2 *Structural and molecular formulae and relative molecular mass*

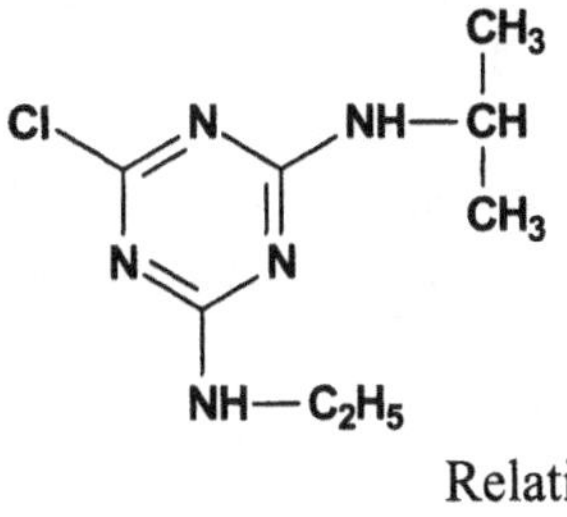

$C_8H_{14}ClN_5$

Relative molecular mass: 215.69

1.1.3 *Chemical and physical properties of the pure substance*

(*a*) *Description*: Colourless powder (Tomlin, 1994)

(*b*) *Melting-point*: 173°C (Lide, 1997)

(*c*) *Density*: 1.187 g/cm^3 at 20°C (Tomlin, 1994)

(*d*) *Spectroscopy data*: Infrared (prism [35712]; grating [13706]) and ultraviolet [16141] spectral data have been reported (Sadtler Research Laboratories, 1980)

(*e*) *Solubility*: Slightly soluble in water (33 mg/L at 20°C); soluble in acetone (31 g/L at 25°C), chloroform (35 g/L at 20°C), dichloromethane (28 g/L at 25°C), diethyl ether (17 g/L at 20°C), ethyl acetate (24 g/L at 25°C), *n*-hexane (0.11 g/L at 25°C), methanol (15 g/L at 25°C), *n*-octanol (10.6 g/L at 25°C) and toluene (6 g/L at 25°C) (Worthing & Walker, 1987; Tomlin, 1994; Budavari, 1996)

(*f*) *Volatility*: Vapour pressure, 0.04 mPa at 20°C (Tomlin, 1994)

(*g*) *Stability*: Forms salts with acids; stable in slightly acidic or basic media; hydrolysed to inactive hydroxy derivative at 70ºC under neutral conditions, more rapidly in alkali or mineral acids (Worthing & Walker, 1987; Tomlin, 1994; Budavari, 1996)

(*h*) *Octanol/water partition coefficient (P)*: log P, 2.61 (Hansch *et al.*, 1995)

(*i*) *Conversion factor*: mg/m^3 = 8.82 × ppm

1.1.4 *Technical products and impurities*

Atrazine is commercially available in various forms, including dry flowable, flowable liquid, flowable suspension concentrate, liquid, water-dispersible granular and wettable powder formulations. The purity of technical-grade atrazine ranges from 92 to 97%. The The impurities include dichlorotriazines, tris(alkylamino)triazines and hydroxytriazines (Tomlin, 1994; Oregon State University, 1996; National Registration Authority for Agricultural and Veterinary Chemicals, 1997; Environmental Protection Agency, 1999). The concentration of active ingredient in most atrazine products registered with the United States Environmental Protection Agency is 43, 80 or 90%; the concentration in other atrazine products ranges from 0.58 to 53.5% (Environmental Protection Agency, 1999).

Trade names for atrazine include A 361; Aatrex; Akticon; Aktikon; Aktinit; Argezin; Atranex; Atrataf; Atrazin; Atrazine; ATZ; Azoprim; Cekuzina-T; CET; Chromozin; Cyazin; Fogard; G 30027; Gesaprim; Griffex; Hungazin; Maizina; Mebazine; Oleogesaprim; Oleogesaprim 200; Primatol; Radazin; Triazine A 1294; Vectal; Wonuk; Zeapos; Zeazin; Zeazine (National Toxicology Program, 1991; Tomlin, 1994; Oregon State University, 1996).

Atrazine may be formulated with many other herbicides, including alachlor, acetochlor, ametryn, amitrole, benoxacor, bentazone, bromoxynil, cyanazine, 2,4-D, dicamba potassium salt, dichlobenil, diuron, glyphosate, imazapyr, imazethapyr, metolachlor, pendimethalin, pyridate and simazine. It is also used in mixtures with these and other herbicides for spraying and is also impregnated into fertilizer (Ahrens, 1994; Tomlin, 1994; Novartis, 1999).

1.1.5 *Analysis*

Methods for the analysis of atrazine in various media are presented in Table 1.

1.2 Production and use

1.2.1 *Production*

Cyanuric chloride is reacted with isopropylamine under basic conditions to form 2,4-dichloro-6-isopropylamino-*s*-triazine, which is then reacted with monoethylamine and dilute caustic to form atrazine (Izmerov, 1982).

Table 1. Selected methods for the analysis of atrazine

Sample matrix	Sample preparation	Assay procedure	Limit of detection	Reference
Formulations	Dissolve in chloroform; centrifuge	GC/FID	NR	Williams (1984)
Drinking-water	Extract in liquid–solid extractor; elute with ethyl acetate and dichloromethane; concentrate by evaporation	GC/ECD GC/MS	0.003 μg/L 0.065 μg/L	Environmental Protection Agency (1995a,b) [Methods 508.1 & 525.2]
	Extract in liquid–liquid extractor (methyl *tert*-butyl ether or pentane)	GC/ECD	0.082 μg/L (MTBE); 0.099 μg/L (pentane)	Environmental Protection Agency (1995c) [Method 551.1]
	Extract with dichloromethane; isolate; extract; dry; concentrate with methyl *tert*-butyl ether	GC/NPD	0.13 μg/L (estimated)	Environmental Protection Agency (1995d) [Method 507]
	Extract with hexane; inject extract	GC/ECD	2.4 μg/L	Environmental Protection Agency (1995e) [Method 505]
Wastewater	Extract with dichloromethane; dry; exchange to hexane	GC/TBD-N	NR	Spectrum Laboratories (1999) [EPA method 619]
	Extract with dichloromethane (liquid sample); extract with dichloromethane:acetone (1:1) (solid sample); inject directly	GC/NPD	NR	Environmental Protection Agency (1994) [Method 8141A]
Forage (all crops)	Extract with chloroform (green forage) or acetonitrile:water (9:1) (dry forage); partition with dichloromethane (dry forage); evaporate to dryness; partition with hexane and acetonitrile; clean-up on alumina column (for all forages)	GC/MCD	0.05-0.1 ppm	Food & Drug Administration (1989)

Table 1 (contd)

Sample matrix	Sample preparation	Assay procedure	Limit of detection	Reference
Urine	Clean-up sample; wash with water; elute with ethyl acetate; remove water and evaporate to dryness; dissolve in acetone	GC/NPD	0.005 ppm	Cheung (1990)

Abbreviations: GC/ECD, gas chromatography/electron capture detection; GC/FID, gas chromatography/flame ionization detection; GC/FPD, gas chromatography/flame photometric detection; GC/MCD, gas chromatography/microcoulometric detection; GC/MS, gas chromatography/mass spectrometry; GC/NPD, gas chromatography/nitrogen-phosphorous detection; GC/TBD-N, gas chromatography/thermionic bead detection-nitrogen mode; NR, not reported

Information available in 1995 indicated that atrazine was produced in Brazil, China, Israel, Italy, Romania, South Africa, Switzerland and the United States (Chemical Information Services, 1995). The world production rate is about 70 000 tonnes per year.

1.2.2 *Use*

Atrazine is used in agriculture as a selective pre- and post-emergence herbicide for annual control of grass and broad-leaved weeds. It has been used on asparagus, bananas, citrus groves, coffee, conifer tree crop areas, forestry, fruit orchards, grasslands, grass crops, guavas, macadamia orchards, maize (corn), oil palms, sorghum, sugar cane, pineapples, roses and vines. It has also been used as a soil sterilant for airfields, parking lots and industrial sites and as an algicide in swimming pools. Recently, many of the uses that contribute residues to water have been reduced or eliminated. In the European Union, where a limit of 0.1 μg/L has been set for all pesticide residues in drinking- and groundwater, the use of atrazine-containing herbicides has been limited mainly to agricultural uses on corn and on sorghum (Council of the European Communities, 1980; Worthing & Walker, 1987; Ahrens, 1994; Tomlin, 1994; Novartis, 1999).

In the United States, atrazine has been a staple for weed control in agriculture over the past 35 years. It is used on approximately 67% of all corn acreage, 65% of sorghum acreage and 90% of sugar-cane acreage and is also used on wheat, guavas, macadamia nuts, conifers and turf and for non-selective use along roads (Ahrens, 1994; Ciba-Geigy AG, 1996; Novartis, 1999). The Environmental Protection Agency estimated that 31–35 million kg (active ingredient) of atrazine were used annually in agricultural crop production in the United States in 1987, 1993 and 1995 (Aspelin, 1997).

1.3 Occurrence

1.3.1 *Natural occurrence*

Atrazine is not known to occur naturally.

1.3.2 *Occupational exposure*

According to the 1981–83 United States National Occupational Exposure Survey (National Institute for Occupational Safety and Health, 1998), approximately 1000 chemical industry workers in the United States were potentially exposed to atrazine. No data were available on the number of agricultural workers exposed. Occupational exposure may occur through dermal contact or inhalation during the manufacture, formulation or application of this herbicide (National Institute for Occupational Safety and Health, 1992).

Ikonen *et al.* (1988) determined the ambient air concentrations of atrazine and the urinary excretion of atrazine metabolites (fully *N*-dealkylated atrazine, i.e. 2-chloro-4,6-diamino-*s*-triazine and 2-chloro-4-ethylamino-6-amino-*s*-triazine) in six Finnish railway workers who filled spraying tank wagons. The air concentration in the personal breathing zone over 7–240 min ranged from 0.24 to 0.89 mg/m^3. The sum of the concentration of the two metabolites in urine samples collected after an 8-h work shift ranged from 30 to 110 μmol/L and was correlated with that of atrazine in the ambient air.

Catenacci *et al.* (1990) determined ambient air levels, skin deposition and urinary excretion of free atrazine over several work shifts in four Italian workers exposed to atrazine during its manufacture and packaging in a production plant. The air concentrations (in 8-h time-weighted average [TWA] personal samples) were 0.07–0.53 mg/m^3, and whole-body skin deposition was 4.1–11 mg/h. Urinary excretion of unmodified atrazine correlated with ambient air concentrations. Maximal excretion rates were found during the work shift and varied between 0.1 and 0.3 μg/h.

In another study, Catenacci *et al.* (1993) evaluated the exposure to atrazine of six Italian herbicide manufacturing workers through personal ambient air measurements, skin pad deposition sampling and determinations of urinary metabolites. Total exposure, reported as a dose, varied from 10 to 700 μmol/work shift, being 10 times higher in baggers than in box operators. Cutaneous exposure was twice as high as by the respiratory route for baggers and 10 times as high for box operators. Urinary excretion of metabolites—bis-dealkylated atrazine (80% of total), deisopropylated atrazine (10%), deethylated atrazine (8%) and unmodified atrazine (1–2%)—accounted for only 1–2% of the external dose and was not correlated to it.

The wide discrepancies between external dose and that accounted for by urinary metabolite excretion may be due to low cutaneous absorption of atrazine (Catenacci *et al.*, 1995). Dermal absorption of atrazine over a 24-h exposure period in volunteers ranged from 1.2 to 5.6%, depending on the dose (Hui *et al.*, 1996). Using these figures and data from the Pesticide Handlers Exposure Database, Breckenridge (1996) estimated the combined occupational exposure to atrazine by inhalation and dermal absorption in a variety of uses, as micrograms of atrazine absorbed per mass of active ingredient used. The estimates range from 0.27 to 158 μg/lb (0.6–350 μg/kg) for 5.6% dermal absorption, depending on the use. The heaviest exposure was that of granular spreaders and handgun operations (27–158 μg/lb active ingredient or 60–350 μg/kg), whereas mixer–loaders (non-handgun), boom applicators, pilots and flaggers had lighter exposure (0.27–4.54 μg/lb active ingredient or 0.6–10 μg/kg).

Information on the use of various atrazine formulations on various crops was combined with the above estimates to yield lifetime average daily doses of atrazine in the treatment of corn, sorghum, sugar-cane and macadamia nuts. These varied from 4×10^{-6} mg/kg bw per day for enclosed-cab ground application on sorghum to 1.6×10^{-3} mg/kg bw per day for some mixer–loader applicators in open cabs on Florida sugar-cane (Lunchick & Selman, 1998).

1.3.3 *Environmental occurrence*

Atrazine and its degradation products occur widely in the global environment as a result of extensive use of atrazine as a pre-and post-emergent herbicide, mainly on maize, sorghum and millet and to a lesser degree on other crops, and as a non-selective herbicide for general weed control. It is found, at generally low levels, in rivers, lakes, estuaries, reservoirs, groundwater and drinking-water. It can also pollute fog and rain when released into the atmosphere during spray application (Thurman *et al.*, 1991, 1992;

Goolsby & Battaglin, 1993; Goolsby *et al.*, 1993; Huber, 1993; Bintein & Devillers, 1996; Schottler & Eisenreich, 1997; Richards & Baker, 1998; Thurman *et al.*, 1998).

(*a*) *Air*

Atmospheric transport and fallout have been implicated in the dispersion of atrazine. Atrazine was detected in ambient air in the region of Paris, France, in 1991 at approximately 0.03 ng/m^3; the maximal concentration in the total atmospheric fallout in rainwater in Paris was 350 ng/L (Chevreuil & Garmouma, 1993). Atrazine was measured at concentrations of < 0.03–2 ng/m^3 in the vapour phase in the Paris area in 1992 and 1993 and at < 5–380 ng/L in fallout in urban and rural sites in the same area. The yearly atmospheric deposition of atrazine was estimated to be 77 μg/m^2 for this area (Chevreuil *et al.*, 1996). The concentration of atrazine in rainwater in Switzerland reached 600 ng/L (Buser, 1990). In rainwater samples in Ohio, United States, in 1985, the concentration of atrazine ranged from undetectable (detection limit, 0.05 μg/L) to 1.0 μg/L, according to season (Richards *et al.*, 1987).

Measurements from aircraft of the concentrations and flux of agrochemicals over Ottawa, Canada, in June 1993 and July 1994 showed concentrations as high as 4.6 ng/m^3 with fluxes ranging from 1.1 to 2.5 ng/m^2 per s (Zhu *et al.*, 1998).

(*b*) *Water*

The concentrations of atrazine in waters receiving runoff from agricultural lands are seasonal, the highest concentrations generally being found during the six weeks to two months after application and lower to undetectable concentrations during the rest of the year. In rivers and streams, the concentrations are highest during runoff after storms in the post-application period (Richards *et al.*, 1987; Richards & Baker, 1998). Typically, atrazine is found more frequently and usually at lower concentrations in groundwater than in surface water. The peak concentrations in impounded water bodies, such as reservoirs, are usually lower than those in rivers and streams; they occur at the same time but may persist for longer because of the longer residence time (Tierney *et al.*, 1998).

(i) *Surface water*

The heaviest use of atrazine in North America is in the midwestern watershed. The United States Geological Survey involved monitoring of residues of atrazine in 76 midwestern reservoirs in 11 states in 1992–93. Atrazine residues were found in 92% of reservoirs, and the 90th percentile of this distribution between early June and the end of July was about 5 μg/L. The concentrations of atrazine in rivers and streams included in an ecological risk assessment of atrazine in North American surface waters rarely exceeded 20 μg/L (Goolsby & Battaglin, 1993; Goolsby *et al.*, 1993; Solomon *et al.*, 1996).

Because atrazine is relatively water soluble, it can be transported in surface runoff after application and may reach groundwater as well. Monitoring of surface waters (Thurman *et al.*, 1991; Squillace & Thurman, 1992; Thurman *et al.*, 1992; Squillace *et al.*, 1993; Thurman *et al.*, 1994, 1998), including the Mississippi River, United States (Pereira

& Rostad, 1990), has shown the widespread presence of atrazine and its dealkylated degradation products, deethylatrazine and deisopropylatrazine. The same compounds are frequently detected in groundwater (Adams & Thurman, 1991; Squillace & Thurman, 1992). Deethylatrazine and deisopropylatrazine are also common degradation products of three other triazine herbicides: simazine, propazine and cyanazine.

Field studies and a regional study of nine rivers in the midwest corn belt of the United States showed that deethylatrazine and deisopropylatrazine occur frequently in surface water that has received runoff from fields treated with atrazine and cyanazine. The concentrations of deethylatrazine and deisopropylatrazine vary with the hydrological conditions and the timing of runoff, with maximum concentrations reaching 5 μg/L. Atrazine was the source of 98% of the deethylatrazine and 75% of the deisopropylatrazine (Thurman *et al.*, 1994).

The concentrations of atrazine in the Minnesota River, United States, exceeded 2000 ng/L, the maximum concentration occurring in mid-June 1990; in 1991, the maximum concentrations in mid-June were 800–900 ng/L. Deethylatrazine was present throughout the year and was detected in 90% of the samples, with maximum concentrations of > 300 ng/L in 1990 and 130 ng/L in 1991. The highest concentration of deisopropylatrazine was 160 ng/L in 1990, and concentrations of 100–200 ng/L were common in June and July 1991 (Schottler *et al.*, 1994). The Minnesota River contributes 1–2 tonnes of atrazine to the Mississippi River; larger drainage basins, such as the Ohio and Missouri Rivers, contribute about 40 and 60 tonnes annually, respectively, to the Mississippi River (Goolsby & Battaglin, 1993; Goolsby *et al.*, 1991, 1993). The annual transport of atrazine into the Gulf of Mexico via the lower Mississippi River and its tributaries was estimated to be 105 tonnes in 1987 and 429 tonnes in 1989, representing less than 2% of the total atrazine application in the entire Mississippi River Basin (Pereira & Rostad, 1990).

Atrazine has been used intensively in the Great Lakes Basin of North America. It has a long half-life in cold aquatic systems of low productivity, such as oligotrophic lakes and groundwater (Ulrich *et al.*, 1994), with an estimated half-life in the Great Lakes exceeding one year (Schottler *et al.*, 1994). It has been suggested that the annual input of atrazine ranges from about 1 tonne in Lake Superior to 10–25 tonnes in Lakes Erie and Ontario. While inputs from tributaries and connecting channels accounted for > 75% of the total load to Lakes Erie, Ontario, Huron and Michigan, atmospheric input accounted for 95% of the atrazine in Lake Superior. The internal degradation rates of atrazine are similar throughout the Great Lakes, approximately 5–10% of the total load being lost annually by internal degradation. The ratios of deethylatrazine to atrazine indicate that 1.5, 0.9, 4 and 5% of the total atrazine is converted to deethylatrazine annually in Lakes Michigan, Ontario, Erie and Huron, respectively (Schottler & Eisenreich, 1997).

Atrazine and deethylatrazine were found in 89–100 % (average, 94%) of samples of water from Sydenham River, Ontario, Canada, collected 30–50 times per year between 1981 and 1987 and in 63–100 % (average, 89%) of paired samples of drinking-water from the town of Dresden, Ontario. The annual mean (± SD) levels of atrazine plus deethylatrazine ranged from 1.3 (± 1.3) to 5.1 (± 10) μg/L in the river water and from 1.1

(± 1.1) to 8.3 (± 36) μg/L in the drinking-water samples. The highest level of atrazine plus deethylatrazine, found in Dresden municipal drinking-water, was 210 μg/L in 1987 (Frank *et al.*, 1990).

Atrazine was one of the most frequently detected pesticides in surface water and sediment samples collected during 1991–95 in a monitoring network that included 27 stations in South Florida canals in the United States. The highest concentration of atrazine found in surface water was 18 μg/L (number of detections, 274), and the highest concentration in sediment was 50 μg/kg (number of detections, 11) (Miles & Pfeuffer, 1997).

In a 12-month study carried out in 18 Swiss lakes and in rain in 1989, both atrazine and deethylatrazine were detected. The occurrence of atrazine in rain during March to October suggested that atmospheric transport was involved and, although a minor contributor to the larger lakes in the midland region, was likely to be the major source of these compounds in the mountain lakes. The concentration of atrazine was lowest (≤ 1 ng/L) in mountain lakes (altitude, > 800 m) and highest (≤ 460 ng/L) in lakes situated in areas with intensive agricultural use of atrazine. Atrazine was found to be rather stable, and it was removed from lakes mainly via outflowing waters rather than by degradation (Buser, 1990).

In the summer of 1991, atrazine was found to be distributed over the whole area of the German Bight of the North Sea at levels of 1–100 ng/L; the highest concentrations were found in the Elbe estuary, reaching 200 ng/L. The River Elbe is the main source of this polluant in this part of the North Sea (Bester & Hühnerfuss, 1993).

Atrazine was detected in a broad range of Mediterranean estuarial waters in a survey made in 1990–91. The areas studied included the Ebro delta on the eastern coast of Spain, the Rhône delta in the south of France, the River Po, Italy (northern Adriatic Sea), the Thermaïkós and Amvrakikós Gulfs in Greece and the Nile Delta in Egypt. The atrazine concentrations (μg/L; limit of detection, < 0.001 μg/L) were: Ebro drainage canal, 0.058–0.308; Ebro River, 0.017–0.190; Ebro delta lagoons, < 0.001–0.057; Rhône River, 0.040–0.291; Rhône delta, 0.017–0.386; River Po, 0.021–0.118; northern Adriatic, < 0.003–0.018; Axios, Loudhias and Aliakmon Rivers, < 0.05–0.70; Thermaïkós Gulf, < 0.05–0.15; Loúros and Árakthos Rivers, < 0.05–0.26; Amvrakikós Gulf, < 0.05–0.80; and Nile Delta, < 0.001 (Readman *et al.*, 1993).

Atrazine was found in 41% of 115 samples at maximum weekly and monthly concentrations of 0.9 and 0.5 μg/L respectively (limit of detection, 0.1 μg/L) at one site in a small agricultural catchment in southern Sweden during 1990–92. At another site in the same general area during 1992–96, atrazine was found in 72% of 95 samples at maximum weekly and monthly concentrations of 3 and 1.5 μg/L, respectively (Kreuger, 1998).

The concentrations (μg/L) and frequency of detection of atrazine in the Arno River in Italy during 1992–95 ranged from a median of 0.06 (maximum, 0.16) (n = 36) with 67% frequency in 1992 to a median of < 0.01 (maximum, 0.07) (n = 51) with a frequency of 4% in 1995 (Griffini *et al.*, 1997).

Atrazine, deethylatrazine and deisopropylatrazine were found in surface and ground-water samples from three sampling sites in the Ebro River. While atrazine and deethyl-atrazine were detected throughout the whole year in the delta waters, deisopropylatrazine was not detected between September and January. Atrazine had the least seasonal variation, remaining at a stable concentration of 0.1 μg/L between March 1992 and March 1993 (Barceló *et al.*, 1996).

A review by the Council of Europe of surveys of pesticide residues in surface waters, conducted principally during the period 1985–92 in the Nordic countries, Netherlands and Germany, found that atrazine and other triazine herbicides were detected at a number of sampling sites throughout the year (Lundbergh *et al.*, 1995).

(ii) *Groundwater*

In a survey of herbicide residues prevalent in groundwater across Iowa (in which some of the most intense application of herbicides occurs in the United States) in 1995, atrazine and deethylatrazine were detected in 41% and 35% of sample, respectively, at maximum concentrations of 2.1 and 0.59 μg/L, respectively (limit of detection, 0.05 μg/L) (Kolpin *et al.*, 1997a).

In 1991, atrazine was detected in 19% of 208 urban wells in nine studies of shallow groundwater that were part of the United States Geological Survey's National Water Quality Assessment Program. The limit of detection was 0.002 μg/L, and the maximum concentration found was 2.3 μg/L (Kolpin *et al.*, 1997b).

In a study of triazine herbicides and their degradation products in near-surface aquifiers in midwestern United States in 1991, involving 837 water samples from 303 wells, the median detectable concentration of atrazine (0.15 μg/L, 158 samples) was almost half that of atrazine plus deethylatrazine and deisopropylatrazine (0.26 μg/L; 197 samples) (Kolpin *et al.*, 1996).

(iii) *Drinking-water*

In an assessment of atrazine in the drinking-water of residents of Ohio, Illinois and Iowa (United States), only small populations were found to be exposed to average concentrations exceeding the Environmental Protection Agency maximum contaminant level of 3 μg/L, and most were exposed to average concentrations of less than 1 μg/L. Large rivers such as the Ohio and Mississippi and most groundwater sources provide water with relatively low concentrations of atrazine; the highest concentrations were found in a few small, groundwater-based public water supplies and private wells. Only 0.25% of the assessed populations in all three states were exposed to concentrations exceeding the maximum contaminant level, and 94–99% of the populations were exposed to < 1 μg/L. In Ohio, with a population of over 10 million people, the average concentrations were 0.07 μg/L from Lake Erie, 0.84 μg/L from other surface water, 0.025 μg/L from public groundwater and 0.052 μg/L from private groundwater (Richards *et al.*, 1995).

In a population-linked assessment of exposure to atrazine in drinking-water supplies in the 21 states of the United States where most atrazine is used, data on community water systems serving 164 million people were summarized for five consecutive years, 1993–97. A community water system was defined as a facility that provides piped water for human consumption to at least 15 service connections around the year; the source of the raw water may be groundwater, surface water (rivers, lakes and reservoirs) or both (Tierney *et al.*, 1998). Atrazine was detected in 7091 (10%) of the samples assessed, with 3% in groundwater (1959 of 57 258 samples), 36% in surface water (4861 of 13 529 samples) and 10% in other water samples (276 of 2776 samples). Of the approximately 125 million people whose exposure to atrazine was measured in this survey, 95 million (75%) had no detectable exposure from the community water systems. When detectable exposures were added to undetectable figures, 112 million (89%) were exposed to mean concentrations of < 0.5 μg/L, and 121 million (97%) were exposed to < 1 μg/L; approximately 3.9 million (3%) were exposed to 1–3 μg/L (Clarkson *et al.*, 1998).

Atrazine was found at concentrations of 0.18–1 μg/L in a representative survey in the United States in 1990–91; 50% of the tested wells had concentrations < 0.28 μg/L (Environmental Protection Agency, 1992). In the United States, persons who obtain potable water from private wells represent about 6% of the population. National groundwater studies have shown that over 98% of private wells have concentrations of < 0.02 μg/L atrazine (Tierney *et al.*, 1998).

In 1988, atrazine was detected at 1–50 ng/L in a number of new wells that serve as sources of drinking-water in the province of Bergamo in northern Italy (Bagnati *et al.*, 1988).

(*c*) *Soil*

Atrazine is degraded in soil by microbial processes and abiotic degradation, yielding deethylatrazine, deisopropylatrazine, hydroxyatrazine and non-extractable residues. Deethylatrazine was the major degradation product from clay-loam and silt-loam plots studied at an experimental field in the Kansas River Valley in the United States in 1989. Deisopropylatrazine was found at significantly lower concentrations than deethylatrazine. Most of the degradation of atrazine occurred in the top metre of soil. The deethylatrazine:atrazine ratio was suggested to be a good indicator of transport of atrazine through the soil (Adams & Thurman, 1991).

Metabolite formation from atrazine and subsequent disappearance were found to be similar in laboratory microcosms and in a field in west Tennessee, United States. The half-life of atrazine was found to be 21 days in the microcosm and 14 days in the field study. Bound residue formation was significant, however, so that the half-life of the chemical may be underestimated (Winkelmann & Klaine, 1991a,b).

In a study of atrazine and its transformation products in surface and subsurface soils from five locations in Iowa, United States, the greatest mobility was seen in sandy and sandy clay–loam subsurface soils, which also had the least organic matter. The mobility relationship of deethylatrazine > atrazine > deisopropylatrazine is consistent with the results of groundwater monitoring (Kruger *et al.*, 1996).

An environmental-fate study conducted in a citrus orchard in Valencia, Spain, in 1993 showed a degradation half-life of 11 days for atrazine, the distribution being highest in the upper layer (0–0.05 m) of soil. Of the four pesticides studied (atrazine, simazine, chlorpyrifos and tetrafidon), atrazine was the most soluble in water and the most mobile. The persistence and mobility of residues are closely related to both climatic conditions and agricultural practices (Redondo *et al.*, 1997).

In field experiments on various subtropical soils in Taiwan, with various soil temperatures and moisture conditions, the deepest movement of atrazine into the soil was 7 cm (Wang *et al.*, 1995, 1996).

In a study in Israel, significant degradation of atrazine (50%) was detected in samples taken from the upper soil (0–25 cm) but none in samples taken from the deepest subsurface soil. Deethylatrazine and deisopropylatrazine were the main degradation products of the upper soil. Inoculation with *Pseudomonas* sp. strain ADP (P.ADP) resulted in 90–100% mineralization of atrazine after 15 days (Shapir & Mandelbaum, 1997).

(*d*) *Food*

No atrazine residue (< 50 μg/kg) was reported in a survey of various food and feeds over the period 1991–92 in 16 428 samples (15 370 surveillance and 1058 compliance) and in the Total Diet Study for 1986–92 in the United States (Food & Drug Administration, 1993). In a further examination of data from the Residue Monitoring Program by the National Food Processors Association, no residues of atrazine, simazine, cyanazine or ametryn were found in 76 973 samples in 1992–94 (Elkins *et al.*, 1998).

Field studies on the metabolism of atrazine in corn and sorghum showed that uptake of residues by plants is relatively low and subsequent metabolism is rapid. The metabolism of atrazine in plants is complex and involves at least 15–20 structures. Direct dietary exposure to atrazine residues in treated crops would be expected to be low and to comprise primarily water-soluble metabolites. There is a little propensity for plant metabolites of atrazine to be transferred to meat, milk or eggs (Ballantine & Simoneaux, 1991).

1.4 Regulations and guidelines

National and regional limits for residues of atrazine in foods are given in Table 2. Occupational exposure limits for atrazine are given in Table 3.

WHO (1993) has established an international guideline for atrazine in drinking-water of 0.002 mg/L. The interim maximum acceptable concentration of atrazine in Canadian drinking-water is 0.005 mg/L (United Nations Environment Programme, 1998). The maximum level of atrazine allowed in primary drinking-water in the United States is 0.003 mg/L (Environmental Protection Agency, 1998). Limits on atrazine residues have been set in the Russian Federation in various matrices: ambient air, maximum allowable concentration (MAC), 0.02 mg/m^3; surface water, MAC, 0.5 mg/L; surface water, MAC for fishing, 0.005 mg/L (United Nations Environment Programme, 1998). Owing to its

Table 2. National and regional pesticide residue limits for atrazine in foods

Country or region	Residue limit (mg/kg)	Commodities
Argentina	0.25	Maize, sorghum, sweet corn
Australia	0. 1[a]	Edible offal (mammalian), maize, sorghum, sugar-cane, sweet corn
	0.02[a]	Lupins
	0.01[a]	Meat, milk, milk products, potatoes, rape-seed
Austria	0.5	Corn
	0.1	Other foods of vegetable origin
Belgium	0.1	All foodstuffs of vegetable origin
Brazil	1.0	Conifers, rubber plants, sisal
	0.2	Corn, sorghum, pineapple, sugar-cane, avocados, bananas, mangos, peaches, apples, citrus fruit, nuts, tea, cocoa, coffee
	0.1	Black pepper
China (Taiwan)	0.25	Field crops, sugar-cane, tropical fruits
Czech Republic	0.1[a]	All products
European Union	0.1	All products
Finland	0.2	Food products
France	0.1	Fruit, vegetables
	0.05	Corn
Germany	0.1	All products of plant origin
Hungary	0.1	All crops
Iceland	0.1	All crops and foodstuffs
India	0.25	Sugar-cane
	0 (nil)	Maize
Ireland	0.1	All products
Israel[b]	15.0	Maize and sorghum fodder
	0.25	Maize and sorghum grain, sweet corn
	0.02	Meat, milk, eggs
Italy	0.5	Corn, sorghum
	0.1	Fruit, garden vegetables
Japan	0.02	Oats, etc. and minor cereals; fruit, vegetables, sugar-cane
Malaysia	1.0	Asparagus, leafy vegetables
	0.25	Corn, millet, sorghum, wheat, pineapple
	0.1	Raisin, sugar-cane
	0.05	Guava
	0.02	Meat, eggs, milk and milk products
	0.01	Potatoes
Mexico	15	Corn (forage), sorghum (forage)
	10	Pineapple (forage)
	5	Wheat (straw)
	0.25	Corn (fresh and grain), pineapple, sorghum (grain), sugar-cane, wheat (grain)

Table 2 (contd)

Country or region	Residue limit (mg/kg)	Commodities
Netherlands	0.1	Corn, fruit, vegetables
	0 (0.05)[c]	Other
Norway	0.1	All products
Singapore	0.1	Citrus fruit, grapes, maize, pineapples, sorghum, sugar-cane, sweet corn
	0.01	Potatoes
South Africa	0.05	Mealies, sorghum, sugar-cane
Spain	0.1	Citrus fruit, fruit with or without shell, seed fruit, stone fruit, berries and small fruit, other fruit, root and tuber vegetables, bulb vegetables, fruit and pepos, vegetables of the genus *Brassica*, fresh aromatic herbs and leafy vegetables, green legumes (fresh), young stalks, fungi, legumes, oilseeds, potatoes, tea, hops, spices, grains, other products for consumption (tobacco, sugar-beets, sugar-cane, other), hay and forage crops, dried products, other edible seeds, other infusions
Switzerland	0.1	Corn
United Kingdom	0.1	All crops and foodstuffs
United States	15[d]	Corn forage or fodder (including field corn, sweet corn, popcorn), sorghum fodder and forage, perennial rye grass
	10[d]	Pineapple fodder and forage
	5[d]	Wheat fodder and straw
	4.0[d]	Range grasses
	0.25[d]	Fresh corn including sweet corn (kernels plus cobs with husks removed), maize grain, macadamia nuts, pineapples, sorghum grain, sugar-cane, sugar-cane fodder and forage, wheat grain
	0.05[d]	Guava
	0.02[d]	Eggs, milk, meat, fat and meat by-products of cattle, goats, hogs, horses, poultry and sheep (negligible residues)
Yugoslavia	0.5	Maize
	0.1	Fruit, vegetables
	0.03	Milk and other dairy products (fat basis)
	0.02	Meat and meat products (fat basis), eggs (shell-free basis)

From Health Canada (1998)

[a] Maximum residue limit set at or about the limit of analytical determination

[b] From State of Israel (1977)

[c] Residues shall be absent; the value in parentheses is the highest concentration at which this requirement is still deemed to have been met.

[d] Atrazine and its metabolites

Table 3. Occupational exposure limits for atrazine

Country	Year	Concentration (mg/m^3)	Interpretation
Australia	1993	5	TWA
Austria	1993	2	TWA
Belgium	1993	5	TWA
Canada	1994	5	TWA
Denmark	1993	2	TWA
Finland	1998	10	TWA
		20	STEL
France	1993	5	TWA
Germany	1998	2 (inhalable fraction of the aerosol)	MAK
Ireland	1997	10	TWA
Netherlands	1997	5	TWA
Russian Federation	1993	2	STEL
Switzerland	1993	2	TWA
United Kingdom	1987	10	TWA
United States			
OSHA (PEL)	1997	5	TWA
NIOSH (REL)	1994	5	TWA
ACGIH[a] (TLV)	1997	5	TWA

From Cook (1987); American Conference of Governmental Industrial Hygienists (ACGIH) (1997; 1998); Deutsches Forschungsgemeinschaft (1998); Occupational Safety and Health Administration (OSHA) (1999)
TWA, time-weighted average; STEL, short-term exposure limit; PEL, permissible exposure limit; REL, recommended exposure limit; TLV, threshold limit value; MAK, maximum workplace concentrations; NIOSH, National Institute for Occupational Safety and Health
[a] The following countries follow the exposure limits suggested by the ACGIH: Bulgaria, Colombia, Jordan, the Republic of Korea, New Zealand, Singapore and Viet Nam

high mobility in soil and its potential to contaminate water, atrazine is banned from use in Italy, Norway and Sweden (National Registration Authority for Agricultural and Veterinary Chemicals, 1997; United Nations Environment Programme, 1998). In 1991, the German government banned all atrazine-containing products (National Registration Authority for Agricultural and Veterinary Chemicals, 1997). In 1993, the United Kingdom banned the use of atrazine in non-agricultural situations, maintaining the agricultural uses on corn (The Pesticide Trust, 1993).

2. Studies of Cancer in Humans

2.1 Cohort studies

On the basis of a retrospective follow-up study of 4388 agricultural chemical production workers in one plant in Alabama, United States, and a study of 1472 workers at a plant in Louisiana, United States, Sathiakumar *et al.* (1996) analysed the mortality pattern among the combined subgroup of 4917 male workers with potential exposure to triazines; 80% were white and 20% were black. The Alabama plant began operation in 1951 and, until the 1980s, manufactured primarily agricultural chemicals, including triazine herbicides and many other pesticides. The Louisiana plant, which started operation in 1970, produced mainly triazine herbicides. The vital status of cohort members was ascertained as of 1 January 1987. Death certificates were used as the source of information on date and cause of death. Periods of employment and associated job title and work area were obtained from company files. By use of a job–exposure matrix constructed by local industrial hygienists, in which job information was converted to information on likelihood of exposure to triazine, cohort members were classified into a group of 2683 (55%) workers who had had definitive or probable exposure and 2234 (45%) who had had possible exposure. Exposure to pesticides other than triazine herbicides was not controlled for in the analysis. The workers were followed-up from the date of starting a triazine-related job up to the date of death, the date of loss to follow-up or 1 January 1987. Overall, 220 deaths were observed, whereas 253 were expected from the mortality rates of the United States male population (standardized mortality ratio [SMR], 0.87; 95% confidence interval [CI], 0.75–0.99). The SMR for all cancer was 1.1 (95% CI, 0.76–1.4) on the basis of 43 observations; five cases were non-Hodgkin lymphomas, with 1.8 expected (SMR, 2.8; 95% CI, 0.91–6.5). Among subjects with definite or probable triazine-related work, 14 cancers were observed (SMR, 0.85; 95% CI, 0.46–1.4), and site-specific cancer analyses yielded no significant findings; three deaths from non-Hodgkin lymphomas were seen when 0.78 were expected (SMR, 3.8; 95% CI, 0.79–11). Two of these three men had had less than one year of employment involving exposure to triazine. Two other cancers of the lymphatic and haematopoietic tissue were seen, when 1.8 were expected. Among men with possible exposure to triazine, 29 cancers were observed (SMR, 1.2; 95% CI, 0.80–1.7), of which two were non-Hodgkin lymphomas when 1.0 was expected. Two cases of soft-tissue sarcoma were also seen among men who had possibly been exposed, with 0.30 expected. Inserting a 10-year latency period into the cancer mortality analysis did not affect the risk estimates substantially. [The Working Group noted that lack of control for exposure to other pesticides reduces the usefulness of this study.]

2.2 Case–control studies

Results of case–control studies of triazines, including atrazine, by cancer site are summarized in Table 4.

Table 4. Case–control studies of triazines, including atrazine, by cancer site

Reference and location	Subjects in the analysis	Exposure contrast	Odds ratio (95% CI)	Comments
Non-Hodgkin lymphoma				
Hoar *et al.* (1986), Kansas, United States	170 white men 948 controls	Ever exposed to triazines versus never worked on a farm	1.9 (0.4–8.0)	Restricted to persons with no use of phenoxyacetic acids
Cantor *et al.* (1992), Iowa–Minnesota, United States	622 white men 1245 controls	Ever used triazines on the farm versus never worked on a farm	1.1 (0.8–1.6)	Adjusted for exposure to other pesticides
		Ever personally handled triazines versus never worked on a farm	1.2 (0.9–1.8)	
Zahm *et al.* (1993a), pooled analysis, United States	993 white men 2918 controls	Ever used atrazine versus never worked on a farm	1.4 (1.1–1.8)	Adjusted for age and state
	636 white male farmers 1901 controls	Ever used atrazine versus never used atrazine	1.2 (0.9–1.7)	Restricted to farming and adjusted for exposure to phenoxyacetic acids and organophosphate insecticides
Zahm *et al.* (1993b), eastern Nebraska, United States	134 white women 707 controls	Ever used triazines versus never worked on a farm	1.2 (0.6–2.6)	
Hodgkin's lymphoma				
Hoar *et al.* (1986), Kansas, United States	121 white men 948 controls	Any herbicide used on a farm versus never worked on a farm	0.9 (0.5–1.6)	Mixed exposure to herbicides
Leukaemia				
Brown *et al.* (1990), Iowa–Minnesota, United States	578 white men 1245 controls	Ever used triazines on a farm versus never worked on a farm	1.1 (0.8–1.5)	Adjusted for exposure to other pesticides

Table 4 (contd)

Reference and location	Subjects in the analysis	Exposure contrast	Odds ratio (95% CI)	Comments
Multiple myeloma				
Brown *et al.* (1993), Iowa, United States	173 white men 650 controls	Any herbicide used on a farm versus never worked on a farm	1.2 (0.8–1.9)	
		Ever having handled atrazine versus never worked on a farm	0.8 (0.4-1.6)	
Soft-tissue sarcoma				
Hoar *et al.* (1986), Kansas, United States	133 white men 948 controls	Any herbicide used on a farm versus never worked on a farm	0.9 (0.5–1.6)	Mixed exposure to herbicides
Ovarian cancer				
Donna *et al.* (1989), Alessandria, Italy	65 women 126 controls	Definite exposure to triazines versus no exposure	2.7 [1.0–6.9]	90% confidence interval; adjusted for reproductive factors but not exposure to other herbicides
		Possible exposure to triazines versus no exposure	1.8 [0.9–3.5]	
Colon cancer				
Hoar *et al.* (1985), Kansas, United States	57 [sex not reported] 948 controls	Exposure to triazines versus never worked on a farm	1.4 (0.2–7.9)	

CI, confidence interval

2.2.1 *Lymphatic and haematopoietic malignancies and soft-tissue sarcoma*

In a case–control study in Kansas, United States, Hoar *et al.* (1986) included 172 histologically confirmed cases of non-Hodgkin lymphoma, 132 of Hodgkin disease and 139 of soft-tissue sarcoma in white men aged 21 years or older during the period 1979–81 (non-Hodgkin lymphoma) and 1976–82 (Hodgkin disease and soft-tissue sarcoma). Cases were identified from the files of a State-wide cancer registry. A total of 1005 control subjects were randomly selected from the background population, with frequency matching by age and vital status. For living cases, controls were selected from a national health care programme (age 65 years or older) or by random-digit dialling (age 64 years or younger); for deceased patients, the controls were selected from Kansas State mortality files. Telephone interviews with subjects or their next-of-kin were completed for 96% of cases and 94% of controls, leaving 170 patients with non-Hodgkin lymphoma, 121 with Hodgkin disease, 133 with soft-tissue sarcoma and 948 control subjects for analysis. The interviews included detailed questions on farming practices, with particular emphasis on use of herbicides and insecticides, including triazines. The main purpose of the study was to test the hypothesis of a link between one or more of the three cancer types under study and exposure to phenoxyacetic acid herbicides on farms. The reference exposure category for calculating the odds ratios was people who had never worked on a farm rather than people never exposed to herbicides on farms. Any use of herbicides was reported for 40 non-Hodgkin lymphoma patients, yielding an odds ratio of 1.6 (95% CI, 0.9–2.6). There was a significant trend in risk with increasing years of herbicide use ($p = 0.02$) and with number of days of exposure per year ($p = 0.0004$). The study showed an association with exposure to triazines, including atrazine (odds ratio, 2.5; 95% CI, 1.2–5.4; 14 exposed cases), and several other herbicides. In the absence of exposure to phenoxyacetic acid, the association with triazines was reduced to 1.9 (95% CI, 0.4–8.0) [or 2.2; 95% CI, 0.4–9.1; conflicting results in table and text]. The odds ratio for non-Hodgkin lymphoma among farmers who did not report use of any herbicides was 1.3 (95% CI, 0.8–2.1). No association was reported between exposure to triazine herbicides and Hodgkin disease or soft-tissue sarcoma. [The Working Group noted that part of the excess risk observed may have been due to the choice of reference category.]

In a subsequent study covering the populations of 66 counties of eastern Nebraska, United States, Zahm *et al.* (1990) included 220 histologically confirmed cases of non-Hodgkin lymphoma diagnosed in white men aged 21 years or older during 1983–86 and 831 white male controls from the general population, frequency matched to cases by age and vital status. Telephone interviews with subjects or their next-of-kin were completed for 201 cases (91%) and 725 control subjects (87%) with collection of information on use of herbicides and insecticides on a farm. Any use of herbicides on a farm [no specification of triazines], in comparison with people who had never lived or worked on a farm, was associated with an increased odds ratio of 1.3 (95% CI, 0.8–2.0) which, in turn, was related mainly to handling phenoxyacetic acids (odds ratio, 1.5; 95% CI, 0.9–2.5).

In another case–control study conducted in Iowa and Minnesota, United States, Cantor *et al.* (1992) studied 780 white men aged 30 years or older, in whom a non-

Hodgkin lymphoma had been newly diagnosed during the period 1980–83. Cases were ascertained from records of the Iowa State Health Registry and a special surveillance of records from Minnesota hospitals and pathology laboratories. In Minnesota, non-Hodgkin lymphoma patients who resided in four large cities at the time of diagnosis were excluded. A control group of white men without a haematopoietic or lymphatic cancer were randomly selected from the same geographic areas and frequency-matched to cases by age, vital status and state of residence, following the same procedures as those described by Hoar *et al.* (1986). Interviews with subjects or their next-of-kin were completed for 694 patients with non-Hodgkin lymphoma (89%) and 1245 controls (approximately 77% response rate); however, only 622 of the cases in interviewed patients were confirmed histologically as non-Hodgkin lymphoma and included in the analysis. Detailed information was sought about socio-demographic variables, life-style factors, occupational history and farming practices, including use of herbicides and insecticides. Farming activities (versus non-farming activities) were associated with a small, but marginally significant increase in risk for non-Hodgkin lymphoma (odds ratio, 1.2; 95% CI, 1.0–1.5), but no trend in risk was seen by first year of work, duration of work or size of the farm. Among those who had worked on a farm, 300 patients (84%) and 603 controls (86%) reported use of at least one herbicide or insecticide, yielding an odds ratio relative to those who had never worked on a farm of 1.2 (95% CI, 0.9–1.4). Any use of triazines, including atrazine, was associated with a slightly increased odds ratio of 1.1 (95% CI, 0.8–1.6), calculated on the basis of 64 exposed cases. [The Working Group noted that part of the excess risk observed may have been due to the choice of reference category.]

To evaluate the relationship between exposure to atrazine in farming and non-Hodgkin lymphoma among white men, Zahm *et al.* (1993a) pooled the data from the three case–control studies conducted in Kansas (Hoar *et al.*, 1986), Iowa–Minnesota (Cantor *et al.*, 1992) and eastern Nebraska (Zahm *et al.*, 1990). In the pooled analysis, data from 993 cases and 2918 controls were included. Overall, 130 patients with non-Hodgkin lymphoma (13%) and 249 controls (9%) had been exposed to atrazine, yielding an odds ratio adjusted for age and state of 1.4 (95% CI, 1.1–1.8). People who had never worked on a farm were used as the unexposed reference category. The age-adjusted odds ratios ranged from a low of 1.2 (95% CI, 0.8–1.8) in Iowa to a high of 2.7 (95% CI, 1.2–5.9) in Kansas. The odds ratio associated with personal handling of atrazine was 1.4 (95% CI, 1.0–1.8; 94 exposed cases). Additional adjustment for any use of phenoxyacetic acid herbicides or organophosphate insecticides, which was restricted to 636 patients with non-Hodgkin lymphoma [64% of all] and 1901 control subjects [65% of all] who reported that they were farmers, reduced the combined odds ratio for non-Hodgkin lymphoma associated with use of atrazine to 1.2 (95% CI, 0.9–1.7). Farmers in Nebraska (the State for which the most detailed information was available on duration and annual frequency of use of atrazine specifically) who had used atrazine for more than 15 years had a twofold risk for non-Hodgkin lymphoma, but the increase disappeared when the analyses were adjusted for use of other herbicides and organophosphate insecticides.

Zahm *et al.* (1993b) studied 206 white women, aged 21 years or older, in 66 counties of eastern Nebraska, United States, in whom histologically confirmed non-Hodgkin lymphoma was diagnosed during the period 1983–86. Cases were identified through the Nebraska Lymphoma Study Group and area hospitals. A total of 824 control subjects were included, frequency-matched on age and vital status, following the same procedures as those described for the study in Kansas (Hoar *et al.*, 1986). Telephone interviews with the women or their next-of-kin were completed for 134 of the initially eligible cases (65%) and 707 of the controls (86%). Detailed information was sought on farming practices, including use of herbicides and insecticides. A total of 119 women [89% of the cases with a completed interview] with non-Hodgkin lymphoma and 471 [67%] controls reported ever having lived or worked on a farm, yielding on odds ratio of 1.0 (95% CI, 0.7–1.4). Any use of triazine herbicides, including atrazine, on the farm was associated with a non-significant risk of 1.2 (95% CI, 0.6–2.6; 12 exposed cases) and personal handling of triazine herbicides with an odds ratio of 2.2 (95% CI, 0.1–32; one exposed case). These estimates were not adjusted for use of other types of herbicide or use of insecticides.

In a case–control study from Iowa and Minnesota, United States, Brown *et al.* (1990) included 669 histologically confirmed cases of leukaemia newly diagnosed among white men aged 30 years or older during 1981–84. Cases were ascertained from records of the Iowa State Health Registry and a special surveillance of records from Minnesota hospitals and pathology laboratories. The control group was the same as that used in the Iowa–Minnesota case–control study of non-Hodgkin lymphoma (Cantor *et al.*, 1992), described above. Personal interviews including detailed questions on farming practices were completed for 578 of the cases (86%) and 1245 controls (77%). Any exposure to triazines, including atrazine, was associated with a slightly increased risk for any type of leukaemia (odds ratio, 1.1; 95% CI, 0.8–1.5; 67 exposed cases). There was a small but significant risk for all types of leukaemia combined (1.2; 95% CI, 1.0–1.5) among persons who lived or worked on a farm; however, the odds ratio for leukaemia among farmers who reported no exposure to pesticides was 1.9 (95% CI, 1.3–2.9).

In a case–control study from Iowa, United States, Brown *et al.* (1993) included 173 white men aged 30 years or older in whom multiple myeloma had been newly diagnosed during 1981–84 and who had been identified from the Iowa Health Registry. The 650 controls included in this study were those used in the case–control studies of non-Hodgkin lymphoma (Cantor *et al.*, 1992) and leukaemia (Brown *et al.*, 1990) in Iowa. The questionnaire was that used in the Iowa–Minnesota study and included detailed questions on occupational history and farming practices. Interviews with subjects or their next-of-kin were completed for 84% of the initially eligible cases and 78% of the controls. Some farming activity was reported by 64% of the patients and 58% of the controls, yielding a non-significantly increased odds ratio of 1.2 (95% CI, 0.8–1.7). The risk for multiple myeloma was not increased among farmers who personally mixed, handled or applied atrazine (odds ratio, 0.8; 95% CI, 0.4–1.6; 12 exposed cases).

2.2.2 *Other sites*

In a hospital-based study in Piedmont, Italy (Donna *et al.*, 1984), 60 women in whom a histologically confirmed primary mesothelial ovarian tumour had been diagnosed during 1974–80 were matched to 127 controls in whom another type of cancer had been diagnosed. Personal interviews including questions on occupational history and exposure to herbicides were completed for 91% of the identified cases and 94% of controls. Exposure to herbicides [no information on exposure to any triazines or to triazines as a group] was regarded as 'definite' in eight cases and no controls and as 'probable' in 10 cases and 14 controls. Definite and probable exposure versus no exposure to herbicides was associated with an odds ratio of 4.4 (95% CI, 1.9–16).

In the population of 143 neighbouring municipalities forming the rural districts of Alessandria Province, Italy, Donna *et al.* (1989) studied all women aged 20–69 years in whom a primary malignant epithelial tumour of the ovary had been diagnosed between 1980 and 1985. Cases were identified from all 18 hospitals serving the area; two controls of the same age were randomly selected for each case from the electoral rolls of the municipalities of the study area. Information on reproductive factors, farming activities and occupational exposure to triazines and other herbicides was collected at interviews conducted at the subjects' homes. The response rates were 94% for cases eligible for the study and 84% for controls, leaving 65 cases and 126 controls for analysis. Interviews were conducted with next-of-kin of 35% of cases and none of the controls. The likelihood of exposure to triazines (definitely exposed, possibly exposed and unexposed) was established blindly by two of the authors independently after all of the interviews had been completed. The odds ratios for ovarian cancer, adjusted for age, number of live births and use of contraceptives were 2.7 (90% CI, 1.0–6.9; seven cases) for definitely exposed and 1.8 (90% CI, 0.9–3.5; 14 cases) for possibly exposed. The odds ratios were slightly higher among individuals with at least 10 years of occupational contact with triazines when compared with those with fewer than 10 years of contact. Restricting the analysis to women who reported having worked in agriculture yielded approximately similar risk estimates associated with exposure to triazine herbicides. [The Working Group noted that the odds ratios for exposure to triazines were of borderline significance and were not adjusted for exposure to other herbicides.]

Hoar *et al.* (1985) reported on a case–control study of 57 histologically confirmed cases [sex unspecified] of colon cancer sampled from among all such cases diagnosed in Kansas, United States, in 1976–82. A total of 948 controls were sampled from the general population. Slightly elevated risks were seen for both farmers who had used herbicides (odds ratio, 1.5; 95% CI, 0.6–4.0; 11 cases) and farmers who had not used herbicides (odds ratio, 1.6; 95% CI, 0.8–3.6). Exposure to triazines was associated with an odds ratio of 1.4 (95% CI, 0.2–7.9), on the basis of two exposed cases.

No data were available on exposure to triazines in general or atrazine in particular and the occurrence of breast cancer.

3. Studies of Cancer in Experimental Animals

3.1 Oral administration

Mouse: Groups of 60 male and 60 female CD-1 mice [age unspecified] were given atrazine (purity, > 96%) in the diet for at least 91 weeks in two separate studies, at concentrations of 0, 10, 300 or 1000 mg/kg of diet (ppm) in the first study and 0, 10, 300, 1500 or 3000 ppm in the second. The survival of treated males was unaffected, but that of female mice receiving 1000 or 3000 ppm atrazine was significantly decreased. Body-weight gain was reduced in male and female mice given 1500 or 3000 ppm atrazine. There was no treatment-related increase in tumour incidence in male or female mice exposed to atrazine in either study (Stevens *et al.*, 1998).

Atrazine was evaluated for carcinogenicity in (C57BL/6×C3H/Anf)F_1 mice and in (C57BL/6×AKR)F_1 mice fed concentrations of 82 mg/kg of diet (21.5 mg/kg bw) (ppm). Atrazine did not increase the incidence of any benign or malignant tumour in these studies (Innes *et al.*, 1969). [The Working Group considered these studies to be inadequate for evaluation since no data were available on the numbers of animals, numbers of dose groups, study duration, observed tumour rates or justification for the low doses used.]

Rat: Groups of 53–56 male and 50–55 female Fischer 344/LATI rats weighing 150–180 g were fed pelleted diets containing 0 (control), 500 (low dose) or 1000 mg/kg of diet (ppm) (high dose) atrazine (purity, 98.9%) during the first eight weeks of the study. Because of toxicity, the high dose was then reduced to 750 ppm and the low dose to 375 ppm. The study was terminated at week 126. The survival of male rats relative to controls was significantly increased at both the high ($p < 0.0001$) and the low ($p = 0.019$) doses. The increased survival of treated female rats was not statistically significant. Female rats had increased incidences of uterine adenocarcinomas (controls, 6/45; low dose, 8/52; high dose, 13/45) and leukaemia and lymphoma (combined) (12/44, 16/52, 22/51), which were significant by the Cochran-Armitage trend test but not by Peto's test for incidental tumours, in which adjustment is made for increased survival observed in treated groups. The overall proportion of animals with benign and malignant uterine tumours was similar in all groups (16/45, 19/52, 17/45). The incidence of primary benign mammary gland tumours was reported to be significantly increased ($p < 0.05$ by Peto's incidental tumour test) in males at the high dose relative to controls (control, 1/48; low dose, 1/51; high dose, 8/53). The mammary gland tumours in males were benign, except for one adenocarcinoma in a male at the high dose (Pintér *et al.*, 1990). [The Working Group noted that the statistical methods used to evaluate the mammary gland tumours were inappropriately applied to the total number of tumours/number of animals examined rather than to the number of tumour-bearing animals/number of animals examined.]

In a critique of the study of Pintér *et al.* (1990), Thakur *et al.* (1998) reported that six of the eight mammary gland tumours in males at the high dose occurred after the last control had died at week 111, and that the significant ($p < 0.0001$) difference in survival between the high-dose and control groups had not been properly taken into account in the evaluation of these tumours. Thakur *et al.* (1998) also noted that the last male at the high dose died at week 136, not week 126, and that Pintér *et al.* (1990) had overlooked a mammary gland fibroma in male controls in their tabulation of tumour rates and subsequent statistical analysis. Thakur *et al.* (1998) concluded that the increase in the incidence of mammary gland tumours in male rats was not significant ($p = 0.8$) when evaluated by a proper statistical analysis with adjustment for survival. [The Working Group concluded that the issue raised by Thakur *et al.* (1998) was valid.]

Atrazine (purity, 97%) was fed to 60 male and 60 female Charles River Fischer Crl:CDF (Fischer 344) rats at concentrations of 10, 70, 200 or 400 mg/kg of diet (ppm) for up to 104 weeks. An additional seven groups of 10 females per dose were treated for and killed at 1, 3, 9, 12, 15, 18 and 24 months. Body-weight gain was reduced in males and females at 400 ppm, but survival was similar in treated and control groups. No significant carcinogenic effects were observed in any group (Wetzel *et al.*, 1994; Stevens *et al.*, 1998; Thakur *et al.*, 1998).

In a similar study, 60 female Sprague-Dawley rats were fed diets containing 0, 70 or 400 ppm atrazine (purity, 97%) for up to 104 weeks, and additional groups of 10 females per dose were treated for and killed at 1, 3, 9, 12, 15, 18 and 24 months. Females at 400 ppm showed a 12% reduction in body-weight gain at 13 weeks and a significant reduction in two-year survival (37%) relative to controls. They also had a statistically significantly ($p < 0.05$) earlier onset of mammary gland tumours relative to controls, although the overall incidences of these neoplasms at the end of the study were similar in the treated and control groups (Wetzel *et al.*, 1994; Stevens *et al.*, 1998).

Groups of 70–90 male and 70–90 female Sprague-Dawley rats were fed diets containing 0, 10, 70, 500 or 1000 ppm atrazine (purity, 96%) for a maximum of 106 weeks. The body-weight gain of animals at 500 and 1000 ppm was significantly reduced. The survival of males at 1000 ppm was significantly increased, and that of females at this dose was significantly decreased. In females, the incidence of mammary gland fibroadenomas was significantly ($p < 0.01$) increased in animals at 1000 ppm (controls, 29/88; 10 ppm, 29/69; 70 ppm, 36/69; 500 ppm, 39/70; 1000 ppm, 45/89), and the incidence of mammary gland adenocarcinomas was significantly ($p < 0.005$) increased in animals at the three highest doses (15/88, 16/69, 27/69, 27/70 and 43/89). In males, the incidence of interstitial-cell tumour of the testis was statistically significantly increased ($p < 0.05$) at 1000 ppm (1/90, 3/70, 2/70, 2/70 and 7/90), but the incidence fell within the historical range for controls at that test laboratory (0–12%) and was attributed in part to the significantly better survival of these animals (Stevens *et al.*, 1994, 1998).

Groups of 49–54 female Sprague-Dawley rats were fed diets containing 0, 10, 100 or 1000 ppm atrazine (purity, 96%) for life. No information on body weight or survival was given. The incidences of mammary gland fibroadenomas were significantly ($p < 0.05$) increased in animals at 10 and 1000 ppm (control, 11/54; 10 ppm, 20/52; 100 ppm, 14/54; 1000 ppm, 22/49), but there was no significant increase in the incidence of malignant mammary gland tumours (11/54, 8/52, 12/54 and 13/49, respectively) (Stevens *et al.*, 1994).

Groups of 29–40 female Sprague Dawley rats culled from the F_2 generation of a two-generation study of reproductive toxicity were fed diets containing atrazine (purity, 97.6%) for up to 104 weeks after exposure *in utero* to 0, 10, 50 or 500 ppm atrazine. No information on body weight or survival was given. The incidences of mammary gland tumours were not increased (controls, 11/30; 10 ppm, 10/40; 50 ppm, 13/40; 500 ppm, 11/29) (Stevens *et al.*, 1994).

Five groups of 80 female Sprague-Dawley rats, eight weeks old, ovariectomized at seven weeks of age and five groups of 80 intact females were fed diets containing 0, 25, 50, 70 or 400 ppm atrazine (purity, at least 96%) for up to 104 weeks. The body-weight gain of both ovariectomized and intact females receiving 400 ppm atrazine was decreased. The survival of ovariectomized females fed 400 ppm atrazine was unaffected, but that of intact females at this dose was significantly reduced. No mammary tumours were found in any group of treated, ovariectomized females; however, the incidence of mammary gland fibroadenomas in the intact females was significantly ($p < 0.05$) increased at the three highest doses after adjustment for survival (16/80, 25/80, 33/78, 29/80 and 25/80), and the incidence of mammary gland carcinomas was significantly ($p < 0.05$) increased in females at 50 and 400 ppm (12/80, 18/80, 20/78, 14/80 and 27/80) (Stevens *et al.*, 1998, 1999).

3.2 Intraperitoneal administration

Mouse: A group of 30 male Swiss mice, four weeks of age, received intraperitoneal injections of 'pure' atrazine in saline every third day for 13 injections (total dose, 0.26 mg/kg bw). Two control groups of 50 mice each were treated with saline or were untreated. The experiment was terminated after 375 days, when all surviving animals were killed. The incidence of lymphomas in the atrazine-treated group (6/30) was significantly ($p < 0.001$) greater than that in the combined control groups (1/100). The six lymphomas in the treated group comprised two histiocytic lymphomas and four plasma-cell lymphomas; one histiocytic lymphoma was found in the untreated control group (Donna *et al.*, 1986). [The Working Group noted that if the histiocytic tumours were sarcomas, they should have been evaluated separately.]

4. Other Data Relevant to an Evaluation of Carcinogenicity and its Mechanisms

4.1 Absorption, distribution, metabolism and excretion

4.1.1 *Humans*

Workers occupationally exposed to atrazine excreted some unchanged atrazine in their urine (Catenacci *et al.*, 1990). The majority of an absorbed dose was recoverable in urine as the fully dealkylated metabolite 2-chloro-4,6-diamino-1,3,5-triazine and the monodealkylated metabolite 2-chloro-4-amino-6-(ethylamino)-1,3,5-triazine which were present in equal amounts; practically none of the other monodealkylated metabolite, 2-chloro-4-amino-6-(isopropylamino)-1,3,5-triazine, was found (Ikonen *et al.*, 1988).

In a study in which gas chromatography was used to identify deethylated, deisopropylated and di-dealkylated atrazine, as well as atrazine itself, in the urine of atrazine manufacture workers, di-dealkylated atrazine represented 80% of the urinary metabolites (Catenacci *et al.*, 1993).

Using a sensitive enzyme-linked immunosorbent assay, Lucas *et al.* (1993) identified a mercapturic acid conjugate of atrazine as the major metabolite in the urine of applicators. Minor metabolites included *N*-dealkylated and *N*-deisopropyl atrazines. No di-dealkylated metabolites were identified, as they would have been expected to degrade during storage, and no hydroxylated conjugates were detected.

4.1.2 *Experimental systems*

Atrazine was well absorbed after oral administration to Fischer 344 rats; the 72-h urinary recoveries were similar (66%) after administration of either 30 mg/kg bw [U-^{14}C]-atrazine in corn oil (Timchalk *et al.*, 1990) or approximately 1.5 mg/kg bw [ring-^{14}C]-atrazine in ethanol (Bakke *et al.*, 1972). Moderate, inversely dose-dependent absorption (3–8% adults; 3–10% juveniles) through the skin was demonstrated in Fischer 344 rats (Shah *et al.*, 1987).

The retention of radiolabel in the carcass of rats ranged from 4% (Timchalk *et al.*, 1990) to 16% (Bakke *et al.*, 1972) 72 h after dosing with [^{14}C]atrazine. The relative retention in tissues was: liver, kidney, lung > heart, brain >> muscle, fat. Less than 0.1% of an oral radioactive dose was detected in expired air (Bakke *et al.*, 1972).

A one-compartment model adequately describes the kinetics of atrazine in the plasma of rats. The plasma concentration peaked 8–10 h after dosing, with an apparent absorption half-time of 2.6 h, and there was first-order elimination with a half-time of 10.8 h. Neither the kinetic characteristics nor the recovery of the dose were affected by concurrent administration of 60 mg/kg bw tridiphane, a herbicidal synergist in plants which blocks glutathione transferase-mediated conjugation (Timchalk *et al.*, 1990).

N-Dealkylation and conjugation with glutathione are the main pathways of metabolism of atrazine in various species *in vivo* and *in vitro* (Böhme & Bär, 1967; Adams *et al.*, 1990; Timchalk *et al.*, 1990). The metabolism of atrazine (and three other triazine herbicides, terbuthylazine, ametryne and terbutryne) has been investigated *in vitro* in liver microsomes from rats, pigs and humans. The principal phase-I reactions in all three species were *N*-monodealkylation, hydroxylation of the isopropyl or *tert*-butyl moiety and sulfoxidation of the substrate. Although all species produced the same type of metabolites, there were species-specific differences in the metabolite ratios (Lang *et al.*, 1996). Subsequent studies have showed that cytochrome P450 1A2 is the major phase-I enzyme involved in the metabolism of *s*-triazines in human liver microsomes (Lang *et al.*, 1997).

The dealkylation product 2-chloro-4,6-diamino-1,3,5-triazine is the major urinary metabolite (64–67%) in rats, others being mercapturates of the mono- and di-dealkylated products (13–14% and 9%, respectively) (Timchalk *et al.*, 1990). Minor metabolic pathways in rats may include alkyl side-chain oxidation (Böhme & Bar, 1967). Oxidative dechlorination to 2-hydroxyatrazine, a metabolite formed in plants (Shimabukuro *et al.*, 1971), did not occur in rat liver homogenates (Dauterman & Muecke, 1974), although Bakke *et al.* (1972) claimed to have found some 2-hydroxyatrazine in rat urine and showed that it was metabolized along pathways similar to those of atrazine.

As there appear to be no remarkable qualitative differences in metabolism among species, the metabolic data do not readily explain the apparent strain-specific development of mammary gland tumours in atrazine-treated Sprague-Dawley rats.

4.2 Toxic effects

4.2.1 *Humans*

No data were available to the Working Group.

4.2.2 *Experimental systems*

The oral LD_{50} of atrazine was reported to be 2000 mg/kg bw in rats [strain not specified] (Ben-Dyke *et al.*, 1970) and 670, 740 and 2300 mg/kg bw in adult female and male, and weanling male Sherman rats, respectively, while the dermal LD_{50} was > 2500 mg/kg bw in Sherman rats of each sex (Gaines & Linder, 1986).

Administration of atrazine by oral gavage at 100–600 mg/kg bw per day to adult male Wistar rats for 7 or 14 days induced both nephrotoxicity and hepatotoxicity (Santa Maria *et al.*, 1986, 1987). The hepatotoxic effects included a dose-related reduction in blood sugar concentration and increases in the activity of serum alanine aminotransferase and alkaline phosphatase and in total serum lipids. Electron micrographs showed degeneration of the smooth endoplasmic reticulum, lipid droplet accumulation and swollen mitochondria. The lowest dose was not toxic to the liver (Santa Maria *et al.*, 1987). Renal toxicity, including dose-related proteinurea, reduced creatinine clearance and increased urinary electrolyte output, was seen at all doses (Santa Maria *et al.*, 1986).

Hormonal imbalances induced by atrazine appears to be significant in the interpretation of possible carcinogenic effects on the mammary gland. Most of the work has been directed towards the effects of atrazine on the hypothalamus–pituitary–gonadal axis. Steroid hormone metabolism was found to be impaired by atrazine, which inhibits 5α-steroid reductase in the anterior pituitary of rats (Kniewald *et al.*, 1979). Subsequently, it was shown in male rats that atrazine (at 120 mg/kg bw per day orally for seven days) increased the wet weight of the anterior pituitary by 60–70%, caused hyperaemia and hypertrophy of the chromophobic cells and reductions of 37, 39 and 46%, respectively, in the activities of 5α-steroid reductase and 3α- and 17β-hydroxysteroid dehydrogenase *in vivo*. The deethylated metabolite was approximately equipotent in reducing 5α-steroid reductase activity after administration *in vivo*. Only 5α-steroid reductase and 17β-hydroxysteroid dehydrogenase were inhibited by either compound in the hypothalamus *in vivo*; deethylatrazine was the more potent inhibitor of these enzymes in the hypothalamus *in vitro* (Babic-Gojmerac *et al.*, 1989).

Subcutaneous administration to Fischer rats of atrazine at 16.6 mg/kg bw from the first day of gestation was reported to increase the conversion of testosterone to 5α-dihydrotestosterone in the anterior hypothalamus of 28-day-old female, but not male, offspring. When 21-day-old offspring were examined after exposure during gestation and lactation, males had a decreased capacity to convert testosterone to either 5α-androstane-3α,17β-diol or 5α-dihydrotestosterone, while no effects were seen in females. In contrast, the number of 5α-dihydrotestosterone receptors in the prostate was enhanced in 21-day-old males exposed during gestation and lactation but not in 28-day-old males exposed only during gestation (Kniewald *et al.*, 1987). Studies *in vitro* have demonstrated inhibition of androgen metabolism by atrazine when incubated with rat pituitary homogenates (Kniewald *et al.*, 1979; Babic-Gojmerac *et al.*, 1989).

Under equilibrium conditions, atrazine was unable to compete with oestradiol for binding to rat uterine oestrogen receptors. Weak competition was noted when the cytosol was preincubated at 25°C prior to incubation with the tracer (Tennant *et al.*, 1994a).

Treatment of adult, ovariectomized Sprague-Dawley rats with up to 300 mg/kg bw atrazine by oral gavage for three days did not increase uterine weight or uterine progesterone concentrations, suggesting lack of oestrogenic potential. When 2 μg/kg bw oestradiol were given by subcutaneous injection in conjunction with an oral dose of 300 mg/kg bw, there was significant inhibition (~25%) of the uterotrophic response (Tennant *et al.*, 1994b). In a similar study, immature female Sprague-Dawley rats were dosed with 0, 50, 150 or 300 mg/kg bw atrazine by gavage for three days. Uterine weight was not increased, but there were significant decreases in uterine progesterone receptor binding activity and peroxidase activity. When atrazine was combined with oestradiol, however, it had no anti-oestrogenic effect on the uterus, but decreases were still observed in uterine progesterone receptor binding and peroxidase activity (Connor *et al.*, 1996). In the same study, atrazine did not affect basal or oestradiol-induced MCF-7 cell proliferation *in vitro* or affect oestradiol-induced luciferase activity in MCF-7 cells transfected with a Gal4-regulated human oestrogen receptor chimaera.

Female Long Evans and Sprague-Dawley rats which had been determined to have regular four-day oestrous cycles received 0, 75, 150 or 300 mg/kg bw per day atrazine by gavage in a suspension of 1% carboxymethylcellulose for 21 days. Atrazine disrupted the regular oestrous cycles in both strains, at all doses in the Long Evans rats but only at 150 or 300 mg/kg per day for a longer period of time in Sprague-Dawley rats. The increased time spent in vaginal dioestrous was associated with elevated serum progesterone and low oestradiol concentrations, indicative of a repetitive pseudopregnancy condition. This hormonal perturbation was not considered to be conducive to the development of mammary tumours, although there was some indication of prolonged oestrous at the lowest dose tested (Cooper *et al.*, 1996).

Sprague-Dawley and Fischer 344 rats were fed atrazine at 0, 10, 70, 200 or 400 mg/kg of diet (ppm), the highest dose being the maximum tolerated dose (resulting in a 10–15% reduction in body-weight gain), for 24 months. Atrazine at 400 ppm lengthened the oestrus cycle of the Sprague-Dawley rats and increased the percentage of days in oestrus (i.e. days under the influence of increased endogenous oestrogen) earlier in life than in controls. This effect was associated with an increased incidence and earlier age of onset of mammary 'tumours' [type not specified] in this sensitive rat strain. Feeding of atrazine at 70 ppm had no effect on these parameters when compared with vehicle-treated controls. The response of Fischer 344 rats to atrazine was clearly different from that of Sprague-Dawley rats, as atrazine at similar doses did not affect circulating oestrogen and prolactin levels, the percentage of days spent in oestrus or the incidence or time of onset of mammary gland neoplasms (Wetzel *et al.*, 1994).

The effects of atrazine on the luteinizing hormone (LH) surge was investigated in female Sprague-Dawley rats. After ovariectomy, the animals received an implanted sustained-release capsule containing oestradiol-17β (4 mg/mL sesame seed oil) and were then given atrazine by gavage at a daily dose of 300 mg/kg bw for three days. The time-course of the LH surge was monitored from 11.00 h on the third day. Control animals had peaks at 18.00 h, whereas treated animals had only a slight increase in LH at 22.00 h. After exposure to 0, 2.5, 5, 40 or 200 mg/kg atrazine for 30 days (the last three days after ovariectomy), the LH surge was delayed and attenuated at the highest dose (Simpkins *et al.*, 1998).

Groups of 80 eight-week-old intact or ovariectomized female Sprague-Dawley rats received atrazine in the diet at concentrations of 0, 25, 50, 70 or 400 ppm. Twenty rats per group were necropsied after 52 weeks of treatment, and the remainder were examined at 104 weeks. No mammary tumours were found in ovariectomized females, whereas the incidence of mammary carcinomas was increased in intact rats at 50 and 400 ppm, and the incidence of fibroadenomas was significantly greater than that in controls at 50, 70 and 400 ppm (Stevens *et al.*, 1998, 1999).

4.3 Reproductive and developmental effects

4.3.1 *Humans*

Data on Ontario farm families from the 1986 Canadian Census of Agriculture were used to assess the effect of exposure of men to pesticides on pregnancy outcome. Use of a number of pesticides and chemicals, including atrazine, in the three-month period preceding a pregnancy was assessed from a questionnaire completed by 1898 couples who conceived during the study period. The use of atrazine itself was not associated with increased odds ratios for miscarriage, pre-term delivery or babies who were small for gestational age, although combinations of activities involving exposure to a variety of chemicals including atrazine generated odds ratios of 2 or greater in some instances (Savitz *et al.*, 1997).

4.3.2 *Experimental systems*

Atrazine was tested for teratogenicity in both natural and buffered waters in the FETAX (frog embryo teratogenicity assay-*Xenopus*). The LD_{50} values for embryos were 100 mg/L in buffered water and 126 mg/L in natural water samples, with corresponding effective concentrations (EC_{50}) for malformations of 33 mg/L and < 8 mg/L, indicating that atrazine is more teratogenic than embryo-lethal in this system. The lowest effective concentrations of atrazine were 11 mg/L in buffered samples and 1.1 mg/L in natural waters (Morgan *et al.*, 1996). [The Working Group noted that the embryotoxic effects occurred only at high concentrations of atrazine approaching its maximal water solubility.] Atrazine was included in a group of pesticides characterized as only slightly toxic after application to developing mallard embryos (Hoffman & Albers, 1984).

It was reported in an abstract that subcutaneous injections of atrazine to neonatal rats on days 4–7 after birth prolonged the period of vaginal opening (Zeljenkova & Vargova, 1996). Daily exposure of adult Fischer rats to 0 or 120 mg/kg bw atrazine by oral gavage in a suspension in paraffin oil for seven days reduced the body weights of both males and females. Fewer treated females had normal oestrous cycles, and the number of days in dioestrous was significantly increased. When both males and females were exposed or when exposed females were mated with unexposed males, fertility was reduced during the first week after exposure, but pregnancy outcome was not affected in those females that became inseminated. No similar effects were observed when only the males were exposed, but atrazine did cause a significant increase in the relative weights of the pituitary and prostate (Šimic *et al.*, 1994).

Groups of 10 adult female Fischer 344 rats received 0 or 120 mg/kg bw per day atrazine by oral gavage six times at two-day intervals, and the oestrous cycle was evaluated during and for 12 days after the treatment period. Two weeks later, they were mated to untreated males, and their offspring were evaluated for spontaneous motor activity at 70 days of age and avoidance conditioning at 72 and 73 days of age. The body weights of the dams were reduced during the treatment period, but no effects were noted on the oestrous cycle, conception or litter size. Female offspring showed increased motor activity, while males had shorter latency times and increased shock avoidance (Peruzovic *et al.*, 1995).

In an evaluation of potential developmental toxicity, groups of 27 CD rats were given atrazine (technical-grade, purity unspecified) at doses of 0, 10, 70 or 700 mg/kg bw per day by gavage on gestation days 6-15. The vehicle was 3% aqueous starch containing 0.5% Tween 80. The dams were necropsied on day 20 of gestation and the fetuses examined for viability, growth and malformations. The incidence of mortality during treatment of dams at the highest dose was 78%; surviving females had reduced body and liver weights at term, but there was no effect on relative liver weight. The rate of post-implantation loss was more than twice that of the controls, and the fetuses of dams that survived this dose showed marked growth retardation. The feed consumption of animals at this dose was significantly reduced throughout the treatment and post-treatment periods. The feed consumption of dams at 70 mg/kg bw per day was slightly but statistically significantly decreased on days 6 and 7, and their body-weight gain was significantly reduced on days 6–10, but all survived to day 20. There were no treatment-related effects on fetal viability, growth or the incidence of external malformations at the low or intermediate doses, although the incidence of several minor skeletal variations was increased in fetuses at the intermediate dose (Infurna *et al.*, 1988).

Groups of 19 New Zealand white rabbits were given doses of 0, 1, 5 or 75 mg/kg bw per day atrazine (technical-grade, purity unspecified) by gavage on gestation days 7–19. The vehicle was 3% aqueous starch containing 0.5% Tween 80. The does were necropsied on day 29 of gestation and the fetuses were examined for viability, growth and malformations. Spontaneous abortions were observed in two does at the high dose and in one doe each at the intermediate and low doses. Does at the high dose had severely reduced feed consumption, reduced body-weight gain, reduced absolute but not relative liver weights, an increased incidence of fetal resorptions and post-implantation loss and decreased fetal body weights of the offspring; in addition, skeletal ossification was noted in this group. There were no dose-related increases in the incidence of malformations (Infurna *et al.*, 1988).

Atrazine was a component of two mixtures designed to mimic the contaminants of groundwater due to agricultural practices that were evaluated for developmental and reproductive toxicity. The mixture contained several other pesticides, fertilizers and other organic substances commonly found in groundwater at two sites in the United States. CD-1 mice were evaluated in a continuous breeding protocol, and a standard study of developmental toxicity was conducted in Sprague-Dawley rats exposed on days 6–20 of gestation. The animals received drinking-water containing the mixtures, in which the concentrations of atrazine were 0, 0.5, 5 and 50 ng/mL (equivalent to 1, 10 and 100 times the median concentration of atrazine at the two sites). In mice, no effects were noted on the reproductive performance of F_0 or F_1 individuals or on spermatogenesis, epididymal sperm concentration, per cent motile sperm, per cent abnormal sperm or the histological appearance of the testis. No evidence of developmental toxicity was observed in rats (Heindel *et al.*, 1994).

4.4 Genetic and related effects

4.4.1 *Humans*

No data were available to the Working Group.

4.4.2 *Experimental systems* (see Table 5 for references)

Atrazine did not induce mutation in bacteriophage, bacteria, *Saccharomyces cerevisiae* or *Nicotiana tabacum*, whereas mutations were induced in *Schizosaccharomyces pombe*, *Aspergillus nidulans*, *Zea mays* and *Drosophila melanogaster*; conflicting results were obtained with *Hordeum vulgare*. In *Drosophila melanogaster*, sex-linked recessive lethal mutations were induced in two studies but not in a third. 6-Thioguanine-resistant mutants were induced in cultured Chinese hamster lung V79 cells, but only in the presence of microsomes from potato, and not in the presence of an exogenous metabolic activation system from rat liver.

Gene conversion was not induced in *A. nidulans*; conflicting results were obtained with *S. cerevisiae*. Mitotic recombination was not increased by atrazine in *S. cerevisiae*, while conflicting results were obtained with *A. nidulans*. Aneuploidy was induced in *Neurospora crassa, A. nidulans* and *D. melanogaster*. An assay for micronucleus induction in *Tradescantia* gave negative results.

Table 5. Genetic and related effects of atrazine

Test system	Results[a]		Dose[b] (LED or HID)	Reference
	Without exogenous metabolic system	With exogenous metabolic system		
Escherichia coli PQ37, SOS repair	–	–	1000 μg/plate	Ruiz & Marzin (1997)
Bacteriophage T4, forward mutation	–	NT	20 μg/plate	Andersen *et al.* (1972)
Bacteriophage, reverse mutation	–	NT	1000 μg/plate	Andersen *et al.* (1972)
Salmonella typhimurium, forward mutation, 8AG[R]	–	–	250	Adler (1980)
Salmonella typhimurium TA100, TA98, TA1535, TA1537, TA1538, reverse mutation	NT	–	5000 μg/plate	Simmon *et al.* (1977)
Salmonella typhimurium TA100, TA98, TA1535, reverse mutation	–	–	100 μg/plate	Lusby *et al.* (1979)
Salmonella typhimurium TA100, TA98, reverse mutation	NT	–	1100 μg/plate	Bartsch *et al.* (1980)
Salmonella typhimurium TA100, TM677, reverse mutation	NT	–[c]	30 000 μg/plate	Sumner *et al.* (1984)
Salmonella typhimurium TA100, TA98, TA97, TA1535, TA1537, TA1538, reverse mutation	–	–	1000 μg/plate	Kappas (1988)
Salmonella typhimurium TA100, reverse mutation	NT	+[c]	NR	Means *et al.* (1988)
Salmonella typhimurium TA100, TA98, TA97, TA102, reverse mutation	–	–	1000 μg/plate	Mersch-Sundermann *et al.* (1988)
Salmonella typhimurium TA100, TA98, TA97, TA1535, TA1537, TA1538, reverse mutation	–	–	1000 μg/plate	Zeiger *et al.* (1988)
Salmonella typhimurium TA100, TA98, TA97, reverse mutation	–	NT	2000 μg/plate	Butler & Hoagland (1989)
Salmonella typhimurium TA100, TA98, TA102, TA1535, TA1537, reverse mutation	–	–	1000 μg/plate	Ruiz & Marzin (1997)
Salmonella typhimurium TA100, TA98, reverse mutation	–	–	1000 μg/plate	Morichetti *et al.* (1992)
Salmonella typhimurium TA1530, TA1531, TA1532, TA1534, *his* G45, reverse mutation (spot test)	–	NT	NR	Seiler (1973)
Salmonella typhimurium (eight unidentified strains), reverse mutation	–	NT	NR	Andersen *et al.* (1972)
Salmonella typhimurium (strains not identified), reverse mutation	–	–	NR	Adler (1980)
Escherichia coli, forward mutation, Amp[R]	–	–	430 μg/plate	Adler (1980)

Table 5 (contd)

Test system	Results[a]		Dose[b] (LED or HID)	Reference
	Without exogenous metabolic system	With exogenous metabolic system		
Saccharomyces cerevisiae, gene conversion	–	+[c]	10	Plewa & Gentile (1976)
Saccharomyces cerevisiae, gene conversion	–	–	2000	Adler (1980)
Saccharomyces cerevisiae, gene conversion	–	–	4000	de Bertoldi *et al.* (1980)
Saccharomyces cerevisiae, mitotic recombination	–	NT	50	Emnova *et al.* (1987)
Saccharomyces cerevisiae, gene conversion (stationary phase cells)	+	NT	64 800	Morichetti *et al.* (1992)
Saccharomyces cerevisiae, gene conversion (logarithmic phase cells)	+	NT	540	Morichetti *et al.* (1992)
Saccharomyces cerevisiae, reverse mutation (stationary phase cells)	–	NT	75 600	Morichetti *et al.* (1992)
Saccharomyces cerevisiae, reverse mutation (logarithmic phase cells)	(+)	NT	2160	Morichetti *et al.* (1992)
Aspergillus nidulans, gene conversion	–	NT	8000	de Bertoldi *et al.* (1980)
Aspergillus nidulans, mitotic recombination	–	+	NR	Adler (1980)
Aspergillus nidulans, mitotic recombination	–	–	1000	Kappas (1988)
Saccharomyces cerevisiae, forward mutation	–	NT	50	Emnova *et al.* (1987)
Schizosaccharomyces pombe, reverse mutation	+	NT	17.5	Mathias (1987)
Schizosaccharomyces pombe, reverse mutation	+	+[c]	70	Mathias (1987)
Aspergillus nidulans, forward mutation	–	+	2500	Benigni *et al.* (1979)
Aspergillus nidulans, aneuploidy	–	+	2000	Benigni *et al.* (1979)
Neurospora crassa, aneuploidy	+	NT	NR	Griffiths (1979)
Hordeum vulgare, mutation	+	NT	1000	Wuu & Grant (1966)
Hordeum vulgare, mutation	–	NT	200	Stroev (1968)
Zea mays, mutation	+	NT	200	Morgun *et al.* (1982)
Zea mays, mutation	+	NT	NR	Plewa (1985)
Nicotiana tabacum, mutation	–	NT	NR[d]	Briza (1989)
Tradescantia paludosa, micronucleus formation	–	NT	200	Ma *et al.* (1984)
Hordeum vulgare, chromosomal aberrations	+	NT	500 (spray)	Wuu & Grant (1967a)
Hordeum vulgare, chromosomal aberrations	–	NT	2000	Müller *et al.* (1972)

Test system	Results[a]		Dose[b] (LED or HID)	Reference
	Without exogenous metabolic system	With exogenous metabolic system		
Vicia faba, chromosomal aberrations	+	NT	400	Wuu & Grant (1967b)
Vicia faba, chromosomal aberrations	–	NT	200	Khudoley *et al.* (1987)
Sorghum sp., chromosomal aberrations	+	NT	NR[d]	Liang & Liang (1972)
Sorghum sp., chromosomal aberrations	–	NT	NR	Müller *et al.* (1972)
Sorghum sp., chromosomal aberrations	+	NT	NR	Lee *et al.* (1974)
Nigella damascena, chromosomal aberrations	–	NT	320	Mathias (1987)
Nigella damascena, chromosomal aberrations	+	NT	40[d]	Mathias (1987)
Zea mays, chromosomal aberrations	–	NT	200	Morgun *et al.* (1982)
Drosophila melanogaster, somatic mutation	+		1000 µg/g feed	Torres *et al.* (1992)
Drosophila melanogaster, somatic mutation	+		200 µg/g feed	Tripathy *et al.* (1993)
Drosophila melanogaster, sex-linked recessive lethal mutation	+		100 µg/g feed	Murnik & Nash (1977)
Drosophila melanogaster, sex-linked recessive lethal mutation	–		2000 µg/g feed	Adler (1980)
Drosophila melanogaster, sex-linked recessive lethal mutation	+		200 µg/g feed	Tripathy *et al.* (1993)
Drosophila melanogaster, dominant lethal mutation	+		100 µg/g feed	Murnik & Nash (1977)
Drosophila melanogaster, aneuploidy	+		100 µg/g feed	Murnik & Nash (1977)
Gene mutation, Chinese hamster lung V79 cells *in vitro*, *hprt* locus	–	–[e]	2000	Adler (1980)
Sister chromatid exchange, Chinese hamster ovary cells *in vitro*	–	–	2000	Adler (1980)
Chromosomal aberrations, Chinese hamster ovary cells *in vitro*	–	–	2000	Adler (1980)
Chromosomal aberrations, Chinese hamster ovary cells *in vitro*	–	NT	250	Ishidate (1988)
DNA damage, human lymphocytes *in vitro*	+	–	100	Ribas *et al.* (1995)
DNA repair exclusive of unscheduled DNA synthesis, human lymphocytes *in vitro*	–	NT	25	Surrallés *et al.* (1995)
Unscheduled DNA synthesis, human EUE cells *in vitro*	–	–[e]	650	Adler (1980)
Sister chromatid exchange, human lymphocytes *in vitro*	–	NT	NR	Ghiazza *et al.* (1984)
Sister chromatid exchange, human lymphocytes *in vitro*	–	–	10	Dunkelberg *et al.* (1994)

Table 5 (contd)

Test system	Results[a]		Dose[b] (LED or HID)	Reference
	Without exogenous metabolic system	With exogenous metabolic system		
Chromosomal aberrations, human lymphocytes *in vitro*	+	NT	0.1	Meisner *et al.* (1992)
Chromosomal aberrations, human lymphocytes *in vitro*	+	NT	1	Meisner *et al.* (1993)
Host-mediated assay, *Escherichia coli* Amp^R in mouse	+		100 po × 1	Adler (1980)
DNA strand breaks, rat stomach, liver and kidney *in vivo*	+		875 po × 1	Pino *et al.* (1988)
DNA strand breaks, rat stomach, liver and kidney *in vivo*	+		350 po × 15	Pino *et al.* (1988)
DNA strand breaks, rat lung *in vivo*	–		875 po × 1	Pino *et al.* (1988)
DNA strand breaks, rat lung *in vivo*	–		350 po × 15	Pino *et al.* (1988)
Rana catesbeiana tadpoles, DNA damage	+		4 μg/mL	Clements *et al.* (1997)
Micronucleus formation, NMRI female mouse bone-marrow cells *in vivo*	+		1400 po × 1	Gebel *et al.* (1997)
Micronucleus formation, NMRI male mouse bone-marrow cells *in vivo*	–		1750 po × 1	Gebel *et al.* (1997)
Chromosome aberrations, mouse bone-marrow cells *in vivo*	–		20 ppm drinking-water × 90 d	Meisner *et al.* (1992)
Dominant lethal effects, mouse spermatids	(+)		1500 po × 1	Adler (1980)
Sperm morphology, mouse	–		600 ip × 4	Osterloh *et al.* (1983)

[a] +, positive; (+), weakly positive; –, negative; NT, not tested

[b] LED, lowest effective dose; HID, highest ineffective dose; unless untherwise stated, in-vitro test, μg/mL; in-vivo test, mg/kg bw per day; NR, not reported; po, oral; d, days; ip, intraperitoneal

[c] Extracts of atrazine-treated *Zea mays*

[d] Commercial pesticide

[e] Positive with potato microsomes at doses up to 3 mmol/L

Dominant lethal effects were induced in *D. melanogaster*. Chromosomal aberrations were induced in the majority of plants studied and in human lymphocytes *in vitro,* but not in cultured rodent cells. Atrazine did not induce sister chromatid exchange or unscheduled DNA synthesis in cultured rodent or human cells. In a single study, it gave rise to DNA damage in human lymphocytes *in vitro*.

Atrazine induced ampicillin-resistant mutations in *Escherichia coli* in a mouse host-mediated assay. In mammals *in vivo*, atrazine induced DNA damage in tadpoles and DNA strand breakage in rat stomach, liver and kidney cells, but not in lung cells, after oral dosing. It weakly induced dominant lethal effects in mouse spermatids but did not induce morphological abnormalities in mouse sperm heads. It did not induce chromosomal aberrations in bone-marrow cells of mice treated *in vivo*, but induced micronuclei in the bone marrow of female mice, but not male mice, treated *in vivo* in one experiment.

4.5 Mechanistic considerations

Several reports on the mode of action of atrazine-induced mammary tumour development in the Sprague-Dawley rat have been published since the last IARC (1991) review (Eldridge *et al.*, 1994a,b; Stevens *et al.*, 1994; Wetzel *et al.*, 1994; Chapin *et al.*, 1996; Connor *et al.*, 1996, 1998; Eldridge *et al.*, 1998; Simpkins *et al.*, 1998; Thakur *et al.*, 1998). Atrazine at high doses in the diet is associated with an increased incidence and/or an earlier onset of mammary gland tumours in female Sprague-Dawley rats; however, it is not tumorigenic in Fischer 344 rats or in CD-1 mice of either sex.

Short- and longer-term studies performed with Sprague-Dawley and Fischer 344 rats have shown that the mammary tumours induced in Sprague-Dawley rats given high doses of atrazine in the diet are likely to be the result of an accelerating effect on normal, age-related perturbations of the oestrous cycle, with a resultant increase in exposure to endogenous oestrogen and prolactin (Eldridge *et al.*, 1994a; Wetzel *et al.*, 1994; Connor *et al.*, 1998; Eldridge *et al.*, 1998; Hauswirth & Wetzel, 1998; Simpkins *et al.*, 1998; O'Connor *et al.*, 1999). Increased exposure to endogenous oestrogen and prolactin most likely leads to the promotion of earlier development of mammary gland tumours (Cutts, 1964; Cutts & Noble, 1964; Manni *et al.*, 1977; Chapin *et al.*, 1996). The lack of effect of atrazine on the incidence of mammary tumours and other evidence of proliferative activity in ovariectomized Sprague-Dawley rats fed the highest dose tested (400 ppm) suggest a non-genotoxic mechanism of action associated with hormonal imbalance. The absence of mutagenicity further supports a non-genotoxic mechanism.

Reproductive senescence in untreated, ageing female Sprague-Dawley rats occurs before mid-life, at which time there is a gradual transition from normal four- to five-day oestrous cycles to extended periods of continuous oestrus (Huang *et al.*, 1978; Lu *et al.*, 1979; Simpkins *et al.*, 1998). The basis for this change appears to involve loss of the capacity of the hypothalamus to mediate the release of sufficient LH from the pituitary gland to induce ovulation (Meites *et al.*, 1977; Wise, 1982, 1984). The early appearance and high spontaneous incidence of mammary gland tumours in untreated, ageing female Sprague-Dawley rats have been attributed to this ageing process (Haseman *et al.,* 1984; McMartin *et al.*, 1992; Simpkins *et al.*, 1998; Stevens *et al.*, 1998). Several studies have demonstrated that administration of atrazine to female Sprague-Dawley rats results in an attenuated LH surge (Simpkins *et al.*, 1998), an increase in the number of days in oestrus (Eldridge *et al.*, 1994a; Wetzel *et al.*, 1994; Eldridge *et al.*, 1998) and histological changes characteristic of extended exposure to endogenous oestrogen (Eldridge *et al.*, 1994a, 1998). Therefore, the mechanism of action appears to involve disruption of the neuroendocrine pathways responsible for the LH surge (Eldridge *et al.*, 1998; Simpkins *et al.*, 1998). The results of studies of carcinogenicity and mode of action indicate that the dose at which this effect occurs in female Sprague-Dawley rats is 70–400 ppm in the diet, whereas dietary exposure of Fischer 344 rats to concentrations as high as 400 ppm has no effect on the incidence of mammary gland neoplasia.

While the details of the disruption of the neuroendocrine pathways that regulate ovulation in Sprague-Dawley rats have not been elucidated, the mechanism probaby does not involve a direct oestrogenic action of atrazine or binding of atrazine and/or its metabolites to the oestrogen receptor. Atrazine did not induce changes in oestrogen-responsive tissues (e.g. increased uterine weight, uterine peroxidase activity or binding to uterine progesterone receptors) in either ovariectomized Sprague-Dawley rats or intact Fischer 344 rats or mice (Tennant *et al.*, 1994b; Connor *et al.*, 1998), and atrazine and its metabolites had no effect on oestrogen receptor binding *in vitro* (Tennant *et al.*, 1994a; Connor *et al.*, 1996, 1998). In fact, atrazine may have weak antioestrogenic activity (Tennant *et al.*, 1994a,b).

The strain difference in the premature onset of mammary tumours (insensitive Fischer 344 rats and sensitive Sprague-Dawley rats) has been attributed to differences in the normal ageing of the reproductive tract in these strains (Eldridge *et al.*, 1994b; Stevens *et al.*, 1994; summarized by Chapin *et al.*, 1996; Eldridge *et al.*, 1998; Thakur *et al.*, 1998). Reproductive cycling begins to decline in female Sprague-Dawley rats of less than one year of age, presumably due to loss of sensitivity of the adrenergic neurons in the hypothalamus that control production of gonadotropin-releasing hormone. This loss of stimulation reduces the release of follicle-stimulating hormone and LH and ultimately delays ovulation. The delayed ovulation, in turn, allows prolonged exposure to oestrogens, with an effect seen as persistent vaginal cornification. In contrast, the adrenergic neurons of female Fischer 344 rats do not lose their sensitivity to oestrogen stimulation, and regular cycling is maintained for a much longer time (Lu *et al.*, 1979; Estes & Simpkins, 1984). Reproductive ageing in this strain of rat is believed to be due to inability to control daily prolactin surges, prolonged activity of the corpora lutea and greater progesterone release. Fischer 344 rats have been reported to have not only lower exposure to endogenous oestrogen and/or prolactin but also a lower spontaneous incidence of mammary gland tumours than Sprague-Dawley rats (van Zwieten *et al.*, 1994; Eldridge *et al.*, 1998). The endocrine milieu of ageing Sprague-Dawley rats thus favours the development of mammary tumours, resulting in the difference in the incidence of spontaneous tumours in ageing females of these two strains.

In women, reproductive senescence is characterized by ovarian depletion, declining oestrogen levels and, eventually, dioestrus (Chapin *et al.*, 1996; Simpkins *et al.,* 1998). While the pattern of reproductive senescence in female Fischer 344 rats is not identical to that of women, Fischer 344 rats share the following features with women, in contrast to female Sprague-Dawley rats: later onset of senescence, low oestrogen concentrations during late life and an ability to control LH secretion during reproductive senescence (Simpkins *et al.*, 1998). The difference in the pattern of reproductive senescence between women (reduced serum oestrogen) and female Sprague-Dawley rats (prolonged elevated serum oestrogen) suggests that the mechanism of action proposed for atrazine-associated mammary tumours in rats would not be operative in humans. The ageing female Sprague-Dawley rat is thus not an appropriate model for the assessment of mammary tumour development in women (Table 6; Chapin *et al.*, 1996).

5. Summary of Data Reported and Evaluation

5.1 Exposure data

Atrazine is a triazine herbicide widely used on a variety of crops, notably maize, sorghum and sugar-cane, for the pre- and post-emergent control of broad-leaved weeds. Occupational exposure may occur through both inhalation and dermal absorption during its manufacture, its formulation and its application by spraying. It is found widely, together with its dealkylated degradation products, in rivers, lakes, estuaries, ground-water and reservoirs. In drinking-water, the levels rarely exceed 1 μg/L. Surveys of various foods and feeds have generally indicated no detectable atrazine residue.

5.2 Human carcinogenicity data

A combined analysis of the results of two cohort studies of agricultural chemical production workers in the United States showed decreased mortality from cancers at all sites combined among the subset of workers who had had definite or probable exposure to triazine. Site-specific analyses in this subset of workers yielded no significant findings; a non-significant increase in the number of deaths from non-Hodgkin lymphoma was seen, but was based on very few observed cases.

A pooled analysis of the results of three population-based case–control studies of men in Kansas, eastern Nebraska and Iowa–Minnesota, United States, in which the risk for non-Hodgkin lymphoma in relation to exposure to atrazine and other herbicides on farms was evaluated, showed a significant association; however, the association was weaker when adjustment was made for reported use of phenoxyacetic acid herbicides or organophosphate insecticides. A sub-analysis of results for farmers in Nebraska, the State in which the most detailed information on atrazine use was available, showed no excess risk for non-Hodgkin lymphoma among farmers who had used atrazine for at least 15 years, after adjustment for use of other pesticides. In a case–control study of non-Hodgkin lymphoma among women in eastern Nebraska, a slight, nonsignificant increase

Table 6. Comparison of reproductive senescence in female rodent strains and women

Parameter	Sprague-Dawley rat	Fischer 344 rat	Women
Start of senescence (% of normal lifespan)	30–40	60–70	60–70
Principal cause of senescence	Hypothalamic failure to stimulate LH/FSH	Hypothalamic failure to control prolactin surges	Depletion of ovarian oocyte content
LH surge capability	Lost	Maintained	Maintained
Predominant cycle pattern	Persistent oestrus	Pseudopregnancy episodes	Menopause (dioestrus)
Oestrogen secretion	Elevated, prolonged	Reduced	Reduced
Oestrogen:progesterone ratio	Elevated	Reduced	Reduced
Prolactin secretion	Persistently elevated	Episodically elevated	Reduced
Spontaneous mammary tumour incidence (lifetime) (%)	30–40	2–5	8–10
Principal known factors that increase mammary tumour risk	Prolactin, oestrogen, chemical mutagens	Prolactin, oestrogen, chemical mutagens	Family history, parity, diet, body weight
Prolactin dependence	High	Median	None

From Chapin *et al.* (1996)
LH, luteinizing hormone; FSH, follicle-stimulating hormone

in risk was seen. In all these studies, farmers tended to have an increased risk for non-Hodgkin lymphoma, but the excess could not be attributed to atrazine.

Less information was available to evaluate the association between exposure to atrazine and other cancers of the lymphatic and haematopoietic tissues. One study of Hodgkin disease in Kansas, one study of leukaemia in Iowa–Minnesota and one study of multiple myeloma from Iowa gave no indication of excess risk among persons handling triazine herbicides.

In a population-based study in Italy, definite exposure to triazines was associated with a two- to threefold increase of borderline significance in the risk for ovarian cancer. The study was small, and potential confounding by exposure to other herbicides was not controlled for in the analysis.

5.3 Animal carcinogenicity data

Atrazine was tested for carcinogenicity in one study in mice by oral administration in the diet. No increase in tumour incidence was observed. It was also tested by oral administration in two studies in Fischer rats and in five studies in Sprague-Dawley rats, including a comparison of intact and ovariectomized females of the latter strain. In Fischer rats, no increase in tumour incidence was observed in one adequate study. The incidence of mammary tumours was increased in intact Sprague-Dawley females in four studies, but no increase was seen in ovariectomized Sprague-Dawley females. Atrazine was also tested by intraperitoneal injection in one study in mice; an increased incidence of lymphomas was reported.

5.4 Other relevant data

N-Dealkylation and conjugation with glutathione are the main metabolic pathways for atrazine in various species *in vivo*. There do not appear to be qualitative differences in the metabolism of atrazine between the strains and species studied that would explain the fact that mammary gland tumours develop in Sprague-Dawley rats but not in Fischer 344 rats or CD-1 mice.

Atrazine has been tested for developmental toxicity in rats and rabbits. No teratogenic effects have been observed. Fetal loss and reduced fetal body weights were seen in rabbits; the incidences of some minor skeletal variants were elevated in exposed fetal rats. No developmental effects were seen in a study of mice and rats exposed to groundwater contaminants that included atrazine.

The evidence from biological assays (e.g. uterine weight, stromal cell proliferation, epithelial cell height) and from in-vitro assays of oestrogen receptors indicates that atrazine does not have intrinsic oestrogenic activity.

Long-term administration of atrazine enhances the onset of reproductive senescence in female Sprague-Dawley (but not Fischer 344) rats, resulting in an earlier onset of persistent oestrus and tissue changes characteristic of long-term exposure to elevated oestrogen levels. Atrazine appears to disrupt neuroendocrine pathways in the hypothalamus by as yet undetermined mechanisms, resulting in attenuation of the luteinizing hormone surge that normally results in ovulation. These hormonal imbalances seen after atrazine administration were associated with an increased incidence and earlier onset of mammary tumours in some but not all studies of carcinogenicity in Sprague-Dawley rats, and not in Fischer 344 rats or CD-1 mice. Ovariectomized Sprague-Dawley rats exposed for two years to the highest dose of atrazine used in the bioassay in which ovariectomized and intact animals were compared did not develop either tumours or other proliferative lesions in the mammary gland.

In contrast to the hormonal changes in Sprague-Dawley rats, reproductive senescence in women is characterized by depletion of the ovarian oocyte content and reduced oestrogen secretion.

No data were available on the genetic and related effects of atrazine in humans. There is weak evidence for genotoxic effects in mammalian cells *in vivo* and *in vitro*. Atrazine was mutagenic in *Drosophila*, yeast and plant cells but was not mutagenic to bacteria. Overall, the results of genotoxicity testing would not appear to bear directly on the strain-specific tumour induction in female Sprague-Dawley rats.

5.5 Evaluation

There is *inadequate evidence* in humans for the carcinogenicity of atrazine.

There is *sufficient evidence* in experimental animals for the carcinogenicity of atrazine.

Overall evaluation

In making its overall evaluation, the Working Group concluded that the mammary tumours associated with exposure to atrazine involve a non-DNA-reactive, hormonally mediated mechanism. In reaching the conclusion, the following evidence was considered:

(a) Atrazine produces mammary tumours (fibroadenomas, adenocarcinomas) only in intact female Sprague-Dawley rats (not in Fischer 344 rats, CD-1 mice or ovariectomized Sprague-Dawley rats) and does not increase the incidences of other tumour types.

(b) Atrazine affects neuroendocrine pathways of the hypothalamus to accelerate the onset of reproductive senescence in female Sprague-Dawley but not Fischer 344 rats.

(c) Atrazine does not have intrinsic oestrogenic activity.

(d) There are critical interspecies differences in the hormonal changes associated with reproductive senescence.

Therefore, there is strong evidence that the mechanism by which atrazine increases the incidence of mammary gland tumours in Sprague-Dawley rats is not relevant to humans.

Atrazine is *not classifiable as to its carcinogenicity to humans (Group 3).*

6. References

Adams, C.D. & Thurman, E.M. (1991) Formation and transport of deethylatrazine in the soil and vadose zone. *J. environ. Qual.*, **20**, 540–547

Adams, N.H., Levi, P.E. & Hodgson, E. (1990) In vitro studies of the metabolism of atrazine, simazine and terbutryn in several vertebrate species. *J. agric. Food Chem.*, **38**, 1411–1417

Adler, I.-D. (1980) A review of the coordinated research effort on the comparison of test systems for the detection of mutagenic effects, sponsored by the EEC. *Mutat. Res.*, **74**, 77–93

Ahrens, W.H., ed. (1994) *Herbicide Handbook*, 7th Ed., Champaign, IL, Weed Science Society of America, pp. 20–23

American Conference of Governmental Industrial Hygienists (ACGIH) (1997) *1997 TLVs® and BEIs®*, Cincinnati, OH, p. 16

American Conference of Governmental Industrial Hygienists (ACGIH) (1998) *TLVs and other Occupational Exposure Values—1998 CD-ROM*, Cincinnati, OH

Andersen, K.J., Leighty, E.G. & Takahashi, M.T. (1972) Evaluation of herbicides for possible mutagenic properties. *J. agric. Food Chem.*, **20**, 649–656

Aspelin, A.L. (1997) *Pesticides Industry Sales and Usage—1994 and 1995 Market Estimates* (EPA Report No. EPA-733/R-97-002), Washington DC, Office of Pesticide Programs

Babic-Gojmerac, T., Kniewald, Z. & Kniewald, J. (1989) Testosterone metabolism in neuro-endocrine organs in male rats under atrazine and deethylatrazine influence. *J. Steroid Biochem.*, **33**, 141–146

Bagnati, R., Benfenati, E., Davoli, E. & Fanelli, R. (1988) Screening of 21 pesticides in water by single extraction with C18 silica bonded phase columns and HRGC-MS. *Chemosphere*, **17**, 59–65

Bakke, J.E., Larson, J.D. & Price, C.E. (1972) Metabolism of atrazine and 2-hydroxyatrazine by the rat. *J. agric. Food Chem.*, **20**, 602–607

Ballantine, L.G. & Simoneaux, B.J. (1991) Pesticide metabolites in food. In: Tweedy, B.G., Dishburger, H.J., Ballantine, L.G., McCarthy, J. & Murphy, J., eds, *Pesticide Residues and Food Safety* (ACS Symposium Series No. 446), Washington DC, American Chemical Society, pp. 96–104

Barceló, D., Chiron, S., Fernandez-Alba, A., Valverde, A. & Alpendurada, M.F. (1996) Monitoring pesticides and metabolites in surface water and groundwater in Spain. In: Meyer, M.T. & Thurman, E.M., eds, *Herbicide Metabolites in Surface Water and Groundwater* (ACS Symposium Series No. 630), Washington DC, American Chemical Society, pp. 237–253

Bartsch, H., Malaveille, C., Camus, A.-M., Martel-Planche, G., Brun, G., Hautefeuille, A., Sabadie, N., Barbin, A., Kuroki, T., Drevon, C., Piccoli, C. & Montesano, R. (1980) Validation and comparative studies on 180 chemicals with *S. typhiumurium* strains and V79 Chinese hamster cells in the presence of various metabolizing systems. *Mutat. Res.*, **76**, 1–50

Ben-Dyke, R., Sanderson, D.M. & Noakes, D.N. (1970) Acute toxicity data for pesticides (1970). *World Rev. Pest Control*, **9**, 119–127

Benigni, R., Bignami, M., Camoni, I., Carere, A., Conti, G., Iachetta, R., Morpurgo, G. & Ortali, V.A. (1979) A new in vitro method for testing plant metabolism in mutagenicity studies. *J. Toxicol. environ. Health*, **5**, 809–819

de Bertoldi, M., Griselli, M., Giovannetti, M. & Barale, R. (1980) Mutagenicity of pesticides evaluted by means of gene conversion in *Saccharomyces cerevisiae* and in *Aspergillus nidulans*. *Environ. Mutag.*, **2**, 359–370

Bester, K. & Hühnerfuss, H. (1993) Triazines in the Baltic and North Sea. *Mar. Pollut. Bull.*, **26**, 423–427

Bintein, S. & Devillers, J. (1996) Evaluating the environmental fate of atrazine in France. *Chemosphere*, **32**, 2441–2456

Böhme, C. & Bär, F. (1967) [The metabolism of triazine herbicides in the animal organism.] *Food Cosmet. Toxicol.*, **5**, 23–28 (in German)

Breckenridge, C. (1996) *Summary of Additional Comments on the Response to the Special Review Position Document for Pesticide Products Containing Atrazine and Simazine*, Suppl. II, Greensboro, NC, Ciba-Geigy Corp.

Briza, J. (1989) Estimation of mutagenicity and metabolic activation after recurrent exposures of *Nicotiana tabacum* L. var. zanthi to 14 pesticides. *Biol. plant.*, **31**, 145–151

Brown, L.M., Blair, A., Gibson, R., Everett, G., Cantor, K.P., Schuman, L.M., Burmeister, L.F., Van Lier, S.F. & Dick, F. (1990) Pesticide exposures and other agricultural risk factors for leukaemia among men in Iowa and Minnesota. *Cancer Res.*, **50**, 6585–6591

Brown, L.M., Burmeister, L.F., Everett, G.D. & Blair, A. (1993) Pesticide exposure and multiple myeloma in Iowa men. *Cancer Causes Control*, **4**, 153–153

Budavari, S., ed. (1996) *The Merck Index*, 12th Ed., Whitehouse Station, NJ, Merck & Co., pp. 147–148

Buser, H.-R. (1990) Atrazine and other *s*-triazine herbicides in lakes and rain in Switzerland. *Environ. Sci. Technol.*, **24**, 1049–1058

Butler, M.A. & Hoagland, R.E. (1989) Genotoxicity assessment of atrazine and some major metabolites in the Ames test. *Bull. environ. Contam. Toxicol.*, **43**, 797–804

Cantor, K.P., Blair, A., Everett, G., Gibson, R., Burmeister, L.F., Brown, L.M., Schuman, L. & Dick, F.R. (1992) Pesticides and other agricultural risk factors for non-Hodgkin's lymphoma among men in Iowa and Minnesota. *Cancer Res.*, **52**, 2447–2455

Catenacci, G., Maroni, M., Cottica, D. & Pozzoli, L. (1990) Assessment of human exposure to atrazine through the determination of free atrazine in urine. *Bull. environ. Contam. Toxicol.*, **44**, 1–7

Catenacci, G., Barbieri, F., Bersani, M., Ferioli, A., Cottica, D. & Maroni, M. (1993) Biological monitoring of human exposure to atrazine. *Toxicol. Lett.*, **69**, 217–222

Catenacci, G., Tringali, S. & Imbriani, M. (1995) [Retrospective study of morbidity in a group occupationally exposed to chlorotriazine herbicides: Preliminary results.] *G. Ital. Med. Lav.*, **17**, 23–26 (in Italian)

Chapin, R.E., Stevens, J.T., Hughes, C.L., Kelce, W.R., Hess, R.A. & Daston, G.P. (1996) Symposium overview: Endocrine modulation of reproduction. *Fundam. appl. Toxicol.*, **29**, 1–17

Chemical Information Services (1995) *Directory of World Chemical Producers 1995/96 Standard Edition*, Dallas, TX, p. 72

Cheung, M.W. (1990) *Analysis of Human Urine to Determine Residues of Atrazine, G-28273, G-28279, and G-30033 Resulting from Oral Ingestion of Atrazine Including Storage Stability Results*, Greensboro, NC, Ciba-Geigy Corp.

Chevreuil, M. & Garmouma, M. (1993) Occurrence of triazines in the atmospheric fallout on the catchment basin of the River Marne (France). *Chemosphere*, **27**, 1605–1608

Chevreuil, M., Garmouma, M., Teil, M.J. & Chesterikoff, A. (1996) Occurrence of organochlorines (PCBs, pesticides) and herbicides (triazines, phenylureas) in the atmosphere and in the fallout from urban and rural stations in the Paris area. *Sci. total Environ.*, **182**, 25–37

Ciba-Geigy AG (1996) *Atrazine and Simazine: A Review of the Issues* [http://www.access.ch/atrazine]

Clarkson, J.R., Hines, N.A., Tierney, T.P., Christensen, B.R. & Mattan, C.M. (1998) *Human Exposure to Atrazine and Simazine via Ground and Surface Drinking Water: Update-IV* (Supplement to EPA MRID No. 44315414), Greensboro, NC, Novartis Crop Protection, pp. 15–21

Clements, C., Ralph, S. & Petras, M. (1997) Genotoxicity of select herbicides in *Rana catesbeiana* tadpoles using the alkaline single-cell gel DNA electrophoresis (comet) assay. *Environ. mol. Mutag.*, **29**, 277–288

Connor, K., Howell, J., Chen, I., Liu, H., Berhane, K., Sciarretta, C., Safe, S. & Zacharewski, T. (1996) Failure of chloro-*s*-triazine-derived compounds to induce estrogen receptor-mediated responses *in vivo* and *in vitro*. *Fundam. appl. Toxicol.*, **30**, 93–101

Connor, K., Howell, J., Safe, S., Chen, I., Liu, H., Berhane, K., Sciarretta, C. & Zacharewski, T. (1998) Failure of chloro-*s*-triazine-derived compounds to induce estrogenic responses *in vivo* and *in vitro*. In: Ballantine, L.G., McFarland, J.E. & Hackett, D.S., eds, *Triazine Herbicides: Risk Assessment* (ACS Symposium Series No. 683), Washington DC, American Chemical Society, pp. 424–431

Cook, W.A., ed. (1987) *Occupational Exposure Limits—Worldwide*, Washington DC, American Industrial Hygiene Association, pp. 18, 128, 162–163

Cooper, R.L., Stoker, T.E., Goldman, J.M,. Parrish, M.B. & Tyrey, L. (1996) Effect of atrazine on ovarian function in the rat. *Reprod. Toxicol.*, **10**, 257–264

Council of the European Communities (1980) Council Directive of 15 July 1980 relating to the quality of water intended for human consumption. *Off. J. Eur. Comm.*, **L229**, 11–29

Cutts, J.H. (1964) Estrone-induced mammary tumors in the rat. II. Effect of alterations in the hormonal environment on tumor induction, behavior, and growth. *Cancer Res.*, **24**, 1124–1130

Cutts, J.H. & Noble, R.L. (1964) Estrone-induced mammary tumors in the rat. I. Induction and behavior of tumors. *Cancer Res.*, **24**, 1116–1123

Dauterman, W.C. & Muecke, W. (1974) *In vitro* metabolism of atrazine by rat liver. *Pestic. Biochem. Physiol.*, **4**, 212–219

Deutsches Forschungsgemeinschaft (1998) *List of MAK and BAT Values 1998* (Report No. 34), Weinheim, Wiley-VCH, p. 26

Donna, A., Betta, P.G., Robutti, F., Crosignani, P., Berrino, F. & Bellingeri, D. (1984) Ovarian mesothelial tumors and herbicides: A case–control study. *Carcinogenesis*, **5**, 941–942

Donna, A., Betta, P.G., Robutti, F. & Bellingeri, D. (1986) Carcinogenicity testing of atrazine: Preliminary report on a 13-month study on male Swiss albino mice treated by intraperitoneal administration. *Med. Lav.*, **8**, 119–121

Donna, A., Crosignani, P., Robutti, F., Betta, P.G., Bocca, R. Mariani, N., Ferrario, F., Fissi, R. & Berrino, F. (1989) Triazine herbicides and ovarian epithelial neoplasms. *Scand. J. Work Environ. Health*, **15**, 47–53

Dunkelberg, H., Fuchs, J., Hengstler, J.G., Klein, E., Oesch, F. & Strüder, K. (1994) Genotoxic effects of the herbicides alachlor, atrazine, pendimethaline, and simazine in mammalian cells. *Bull. environ. contam. Toxicol.*, **52**, 498–504

Eldridge, J.C., Fleenor-Heyser, D.G., Extrom, P.C., Wetzel, L.T., Breckenridge, C.B., Gillis, J.H., Luempert, L.G., III & Stevens, J.T. (1994a) Short-term effects of chlorotriazines on estrus in female Sprague-Dawley and Fischer 344 rats. *J. Toxicol. environ. Health*, **43**, 155–167

Eldridge, J.C., Tennant, M.K., Wetzel, L.T., Breckenridge, C.B. & Stevens, J.T. (1994b) Factors affecting mammary tumor incidence in chlorotriazine-treated female rats: Hormonal properties, dosage, and animal strain. *Environ. Health Perspectives*, **102** (Suppl. 11), 29–36

Eldridge, J.C., McConnell, R.F., Wetzel, L.T. & Tisdel, M.O. (1998) Appearance of mammary tumors in atrazine-treated female rats: Probable mode of action involving strain-related control of ovulation and estrous cycling. In: Ballantine, L.G., McFarland, J.E. & Hackett, D.S., eds, *Triazine Herbicides: Risk Assessment* (ACS Symposium Series No. 683), Washington DC, American Chemical Society, pp. 414–423

Elkins, E.R., Lyon, R.S. & Jarman, R. (1998) Pesticides residues in processed foods: Not a food safety concern. In: Ballantine, L.G., McFarland, J.E. & Hackett, D.S., eds, *Triazine Herbicides: Risk Assessment* (ACS Symposium Series No. 683), Washington DC, American Chemical Society, pp. 116–122

Emnova, E.E., Merenyuk, G.V. & Curkan, L.G. (1987) Genetic activity of sim-triazine herbicides on *Saccharomyces cerevisiae. Tsitol. Genet.*, **21**, 127–131

Environmental Protection Agency (1992) *Another Look. National Survey of Pesticides in Drinking Water Wells. Phase II Report* (EPA 579/09-91-020; NTIS PB 91-125765), Washington DC, Office of Water Quality & Office of Pesticides and Toxic Substances

Environmental Protection Agency (1994) Method 8141A. Organophosphorus compounds by gas chromatography: Capillary column technique [Rev. 1]. In: *Test Methods for Evaluating Solid Waste—Physical/Chemical Methods* (US EPA No. SW-846), Washington DC, Office of Solid Waste

Environmental Protection Agency (1995a) Method 508.1. Determination of chlorinated pesticides, herbicides, and organohalides by liquid–solid extraction and electron capture gas chromatography [Rev. 2.0]. In: *Methods for the Determination of Organic Compounds in Drinking Water* (EPA Report No. EPA-600/4-88/039), Cincinnati, OH, Environmental Monitoring Systems Laboratory

Environmental Protection Agency (1995b) Method 525.2. Determination of organic compounds in drinking water by liquid–solid extraction and capillary column gas chromatography/mass spectrometry [Rev. 2.0]. In: *Methods for the Determination of Organic Compounds in Drinking Water* (EPA Report No. EPA-600/4-88/039), Cincinnati, OH, Environmental Monitoring Systems Laboratory

Environmental Protection Agency (1995c) Method 551.1. Determination of chlorination disinfection byproducts, chlorinated solvents, and halogenated pesticides/herbicides in drinking water by liquid–liquid extraction and gas chromatography with electron-capture detection [Rev. 1.0]. In: *Methods for the Determination of Organic Compounds in Drinking Water* (EPA Report No. EPA-600/4-90/020), Cincinnati, OH, Environmental Monitoring Systems Laboratory

Environmental Protection Agency (1995d) Method 507. Determination of nitrogen- and phosphorus-containing pesticides in water by gas chromatography with a nitrogen-phosphorus detector [Rev. 2.1]. In: *Methods for the Determination of Organic Compounds in Drinking Water, Supplement III* (EPA Report No. EPA-600/R-95/131; US NTIS PB95-261616), Cincinnati, OH, Environmental Monitoring Systems Laboratory

Environmental Protection Agency (1995e) Method 505. Analysis of organohalide pesticides and commercial polychlorinated biphenyl (PCB) products in water by microextraction and gas chromatography [Rev. 2.1]. In: *Methods for the Determination of Organic Compounds in Drinking Water* (EPA Report No. EPA-600/4-88/039), Cincinnati, OH, Environmental Monitoring Systems Laboratory

Environmental Protection Agency (1998) *Drinking Water and Health, National Primary Drinking Water Regulations, Technical Factsheet on Atrazine*, Washington DC, Office of Ground Water and Drinking Water [http://www.epa.gov/OGWDW/dwh/t-soc/atrazine.html]

Environmental Protection Agency (1999) *California Environmental Protection Agency—Department of Pesticide Regulation: USEPA/OPP Pesticide Product Database Query* [http://www.cdpr.ca.gov/docs/epa/m2.htm]

Estes, K.S. & Simpkins, J.W. (1984) Age-related alterations in dopamine and norepinephrine activity within microdissected brain regions of ovariectomized Long Evans rats. *Brain Res.*, **298**, 209–218

Food & Drug Administration (1989) Atrazine. In: *Pesticide Analytical Manual*, Vol. II, *Methods Which Detect Multiple Residues*, Washington DC, United States Department of Health and Human Services, pp. 1–7

Food & Drug Administration (1993) FDA monitoring program. *J. Assoc. off. anal. Chem. int.*, **76**, 127A–148A

Frank, R., Clegg, B.S., Sherman, C. & Chapman, N.D. (1990) Triazine and chloroacetamide herbicides in Sydenham River water and municipal drinking water, Dresden, Ontario, Canada, 1981–1987. *Arch. environ. Contam. Toxicol.*, **19**, 319–324

Gaines, T.B. & Linder, R.E. (1986) Acute toxicity of pesticides in adult and weanling rats. *Fundam. appl. Toxicol.*, **7**, 299–308

Gebel, T., Kevekordes, S., Pav, K., Edenharder, R. & Dunkelberg, H. (1997) In vivo genotoxicity of selected herbicides in the mouse bone-marrow micronucleus test. *Arch. Toxicol.*, **71**, 193–197

Ghiazza, G., Zavarise, G., Lanero, M. & Ferraro, G. (1984) SCE (sister chromatid exchanges) induced in chromosomes of human lymphocytes by trifluralin, atrazine and simazine. *Bull. Soc. ital. Biol. sper.*, **60**, 2149–2153

Goolsby, D.A. & Battaglin, W.A. (1993) Occurrence, distribution and transport of agricultural chemicals in surface waters of the midwestern United States. In: Goolsby, D.A., Boyer, L.L. & Mallard, G.E., eds, *Selected Papers on Agricultural Chemicals in Water Resources of the Midcontinental United States* (Open File Report 93-418), Denver, CO, United States Geological Survey, pp. 1–25

Goolsby, D.A., Coupe, R.L. & Markovchick, D.J. (1991) *Distribution of Selected Herbicides and Nitrate in the Mississippi River and its Major Tributaries: April through June, 1991* (United States Geological Survey, Water Resources Investigation Report No. 91-4163), Denver, CO, United States Geological Survey

Goolsby, D.A., Battaglin, W.A., Fallon, J.D., Aga, D.S. Kolpin, D.W. & Thurman, E.M. (1993) Persistence of herbicides in selected reservoirs in the midwestern United States: Some preliminary results. In: Goolsby, D.A., Boyer, L.L. & Mallard, G.E., eds, *Selected Papers on Agricultural Chemicals in Water Resources of the Midcontinental United States* (Open File Report 93-418), Denver, CO, United States Geological Survey, pp. 51–63

Griffini, O., Bao, M.L., Barbieri, C., Burrini, D. & Pantani, F. (1997) Occurrence of pesticides in the Arno River and in potable water—A survey of the period 1992–1995. *Bull. environ. Contam. Toxicol.*, **59**, 202–209

Griffiths, A.J.F. (1979) *Neurospora* prototroph selection system for studying aneuploid production. *Environ. Health Perspectives*, **31**, 75–80

Hansch, C., Leo, A. & Hoekman, D. (1995) *Exploring QSAR: Hydrophobic, Electronic, and Steric Constants*, Washington DC, American Chemical Society, p. 48

Haseman, J.K., Huff, J. & Boorman, G.A. (1984) Use of historical control data in carcinogenicity studies in rodents. *Toxicol. Pathol.*, **12**, 126–135

Hauswirth, J.W. & Wetzel, L.T. (1998) Toxicity characteristics of the 2-chlorotriazines atrazine and simazine. In: Ballantine, L.G., McFarland, J.E. & Hackett, D.S., eds, *Triazine Herbicides: Risk Assessment* (ACS Symposium Series No. 683), Washington DC, American Chemical Society, pp. 370–383

Health Canada (1998) *Maximum Residue Limits*, Pest Management Regulatory Agency [http://www.hc-sc.gc.ca/pmra-arla/qinter3-e.html]

Heindel, J.J., Chapin, R.E., Gulati, D.K., George, J.D., Price, C.J., Marr, M.C., Myers, C.B., Barnes, L.H., Fail, P.A., Grizzle, T.B., Schwetz, B.A. & Yang, R.S.H. (1994) Assessment of the reproductive and developmental toxicity of pesticide/fertilizer mixtures based on confirmed pesticide contamination in California and Iowa groundwater. *Fundam. appl. Toxicol.*, **22**, 605–621

Hoar, S.K., Blair, A., Holmes, F.F., Boysen, C. & Robel, R.J. (1985) Herbicides and colon cancer (Letter). *Lancet*, **i**, 1277–1278

Hoar, S.K., Blair, A., Holmes, F.F., Boysen, C.D., Robel, R.J., Hoover, R. & Fraumeni, J.F. (1986) Agricultural herbicide use and risk of lymphoma and soft-tissue sarcoma. *J. Am. med. Assoc.*, **256**, 1141–1147

Hoffman, D.J. & Albers, P.H. (1984) Evaluation of potential embryotoxicity and teratogenicity of 42 herbicides, insecticides and petroleum contaminants to mallard eggs. *Arch. environ. Contam. Toxicol.*, **13**, 15–27

Huang, H.H., Steger, R.W., Bruni, J.F. & Meites, J. (1978) Patterns of sex steroid and gonadotropin secretion in aging female rats. *Endocrinology*, **103**, 1855–1859

Huber, W. (1993) Ecotoxicological relevance of atrazine in aquatic systems. *Environ. Toxicol. Chem.*, **12**, 1865–1881

Hui, X., Wester, R., Mailbach, H.I., Gilman, S.D., Gee, S.J., Hammock, B.D., Simoneaux, B., Breckenridge, C. & Kahrs, R. (1996) *In Vivo Percutaneous Absorption of Atrazine in Man*, Greensboro, NC, Ciba-Geigy Corp.

IARC (1991) *IARC Monographs on the Evaluation of Carcinogenic Risks to Humans*, Vol. 53, *Occupational Exposures in Insecticide Application, and Some Pesticides*, Lyon, pp. 441–466

Ikonen, R., Kangas, J. & Savolainen, H. (1988) Urinary atrazine metabolites as indicators for rat and human exposure to atrazine. *Toxicol. Lett.*, **44**, 109–112

Infurna, R., Levy, B., Meng, C., Yau, E., Traina, V., Rolofson, G., Stevens, J. & Barnett, J. (1988) Teratological evaluations of atrazine technical, a triazine herbicide, in rats and rabbits. *J. Toxicol. environ. Health*, **24**, 307–319

Innes, J.R.M., Ulland, B.M., Valerio, M.G., Petrucelli, L., Fishbein, L., Hart, E.R., Pallota, A.J., Bates, R.R., Falk, H.L., Gart, J.J., Klein, M., Mitchell, I. & Peters, J. (1969) Bioassay of pesticides and industrial chemicals for tumorigenicity in mice: A preliminary note. *J. natl Cancer Inst.*, **42**, 1101–1114

Ishidate, M., Jr (1988) *Data Book of Chromosmal Aberration Test In Vitro*, rev. Ed., New York, Elsevier

Izmerov, N.F., ed. (1982) *International Register of Potentially Toxic Chemicals, Scientific Reviews of Society Literature on Toxicity of Chemicals: Atrazine* (Issue 18), Moscow, Centre of International Projects, United Nations Environment Programme

Kappas, A. (1988) On the mutagenic and recombinogenic activity of certain herbicides in *Salmonella typhimurium* and *Aspergillus nidulans*. *Mutat. Res.*, **204**, 615–621

Khudoley, V.V., Mizgireuv, I. & Pliss, G.B. (1987) The study of mutagenic activity of carcinogens and other chemical agents with *Salmonella typhimurium* assays: Testing of 126 compounds. *Arch. Geschwulstforsch.*, **57**, 453–462

Kniewald, J., Mildner, P. & Kniewald, Z. (1979) Effects of *s*-triazine herbicides on hormone-receptor complex formation, 5α-reductase and 3α-hydroxysteroid dehydrogenase activity at the anterior pituitary level. *J. Steroid Biochem.*, **11**, 833–838

Kniewald, J., Peruzovic, M., Gojmerac, T., Milkovic, K. & Kniewald, Z. (1987) Indirect influence of s-triazines on rat gonadotropic mechanism at early postnatal period. *J. Steroid Biochem.*, **27**, 1095–1100

Kolpin, D.W., Thurman, E.M. & Goolsby, D.A. (1996) Occurrence of selected pesticides and their metabolites in near-surface aquifers of the midwestern United States. *Environ. Sci. Technol.*, **30**, 335–340

Kolpin, D.W., Kalkhoff, S.J., Goolsby, D.A., Sneck-Fahrer, D.A. & Thurman, E.M. (1997a) Occurrence of selected herbicides and herbicide degradation products in Iowa's ground water, 1995. *Ground Water*, **35**, 679–688

Kolpin, D.W., Squillace, P.J., Zogorski, J.S. & Barbash, J.E. (1997b) Pesticides and volatile organic compounds in shallow urban groundwater of the United States. In: Chilton, J., ed., *Ground Water in the Urban Environment: Problems, Processes and Management*, Rotterdam, A.A. Balkema, pp. 469–474

Kreuger, J. (1998) Pesticides in stream water within an agricultural catchment in southern Sweden. *J. total Environ.*, **216**, 227–251

Kruger, E.L., Zhu, B. & Coates, J.R. (1996) Relative mobilities of atrazine, five atrazine degradates, metolachlor, and simazine in soils of Iowa. *Environ. Sci. Technol.*, **15**, 691–694

Lang, D., Criegee, D., Grothusen, A., Saalfrank, R.W. & Böcker, R.H. (1996) *In vitro* metabolism of atrazine, terbuthylazine, ametryne, and terbutryne in rats, pigs, and humans. *Drug Metab. Disposition*, **24**, 859–865

Lang, D., Rettie, A.E. & Böcker, R.H. (1997) Identification of enzymes involved in the metabolism of atrazine, terbuthylazine, ametryne, and terbutryne in human liver microsomes. *Chem. Res. Toxicol.*, **10**, 1037–1044

Lee, K.C., Rao, G.M., Barnett, F.L. & Liang, G.H. (1974) Further evidence of meiotic instability induced by atrazine in grain sorghum. *Cytologia*, **39**, 697–702

Liang, G.H. & Liang, Y.T.S. (1972) Effects of atrazine on chromosomal behavior in sorghum. *Can. J. Genet. Cytol.*, **14**, 423–427

Lide, D.R., ed. (1997) *CRC Handbook of Chemistry and Physics*, 78th Ed., Boca Raton, FL, CRC Press, p. 3-15

Lu, K.H., Hopper, B.R., Vargo, T.M. & Yen, S.S.C. (1979) Chronological changes in sex steroid, gonadotropin and prolactin secretion in aging female rats displaying different reproductive states. *Biol. Reprod.*, **21**, 193–203

Lucas, A.D., Jones, A.D., Goodrow, M.H., Saiz, S.G., Blewett, C., Seiber, J.N. & Hammock, B.D. (1993) Determination of atrazine metabolites in human urine: Development of a biomarker of exposure. *Chem. Res. Toxicol.*, **6**, 107–116

Lunchick, C. & Selman, F. (1998) The assessment of worker exposure to atrazine and simazine: A tiered approach. In: Ballantine, L.G., McFarland, J.F. & Hackett, D.S., eds, *Triazine Herbicides: Risk Assessment* (ACS Symposium Series No. 683), Washington DC, American Chemical Society, pp. 141–155

Lundbergh, I., Kreuger, J. & Johnson, A. (1995) *Pesticides in Surface Waters*, Strasbourg, Council of Europe Press, pp. 5–55

Lusby, A.F., Simmons, Z. & McGuire, P.M. (1979) Variation in mutagenicity of s-triazine compounds tested on four Salmonella strains. *Environ. Mutag.*, **1**, 287–290

Ma, T., Harris, M.M., Anderson, V.A., Ahmed, I., Mohammad, K., Bare, J.L. & Lin, G. (1984) Tradescantia-micronucleus (Trad-MCN) tests on 140 health-related agents. *Mutat. Res.*, **138**, 157–167

Manni, A., Trujillo, J.E. & Pearson, O.H. (1977) Predominant role of prolactin in stimulating the growth of 7,12-dimethylbenz(a)anthracene-induced rat mammary tumor. *Cancer Res.*, **37**, 1216–1219

Mathias, M. (1987) Comparison of the genotoxic activity of two preparations of atrazine in the yeast *Schizosaccharomyces pombe* and the plant *Nigella damascena. Bull. Soc. R. Sci. Liège*, **56**, 425–432

McMartin, D.N., Sahota , P.S., Gunson, D.E., Han Hsu, H. & Spaet, R.H. (1992) Neoplasms and related proliferative lesions in control Sprague-Dawley rats from carcinogenicity studies. Historical data and diagnostic considerations. *Toxicol. Pathol.*, **20**, 212–225

Means, J.C., Plewa, M.J. & Gentile, J.M. (1988) Assessment of the mutagenicity of fractions from *s*-triazine-treated *Zea mays. Mutat. Res.*, **197**, 325–336

Meisner, L.F., Belluck, D.A. & Roloff, B.D. (1992) Cytogenetic effects of alachlor and/or atrazine *in vivo* and *in vitro*. *Environ. mol. Mutag.*, **19**, 77–82

Meisner, L.F., Roloff, B.D. & Belluck, D.A. (1993) In vitro effects of N-nitrosoatrazine on chromosome breakage. *Arch. environ. Contam. Toxicol.*, **24**, 108–112

Meites, J., Huang, H.H. & Simpkins, J.W. (1977) Recent studies on neuroendocrine control of reproductive senescence in the rats. In: Schneider, E.L., ed., *The Aging Reproduction System*, New York, Raven Press, pp. 213–235

Mersch-Sundermann, V., Dickgiesser, N., Hablizel, Y. & Gruber, B. (1988) Examination of mutagenicity of organic microcontaminations on the environment. I. Communication: The mutagenicity of selected herbicides and insecticides with the Salmonella-microsome-test (Ames test) in consideration of the pathogenetic potence of contaminated ground- and drinking-water. *Zbl. Bakt. Hyg., I. Abt. Orig. B*, **186**, 247–260

Miles, C.J. & Pfeuffer, R.J. (1997) Pesticides in canals of south Florida. *Arch. environ. Contam. Toxicol.*, **32**, 337–345

Morgan, M.K., Scheuerman, P.R. & Bishop, C.S. (1996) Teratogenic potential of atrazine and 2,4-D using FETAX. *J. Toxicol. environ. Health*, **48**, 151–168

Morgun, V.V., Logvinenko, V.F., Merezhinskii, T.G. & Lapina, T.V. (1982) Cytogenetic and genetic activity of the herbicides atrazine, simazin, prometrin, and linuron. *Cytol. Genet. (USSR)*, **16**, 42–45

Morichetti, E., Della Croce, C., Rosellini, D., Bronzetti, G. & Soldani G. (1992) Genetic and biochemical studies on a commercial preparation of atrazine. *Toxicol. environ. Chem.*, **37**, 35–41

Müller, A., Ebert, E. & Gast, A. (1972) Cytogenetic studies with atrazine (2-chloro-4-ethylamino-6-isopropylamino-*s*-triazine) on plants. *Experientia*, **28**, 704–705

Murnik, M.R. & Nash, C.L. (1977) Mutagenicity of the triazine herbicides atrazine, cyanazine, and simazine in *Drosophila melanogaster*. *J. Toxicol. environ. Health*, **3**, 691–697

National Institute for Occupational Safety and Health (1992) *Occupational Safety and Health Guideline for Atrazine*, Cincinnati, OH, pp. 1–6

National Institute for Occupational Safety and Health (1998) *National Occupational Exposure Survey (1981–1983)*, Cincinnati, OH

National Registration Authority for Agricultural and Veterinary Chemicals (NRA) (1997) *Review Summary on the NRA Review of Atrazine*, Canberrra

National Toxicology Program (1991) *NTP Chemical Repository Data Sheet: Atrazine*, Research Triangle Park, NC

Novartis (1999) *Crop Protection Products* [http://www.cp.novartis.com/d_frame.htm]

Occupational Safety and Health Administration (1999) *OSHA Chemical Sampling Information* [http://www.osha-slc.gov:80/OCIS/toc_chemsamp.html]

O'Connor, J.C., Plowchalk, D.R., Van Pelt, C.S., Davis, L.G. & Cook, J.C. (1999) Role of prolactin (PRL) in triazine-mediated rat mammary tumors. *Toxicol. Sci.* (in press)

Oregon State University (1996) *EXTOXNET (Extension Toxicology Network/Pesticide Information Profiles): Atrazine* [http://ace.ace.orst.edu/info/extoxnet/pips/atrazine.htm]

Osterloh, J., Letz, G., Pond, S. & Becker, C. (1983) An assessment of the potential testicular toxicity of 10 pesticides using the mouse-sperm morphology assay. *Mutat. Res.*, **116**, 407–415

Pereira, W. & Rostad, C.E. (1990) Occurrence, distributions and transport of herbicides and their degradation products in the lower Mississippi River and its tributaries. *Environ. Sci. Technol.*, **24**, 1400–1406

Peruzovic, M., Kniewald, J., Capkun, V. & Milkovic, K. (1995) Effect of atrazine ingested prior to mating on rat females and their offspring. *Acta physiol. hung.*, **83**, 79–89

Pino, A., Muara, A. & Grillo, P. (1988) DNA damage in stomach, kidney, liver and lung of rats treated with atrazine. *Mutat. Res.*, **209**, 145–147

Pintér, A., Török, G., Börzsönyi, M., Surján, A., Csík, M., Kelecsényi, Z. & Kocsis, Z. (1990) Long-term carcinogenicity bioassay of the herbicide atrazine in F344 rats. *Neoplasma*, **37**, 533–544

Plewa, M.J. (1985) Plant genetic assays and their use in studies on environmental mutagenesis in developing countries. *Basic Life Sci.*, **34**, 249–268

Plewa, M.J. & Gentile, J.M. (1976) Mutagenicity of atrazine: A maize-microbe bioassay. *Mutat. Res.*, **38**, 287–292

Readman, J.W., Albanis, T.A., Barcelo, D., Galassi, S., Tronczynski, J. & Gabrielides, G.P. (1993) Herbicide contamination of Mediterranean estuarine waters: Results from a MED POL pilot survey. *Marine Pollut. Bull.*, **26**, 613–619

Redondo, M.J., Ruiz, M.J., Font, G. & Boluda, R. (1997) Dissipation and distribution of atrazine, simazine, chlorpyrifos and tetradifon residues in citrus orchard soil. *Arch. environ. Contam. Toxicol.*, **32**, 346–352

Ribas, G., Frenzilli, G., Barale, R. & Marcos, R. (1995) Herbicide-induced DNA damage in human lymphocytes evaluated by the single-cell gel electrophoresis (SCGE) assay. *Mutat. Res.*, **344**, 41–54

Richards, R.P. & Baker, D.B. (1998) Triazines in waters of the midwest: exposure patterns. In: Ballantine, L.G., McFarland, J.E. & Hackett, D.S., eds, *Triazine Herbicides: Risk Assessment* (ACS Symposium Series No. 683), Washington DC, American Chemical Society, pp. 336–346

Richards, R.P., Kramer, J.W., Baker, D.B. & Krieger, K.A. (1987) Pesticides in rainwater in the northeastern United States. *Nature*, **327**, 129–131

Richards, R.P., Baker, D.B., Christensen, B.R. & Tierney, D.P. (1995) Atrazine exposures through drinking water: Exposure assessments for Ohio, Illinois and Iowa. *Environ. Sci. Technol.*, **29**, 406–412

Ruiz, M.J. & Marzin, D. (1997) Genotoxicity of six pesticides by Salmonella mutagenicity test and SOS chromotest. *Mutat Res.*, **390**, 245–255

Sadtler Research Laboratories (1980) *Sadtler Standard Spectra 1980. Cumulative Index*, Philadelphia, PA

Santa Maria, C., Vilas, M.G., Muriana, F.G. & Relimpio, A. (1986) Subacute atrazine effects on rat renal function. *Bull. environ. Contam. Toxicol.*, **36**, 325–331

Santa Maria, C., Moreno, J. & Lopez-Campos, J.L. (1987) Hepatotoxicity induced by the herbicide atrazine in the rat. *J. appl. Toxicol.*, **7**, 373–378

Sathiakumar, N., Delzell, E. & Cole, P. (1996) Mortality among workers at two triazine herbicide manufacturing plants. *Am. J. ind. Med.*, **29**, 143–151

Savitz, D.A., Arbuckle, T., Kaczor, D. & Curtis, K.M. (1997) Male pesticide exposure and pregnancy outcome. *Am. J. Epidemiol.*, **146**, 1025–1036

Schottler, S.P. & Eisenreich, S.J. (1994) Herbicides in the great Lakes. *Environ. Sci. Technol.*, **28**, 2228–2232

Schottler, S.P. & Eisenreich, S.J. (1997) Mass balance model to quantify atrazine sources, transformation rates, and trends in the Great Lakes. *Environ. Sci. Technol.*, **31**, 2616–2625

Schottler, S.P., Eisenreich, S.J. & Capel, P.D. (1994) Atrazine, alachlor and cynazine in a large agricultural river system. *Environ. Sci. Technol.*, **28**, 1079–1089

Seiler, J.P. (1973) A survey on the mutagenicity of various pesticides. *Experientia*, **29**, 622–623

Shah, P.V., Fisher, H.L., Sumler, M.R., Monroe, R.J., Chernoff, N. & Hall, L.L. (1987) Comparison of the penetration of 14 pesticides through the skin of young and adult rats. *J. Toxicol. environ. Health*, **21**, 353–366

Shapir, N. & Mandelbaum, R.T. (1997) Atrazine degradation in subsurface soil by indigenous and introduced microorganisms. *J. agric. Food Chem.*, **45**, 4481–4486

Shimabukuro, R.H., Frear, D.S., Swanson, H.R. & Walsh, W.C. (1971) Glutathione conjugation. An enzymatic basis for atrazine resistance in corn. *Plant Physiol.*, **47**, 10–14

Šimic, B.S., Kniewald, J. & Kniewald, Z. (1994) Effect of atrazine on reproductive performance in the rat. *J. appl. Toxicol.*, **14**, 401–404

Simmon, V.F., Kauhanen, K. & Tardiff, R.G. (1977) Mutagenic activity of chemicals identified in drinking water. In: Scott, D., Bridges, B.A. & Sobels, F.H., eds, *Progress in Genetic Toxicology: Developments in Toxicology and Environmental Science*, Vol. 2, Amsterdam, Elsevier, pp. 249–258

Simpkins, J.W., Eldridge, J.C. & Wetzel, L.T. (1998) Role of strain-specific reproductive patterns in the appearance of mammary tumors in atrazine-treated rats. In: Ballantine, L.G., McFarland, J.E. & Hackett, D.S., eds, *Triazine Herbicides: Risk Assessment* (ACS Symposium Series No. 683), Washington DC, American Chemical Society, pp. 399–413

Solomon, K.R., Baker, D.B., Richards, R.P., Dixon, K.R., Klaine, S.J., La Point, T.W., Kendall, R.J., Weisskopf, C.P., Giddings, J.M., Giesy, J.P., Hall, L.W., Jr & Williams, W.M. (1996) Ecological risk assessment of atrazine in North American surface waters. *Environ. Toxicol. Chem.*, **15**, 31–76

Spectrum Laboratories (1999) *EPA Method 619* [http://www.speclab.com/compound/m619/htm]

Squillace, P.J. & Thurman, E.M. (1992) Herbicide transport in rivers: Importance of hydrology and geochemistry in nonpoint-source contamination. *Environ. Sci. Technol.*, **26**, 538–545

Squillace, P.J., Thurman, E.M. & Furlong, E.T. (1993) Ground water as a nonpoint-source of atrazine and deethylatrazine in a river during base flow conditions. *Water Resources Res.*, **29**, 1719–1729

State of Israel (1977) *Pesticide Residue Tolerances in Israel*, Tel Aviv, Ministry of Agriculture, Plant Protection Department, p. 26

Stevens, J.T., Breckenridge, C.B., Wetzel, L.T., Gillis, J.H., Luempert, L.G., III & Eldridge, J.C. (1994) Hypothesis for mammary tumorigenesis in Sprague-Dawley rats exposed to certain triazine herbicides. *J. Toxicol. environ. Health*, **43**, 139–153

Stevens, J.T., Breckenridge, C.B., Wetzel, L., Thakur, A.K., Liu, C., Werner, C., Luempert, L.G. & Eldridge, J.C. (1998) Risk characterization for atrazine: Oncogenicity profile. *J. Toxicol. environ. Health*, **55**, 101–141

Stevens, J.T., Breckenridge, J.C. & Wetzel, L. (1999) A risk characterization for atrazine: Oncogenicity profile. *J. Toxicol. environ. Health*, **56**, 69–109

Stroev, V.S. (1968) Mutagenic effect of herbicides on barley. *Sov. Genet.*, **4**, 1539–1542

Sumner, D.D., Cassidy, J.E., Szolics, I.M., Marco, G.J., Bakshi, K.S. & Brusick, D.J. (1984) Evaluation of the mutagenic potential of corn (*Zea mays* L.) grown in untreated and atrazine (AAtrex®) treated soil in the field. *Drug chem. Toxicol.*, **7**, 243–257

Surrallés, J., Xamena, N., Creus, A. & Marcos, R. (1995) The suitability of the micronucleus assay in human lymphocytes as a new biomarker of excision repair. *Mutat Res.*, **342**, 43–59

Tennant, M.K., Hill, S.D., Eldridge, J.C., Wetzel, T.L., Breckenridge, C.B. & Stevens, J.T. (1994a) Chloro-*s*-triazine antagonism of estrogen action: Limited interaction with estrogen receptor binding. *J. Toxicol. environ. Health*, **43**, 197–211

Tennant, M.K., Hill, S.D., Eldridge, J.C., Wetzel, T.L., Breckenridge, C.B. & Stevens, J.T. (1994b) Possible antiestrogenic properties of chloro-*s*-triazines in rat uterus. *J. Toxicol. environ. Health*, **43**, 183–196

Thakur, A.K., Wetzel, L.T., Voelker, R.W. & Wakefield, A.E. (1998) Results of a two-year oncogenicity study in Fischer 344 rats with atrazine. In: Ballantine, L.G., McFarland, J.E. & Hackett, D.S., eds, *Triazine Herbicides: Risk Assessment* (ACS Symposium Series No. 683), Washington DC, American Chemical Society, pp. 384–398

The Pesticide Trust (1993) Atrazine and simazine: Restrictions now effective. *Pestic. News*, **21**

Thurman, E.M., Goolsby, D.A., Meyer, M.T. & Kolpin, D.W. (1991) Herbicides in surface waters of the midwestern United States: The effect of spring flush. *Environ. Sci. Technol.*, **25**, 1794–1796

Thurman, E.M., Goolsby, D.A., Meyer, M.T., Mills, M.S., Pomes, M.L. & Kolpin, D.W. (1992) A reconnaissance study of herbicides and their metabolites in surface water of the midwestern United States using immunoassay and gas chromatography/mass spectrometry. *Environ. Sci. Technol.*, **26**, 2440–2447

Thurman, E.M., Meyer, M.T., Mills, M.S., Zimmerman, L.R., Perry, C.A. & Goolsby, D.A. (1994) Formation and transport of deethylatrazine and deisopropylatrazine in surface waters. *Environ. Sci. Technol.*, **28**, 2267–2277

Thurman, E.M., Kolpin, D.W., Goolsby, D.A. & Meyer, M.T. (1998) Source and transport of desethylatrazine and deisopropylatrazine to ground water of the midwestern United States. In: Ballantine, L.G., McFarland, J.E. & Hackett, D.S., eds, *Triazine Herbicides: Risk Assessment* (ACS Symposium Series No. 683), Washington DC, American Chemical Society, pp. 189–207

Tierney, D.P., Clarkson, J.R., Christensen, B.R. Golden, K.A. & Hines, N.A. (1998) Exposure to the herbicides atrazine and simazine in drinking water. In: Ballantine, L.G., McFarland, J.E. & Hackett, D.S., eds, *Triazine Herbicides: Risk Assessment* (ACS Symposium Series No. 683), Washington DC, American Chemical Society, pp. 252–265

Timchalk, C., Dryzga, M.D., Langvardt, P.W., Kastl, P.E. & Osborne, D.W. (1990) Determination of the effect of tridiphane on the pharmacokinetics of [^{14}C]-atrazine following oral administration to male Fischer 344 rats. *Toxicology*, **61**, 27–40

Tomlin, C., ed. (1994) *The Pesticide Manual*, 10th Ed., Thornton Heath, British Crop Protection Council/Cambridge, The Royal Society of Chemistry, pp. 51–52

Torres, C., Ribas, G., Xamena, N., Creus, A. & Marcos, R. (1992) Genotoxicity of four herbicides in the Drosophila wing spot test. *Mutat. Res.*, **280**, 291–295

Tripathy, N.K., Routray, P.K, Sahu, G.P. & Anandkumar, A. (1993) Atrazine, a triazine herbicide, is genotoxic in the Drosophila somatic and germ line cells. *Biol. zent. Bl.*, **112**, 312–318

Ulrich, M.M., Müller, S.R., Singer, H.P., Imboden, D.M. & Schwartzenbach, R.P. (1994) Input and dynamic behavior of the organic pollutants tetrachloroethene, atrazine, and NTA in a lake: A study combining mathematical modelling and field measurements. *Environ. Sci. Technol.*, **28**, 1674–1685

United Nations Environment Programme (1998) *UNEP Chemicals (IRPTC) Data Bank Legal File, Recommendations and Legal Mechanisms*, Geneva, WHO [http://irptc.unep.ch/irptc]

Wang, Y.S., Duh, J.R., Liang, Y.F. & Chen, Y.L. (1995) Dissipation of three *s*-triazine herbicides, atrazine, simazine and ametryn, in subtropical soils. *Bull. environ. Contam. Toxicol.*, **55**, 351–358

Wang, Y.S., Duh, J.R., Lin, K.Y. & Chen, Y.L. (1996) Movement of three *s*-triazine herbicides, atrazine, simazine and ametryn, in subtropical soils. *Bull. environ. Contam. Toxicol.*, **57**, 743–750

Wetzel, L.T., Luempert, L.G., III, Breckenridge, C.B., Tisdel, M.O., Stevens, J.T., Thakur, A.K., Extrom, P.J. & Eldridge, J.R. (1994) Chronic effects of atrazine on estrous and mammary gland tumor formation in female Sprague-Dawley and Fischer 344 rats. *J. Toxicol. environ. Health*, **43**, 169–182

WHO (1993) *Guidelines for Drinking Water Quality*, 2nd Ed., Vol. 1, *Recommendations*, Geneva, pp. 77–78

Williams, S., ed. (1984) *Official Methods of Analysis of the Association of Official Analytical Chemists*, Arlington, VA, pp. 145–146

Winkelmann, D.A. & Klaine, S.J. (1991a) Degradation and bound residue formation of atrazine in a western Tennessee soil. *Environ. Toxicol. Chem.*, **10**, 335–345

Winkelmann, D.A. & Klaine, S.J. (1991b) Degradation and bound residue formation of four atrazine metabolites, deethylatrazine, deisopropylatrazine, dealkylatrazine and hydroxy-atrazine, in a western Tennessee soil. *Environ. Toxicol. Chem.*, **10**, 347–354

Wise, P.M. (1982) Norepinephrine and dopamine activity in microdissected brain areas of the middle-aged and young rat on proestrus. *Biol. Reprod.*, **27**, 562–574

Wise, P.M. (1984) Estradiol-induced daily luteinizing hormone and prolactin surges in young and middle-aged rats: Correlations with age-related changes in pituitary responsiveness and catecholamine turnover rates in microdissected brain areas. *Endocrinology*, **115**, 801–809

Worthing, C.R. & Walker, S.B., eds. (1987) *The Pesticide Manual: A World Compendium*, 8th Ed., Thornton Heath, British Crop Protection Council, pp. 36–37

Wuu, K.D. & Grant, W.F. (1966) Morphological and somatic chromosomal aberrations induced by pesticides in barley (*Hordeum vulgare*). *Can. J. Genet. Cytol.*, **8**, 481–501

Wuu, K.D. & Grant, W.F. (1967a) Chromosomal aberrations induced by pesticides in meiotic cells of barley. *Cytologia*, **32**, 31–41

Wuu, K.D. & Grant, W.F. (1967b) Chromosomal aberrations induced in somatic cells of *Vicia faba* by pesticides. *Nucleus*, **10**, 37–46

Zahm, S.H., Weisenburger, D.D., Babbit, P.A., Saal, R.C., Vaught, J.B., Cantor, K.P. & Blair, A. (1990) A case–control study of non-Hodgkin's lymphoma and the herbicide 2,4-dichlorophenoxyacetic acid (2,4-D) in eastern Nebraska. *Epidemiol. Res.*, **1**, 349–356

Zahm, S.H., Weisenburger, D.D., Cantor, K.P., Holmes, F.F. & Blair, A. (1993a) Role of the herbicide atrazine in the development of non-Hodgkin's lymphoma. *Scand. J. Work Environ. Health*, **19**, 108–114

Zahm, S.H., Weisenburger, D.D., Saal, R.C., Vaught, J.B., Babbit, P.A. & Blair, A. (1993b) The role of agricultural pesticide use in the development of non-Hodgkin's lymphoma in women. *Arch. environ. Health*, **48**, 353–358

Zeiger, E., Anderson, B., Haworth, S., Lawlor, T. & Mortelmans, K. (1988) Salmonella mutagenicity tests: IV. Results from the testing of 300 chemicals. *Environ. mol. Mutag.*, **11**, 1–158

Zeljenkova, D. & Vargova, M. (1996) Possible estrogenic effects of some herbicides (Abstract). *Teratology*, **53**, 39A

Zhu, T., Desjardins, R.L., MacPherson, J.I., Pattey, E. & St Amour, G. (1998) Aircraft measurements of the concentrations and flux of agrochemicals. *Environ. Sci. Technol.*, **32**, 1032–1038

van Zwieten, M.J., HogenEsch, H., Majka, J.A. & Boorman, G.A. (1994) Nonneoplastic and neoplastic lesions of the mammary gland. In: Mohr, U., Dungworth, D.L. & Capen, C.C., eds, *Pathobiology of the Aging Rat*, Vol. 2, *Nervous System and Special Sense Organs, Endocrine System, Digestive System, Integumentary System, and Mammary Gland, Musculoskeletal System and Soft Tissue, and General Aspects*, Washington DC, ILSI Press, pp. 459–475

BUTYL BENZYL PHTHALATE

This substance was considered by previous working groups, in 1981 (IARC, 1982) and 1987 (IARC, 1987). Since that time, new data have become available, and these have been incorporated into the monograph and taken into consideration in the present evaluation.

1. Exposure Data

1.1 Chemical and physical data

1.1.1 *Nomenclature*

Chem. Abstr. Serv. Reg. No.: 85-68-7
Deleted CAS Reg. No.: 58128-78-2
Chem. Abstr. Name: 1,2-Benzenedicarboxylic acid, butyl phenylmethyl ester
IUPAC Systematic Name: Phthalic acid, benzyl butyl ester
Synonyms: BBP; benzyl butyl phthalate; benzyl *n*-butyl phthalate

1.1.2 *Structural and molecular formulae and relative molecular mass*

O
||
C—O—$(CH_2)_3$—CH_3

C—O—CH_2—
||
O

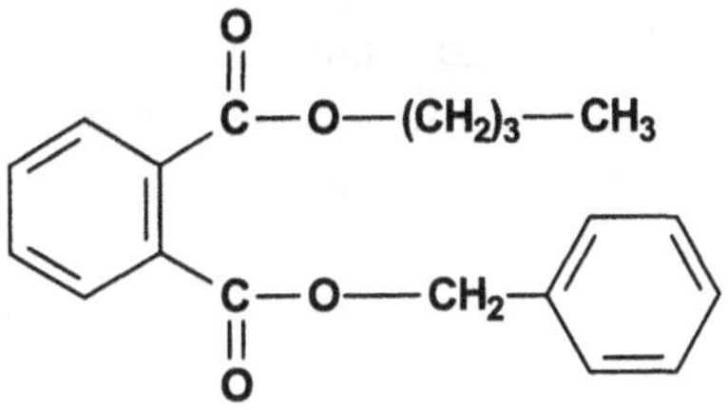

$C_{19}H_{20}O_4$ Relative molecular mass: 312.4

1.1.3 *Chemical and physical properties of the pure substance* (from Verschueren, 1996, except where noted)

(*a*) *Description*: Clear, oily liquid
(*b*) *Boiling-point*: 370°C
(*c*) *Melting-point*: < –35°C
(*d*) *Density*: 1.1 g/cm³ at 25°C
(*e*) *Solubility*: Slightly soluble in water
(*f*) *Volatility*: Vapour pressure, 1.14 mPa at 20°C; relative vapour density (air = 1), 10.8 (National Toxicology Program, 1991)
(*g*) *Octanol/water partition coefficient (P)*: log P, 4.91
(*h*) *Conversion factor*: mg/m³ = 12.78 × ppm

1.2 Production and use

Information available in 1995 indicated that butyl benzyl phthalate was produced in 12 countries worldwide (Chemical Information Services, 1995).

Butyl benzyl phthalate is used as a plasticizer for polyvinyl chloride in vinyl floor tiles, vinyl foam and carpet backing, in cellulosic resins, and as an organic intermediate. It has also been used as a solvent and fixative in perfume (National Toxicology Program, 1991; Lewis, 1993).

1.3 Occurrence

1.3.1 *Natural occurrence*

Butyl benzyl phthalate is not known to occur naturally.

1.3.2 *Occupational exposure*

According to the 1981–83 National Occupational Exposure Survey (National Institute for Occupational Safety and Health, 1998), approximately 330 000 workers in the United States were potentially exposed to butyl benzyl phthalate. Occupational exposure may occur during its production and in its use as a plasticizer in polyvinyl chloride products such as vinyl floor tiles.

1.3.3 *Environmental occurrence*

According to the United States Environmental Protection Agency Toxic Chemical Release Inventory for 1987, 147 000 kg butyl benzyl phthalate were released into the air, 860 kg were discharged into water, and 3900 kg were released onto the land from manufacturing and processing facilities in the United States. By 1993, 170 000 kg were released into air, 620 kg were discharged into water, 38 kg were disposed of by underground injection, and 1200 kg were released onto the land (National Library of Medicine, 1998a).

Butyl benzyl phthalate has been detected in surface water, groundwater and drinking-water in many locations at levels generally well below 10 μg/L. Concentrations lower than 0.1 μg/m^3 have been found in indoor air due to release from products such as vinyl flooring, caulks and adhesives and carpets. It also has been detected at parts per million in a few foods (Solutia, 1998; National Library of Medicine, 1998b).

1.4 Regulations and guidelines

The time-weighted average exposure limits for exposure to butyl benzyl phthalate in workplace air are 3 mg/m^3 in Sweden and 5 mg/m^3 in Ireland and the United Kingdom (International Labour Office, 1991; National Library of Medicine, 1998c).

No international guidelines for butyl benzyl phthalate in drinking-water have been established (WHO, 1993).

2. Studies of Cancer in Humans

No data were available to the Working Group.

3. Studies of Cancer in Experimental Animals

Previous evaluation

Butyl benzyl phthalate was tested in mice and in female rats by oral administration and in male mice by intraperitoneal injection. A somewhat increased incidence of monocytic leukaemias was reported in female rats. In mice, no increased incidence of tumours was observed (IARC, 1982).

New studies

3.1 Oral administration

Rat: Groups of 60 male and 60 female Fischer 344/N rats, six weeks of age, were fed diets containing 0, 3000, 6000 or 12 000 mg/kg (ppm) (males) and 0, 6000, 12 000 or 24 000 mg/kg (females) butyl benzyl phthalate (purity, > 99.5%) for 105 weeks. Ten rats per group were killed at 15 months. A decrease in body-weight gain was dose-related, especially in females at the high dose. There was no effect on survival. Male rats had an increased incidence of pancreatic acinar-cell adenomas (control, 3/50; low dose, 2/49; intermediate dose, 3/50; high dose, 10/50; $p < 0.016$); one pancreatic acinar-cell carcinoma was seen in a male at the high dose. The prevalence of focal hyperplasia of the pancreas was also increased in males in a dose-related manner (4/50, 7/49, 9/50, 12/50). Urinary bladder transitional-cell hyperplasia [type not specified] was seen in 4/50, 0/50, 1/50 and 10/50 females in the four groups, respectively (National Toxicology Program, 1997a). [The Working Group noted that no bladder lesions were seen in a 90-day study.]

A further study was conducted with animals on restricted diets in an effort to evaluate the effect of weight-matched control groups on the sensitivity of the bioassay. The aim was to achieve a body weight reduction of about 15% in comparison with rats fed *ad libitum*. Groups of 50 male and 50 female Fischer 344/N rats, six weeks of age, were fed diets containing concentrations of 0, 12 000 (males) or 24 000 (females) mg/kg (ppm) butyl benzyl phthalate for either 24 or 30–32 months and killed at those times. Body-weight depression was observed in females but not males; the rate of survival of male rats was slightly decreased. There was no increase in the incidence of pancreatic tumours at either 24 or 30–32 months. The incidence of urinary bladder papillomas or carcinomas was marginally increased in female rats (6/50 versus 1/49; $p = 0.077$) at 32 months; four of these females had bladder carcinomas, with none in controls ($p > 0.079$ by the Kaplan-Meier test after adjustment for intercurrent mortality). The incidence of bladder hyperplasia was also increased in females at 24 months (14/50 versus 0/50 in controls) and at 32 months (16/50 versus 0/49) (National Toxicology Program, 1997b).

3.2 Administration with known carcinogens or modifying agents

Groups of 27 female Sprague-Dawley rats, 43 days of age, were given butyl benzyl phthalate [purity unspecified] at doses of 250 or 500 mg/kg bw intragastrically in corn oil, daily for seven days before intragastric administration of 31 mg/kg bw dimethylbenz-[*a*]anthracene (DMBA) in corn oil at 50 days of age. After 15 weeks, the rats were killed and the mammary tumour incidences determined. Administration of butyl benzyl phthalate did not affect body-weight gain. The incidence of palpable mammary tumours was significantly inhibited by pretreatment with butyl benzyl phthalate, by 58 and 71% at 250 and 500 mg/kg bw, respectively ($p < 0.05$). The number of adenocarcinomas per rat was also significantly reduced, being 4.0 with DMBA alone, 1.6 with 250 mg/kg bw butyl benzyl phthalate and 1.2 with 500 mg/kg bw ($p < 0.05$) (Singletary *et al.*, 1997).

4. Other Data Relevant to an Evaluation of Carcinogenicity and its Mechanisms

4.1 Absorption, distribution, metabolism and excretion

4.1.1 *Humans*

No data were available to the Working Group.

4.1.2 *Experimental systems*

A few studies on the absorption, distribution, metabolism and excretion of butyl benzyl phthalate have been conducted in rats, and one study has been performed in beagle dogs. Initial metabolism involves cleavage of one ester, as shown by the studies described below. After dosing by gavage of male Fischer 344 rats with 2, 20 or 200 mg/kg bw [ring-^{14}C]butyl benzyl phthalate, 62–72 and 13–15% of the dose was excreted in urine and faeces, respectively, within 24 h. By 96 h, 92–98% of the dose had been eliminated, 71–80 and 18–23% being eliminated in urine and faeces, respectively. The radiolabel found in urine was associated with monophthalates (22–42% of the dose), monophthalate glucuronide conjugates (14–21% of the dose) and unknown metabolites. At a dose of 2000 mg/kg bw, 22 and 72% were eliminated after 96 h in urine and faeces, respectively. The increased faecal elimination at this high dose relative to excretion in urine may represent incomplete absorption of butyl benzyl phthalate. After intravenous administration of a 20-mg/kg bw dose, [ring-^{14}C]butyl benzyl phthalate was rapidly distributed to the tissues, and the radiolabel was eliminated with a half-life of around 6 h in all tissues. Some 55% of an intravenous 20-mg/kg bw dose was excreted in the bile after 4 h. Analysis of the bile revealed the presence of mono-*n*-butyl phthalate and monobenzyl phthalate glucuronides, representing 26 and 13% of the dose, respectively; trace amounts of the free monoesters, representing 1.1 and 0.9% of the dose, respectively; and unknown metabolites (14% of the dose), but no parent butyl benzyl phthalate. This study demonstrates that butyl benzyl phthalate is rapidly metabolized in rats; the metabolites are excreted in the bile and, after enterohepatic circulation, are eliminated in the urine. Mono-*n*-butyl phthalate is formed in large amounts, mono-*n*-butyl and monobenzyl phthalates accounting for 44 and 16% of a 20-mg/kg bw intravenous dose, respectively (Eigenberg *et al.*, 1986).

Similarly, when male Wistar-Imamichi rats were given 3.6 mmol/kg bw (about 1100 mg/kg bw) of butyl benzyl phthalate orally for three days, both free and glucuronide conjugated (ratio, about 7:3) butyl benzyl phthalate monoester metabolites were excreted in the urine. The ratio of mono-*n*-butyl phthalate to monobenzyl phthalate was about 5:3 (Mikuriya *et al.*, 1988).

After dermal application of 157 μmol/kg bw (about 49 mg/kg bw) [ring-^{14}C]butyl benzyl phthalate to the shaved skin of male Fischer 344 rats, some 30% of the dose was excreted in the urine and faeces within seven days; 45% of the dose was found in the skin at the application site, 6.3% in the plastic cap used to occlude the skin and 4.6% in muscle and < 1% in other tissues (Elsisi *et al.*, 1989).

Beagle dogs were given a 5-g/kg bw oral dose of butyl benzyl phthalate divided over a 4-h period. Unchanged butyl benzyl phthalate in the faeces comprised 88–91% of the dose. While butyl benzyl phthalate was not present in the urine, some 4.2% of the dose was present as phthalic acid (Erickson, 1965).

4.2 Toxic effects

4.2.1 *Humans*

Butyl benzyl phthalate has been reported to be slightly irritating to the skin, eye and mucous membranes and to depress the central nervous system (Gosselin *et al.*, 1984). In a patch test with 200 volunteers, which involved 15 daily applications over a three-week period, Hammond *et al.* (1987) observed neither primary irritation nor sensitization reactions.

4.2.2 *Experimental systems*

The oral LD_{50} of butyl benzyl phthalate administered in corn oil to male and female Fischer 344 rats was reported to be 2.3 g/kg bw and that in male and female $B6C3F_1$ mice to be 6.2 and 4.2 g/kg bw, respectively (National Toxicology Program, 1982). In male Sprague-Dawley rats, the oral LD_{50} of butyl benzyl phthalate administered in undiluted form was 20 g/kg (Hammond *et al.*, 1987). In Swiss Webster mice, the intraperitoneal LD_{50} of butyl benzyl phthalate was 3.2 g/kg (Calley *et al.*, 1966). The dermal LD_{50} in rabbits was reported to be > 10 g/kg (Hammond *et al.*, 1987).

Like other phthalate diesters, butyl benzyl phthalate increases the weight of the liver in rats. When administered at dietary levels of 0.6, 1.2 or 2.5% for 21 days to male and female Fischer 344 rats, butyl benzyl phthalate produced hepatic peroxisome proliferation, with weak induction of peroxisomal activity (palmitoyl-coenzyme A oxidation) in both males and females. Microsomal activites (lauric acid 12-hydroxylase) were strongly induced in males but hardly at all in females. Ultrastructural examination of liver sections revealed an increase in the numbers of peroxisomes (Barber *et al.*, 1987).

Many chemicals are known to produce hepatic peroxisome proliferation in rats and/or mice, and the characteristics of rodent peroxisome proliferators have been described elsewhere (Bentley *et al.*, 1993; Ashby *et al.*, 1994; Lake, 1995a,b; IARC, 1995; Cattley *et al.*, 1998). Butyl benzyl phthalate was less potent than di(2-ethylhexyl)phthalate and some branched-chain phthalate diesters in producing hepatic peroxisome proliferation in rats (Barber *et al.*, 1987; Lin, 1987). In comparison with rodent peroxisome proliferators in general, butyl benzyl phthalate is only a weak agent (Barber *et al.*, 1987; Ashby *et al.*, 1994; IARC, 1995). While an association between peroxisome proliferation and liver tumour formation in rodents has been reported (Ashby *et al.*, 1994), weak peroxisome proliferators do not necessarily produce liver tumours in rats or mice after chronic administration (Bentley *et al.*, 1993; Lake, 1995a).

Butyl benzyl phthalate was one of several phthalates tested for oestrogenic activity in a recombinant yeast cell line containing the human oestrogen receptor gene, which was expressed in such a way that it controlled expression of the reporter gene *lacZ*. The maximum induction of *lacZ* via the human oestrogen receptor was 50% that caused by oestradiol-17β, while the relative potency was 0.000001. Comparable results were obtained in a similar test for proliferation of the oestrogen-responsive human breast cancer cell lines MCF-7 and ZR-75 (Harris *et al.*, 1997).

The oestrogenic activity of phthalates was further investigated *in vitro* in competitive ligand-binding assays, in assays for yeast and mammalian gene expression and *in vivo* in a uterotrophic assay. Butyl benzyl phthalate competed weakly for oestrogen receptor binding (the concentration causing 50% inhibition being 36 μmol/L in comparison with 1.3 nmol/L for oestradiol), induced luciferase activity in transfected MCF-7 cells and stably transfected HeLa cells at a concentration of 10 μmol/L and weakly supported oestrogen-inducible growth in yeast cells (also at 10 μmol/L), but did not demonstrate any oestrogenic activity in mammals *in vivo* (Zacharewski *et al.*, 1998).

4.3 Reproductive and developmental effects

4.3.1 *Humans*

No data were available to the Working Group.

4.3.2 *Experimental systems*

Butyl benzyl phthalate was tested for developmental toxicity by dietary administration in rats and mice (Schwetz & Harris, 1993). In Sprague-Dawley rats exposed on days 6–15 of gestation to concentrations of 0.5–2%, maternal and developmental toxicity were observed at ≥ 1.25%. The developmental effects reported included an increased incidence of malformations and variations at 1.25% and embryonic death, reduced fetal body weights and an increased incidence of malformations and variations at 2%. In CD-1 mice exposed on days 6–15 of gestation to concentrations of 0.1–1.25%, maternal and developmental toxicity were reported at 1.25%. The developmental effects included embryonic death, reduced fetal weight and an increased incidence of malformations and variations. [The Working Group noted that only summary data of these National Toxicology Program studies were reported in the published literature.]

Groups of 10 adult male Fischer 344 rats were fed diets containing 0, 0.625, 1.25, 2.5 or 5% butyl benzyl phthalate (purity, > 98%) for 14 days. Rats exposed to the two higher doses were weak and lethargic and showed reduced body-weight gain and reduced weights of the testes, epididymides, prostate and seminal vesicle. The changes in organ weights persisted after correction for differences in body weight, except for that of the prostate, and were accompanied by dose-related atrophy of the testes and epididymides. Isolated sperm granulomas were found at the two highest doses (Agarwal *at al.*, 1985).

Groups of 15–18 Wistar rats received diets containing 0, 0.25, 0.5, 1 or 2% butyl benzyl phthalate on days 0–20 of gestation, providing daily intakes estimated to be 0, 180, 380, 650 and 970 mg/kg bw, respectively. Maternal food consumption and body-weight gain were reduced at the two higher doses, and the litters of dams at the highest dose were resorbed. The body weights of pups at all but the lowest dose were reduced. No increase in the incidence of anomalies or malformations in the fetuses was observed (Ema *et al.*, 1990). To determine whether the embryolethality was the result of reduced food consumption, a pair-feeding study was conducted in which pregnant rats received the same amount of diet consumed by the rats given 2% butyl benzyl phthalate. Although effects of the dietary reduction were observed, complete resorption was not seen in any of the pair-fed rats (Ema *et al.*, 1991). When exposure to 2% was limited to days 0–11 or 11–20 of pregnancy, complete resorptions were seen only in the former group, while reduced fetal body weights, cleft palate and fused sternebrae were observed in the group exposed during days 11–20 (Ema *et al.*, 1992a). When exposure was restricted to days 0–7, 7–16 or 16–20, increased resorptions in comparison with pair-fed rats were present only in groups exposed to 2.0% butyl benzyl phthalate on days 0–7 or 7–16, while reduced fetal body weights were present in all treated groups; malformations (cleft palate and fused sternebrae) were present only in the group exposed on days 7–16 of gestation (Ema *et al.*, 1992b). In rats exposed to butyl benzyl phthalate by gavage at a dose of 0, 0.5, 0.75 or 1 g/kg bw daily on days 7–15, maternal lethality was seen at the highest dose and reduced body-weight gain and an increased incidence of resorptions at the two higher doses; complete resorption was observed at 1 g/kg bw. Reduced fetal weight and an increased incidence of cleft palate, fused ribs and dilated renal pelves were found at 0.75 mg/kg bw (Ema *et al.*, 1992c). In an effort to define further the critical period for induction of teratogenicity by butyl benzyl phthalate, groups of rats were gavaged with 0.6, 0.75 or 1 g/kg bw daily on days 7–9, 10–12 or 13–15 of gestation. Exposure during any period resulted in dose-related increases in the rate of resorptions. Decreases in fetal body weight were observed only in groups exposed on days 7–9 or 10–12 of gestation, while malformations were present in fetuses exposed on days 7–9 or 13–15 (Ema *et al.*, 1993). Post-implantation loss after dietary exposure to 2% butyl benzyl phthalate was seen as early as gestation day 11 and appeared to be related to reduced maternal plasma progesterone concentrations and impaired luteal function (Ema *et al.*, 1994). The spectra of phase-specific effects on fetal development induced by metabolites of butyl benzyl phthalate (mono-*n*-benzyl phthalate and mono-*n*-butyl phthalate) and a related phthalate (di-*n*-butyl phthalate) were similar to that of butyl benzyl phthalate itself (Ema *et al.*, 1995, 1996a,b,c).

Butyl benzyl phthalate was given to female Wistar rats [number not specified] in the drinking-water at a concentration of 0 or 1000 μg/L two weeks before mating, during gestation and throughout three weeks of lactation. Treatment had no effect on litter size at birth, but male offspring were significantly larger on day 22. By days 90–95, the body weights were similar to those of controls, but the relative weight of the testes was reduced. There were no effects on testicular tissue, but butyl benzyl phthalate-treated males had a significantly reduced daily rate of sperm production (Sharpe *et al.*, 1995). A recent note from the authors, however, reported an unexplained temporal decrease in absolute testicular weight in control animals in their breeding colony. This decrease appeared to be at least as large as the effects seen with diethylstilboestrol, which had been used as a positive control in the studies of developmental toxicity (Sharpe *et al.*, 1998).

Butyl benzyl phthalate was administered in the drinking-water to AP rats at a concentration of 0 or 1000 μg/L, the latter resulting in an estimated exposure to 180 μg/kg bw per day, during gestation and lactation. The weight of male pups at birth was significantly increased, as was the anogenital distance in males on day 2; female pups showed slightly earlier vaginal opening. Butyl benzyl phthalate had no significant effect on male body weights at day 90 or 137, however, nor were there effects on testicular weight, caudal or testicular sperm counts or the degree of positivity of pituitary cells for follicular-stimulating hormone (Ashby *et al.*, 1997).

Butyl benzyl phthalate (purity, 98%) was evaluated for reproductive toxicity in the OECD 421 screening protocol. Groups of 10 WU rats, 10–11 weeks of age, were exposed for 29 days (males) or from 14 days before mating to six days *post partum* (females) to 0, 250, 500 or 1000 mg/kg bw per day by oral gavage. Mating, fertility and the viability and growth of the offspring were examined, and the reproductive tracts of the parental animals were assessed histologically. The body-weight gain of males at the high dose was reduced during treatment, while that of females was reduced during gestation. The numbers of animals that became pregnant were nine, eight, seven and four, with increasing dose. The litter size of dams at the high dose was significantly reduced at parturition, while the average pup weight at birth was reduced at the two higher doses. No dose-related anomalies were observed. At the high dose, the offspring had reduced testicular weights, while the parental males showed degeneration and Leydig-cell hyperplasia (Piersma *et al.*, 1995).

Groups of 10–14 Wistar rats received 0, 250, 500, 750 or 1000 mg/kg bw per day butyl benzyl phthalate (purity, 98.2%) by oral gavage on days 0–8 of gestation or pseudogestation. The high dose was lethal to 2/14 pregnant females, and the body-weight gain was lower in all treated groups during exposure. A dose-related increase was seen in the percentage of females that did not become pregnant, and the numbers of implantation sites and fetal body weights at term were decreased. Similar overt toxicity was seen in pseudopregnant females exposed to butyl benzyl phthalate, which also had dose-related reductions in ovarian and uterine weights. The authors concluded that altered ovarian and/or uterine function may contribute to the embryotoxicity of butyl benzyl phthalate (Ema *et al.*, 1998).

Butyl benzyl phthalate did not affect uterine vascular permeability in ovarectomized Swiss mice 4 h after subcutaneous administration of 10^{-4} mol [31 mg/mouse], nor did it inhibit oestradiol-stimulated increases in uterine vascular permeability (Milligan *et al.*, 1998).

4.4 Genetic and related effects

4.4.1 *Humans*

No data were available to the Working Group.

4.4.2 *Experimental systems* (see Table 1 for references)

Butyl benzyl phthalate did not induce gene mutation in *Salmonella typhimurium* strains TA100, TA1535, TA1537 or TA98 with or without addition of an exogenous metabolic activation system. In single studies, it did not induce sex-linked recessive lethal mutation in *Drosophila,* gene mutation at the *tk* locus in mouse lymphoma L5178Y cells or sister chromatid exchange or chromosomal aberrations in Chinese hamster ovary cells *in vitro*. In one study, butyl benzyl phthalate given as a single intraperitoneal injection did not induce sister chromatid exchange in the bone marrow of male B6C3F1 mice. After a standard harvest time of 17 h, chromosomal aberrations were induced in the bone marrow of these mice; there was no increase in in the incidence of aberrations when a delayed harvest time of 36 h was used.

5. Summary of Data Reported and Evaluation

5.1 Exposure data

Exposure to butyl benzyl phthalate occurs during its production and use as a plasticizer, mainly in polyvinyl chloride products. It has been detected at low levels in indoor air, water and a few foods.

5.2 Human carcinogenicity data

No data were available to the Working Group.

5.3 Animal carcinogenicity data

Butyl benzyl phthalate was tested for carcinogenicity by oral administration in one experiment in mice and three experiments in rats, including two studies with dietary restriction. No increase in the incidence of tumours was observed in mice. A marginal increase in the incidence of bladder tumours was observed in female rats after 32 months of dietary restriction. An increased incidence of benign pancreatic tumours was seen in one conventional study in male rats, but not after dietary restriction, despite extension of the period of dosing to 32 months.

Table 1. Genetic and related effects of butyl benzyl phthalate

Test system	Result[a]		Dose[b] (LED or HID)	Reference
	Without exogenous metabolic system	With exogenous metabolic system		
Salmonella typhimurium TA100, TA98, reverse mutation	–	–	1000 μg/plate	Kozumbo *et al.* (1982)
Salmonella typhimurium TA100, TA98, TA1535, TA1537, reverse mutation	–	–	11 550 μg/plate	Zeiger *et al.* (1985)
Drosophila melanogaster, sex-linked recessive lethal mutation	–		50 000 ppm feed	Valencia *et al.* (1985)
Gene mutation, mouse lymphoma L5178Y cells, *tk* locus *in vitro*	–	–	67	Myhr & Caspary (1991)
Sister chromatid exchange, Chinese hamster ovary cells *in vitro*	–	–	1250	Galloway *et al.* (1987)
Chromosomal aberrations, Chinese hamster ovary cells *in vitro*	–	–	1250	Galloway *et al.* (1987)
Sister chromatid exchange, male B6C3F$_1$ mouse bone-marrow cells *in vivo*	–		2500 ip × 1	National Toxicology Program (1997a)
Chromosomal aberrations, male B6C3F$_1$ mouse bone-marrow cells *in vivo*	(+)		5000 ip × 1	National Toxicology Program (1997a)

[a] (+), weakly positive; –, negative

[b] LED, lowest effective dose; HID, highest ineffective dose; unless otherwise stated, in-vitro tests, μg/mL; in-vivo tests, mg/kg bw per day; ip, intraperitoneal

In one study in rats, butyl benzyl phthalate inhibited mammary carcinogenesis produced by prior administration of 7,12-dimethylbenz[*a*]anthracene.

5.4 Other relevant data

Butyl benzyl phthalate is hydrolysed in the gastrointestinal tract to mono-*n*-butyl phthalate and monobenzyl phthalate, which are absorbed, further metabolized, glucuronidated and excreted in the urine. Butyl benzyl phthalate weakly stimulated hepatic peroxisome proliferation. Although the compound binds weakly to oestrogen receptors *in vitro*, it had no oestrogenic activity *in vivo* in tests which included uterotropic effects and vaginal cornification.

Butyl benzyl phthalate has been tested for developmental toxicity in mice by administration in the diet and in rats by administration in the diet, by gavage and in drinking-water. Malformations and embryonic deaths were observed in both species, generally at maternally toxic doses. In rats, alterations in ovarian and/or uterine function appeared to be involved in the decreased embryonic viability. Testicular toxicity has been observed in male rats exposed to butyl benzyl phthalate.

No data were available on the genetic and related effects of butyl benzyl phthalate in humans. Butyl benzyl phthalate was not genotoxic in experimental systems, except for weak clastogenicity in bone-marrow cells of mice treated *in vivo* in one study.

5.5 Evaluation

There is *inadequate evidence* in humans for the carcinogenicity of butyl benzyl phthalate.

There is *limited evidence* in experimental animals for the carcinogenicity of butyl benzyl phthalate.

Overall evaluation

Butyl benzyl phthalate is *not classifiable as to its carcinogenicity to humans (Group 3).*

6. References

Agarwal, D.K., Maronpot, R.R., Lamb J.C., IV & Kluwe, W.M. (1985) Adverse effects of butyl benzyl phthalate on the reproductive and hematopoietic systems of male rats. *Toxicology*, **35**, 189–206

American Conference of Governmental Industrial Hygienists (1998) *TLVs and Other Occupational Exposure Values—1998 CD-ROM*, Cincinnati, OH

Ashby, J., Brady, A., Elcombe, C.R., Elliott, B.M., Ishmael, J., Odum, J., Tugwood, J.D., Kettle, S. & Purchase, I.F.H. (1994) Mechanistically-based human hazard assessment of peroxisome proliferator-induced hepatocarcinogenesis. *Hum. exp. Toxicol.*, **13** (Suppl. 2), S1–S117

Ashby, J., Tinwell, H., Lefevre, P.A., Odum, J., Paton, D., Millward, S.W., Tittensor, S. & Brooks, A.N. (1997) Normal sexual development of rats exposed to butyl benzyl phthalate from conception to weaning. *Regul. Toxicol. Pharmacol.*, **26**, 102–118

Barber, E.D., Astill, B.D., Moran, E.J., Schneider, B.F., Gray, T.J.B., Lake, B.G. & Evans, J.G. (1987) Peroxisome induction studies on seven phthalate esters. *Toxicol. ind. Health*, **3**, 7–24

Bentley, P., Calder, I., Elcombe, C., Grasso, P., Stringer, D. & Wiegand, H.-J. (1993) Hepatic peroxisome proliferation in rodents and its significance for humans. *Food chem. Toxicol.*, **31**, 857–907

Calley, D., Autian, J. & Guess, W.L. (1966) Toxicology of a series of phthalate esters. *J. pharm. Sci.*, **55**, 158–162

Cattley, R.C., DeLuca, J., Elcombe, C., Fenner-Crisp, P., Lake, B.G., Marsman, D.S., Pastoor, T.A., Popp, J.A., Robinson, D.E., Schwetz, B., Tugwood, J. & Wahli, W. (1998) Do peroxisome proliferating compounds pose a hepatocarcinogenic hazard to humans? *Regul. Toxicol. Pharmacol.*, **27**, 47–60

Chemical Information Services (1995) *Directory of World Chemical Producers 1995/96 Standard Edition*, Dallas, TX, p. 86

Eigenberg, D.A., Bozigian, H.P., Carter, D.E. & Sipes, I.G. (1986) Distribution, excretion, and metabolism of butylbenzyl phthalate in the rat. *J. Toxicol. environ. Health*, **17**, 445–456

Elsisi, A.E., Carter, D.E. & Sipes, I.G. (1989) Dermal absorption of phthalate diesters in rats. *Fundam. appl. Toxicol.*, **12**, 70–77

Ema, M., Murai, T., Itami, T. & Kawasaki, H. (1990) Evaluation of the teratogenic potential of the plasticizer butyl benzyl phthalate in rats. *J. appl. Toxicol.*, **10**, 339–343

Ema, M., Itami, T. & Kawasaki, H. (1991) Evaluation of the embryolethality of butyl benzyl phthalate by conventional and pair-feeding studies in rats. *J. appl. Toxicol.*, **11**, 39–42

Ema, M., Itami, T. & Kawasaki, H. (1992a) Embryolethality and teratogenicity of butyl benzyl phthalate in rats. *J. appl. Toxicol.*, **12**, 179–183

Ema, M., Itami, T. & Kawasaki, H. (1992b) Effect of period of exposure on the developmental toxicity of butyl benzyl phthalate in rats. *J. appl. Toxicol.*, **12**, 57–61

Ema, M., Itami, T. & Kawasaki, H. (1992c) Teratogenic evaluation of butyl benzyl phthalate in rats by gastric intubation. *Toxicol. Lett.*, **61**, 1–7

Ema, M., Itami, T. & Kawasaki, H. (1993) Teratogenic phase specificity of butyl benzyl phthalate in rats. *Toxicology*, **79**, 11–19

Ema, M., Kurosaka, R., Amano, H. & Ogawa, Y. (1994) Embryolethality of butyl benzyl phthalate during early pregnancy in the rat. *Reprod. Toxicol.*, **8**, 231–236

Ema, M., Kurosaka, R., Amano, H. & Ogawa, Y. (1995) Comparative developmental toxicity of *n*-butyl benzyl phthalate and di-*n*-butyl phthalate in rats. *Arch. environ. Contam. Toxicol.*, **28**, 223–228

Ema, M., Harazono, A., Miyawaki, E. & Ogawa, Y. (1996a) Characterization of developmental toxicity of mono-*n*-benzyl phthalate in rats. *Reprod. Toxicol.*, **10**, 365–372

Ema, M., Kurosaka, R., Harazono, A., Amano, H. & Ogawa, Y. (1996b) Phase specificity of developmental toxicity after oral administration of mono-*n*-butyl phthalate in rats. *Arch. environ. Contam. Toxicol.*, **31**, 170–176

Ema, M., Harazono, A., Miyawaki, E. & Ogawa, Y. (1996c) Developmental toxicity of mono-*n*-benzyl phthalate, one of the metabolites of the plasticizer *n*-butyl benzyl phthalate in rats. *Toxicol. Lett.*, **86**, 19–25

Ema, M., Miyawaki, E. & Kawahima, K. (1998) Reproductive effects of butyl benzyl phthalate in pregnant and pseudopregnant rats. *Reprod. Toxicol.*, **12**, 127–132

Erickson, N.G. (1965) The metabolism of diphenyl phthalate and butylbenzyl phthalate in the beagle dog. *Diss. Abstr.*, **26**, 3014–3015

Galloway, S.M., Armstrong, M.J., Reuben, C., Colman, S., Brown, B., Cannon, C., Bloom, A.D., Nakamura, F., Ahmed, M., Duk, S., Rimpo, J., Margolin, B.H., Resnick, M.A., Anderson, B. & Zeiger, E. (1987) Chromosome aberrations and sister chromatid exchanges in Chinese hamster ovary cells: Evaluations of 108 chemicals. *Environ. mol. Mutag.*, **10** (Suppl. 10), 1–175

Gosselin, R.E., Smith, R.P., Hodge, H.C. & Braddock, J.E. (1984) *Clinical Toxicology of Commercial Products*, 5th Ed., Baltimore, MD, Williams & Wilkins, p. II-204

Hammond, B.G., Levinskas, G.J., Robinson, E.C. & Johannsen, F.R. (1987) A review of the sub-chronic toxicity of butyl benzyl phthalate. *Toxicol. ind. Health*, **3**, 79–98

Harris, C.A., Henttu, P., Parker, M.G. & Sumpter, J.P. (1997) The estrogenic activity of phthalate esters *in vitro*. *Environ. Health Perspectives*, **105**, 802–811

IARC (1982) *IARC Monographs on the Evaluation of the Carcinogenic Risk of Chemicals to Humans*, Vol. 29, *Some Industrial Chemicals and Dyestuffs*, Lyon, pp. 193–201

IARC (1987) *IARC Monographs on the Evaluation of Carcinogenic Risks to Humans*, Suppl. 7, *Overall Evaluations of Carcinogenicity: An Updating of* IARC Monographs *Volumes 1 to 42*, Lyon, p. 59

IARC (1995) *Peroxisome Proliferation and its Role in Carcinogenesis. Views and Expert Opinions of an IARC Working Group* (IARC Technical Report No. 24), Lyon

International Labour Office (1991) *Occupational Exposure Limits for Airborne Toxic Substances*, 3rd Ed. (Occupational Safety and Health Series No. 37), Geneva, pp. 62–63

Kozumbo, W.J., Kroll, R. & Rubin, R.J. (1982) Assessment of the mutagenicity of phthalate esters. *Environ. Health Perspectives*, **45**, 103–109

Lake, B.G. (1995a) Mechanisms of hepatocarcinogenicity of peroxisome-proliferating drugs and chemicals. *Ann. Rev. Pharmacol. Toxicol.*, **35**, 483–507

Lake, B.G. (1995b) The biology and molecular consequences of peroxisome proliferation in experimental animals and humans. In: *Peroxisome Proliferation and its Role in Carcinogenesis* (IARC Technical Report No. 24), Lyon, pp. 19–40

Lewis, R.J., Jr (1993) *Hawley's Condensed Chemical Dictionary*, 12th Ed., New York, Van Nostrand Reinhold Co., p. 183

Lin, L.I.-K. (1987) The use of multivariate analysis to compare peroxisome induction data on phthalate esters in rats. *Toxicol. ind. Health*, **3**, 25–48

Mikuriya, H., Ikemoto, I. & Tanaka, A. (1988) Urinary metabolites contributing to testicular damage induced by butylbenzyl phthalate. *Jikeikai med. J.*, **35**, 403–409

Milligan, S.R., Balasubramanian, A.V. & Kalita, J.C. (1998) Relative potency of xenobiotic estrogens in an acute *in vivo* mammalian assay. *Environ. Health Perspectives*, **106**, 23–26

Myhr, B.C. & Caspary, W.J. (1991) Chemical mutagenesis at the thymidine kinase locus in L5178Y mouse lymphoma cells: Results for 31 coded compounds in the National Toxicology Program. *Environ. mol. Mutag.*, **18**, 51–83

National Institute for Occupational Safety and Health (1998) *National Occupational Exposure Survey (1981–83)*, Cincinnati, OH

National Library of Medicine (1988a) *Toxic Chemical Release Inventory 1987 & 1996* (TRI87 & TRI96), Bethesda, MD

National Library of Medicine (1998b) *Hazardous Substances Data Bank (HSDB)*, Bethesda, MD [Record No. 2107]

National Library of Medicine (1998c) *Registry of Effects of Toxic Substances (RTECS)*, Bethesda, MD [Record No. 32]

National Toxicology Program (1982) *Carcinogenesis Bioassay of Butyl Phthalate (CAS No. 85-68-7) in F344/N Rats and B6C3F$_1$ Mice (Feed Study)* (NTP-80-25; NIH Publ. No. 82-1769), Research Triangle Park, NC

National Toxicology Program (1991) *NTP Chemical Repository Data Sheet: Butyl Benzyl Phthalate*, Research Triangle Park, NC

National Toxicology Program (1997a) *Carcinogen Bioassay of Butyl Benzyl Phthalate (CAS No. 85-68-7) in F344 Rats and B6C3F1 Mice (Feed Studies)* (Tech. Rep. Ser. No. 458; NIH Publ. No. 97-3374), Research Triangle Park, NC

National Toxicology Program (1997b) *Effect of Dietary Restriction on Toxicology and Carcinogenesis in F344/N Rats and B6C3F$_1$ Mice* (Tech. Rep. Ser. No. 460), Research Triangle Park, NC [Draft]

Piersma, A., Verhoef, A. & Dortant, P.M. (1995) Evaluation of the OECD 421 reproductive toxicity screening test protocol using butyl benzyl phthalate. *Toxicology*, **99**, 191–197

Schwetz, B.A & Harris, M.W. (1993) Developmental toxicology: Status of the field and contribution of the National Toxicology Program. *Environ. Health Perspectives*, **100**, 269-282

Sharpe, R.M., Fisher, J.S., Millar, M.M., Jobling, S. & Sumpter, J.P. (1995) Gestational and lactational exposure of rats to xenoestrogens results in reduced testicular size and sperm production. *Environ. Health Perspectives*, **103**, 1136–1143

Sharpe, R.M., Turner, K.J. & Sumpter, J.P. (1998) Endocrine disruptors and testis development. *Environ. Health Perspectives*, **106**, A220–A221

Singletary, K., MacDonald, C. & Wallig, M. (1997) The plasticizer benzyl butyl phthalate (BBP) inhibits 7,12-dimethylbenz[a]anthracene-induced rat mammary DNA adduct formation and tumorigenesis. *Carcinogenesis*, **18**, 1669–1673

Solutia (1998) *Summary of Potential Exposures to Butyl Benzyl Phthalate*, St Louis, MO

Valencia, R., Mason, J.M., Woodruff, R.C. & Zimmering, S. (1985) Chemical mutagenesis testing in Drosophila. III. Results of 48 coded compounds tested for the National Toxicology Program. *Environ. Mutag.*, **7**, 325–348

Verschueren, K. (1996) *Handbook of Environmental Data on Organic Chemicals*, 3rd Ed., New York, Van Nostrand Reinhold Co., pp. 372–375

WHO (1993) *Guidelines for Drinking Water Quality*, 2nd Ed., Vol. 1, *Recommendations*, Geneva

Zacharewski, T.R., Meek, M.D., Clemons, J.H., Wu, Z.F., Fielden, M.R. & Matthews, J.B. (1998) Examination of the *in vitro* and *in vivo* estrogenic activities of eight commercial phthalate esters. *Toxicol. Sci.*, **46**, 282–293

Zeiger, E., Haworth, S., Mortelmans, K. & Speck, W. (1985) Mutagenicity testing of di(2-ethylhexyl)phthalate and related chemicals in Salmonella. *Environ. Mutag.*, **7**, 213–232

CHLOROFORM

This substance was considered by previous working groups, in 1971 (IARC, 1972), 1978 (IARC, 1979) and 1987 (IARC, 1987). Since that time, new data have become available, and these have been incorporated into the monograph and taken into consideration in the present evaluation.

1. Exposure Data

1.1 Chemical and physical data

1.1.1 *Nomenclature*

Chem. Abstr. Serv. Reg. No.: 67-66-3
Deleted CAS Reg. No.: 8013-54-5
Chem. Abstr. Name: Trichloromethane
IUPAC Systematic Name: Chloroform
Synonyms: HCC 20; R 20; R 20 (refrigerant); trichloroform

1.1.2 *Structural and molecular formulae and relative molecular mass*

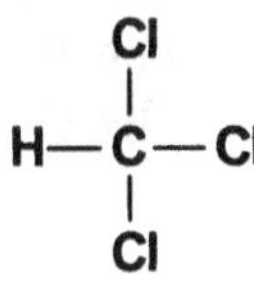

$CHCl_3$ Relative molecular mass: 119.38

1.1.3 *Chemical and physical properties of the pure substance*

(*a*) *Description*: Colourless liquid with characteristic odour (Budavari, 1996)
(*b*) *Boiling-point*: 61.1°C (Lide, 1997)
(*c*) *Melting-point*: –63.6°C (Lide, 1997)
(*d*) *Density*: 1.4832 g/cm^3 at 20°C (Lide, 1997)
(*e*) *Solubility*: Slightly soluble in water; miscible in ethanol and ethyl ether; soluble in acetone (Lide, 1997)
(*f*) *Volatility*: Vapour pressure, 21.3 kPa at 20°C; relative vapour density (air = 1), 4.12 (National Toxicology Program, 1991)
(*g*) *Octanol/water partition coefficient (P)*: log P, 1.97 at 20°C (Verschueren, 1996)
(*h*) *Conversion factor*: mg/m^3 = 4.88 × ppm

1.2 Production and use

Worldwide commercial production of chloroform amounted to about 440 000 tonnes in 1987. Significant amounts are also produced as by-products in the chlorination of water and in the bleaching of paper pulp (WHO, 1994). Information available in 1995 indicated that chloroform was produced in 19 countries (Chemical Information Services, 1995). The volume of commercial production of chloroform in the United States was approximately 229 000 tonnes in 1991 and 216 000 tonnes in 1993 (International Trade Commission, 1991, 1993).

Chloroform is used in pesticide formulations, as a solvent and as a chemical intermediate. Its use as an anaesthetic and in proprietary medicines is banned in some countries (WHO, 1994). Chloroform is used as a solvent for fats, oils, rubber, alkaloids, waxes, gutta-percha and resins; as a cleansing agent; in fire extinguishers to lower the freezing temperature of carbon tetrachloride; and in the rubber industry (Budavari, 1996). It is used in the manufacture of fluorocarbon plastics, resins, refrigerants and propellants. It has been used as an analgesic, muscle relaxant, carminative, flavouring agent, preservative, bactericide, heat-transfer medium and as a counter-irritant in liniments (National Toxicology Program, 1991).

1.3 Occurrence

1.3.1 *Natural occurrence*

Chloroform is not known to occur naturally.

1.3.2 *Occupational exposure*

According to the 1981–83 National Occupational Exposure Survey (National Institute for Occupational Safety and Health, 1998), approximately 96 000 workers in the United States were potentially exposed to chloroform. Occupational exposure to chloroform may occur during its production and during its use as a solvent and chemical intermediate.

1.3.3 *Environmental occurrence*

The concentrations of chloroform found in the oceans in remote regions are typically several nanograms per litre. In coastal waters, inland rivers, lakes and groundwater, the concentrations range from several nanograms per litre in rural and remote areas up to 100 μg/L or more in areas directly affected by industrialized sources. In drinking-water treated by chlorination, the concentrations are typically 10–100 μg/L (WHO, 1994; National Library of Medicine, 1998a).

The reported concentrations of chloroform in ambient air range from < 1 μg/m^3 in remote regions to around 10 μg/m^3 in urban areas. Indoor air concentrations in residences and offices can be higher, and the average concentration in the air above indoor swimming pools has been reported to be about 100 μg/m^3 (WHO, 1994).

Chloroform has also been detected in a variety of foods at concentrations of < 1 to 90 μg/kg (WHO, 1994).

On the basis of estimates of mean exposure from various media, the general population is exposed to chloroform principally in food (approximately 1 μg/kg bw per day), drinking-water (approximately 0.5 μg/kg bw per day) and indoor air (0.3–1 μg/kg bw per day). The estimated intake from outdoor air is considerably less (0.01 μg/kg bw per day). The estimated total intakes of individuals living in dwellings supplied with tap-water containing relatively high concentrations of chloroform may be up to 10 μg/kg bw per day (WHO, 1994).

According to the United States Environmental Protection Agency Toxic Chemical Release Inventory for 1987, 12 000 000 kg of chloroform were released into the air, 560 000 kg were discharged into water, 7000 kg were disposed of by underground injection, and 18 000 kg were released onto the land from manufacturing and processing facilities in the United States. By 1996, 4 200 000 kg were released into the air, 150 000 kg were discharged into water, 21 000 kg were disposed of by underground injection, and 15 000 kg were released onto the land (National Library of Medicine, 1998b).

1.4 Regulations and guidelines

The American Conference of Governmental Industrial Hygienists (1997) has recommended 49 mg/m^3 as the 8-h time-weighted average threshold limit value for occupational exposure to chloroform in workplace air. Values of 9.8–240 mg/m^3 have been used as standards or guidelines in other countries (International Labour Office, 1991).

WHO (1993) has established an international drinking-water guideline for chloroform of 200 μg/L.

2. Studies of Cancer in Humans

2.1 Ecological studies

In some ecological studies, chloroform or total trihalomethane concentrations in drinking-water or surrogate exposure indicators, such as plain chlorination of drinking-water, were correlated with cancer mortality or incidence, but the site-specific excess risks were inconsistent across studies. The results of such studies are not presented here, as ecological studies suffer from several drawbacks, deriving from the impossibility of linking exposure to the end-point at the individual level; further limitations of ecological studies are described in the Preamble. In addition, exposure was usually assessed on the basis of cross-sectional sampling. Although the risk estimates derived in ecological studies are usually adjusted for some sociodemographic parameters at the geographical level, ample possibility is left for uncontrolled confounding.

2.2 Cohort studies

These studies are summarized in Table 1.

Wilkins and Comstock (1981) followed-up 14 553 male and 16 227 female residents over 25 years of age of Washington County, MD (United States) using data from a census

Table 1. Cohort studies of chloroform exposure or water chlorination and cancer

Reference	Population/ follow-up	Sex	Exposure	Cancer site	RR	95% CI	Comments
Wilkins & Comstock (1981)	Washington County, MD, USA, 1963–75	14 583 men and 16 247 women	Surface and chlorination (average, 107 µg/L chloroform) versus deep well and no chlorination	*Incidence in men*			Adjustment for age, marital status, education, smoking, church attendance, adequacy of housing, persons per room
				Liver	0.71	0.19–3.5	
				Kidney	0.78	0.27–2.7	
				Bladder	1.8	0.80–4.8	
				Incidence in women			
				Liver	1.8	0.64–6.8	
				Kidney	1.0	0.26–6.0	
				Bladder	1.6	0.54–6.3	
				Mortality, men and women			
				Liver	3.0	0.92–15	
				Kidney	2.8	0.7–23	
				Breast	2.3	1.2–4.9	
				Bladder	2.2	0.7–9.4	
				Oesophagus	1.8	0.5–8.7	
				Cervix	1.7	0.6–6.7	
				Leukaemia	1.6	0.9–3.1	
				Rectum	1.4	0.7–3.2	
				Ovary	1.3	0.4–4.9	
				Lung	1.0	0.6–1.6	
				Colon	0.9	0.6–1.4	
				Prostate	0.9	0.4–2.1	
				Stomach	0.6	0.3–1.4	
Doyle *et al.* (1997)	Iowa Women's Health Study (28 237), 1963–75	Women	Chloroform concentration from statewide survey of water supplies	Colon	1.7	1.1–2.5	RR for highest categories (> 13 µg/L; *p* (trend) < 0.05); adjustment for a number of factors (see text)
				Lung	1.2	0.7–2.0	
				Melanoma	1.1	0.4–3.2	
				All cancers	1.2	1.0–1.5	

RR, relative risk; CI, confidence interval

conducted in 1963. Cancer incidence and mortality rates in 1963–75 were assessed in two subcohorts: people exposed to chlorinated surface water (average chloroform concentration, 107 μg/L) and users of water from deep wells with no chlorination. Risk ratios were calculated by contrasting the two cohorts, with adjustment for age, marital status, education, smoking, church attendance, adequacy of housing and number of persons per room. Incidence rates were reported for several subsites of cancer. No significant elevations or deficits were seen for cancers of the liver, kidney or urinary bladder in either men or women who drank chlorinated surface water. The only significant excess risk was reported for death from breast cancer (relative risk, 2.7; 95% confidence interval [CI], 1.2–4.9), and excesses of borderline significance were found for liver cancer (relative risk, 3.0; 95% CI, 0.92–15).

The cohort involved in the Iowa Women's Health Study in the United States, consisting of 41 836 women aged 55–69 in 1986, was followed-up for cancer incidence through 31 December 1993 (Doyle *et al.*, 1997). The source of the drinking-water for each cohort member was assessed from a mail survey in 1989. Women who reported having drunk municipal or private well-water for less than the past 10 years were excluded. Data on 252 municipal water supplies in 1979 and 856 municipal water systems in 1986–87 were used to assess exposure. All women who lived in the same community and reported drinking municipal water were assigned the same concentration of trihalomethanes, including chloroform. The chloroform concentrations in 1986–87 were categorized as below the detection limit (reference) or 1–2, 3–13 and 14–287 μg/L. The incidences of a number of cancers were estimated in the categories. Significantly increasing trends over the categories were observed for cancers of the colon (risk ratio for highest versus lowest category, 1.7 [95% CI, 1.1–2.5]; $p < 0.01$ for trend), lung (1.8 [95% CI, 0.97–2.6]; $p = 0.025$ for trend), melanoma (3.4 [95% CI, 1.3–8.6]; $p = 0.049$ for trend) and all cancers (1.2 [95% CI, 1.0–1.5]; $p < 0.01$ for trend) after adjustment for some potential confounding variables. The excess of cancers at all sites was driven predominantly by excess incidences of cancers of the colon, lung and endometrium and malignant melanoma. All of the relative risks were adjusted for age, education, smoking, physical activity, fruit and vegetable intake, total energy intake, body mass index and waist-to-hip ratio.

2.3 Case–control studies

These studies are summarized in Table 2.

2.3.1 *Multiple sites*

Brenniman *et al.* (1980) studied 3208 deceased cases of gastrointestinal and urinary tract cancers and 43 666 non-cancer deaths as controls in Illinois (United States). All of the deaths were extracted from state death certificate tapes over the period 1973–76 and classified according to residence in communities served by chlorinated or unchlorinated groundwater on the basis of data obtained from water-treatment plants by referring to the 1963 inventory of municipal water facilities. Populations using surface water supplies and those living in Cook County (mostly Chicago) were excluded. Slight excesses (odds

Table 2. Case–control studies of chloroform exposure or water chlorination and cancer

Reference	Population	Sex	Exposure	Cancer site		Odds ratio	95% CI or *p* value	Comments
Multiple sites								
Brenniman *et al.* (1980)	Illinois, USA; 3208 deaths 1973–76 from gastrointestinal and urinary-tract cancers; 43 666 non-cancer controls	Men and women	Chlorinated/unchlorinated water supplies based on residence	Oesophagus	Men	0.9	NS	
					Women	1.1	NS	
				Stomach	Men	0.9	NS	
					Women	1.1	NS	
				Colon/rectum	Men	1.1	NS	
					Women	1.2	< 0.05	
				Colon	Men	1.0	NS	
					Women	1.2	NS	
				Rectum	Men	1.1	NS	
					Women	1.3	NS	
				Liver	Men	0.9	NS	
					Women	1.1	NS	
				Gall-bladder	Men	0.6	NS	
					Women	1.2	NS	
				Digestive (excl. liver)				
					Men	1.0	NS	
					Women	1.1	< 0.05	
				Urinary bladder	Men	1.1	NS	
					Women	0.7	NS	
				All gastrointestinal and urinary				
				Total	Men			
					Women	1.0	NS	
				SMSA	Men	1.1	NS	
					Women	1.0	NS	
				Urban	Men	1.3	< 0.05	
					Women	1.0	NS	
						1.3	< 0.25	
				Rural	Men	1.1	NS	
					Women	1.3	NS	

Table 2 (contd)

Reference	Population	Sex	Exposure	Cancer site		Odds ratio	95% CI or *p* value	Comments
Multiple sites (contd)								
Alavanja *et al.* (1980)	New York State, USA, 7 counties 3446 from gastro-intestinal and urinary-tract cancers; 3444 matched controls. Unknown number of cases of lung cancer	Men and women	Chlorination/no chlorination at usual place of residence	All gastrointestinal and urinary				
				Total	Men	2.1	< 0.005	
					Women	1.4	< 0.005	
				Urban	Men	3.6	< 0.005	
					Women	2.2	< 0.005	
				Lung				
				Total	Men	1.8	< 0.005	
					Women	1.5	NS	
				Urban	Men	3.2	< 0.005	
					Women	2.9		
				Oesophagus	Men	2.4	< 0.05	
					Women	1.3	NS	
				Stomach	Men	1.7	< 0.025	
					Women	2.2	< 0.025	
				Colon	Men	2.0	< 0.005	
					Women	1.3	NS	
				Rectum	Men	2.3	< 0.005	
					Women	1.3	NS	
				Liver and kidney				
					Men	2.8	< 0.005	
					Women	1.5	NS	
				Pancreas	Men	2.6	< 0.005	
					Women	1.3	NS	
				Urinary bladder	Men	2.0	< 0.005	
					Women	0.8	NS	
				Total	Men	2.1	< 0.005	
					Women	1.4	< 0.005	

Table 2 (contd)

Reference	Population	Sex	Exposure	Cancer site	Odds ratio	95% CI or *p* value	Comments
Multiple sites (contd)							
Gottlieb	Louisiana, USA	Men and	Chlorination/no chlori-	Rectum	1.8	1.3–2.6	
et al. (1981,	11 349 deaths from	women	nation of water source	Lung	1.4	1.0–1.8	
1982);	cancer; 22 698 non-		at death	Breast	1.5	1.2–2.0	
Gottlieb &	cancer deaths		Chlorination level	Rectum	1.3	0.9–1.8	Low (< 1.09 ppm)
Carr (1982)					1.7	1.2–2.4	High (> 1.09 ppm)
Kanarek &	Wisconsin, USA	Women	Chlorinated/unchlori-	Oesophagus	0.30	NS	Multiple adjustments
Young	[numbers not given]		nated water supplies	Stomach	1.3	NS	
(1982)				Colon	1.5	< 0.02	
				Rectum	1.6	NS	
				Liver	1.3	NS	
				Pancreas	1.5	NS	
				Kidney	0.5	NS	
				Urinary bladder	1.4	NS	
				Lung	0.7	0.6	
				Brain	4.7	< 0.03	
				Breast	0.8	NS	
			Organic contamination and chlorination	Colon	1.8	0.03	
			Chlorinated surface water		2.8	0.01	
			Purified chlorinated		1.7	0.01	
			Unpurified chlorinated		1.5	0.05	
			Organic contamination and chlorination	Brain	6.9	0.03	
			Unpurified chlorinated		4.4	0.04	

Table 2 (contd)

Reference	Population	Sex	Exposure	Cancer site	Odds ratio	95% CI or p value	Comments
Multiple sites (contd)							
Siemiatycki (1991)	Montréal, Canada 99 oesophageal cancer, 251 stomach cancer, 497 colon cancer, 257 rectal cancer, 116 pancreatic cancer, 857 lung cancer, 449 prostate cancer, 484 bladder cancer, 177 kidney cancer, 103 skin melanoma, 215 non-Hodgkin lymphoma	Men	Chloroform, occupational	Prostate	4.0	1.4–12	90% CI; multiple adjustments
				Lung	8.8	1.2–65	French Canadians
Colon/rectum							
Lawrence *et al.* (1984)	New York State (USA) teachers, deaths 395 cases, 395 controls	Women	Chlorinated/unchlorinated water supplies	Colorectal cancer	1.1	0.8–1.4	90% CI
Young *et al.* (1987)	Wisconsin, USA 347 cases; 639 cancer controls; 611 population controls	Men and women	Cumulative trihalomethane (mg), population controls	Colon			Response rate, 65%; results for general population controls are presented
				Over lifetime			
				< 100	1.0		
				100–300	1.1	0.7–1.8	
				> 300	0.73	0.4–1.2	
				Over past 10 years			
				< 33	1.0		
				33–99	0.9	0.5–1.5	
				> 99	1.0	0.4–2.3	

Table 2 (contd)

Reference	Population	Sex	Exposure	Cancer site	Odds ratio	95% CI or *p* value	Comments
Urinary bladder							
Cantor *et al.* (1987)	USA; 2805 cases; 5258 population controls	Men and women	Years of residence with chlorinated surface drinking-water source	*Men, low consumption (below median)*			Newly diagnosed cases; interviews
				Never	1.0		
				≥ 60 years	0.8	0.5–1.5	*p* trend = 0.7
				Women, low consumption (below median)			
				Never	1.0		
				≥ 60 years	1.7	0.7–4.0	*p* trend = 0.4
				Men, high consumption (above median)			
				Never	1.0		
				≥ 60 years	1.2	0.7–2.1	*p* trend = 0.4
				Women, high consumption (above mean)			
				Never	1.0		
				≥ 60 years	3.2	1.2–8.7	*p* trend = 0.02
			Nonsmokers only	*Men, low consumption (below median)*			
				Never	1.0		
				≥ 60 years	1.3	0.4–4.4	*p* trend = 0.6
				Women, low consumption (below median)			
				Never	1.0		
				≥ 60 years	4.3	1.3–14	*p* trend = 0.02

Table 2 (contd)

Reference	Population	Sex	Exposure	Cancer site	Odds ratio	95% CI or *p* value	Comments
Urinary bladder (contd)							
Cantor *et al.* (1987) (contd)				*Men, high consumption (above median)*			
				Never	1.0		
				≥ 60 years	3.7	1.1–12	*p* trend = 0.02
				Women, high consumption (above median)			
				Never	1.0		
				≥ 60 years	3.6	0.8–15	*p* trend = 0.2
Zierler *et al.* (1988)	Massachusetts, USA; mortality; 614 cases, 1074 population controls	Men and women	Chlorine versus chloramine by residence	Crude analysis	1.3	1.1–1.7	Lifetime exposure
					1.2	1.0–1.5	Usual exposure
				Adjusted analysis	1.6	1.2–2.1	Lifetime exposure
					1.4	1.1–1.8	Usual exposure See text for adjustment
McGeehin *et al.* (1993)	Colorado; USA; 261 cases, 327 population controls	Men and women	Crude analysis by years of exposure to chlorinated water and by smoking status	*Nonsmokers*			Telephone interviews with subjects for residential and water source histories; water utility data
				0 years	1.0		
				1–11 years	0.8	0.2–2.4	
				12–34 years	0.9	0.3–2.3	
				> 34 years	2.9	1.2–7.4	
				Smokers			
				0 years	1.0		
				1–11 years	0.8	0.4–1.4	
				12–34 years	1.4	0.8–2.4	
				> 34 years	2.1	1.1–3.8	
			Adjusted analysis by years of exposure to chlorinated water	0 years	1.0		See text for adjustments
				1–10 years	0.7	0.4–1.3	*p* for trend < 0.01
				11–20 years	1.4	0.8–2.5	
				21–30 years	1.5	0.8–2.9	
				> 30 years	1.8	1.1–2.9	

Table 2 (contd)

Reference	Population	Sex	Exposure	Cancer site	Odds ratio	95% CI or *p* value	Comments
Urinary bladder (contd)							
Cantor *et al.* (1998)	Iowa, USA 1123 cases 1983 controls	Men and women	Total lifetime trihalomethanes (g) Highest category (≥ 2.42)	 Men Women	 1.8 0.6	 1.2–2.7 0.3–1.4	Multiple adjustments *p* for trend = 0.05 *p* for trend, NS
			Lifetime average total trihalomethanes (µg/L) Highest category (≥ 46.4)	Men Women	1.5 0.6	1.0–2.4 0.3–1.3	*p* for trend = 0.02 *p* for trend = 0.33
Colorectal cancer							
Hildesheim *et al.* (1998)	Iowa, USA 560 colon cancers 537 rectal cancers 1983 controls with information on water use	Men and women	Total lifetime trihalomethanes (g) Highest category (≥ 2.42)	Colon Rectum	1.1 1.6	0.7–1.8 1.0–2.6	*p* for trend, NS *p* for trend = 0.08
			Lifetime average total trihalomethanes (g/L) Highest category (≥ 46.4)	Colon Rectum	1.1 1.7	0.7–1.6 1.1–2.6	*p* for trend, NS *p* for trend = 0.01
Brain cancer							
Heineman *et al.* (1994)	Southern Louisiana, New Jersey, Philadelphia, USA; 300 cases 320 controls	Men	Chloroform (occupational)	Astrocytic brain Duration of exposure			
				Never	1.0		
				2–20 years	0.8	0.4–1.4	
				≥ 21 years	2.3	0.8–6.6	*p* for trend, NS

Table 2 (contd)

Reference	Population	Sex	Exposure	Cancer site	Odds ratio	95% CI or *p* value	Comments
Brain cancer (contd)							
Heineman *et al.* (1994) (contd)				Cumulative exposure score			
				0			
				Low	1.0		
				Medium	0.8		0.4–1.6
				High	1.3		0.6–2.9
					1.8		0.4–7.8
							p for trend, NS
				Averate intensity			
				0	1.0		
				Low-medium	1.0		0.6–1.7
				High	1.4		0.4–5.2

CI, confidence interval; NS, not significant ($p > 0.05$); SMSA, standard metropolitan statistical area ratio, 1.2, $p < 0.05$) were found in chlorinated communities for cancers of the colon and rectum combined and for cancers of the total digestive tract only in women. The odds ratios were adjusted for age, sex, urban or rural residence and standard metropolitan statistical area or other areas. The odds ratios for total gastrointestinal and urinary tract cancers were significantly elevated only among women in standard metropolitan statistical areas (odds ratio, 1.3; $p \leq 0.025$) and women in urban areas (odds ratio, 1.2; $p \leq 0.05$). [The Working Group noted that the chloroform concentrations in drinking-water were not given.]

Alavanja *et al.* (1980) reported on a case–control study of 3446 deaths from gastro-intestinal and urinary tract cancers conducted in seven counties in New York State (United States) selected for a low rate of immigration and no major change in the source or distribution of water supply during the preceding 15 years. The counties were then classified according to whether the predominant source of drinking-water was chlorinated groundwater, chlorinated surface water or unchlorinated groundwater. The cases and 3444 matched controls and their 'usual place of residence' were identified from New York State death certificates for the period 1968–70. Each residence was classified into one of three exposure categories defined by the drinking-water source of the county. Raised odds ratios, most of which were significant, were observed for cancers of the oesophagus, stomach, large intestine, rectum, liver and kidney, pancreas and urinary bladder (see Table 2). The odds ratios consistently exceeded unity in people of each sex, with one exception: 0.82 for bladder cancer in women. Mortality from lung cancer was also studied [number of deaths not reported], and significantly raised odds ratios ($p < 0.005$) were found for men (odds ratio, 1.8) and in urban areas (odds ratio, 3.2). [The Working Group noted that it is not clear which confounders were adjusted for and that the chloroform concentrations in the drinking-water were not given.]

Gottlieb *et al.* (1981), Gottlieb and Carr (1982) and Gottlieb *et al.* (1982) conducted a multisite case–control study between 1960 and 1975 in parishes in South Louisiana (United States). Cancer deaths were compared with non-cancer deaths individually matched on age, sex, race and year of death. Use of a chlorinated water source at the residence at the time of death was the exposure indicator. Excesses were found for rectal cancer (odds ratio, 1.8; 95% CI, 1.3–2.6), lung cancer (odds ratio, 1.4; 95% CI, 1.0–1.8) and breast cancer (odds ratio, 1.5; 95% CI, 1.2–2.0) in association with concentrations of chlorine greater than or less than 1.09 ppm when compared with no chlorination. There was a suggestion of an exposure–response gradient for rectal cancer only. [The Working Group noted that the chloroform concentrations were not given.]

A multisite case–control study was conducted of deaths from cancer and other causes among white women who had lived for 15–20 years before their death in 28 counties in Wisconsin (United States). Counties with less than a 10% population increase attributed to immigration over the previous 20 years and with both chlorinated and unchlorinated water supplies were selected (Young *et al.*, 1981; Kanarek & Young, 1982). Data from all 202 waterworks and the 1970 Wisconsin Waterworks Survey were used to obtain longitudinal data on chlorine concentrations and other water characteristics. Cases of cancers of the oesophagus, stomach, colon, rectum, liver, pancreas, urinary bladder, kidney, lung, brain and breast and controls were ascertained during a follow-up period in 1972–77. The results were presented as contrasts between chlorinated and unchlorinated water; urbanization, marital status, occupation, age, organic contamination of water, water purification and source depth were included in logistic models. Significant ($p < 0.05$) excess odds ratios were found for cancers of the colon (odds ratio, 1.5; $p < 0.02$) and brain (odds ratio, 4.7; $p < 0.03$). For colon cancer, interactions were found between chlorination and water with organic contamination (odds ratio, 1.8; $p = 0.03$), surface water (odds ratio, 2.8; $p < 0.01$) and purified water (odds ratio, 1.8; $p < 0.01$). Similarly, excesses were observed for brain cancer in association with exposure jointly to chlorination and organic contamination (odds ratio, 6.9; $p = 0.03$) and unpurified water (odds ratio, 4.4; $p = 0.04$). [The Working Group noted that the chloroform concentrations in drinking-water were not given.]

A population-based case–control study of cancer associated with occupational exposure among male residents of Montréal, Canada, aged 35–70, included histologically confirmed cases of several types of cancer, newly diagnosed between 1979 and 1985 in 19 major hospitals (Siemiatycki, 1991). Interviews were carried out with 3730 cancer patients (response rate, 82%) and 533 age-stratified controls from the general population (response rate, 72%). The main cancer sites included were: oesophagus (99 cases), stomach (251 cases), colon (497 cases), rectum (257 cases), pancreas (116 cases), lung (857 cases), prostate (449 cases), bladder (484 cases), kidney (177 cases), skin melanoma (103 cases) and non-Hodgkin lymphoma (215 cases). For each site of cancer analysed, two controls were available: a population control and a control selected from among cases of cancer at the other sites. The interview was designed to obtain lifetime job histories and information on potential confounders. Each job was reviewed by a team of chemists and industrial hygienists who translated the jobs into occupational exposures using a checklist of 293 substances found in the workplace. Chloroform was one of the substances. About 0.7% of the subjects had ever been exposed to chloroform. Among the main occupations to which exposure to chloroform was attributed were nurses' aides and orderlies, dental prosthesis makers and laboratory technicians. No excess risks were seen for cancers at most of the sites examined; however, the odds ratio for prostate cancer, based on six exposed cases, was 4.0 (90% CI, 1.4–12), and the odds ratio for lung cancer among French Canadians, based on six exposed cases, was 8.8 (90% CI, 1.2–65). [The Working Group noted the limited power and the exploratory nature of the study.]

2.3.2 *Cancers of the colon and rectum*

Lawrence *et al.* (1984) reported the results of a study of 395 deaths from colorectal cancer (319 colon, 76 rectal) and 395 deaths from other causes that occurred during 1962–78 among white women teachers in New York State (United States). Cases and controls were matched on age and year of death. A crude analysis for the colorectal cancer risk of teachers who were exposed to chlorinated surface water or who were unexposed (exposed to groundwater containing little or no trihalomethanes) resulted in an odds ratio of 1.1 (90% CI, 0.79–1.4). An additional analysis with adjustment for water source type, population density at place of residence, marital status and the matching variables gave a similar result.

On the basis of their previous findings of an excess risk for colon cancer associated with exposure to chlorinated water supplies (Kanarek & Young, 1982; see section 2.3.1), Young *et al.* (1987) conducted a case–control study of 347 incident cases of colon cancer and 639 cancer controls, excluding gastrointestinal and urinary tract cancers, identified in the Wisconsin cancer reporting system. A group of 611 population controls was also used. White men and women in whom colon cancer had been diagnosed when they were aged 35–90 were considered eligible. The overall response rate to a self-administered questionnaire on background variables, past water sources, water-drinking and bathing habits, home treatment of tap water, and medical, occupational, social and lifestyle histories was 65%. The exposure of each study subject to trihalomethanes was estimated from an algorithm based on the results of a survey of 81 Wisconsin water supplies, historical data from water facilities, the residential history of the subjects, data on individual water use and other information. Average trihalomethane concentrations of 10–40 μg/L or > 40 μg/L at the place of residence in 1951–81 were not associated with an excess risk for colon cancer, when compared with exposure to < 10 μg/L. A similar result was found with cumulative lifetime exposure to trihalomethanes (in milligrams) over the past 30, over the past 20 and over the past 10 years of exposure.

2.3.3 *Urinary bladder cancer*

Cantor *et al.* (1987) interviewed 2805 patients with urinary bladder cancer aged 21–84 years at the time of diagnosis and 5258 population controls in a case–control study in 10 geographical areas in the United States. The cases were newly diagnosed and histologically confirmed during 1977–78. Controls were frequency matched on sex, age and geographical area. All subjects were administered a questionnaire at home by trained interviewers, which included questions on consumption of tap water during a typical week one year before the interview. A lifetime residential history, with water sources, was ascertained. A total of 1102 water utilities were visited, and utility personnel were interviewed; the water sources were then categorized for chlorination status (chlorination/no chlorination) during various periods. The residential histories of the subjects were linked with year-by-year water source and data on treatment. Logistic regression models with adjustment for sex, age, study area, smoking, high-risk occupation and population size were used with various indicators of water quality. The only significant trends ($p = 0.02$) with duration of residence with a chlorinated surface drinking-water source were found for women whose tap-water consumption was above the median, for nonsmoking women whose tap-water consumption was below the median and for nonsmoking men whose consumption was above the median. [The Working Group noted that the chloroform concentrations in the drinking-water were not given.]

Zierler *et al.* (1988) reported the results of a study of 614 persons with urinary bladder cancer who had died after the age of 44 years during 1978–84 while resident in

Massachusetts (United States) and whose drinking-water had been disinfected with either chlorine or chloramine. Chloramination results in substantially lower concentrations of trihalomethanes than chlorination (Lykins & Koffskey, 1986) and has been used in Massachusetts since 1938. A total of 1074 controls were selected from among persons who had died from cardiovascular disease, cerebrovascular disease, chronic obstructive pulmonary disease or lymphatic cancer. Data on water treatment were obtained from the Massachusetts Water Resources Authority, the United States Environmental Protection Agency and the State Division of Water Supply in the Department of Environmental Quality Engineering. Residence in communities with chlorinated drinking-water was contrasted with residence in communities with chloraminated drinking-water. Information was obtained for each deceased person on his or her residential and smoking history, and mortality odds ratios were calculated. About one-half of the eligible cases and controls were excluded, predominantly because informants could not be located. The crude mortality odds ratio for bladder cancer associated with lifetime exposure to chlorine versus chloramine was 1.3 (95% CI, 1.1–1.7), and that for usual exposure to chlorine versus chloramine was 1.2 (95% CI, 1.0–1.5). Adjustment for age, sex, cigarette pack–years and residence in a community in which at least 3% of the working population had jobs in industries in which there is a high risk for bladder cancer resulted in an odds ratio of 1.6 (95% CI, 1.2–2.1) for lifetime and 1.4 (95% CI, 1.1–1.8) for usual exposure. [The Working Group noted that the concentrations of chloroform in the drinking-water were not given and the possibility of selection bias due to the exclusion of about one-half of the study subjects.]

A population-based study of 327 histologically verified cases of urinary bladder cancer from the State cancer registry matched to 261 controls with other cancers was conducted in Colorado (United States) during 1990–91 (McGeehin *et al.*, 1993). Telephone interviews were used to obtain individual residential and water source histories from living patients and controls; the responses were 78% and 75%, respectively. These data were linked to data from water utilities and the Colorado Department of Health records. More than 34 years of exposure to chlorinated water, contrasted with no such exposure, was associated with increased risks in both nonsmokers (crude odds ratio, 2.9; 95% CI, 1.2–7.4) and smokers (odds ratio, 2.1; 95% CI, 1.1–3.8). Adjustment for coffee consumption, smoking, tap-water intake, family history of urinary bladder cancer, sex and medical history of urinary bladder infection or kidney stones resulted in odds ratios that increased with lifetime years of exposure to chlorinated water, to 1.8 (95% CI, 1.1–2.9) for the highest category (> 30 years) of exposure. The total lifetime trihalomethane concentration was calculated for each subject as a time-weighted mean from data for each water system in Colorado in 1989. The mean lifetime concentration was 620 μg/L for cases and 420 μg/L for controls ($p < 0.001$). [The Working Group noted that the chloroform concentrations were not given.]

Cantor *et al.* (1998) reported on a case–control study of bladder cancer among residents of Iowa (United States) aged 40–85 years. Patients with histologically confirmed bladder cancer were identified through the State Health Registry of Iowa, supplemented by a rapid reporting system, during 1986–89. Patients, controls and proxies were sent a questionnaire and interviewed by telephone in order to obtain demographic data, smoking history, occupational history, further indicators of lifestyle and medical conditions and the frequency of consumption as an adult inside and outside the home of beverages containing tap-water and other beverages. Lifetime residential histories were recorded, and the water source at each place was identified. For 10% of the patients and none of the controls, the interviews were conducted with proxies. All 280 Iowa water utilities that served at least 1000 persons were contacted for historical information, and at each utility an interviewer collected one or two samples from the clear well where the water enters the distribution system or from nearby in the system. The concentration of total trihalomethanes (grams) and the lifetime average trihalomethane concentration (μg/L) were calculated for 1123 cases and 1983 controls. The logistic regression models included adjustment for age, study period, level of education, high-risk occupation and cigarette smoking. The risk increased significantly with increasing total lifetime dose of trihalomethanes and lifetime average total trihalomethane concentration in men but not in women. The odds ratio for men in the highest total lifetime trihalomethane category (over 2.4 g) was associated with an odds ratio of 1.8 (95% CI, 1.2–2.7), the trend over six increasing categories being significant at $p = 0.05$; for the highest lifetime concentration (> 46 μg/L), the odds ratio was 1.5 (95% CI, 1.0–2.4; p for trend = 0.02). The corresponding odds ratios for women were 0.6 (95% CI, 0.3–1.4) and 0.6 (95% CI, 0.3–1.3).

2.4 Colorectal cancer

Hildesheim *et al.* (1998) reported on a case-control study of colon and rectal cancer among residents of Iowa, United States, aged 40–85 years. Patients with histologically confirmed cancers of the colon and rectum were identified through the State Health Registry of Iowa during 1986–87; the controls, the mailed questionnaire and the telephone interview were the same as those in the study of Cantor *et al.* (1998; see section 2.3.3). The concentration of total trihalomethanes (g) and the lifetime average trihalomethane concentrations (μg/L) were calculated for 560 colon cancer patients, 537 rectal cancer patients and 1983 controls from data on water samples and from interviews. About 15% of the patients were interviewed by proxy. The logistic regression models included adjustment for sex, age, study period, education, high-risk occupation and cigarette smoking. There was a suggestion of a trend of increasing risk for rectal cancer with lifetime concentration of trihalomethanes (odds ratio for the highest category (≥ 2.4 g), 1.6; 95% CI, 1.0–2.6; p for trend, 0.08) and for average lifetime concentration of trihalomethanes (odds ratio for the highest category (≥ 46 μg/L), 1.7; 95% CI, 1.1–2.6; p for trend, 0.01). No such trend was observed for colon cancer.

2.5 Brain cancer

Heineman *et al.* (1994) reported on occupational exposures to chlorinated aliphatic hydrocarbons and the risk for astrocytic brain cancer. A total of 300 cases of histologically confirmed brain tumours in deceased white men and 320 deceased population controls were identified in southern Lousiana, New Jersey and Philadelphia (United States) during 1978–81. The controls were frequency matched with the cases by age and area of death. Lifelong occupational histories were obtained by interviewing next-of-kin. Each job title was converted into period-specific probabilities and intensities of exposures to seven chlorinated hydrocarbon compounds, including chloroform. The logistic regression models included adjustment for age, study area and employment in electronics-related occupations or industries. Analyses by duration of exposure, cumulative exposure score and average intensity showed little indication of an association between exposure to chloroform and brain cancer.

3. Studies of Cancer in Experimental Animals

Previous evaluation

Chloroform was tested in three experiments in mice and in one in rats by oral administration. It produced hepatocellular adenomas and carcinomas in mice, malignant kidney tumours in male rats and tumours of the thyroid in female rats. Chloroform was also tested in one experiment by subcutaneous injection and in one by intraperitoneal injection in mice: these experiments were considered to be inadequate (IARC, 1979).

New studies

3.1 Oral administration

Mouse: Groups of female B6C3F$_1$ mice, 8.5 weeks of age, were given chloroform (pesticide quality, distilled to separate out diethylcarbonate) in distilled drinking-water at concentrations of 0 (control), 0 (matched control), 200, 400, 900 or 1800 mg/L (ppm) for 104 weeks, the numbers of mice per group being 430, 50, 430, 150, 50 and 50, respectively. Analysis of chloroform in the drinking-water indicated that the concentrations were maintained to an average of 93% or more of the target concentration over a four-day interval; these concentrations resulted in time-weighted average doses of 0, 0, 34, 65, 130 and 260 mg/kg bw, respectively. Survival was affected at the higher doses, with a 25% incidence of early deaths at 900 and 1800 mg/L. Survival of animals beyond the initial period did not differ significantly between groups. Chloroform did not increase the tumour incidence (Jorgenson *et al.*, 1985).

Groups of 35 male B6C3F$_1$ mice, approximately 30 days of age, were given chloroform [purity not specified] in deionized drinking-water at concentrations of 0, 600 or 1800 mg/L (ppm) until they were killed at 52 weeks. This treatment did not increase the incidence of liver or lung tumours (Klaunig *et al.*, 1986). [The Working Group noted that these were the control groups for a two-stage initiation–promotion study.]

Groups of 52 male and 52 female ICI mice, not more than 10 weeks of age, were given chloroform in toothpaste by oral gavage at doses of 17 or 60 mg/kg bw per day for 80 weeks followed by a further 16–24 weeks without treatment. A vehicle control group of 104 males and 104 females received 1 mL/kg bw per day of unflavoured toothpaste by oral gavage. The survival of males beyond 60 weeks decreased to 10–30%, and that of females beyond 50 weeks to 10–20%. Chloroform increased the incidence of renal tubule tumours (adenomas and carcinomas) in males at the high dose (Table 3). This experiment was repeated under the same conditions with a group of 52 male mice that received chloroform at 60 mg/kg bw per day; 52 males served as untreated controls, and a control group of 260 male mice received the toothpaste base. Chloroform again increased the incidence of renal tubule tumours (adenomas and carcinomas; Table 3). In a third experiment under the same conditions, groups of 52 male mice of the ICI, C57BL, CBA and CF1 strains received either 60 mg/kg bw per day of chloroform in toothpaste base by oral gavage or 1 mL/kg bw per day of toothpaste alone; an additional group of 100 ICI males was untreated, and groups of 52 males received chloroform at 0 or 60 mg/kg bw day in arachis oil. Chloroform produced renal tubule tumours (adenomas and carcinomas) only in ICI strain males, with the highest incidence in the group receiving chloroform in arachis oil (Table 3; Roe *et al.*, 1979).

Rat: Groups of 25 male and 25 female Sprague-Dawley rats (males weighing 180–240 g and females weighing 130–175 g received chloroform at concentrations of 15, 75 or 165 mg/kg bw per day, on six days per week, in toothpaste base by oral gavage. A control group of 75 males and 75 females received 1 mL/kg bw per day of toothpaste

Table 3. Incidence of renal tubule adenomas and carcinomas in ICI mice exposed orally to chloroform

Treatment	Sex	Incidence of renal tumours
Toothpaste	Male	0/72
17 mg/kg bw per day chloroform		0/37
60 mg/kg bw per day chloroform		8/38
Toothpaste	Female	0/59
17 mg/kg bw per day chloroform		0/35
60 mg/kg bw per day chloroform		0/38
None	Male	1/48
Toothpaste (1)		6/237
Toothpaste (2)		2/51
60 mg/kg bw per day chloroform		9/49
None	Male	0/83
Toothpaste		1/49
Arachis oil		1/50
60 mg/kg bw per day chloroform in toothpaste		5/47
60 mg/kg bw per day chloroform in arachis oil		12/48

From Roe *et al.* (1979)

base. Because of poor survival in all groups due to intercurrent disease, the study was terminated after one year. There was no increase in tumour incidence. In a second experiment, groups of 50 male (weighing 180–240 g) and 50 female (weighing 130–175 g) Sprague-Dawley rats were given chloroform at a concentration of 0 or 60 mg/kg bw per day, on six days per week, in 1 mL/kg bw of toothpaste by oral gavage for 80 weeks and observed for a further 15 weeks. Chloroform did not increase the tumour incidence (Palmer *et al.*, 1979).

Groups of 26 and 32 male and 22 and 45 female weanling Wistar rats [age unspecified] were given chloroform [purity not specified] in the drinking-water at a concentration of 0 or 2.9 g/L, respectively, for 72 weeks, when the dose was halved to 1.45 g/L for the remaining weeks because of increased consumption of water. The animals were necropsied when found dead or moribund. Controls of each sex survived for approximately 145 weeks, while those exposed to chloroform survived for approximately 185 weeks. Chloroform produced neoplastic nodules in the livers of 10 female rats, representing a 25% incidence compared with 0% in the control group (Tumasonis *et al.*, 1987).

Groups of male Osborne-Mendel rats, seven weeks of age, were given chloroform (pesticide quality) in drinking-water at concentrations of 0 (control), 0 (matched control), 200, 400, 900 or 1800 mg/L (ppm) for 104 weeks, the numbers of rats per group being 330, 50, 330, 150, 50 and 50, respectively. Analysis of chloroform in the drinking-water indicated that the concentrations were maintained to an average of 93% or more of the target concentration over a four-day interval; these concentrations resulted in time-weighted average doses of 19, 38, 81 and 160 mg/kg bw, respectively. The survival of these groups at 104 weeks was 12, 25, 29, 60 and 66%, respectively. Chloroform produced a statistically significant ($p < 0.01$) increase in the incidence of renal tubule tumours (adenomas and carcinomas) at the highest dose: control, 5/301; matched controls, 1/50; 200 mg/L, 6/313; 400 mg/L, 7/148; 900 mg/L, 3/48; and 1800 mg/L, 7/50 (Jorgensen *et al.*, 1985).

Dog: Groups of 8–16 male and 8–16 female pure-bred beagle dogs, 18–24 weeks of age, were given chloroform [purity not specified] in a toothpaste base orally by gelatin capsule at concentrations of 0, 15 or 30 mg/kg bw per day, on seven days per week for at least seven years. One group of eight males and eight females was untreated, and another control group received an alternative toothpaste. Survival was excellent, with 84/96 animals still alive after seven years. Exposure to chloroform was not associated with any increase in tumour incidence (Heywood *et al.*, 1979).

3.2 Inhalation

Mouse: Groups of 50 male and 50 female BDF_1 mice, six weeks of age, were given chloroform (purity, > 99%) in air by inhalation for 6 h per day on five days per week for 104 weeks at concentrations of 0, 5, 30 or 90 ppm. The 30- and 90-ppm doses were acutely lethal to the mice; thus, mice were first exposed to 5 ppm for two weeks, then to 10 ppm for two weeks (and, in the 90 ppm group, then 30 ppm for a further two weeks) before the 30 and 90 ppm concentrations were maintained. Under these conditions, chloroform produced renal tubular tumours (adenomas and carcinomas) in male mice at the two highest concentrations: control, 0/50; low-dose, 1/50; mid-dose, 7/50; high-dose, 12/48 (Nagano *et al.*, 1998).

Rat: Groups of 50 male and 50 female Fischer 344 rats, six weeks of age, were given chloroform (purity, 99%) in air by inhalation for 6 h per day on five days per week for 104 weeks at concentrations of 0, 10, 30 or 90 ppm. Chloroform did not increase the incidence of tumours (Nagano *et al.*, 1998).

3.3 Administration with known carcinogens

Mouse: Groups of 23–39 male and 25–45 female CD-1 Swiss mice, 15 days of age, were given a single intraperitoneal injection of 0, 5 or 20 mg/kg bw *N*-ethyl-*N*-nitrosourea (ENU) in 1 mol/L sodium acetate. At five weeks of age, the mice either received no further treatment or were given chloroform (purity, > 99%) in the drinking-water at a concentration of 1800 mg/L (ppm) for the next 46 weeks (i.e. until 51 weeks of age). All mice were killed at 52 weeks of age. Chloroform did not alter the incidence of ENU-initiated lung tumours in mice of either sex nor of liver tumours in female mice. Chloroform decreased the incidence of ENU-initiated liver tumours in male mice by approximately one-half (Pereira *et al.*, 1985).

Rat: In a two-stage model of liver carcinogenesis, groups of 12 male Sprague-Dawley rats weighing 225–275 g received a two-thirds partial hepatectomy followed 20–22 h later by a single oral gavage dose of 1.5 mmol/kg bw chloroform [purity not specified] in tricaprylin, or 0.5 mmol/kg bw *N*-nitrosodiethylamine (NDEA) in distilled water as a positive control. Three days later, sodium phenobarbital was added at a concentration of 500 mg/L (ppm) to the drinking-water for 47 days, and the animals were killed six days later. Chloroform did not increase the incidence of γ-glutamyltranspeptidase-positive foci of hepatocellular alteration in either the partially hepatectomized or the intact rats (Pereira *et al.*, 1982).

In the promotion part of the above two-stage model of liver carcinogenesis, groups of 15 or 16 male Sprague-Dawley rats weighing 225–275 g were given by gavage an initiating dose of NDEA in distilled water, and three days later either an oral gavage dose of 1.5 mmol/kg bw chloroform [purity not specified] in tricaprylin twice weekly for 53 days, 2 mL/kg bw tricaprylin alone or 500 mg/L (ppm) of sodium barbital in the drinking-water as a positive control. Rats were killed four to five days after the 53 days of promotion regimen. Chloroform did not statistically significantly increase the incidence of γ-glutamyltranspeptidase-positive foci of hepatocellular alteration (Pereira *et al.*, 1982).

In a two-stage initiation–promotion model of liver carcinogenesis, groups of four to six female Sprague-Dawley rats, three weeks of age, received a single oral gavage dose of 8 mg/kg bw NDEA followed one week later by an oral gavage dose of 25, 100, 200 or 400 mg/kg bw chloroform (purity, 99%) twice weekly for 11 consecutive weeks, at which time the surviving animals were killed. These doses of chloroform were also administered to groups that had not been initiated with NDEA. Chloroform increased the incidence of adenosine-5′-triphosphatase-deficient, γ-glutamyltranspeptidase-positive and glycogen-positive foci of hepatocellular alteration in the NDEA-initiated groups, but not in the uninitiated groups (Deml & Oesterle, 1985, 1987).

In a rat model of gastrointestinal carcinogenesis, groups of 40 male Fischer 344 rats, seven weeks of age, received a subcutaneous injection of 200 mg/kg bw 1,2-dimethylhydrazine, followed seven days later by administration of chloroform (preservative-free grade) at concentrations of 900 or 1800 mg/L in drinking-water for 39 weeks, at which time all the surviving animals were killed. Survival was 98–100%. Chloroform produced a statistically significant ($p < 0.001$) reduction in the incidence of gastrointestinal tract tumours (including those of the stomach, duodenum, jejunum, caecum and colon); when the incidence of colon tumours was analysed independently, it was significantly reduced ($p < 0.001$) at both doses (Daniel *et al.*, 1989).

In a two-stage initiation–promotion model of liver carcinogenesis, groups of 11 or 12 male Fischer 344 rats weighing 150–160 g were subjected to a partial (67%) hepatectomy followed 18 h later by a single oral gavage dose of either 0.5 mmol/kg bw NDEA in saline or 2 mL/kg bw sterile saline. Two weeks after the hepatectomy, the groups were given water containing 500 mg/L (ppm) phenobarbital or 1800 mg/L chloroform (preservative-free high-performance liquid chromatography-grade), drinking-water containing both phenobarbital at concentrations of 650, 700, 800 or 950 mg/L and chloroform at concentrations of 200, 400, 900 or 1800 mg/L, or distilled water alone, for the next 12 weeks, at which time all the surviving animals were killed. Chloroform reduced the number of γ-glutamyltranspeptidase-positive and glutathione-*S*-transferase (placental form)-positive foci of hepatocellular alteration in a dose-related manner (Reddy *et al.*, 1992).

4. Other Data Relevant to an Evaluation of Carcinogenicity and its Mechanisms

4.1 Absorption, distribution, metabolism and excretion

4.1.1 *Humans*

After inhalation of approximately 5 mg [^{38}Cl]chloroform, ~ 80% of the chloroform was found to have been absorbed (Morgan *et al.*, 1970). Eight volunteers expired 18–67% of an oral dose of 500 mg [^{13}C]chloroform (in capsules of olive oil) unchanged; in two subjects, about half of the dose was eliminated in the expired air as $^{13}CO_2$. The decline in the concentration of chloroform in blood was described by a two-compartment model, with initial and second-phase half-lives of 14 and 90 min, respectively, averaged over four subjects (Fry *et al.*, 1972).

The uptake and elimination of inhaled chloroform (2–2.5% v/v in air) by eight patients during general anaesthesia was rapid, with an average blood concentration of about 175 mg/L (Poobalasingham & Payne, 1978). Smith *et al.* (1973) reported that concentrations of 70–165 mg of chloroform per litre of blood produced adequate surgical anaesthesia; at a concentration of 50 mg/L, patients became responsive again. One hour after anaesthesia was terminated, the arterial chloroform concentration was 20–40 mg/L.

Chloroform has been detected *post mortem* in tissue samples from various organs at concentrations of 1–68 μg/kg wet tissue, the concentration in body fat being the highest (McConnell *et al.*, 1975). When subjects inhaled a mixture of oxygen/nitrogen (20/80) containing less than 0.025 μg/L chloroform, traces up to 11 μg/h per subject were found in expired air (Conkle *et al.*, 1975).

After chloroform was applied to the forearm of male volunteers aged 23–36, and exhaled air and urine were collected and analysed, absorption of chloroform was ~7.8% after application of 50 μg in water and ~1.6% after application of 250 μg in ethanol. More than 94% of the absorbed dose was excreted via the lungs between 15 min and 2 h after dosing, 69 and 88% of which was CO_2 after application in ethanol and water, respectively (Dick *et al.*, 1995).

Cytochrome P450 (CYP) 2E1 was shown to be a major enzyme in the oxidation of chloroform in human liver microsomes (Guengerich *et al.*, 1991).

4.1.2 *Experimental systems*

Chloroform is rapidly absorbed and distributed to all organs, with relatively high concentrations in nervous tissue (Von Oettingen, 1964). After intraduodenal injection of [^{14}C]chloroform to rats, 70% of the radiolabel was associated with unchanged chloroform in the expired air and 4% with CO_2 after 18 h. In an experiment with tissue slices *in vitro*, the liver and, to a much lesser extent, the kidney were the main organs in which CO_2 was formed (Paul & Rubinstein, 1963). Mink *et al.* (1986) administered [^{14}C]chloroform by intragastric intubation to fasted male Sprague-Dawley rats (100 mg/kg bw) and male B6C3F$_1$ mice (150 mg/kg bw) and found that the majority of the compound was eliminated in expired air through the lungs of both species within 8 h. The mice eliminated 40–81% of the total dose as $^{14}CO_2$ and 5–26% as the parent compound, whereas the rats exhaled 4–18% as $^{14}CO_2$ and 41–67% as unmetabolized chloroform.

The blood concentrations in male Fischer 344 rats during 24-h dermal exposure to pure chloroform peaked after 4–8 h at 52 μg/mL and remained constant for the duration of the exposure (Morgan *et al.*, 1991).

[^{14}C]Chloroform in olive oil given periodically to mice, rats and monkeys (60 mg/kg bw) was completely absorbed, since 93–98% of the radiolabel was recovered from exhaled air, urine, faeces and the carcass. Most of the dose was excreted unchanged by monkeys, as $^{14}CO_2$ by mice and as a mixture of the two by rats. Three metabolites were detected in the urine of rats and mice, one of which was identified as urea (Brown, D.M. *et al.*, 1974; Taylor *et al.*, 1974).

A study of the tissue distribution of chloroform in three strains of mice (CF/LP, CBA and C57) by whole-body autoradiography after oral dosing with 60 mg/kg bw [^{14}C]chloroform showed the greatest amounts of radiolabel in liver and kidneys, with significant amounts in the renal cortex but not the medulla of male mice. In female mice, the highest levels of radiolabel were found in the liver, intestine and bladder with much less in kidney (Taylor *et al.*, 1974). No sex differences in renal binding were found in rats or monkeys (Brown, D.M. *et al.*, 1974).

In male Wistar rats, the integrated area under the blood concentration–time curve after oral administration of chloroform at 75 mg/kg bw in water was 8.7 times greater than after administration in vegetable oil. In both cases, chloroform was well absorbed, peak blood concentrations being reached approximately 6 min after administration; uptake from aqueous solution gave rise to higher peak blood concentrations (Withey *et al.*, 1983). In male Fischer 344 rats, administration of chloroform in a low-dose volume (2 mL/kg bw) of either corn oil or 2% emulphor:water did not appear to affect the absorption or tissue dosimetry of chloroform; however, in B6C3F$_1$ mice treated with chloroform in a high-dose volume (10 mL/kg bw) of the vehicle, these parameters were affected by the vehicle used (Dix *et al.*, 1997).

The fraction of the dose exhaled as unchanged chloroform did not increase proportionately to that administered in either male Osborne-Mendel rats or male B6C3F$_1$ mice exposed to 90, 360 or 1040 ppm [440, 1800 or 5100 mg/m^3] or 10, 90 or 360 ppm [49, 440 or 1800 mg/m^3] [^{14}C]chloroform for 6 h, respectively. $^{14}CO_2$ was the major metabolite exhaled. The data indicate metabolic saturation at the higher doses (Corley *et al.*, 1990).

The metabolism of chloroform has been extensively reviewed (Hathway, 1974; Charlesworth, 1976; Pohl, 1979; Davidson *et al.*, 1982). There is considerable evidence for the metabolism of chloroform to phosgene (Mansuy *et al.*, 1977; Pohl *et al.*, 1977, 1979, 1980). The finding of 2-oxo-thiazolidine-4-carboxylic acid (4-carboxy-thiazolidine-2-one) in incubates is strong evidence for the formation of phosgene, as the reactive metabolite phosgene is formed by mixed-function oxidation of chloroform to trichloromethanol after dehydrochlorination (Mansuy *et al.*, 1977; Pohl *et al.*, 1977, 1980). Phosgene reacts with water to give CO_2 and HCl, which explains the presence of CO_2 as a metabolite *in vivo* in a number of studies. Phosgene also reacts with tissue nucleophiles to form covalently bound products (Mansuy *et al.*, 1977; Pohl *et al.*, 1980). In phenobarbital-treated rats, liver necrosis was observed only with doses of chloroform high enough to decrease the concentration of reduced glutathione in liver (Docks & Krishna, 1976). Chloroform depletes liver glutathione by reacting with it (Pohl *et al.*, 1980, 1981). Covalent binding of [^{14}C]chloroform-derived radiolabel to microsomal proteins *in vitro* was inhibited by cysteine (Pohl *et al.*, 1977).

Chloroform is metabolized to a greater extent in mice than in rats (Mink *et al.*, 1986). More covalent binding of [^{14}C]chloroform metabolites to liver and kidney proteins *in vivo* was seen in B6C3F$_1$ mice than in Osborne-Mendel rats. The uptake of chloroform by male B6C3F$_1$ mice in a closed chamber was more rapid than that by male Fischer 344 rats after exposure to initial concentrations of chloroform ranging from 1000 to 5000 ppm [4900–25 000 mg/m^3] and 103–2581 ppm [510–13 000 mg/m^3], respectively (Corley *et al.*, 1990). This difference was attributed to the higher rate of chloroform metabolism in mice.

The metabolism of chloroform to phosgene in mouse kidney has been implicated as the reactive pathway, as in the liver (Branchflower *et al.*, 1984). Strain differences in sensitivity to chloroform-induced nephrotoxicity correlate with the ability of the kidney to metabolize chloroform. Chloroform metabolism in renal cortical slices from male, but not female, ICR mice was found to be responsible for the sensitivity of male mice to chloroform-induced nephrotoxicity (Smith & Hook, 1983, 1984). Homogenates of kidney from male DBA/2J mice metabolized chloroform twice as fast as those from C57BL/6J mice (Pohl *et al.*, 1984), and covalent binding of chloroform to renal microsomes was much greater in male DBA mice than in male C57BL/6 mice, consistent with the sensitivity of the DBA strain to chloroform-induced nephrotoxicity (Clemens *et al.*, 1979).

Purified CYP 2El in the presence of liver microsomes prepared from acetone-induced rats metabolized chloroform (Brady *et al.* 1989; Guengerich *et al.*, 1991).

Testai and Vittozzi (1986) demonstrated that reductive biotransformation of chloroform takes place in rat microsomes *in vitro* and is dependent on inducible P450 enzymes. Reductive metabolism was negligible with microsomes from uninduced animals. The results of several investigations suggest that reductive metabolism of chloroform *in vivo* would be significant only at high concentrations of chloroform (5 mmol/L) under very low pO_2 (0–1%) and would be totally inhibited by the presence of higher concentrations of oxygen (Luke *et al.*, 1988; De Curtis *et al.*, 1994; Gemma *et al.*, 1996).

4.1.3 *Comparison of humans and rodents*

The metabolism of chloroform in human and rat (male Sprague-Dawley) liver microsomes *in vitro* is similar. The kinetics in the two species were quite similar, but less total irreversible binding was seen in human samples. Cysteine inhibited covalent binding of chloroform metabolites to macromolecules in both human and rat microsomes (Cresteil *et al.*, 1979).

The metabolism of ^{14}C[chloroform] in liver and kidney microsomes prepared from male Fischer 344 rats, Osborne-Mendel rats, B6C3F$_1$ mice, Syrian golden hamsters and humans was measured by trapping formed $^{14}CO_2$. The order of the rate of [^{14}C]chloroform metabolism in liver microsomes was hamster > mouse > rat > human. Microsomes prepared from the kidneys of the various species were less active than liver microsomes. The metabolism of [^{14}C]chloroform in kidney microsomes was greatest in mice (B6C3F$_1$) followed by hamster > rat > human, no activity being detected in human kidney microsomes (Corley *et al.* 1990). Amet *et al.* (1997) detected CYP 2E1 in human liver but not in kidney.

Mice were exposed on day 11, 14 or 17 of gestation to [^{14}C]chloroform for 10-min in an all-glass chamber in which 100 μCi were mixed with maize oil and gently heated. The radiolabel was observed to cross the placenta. In mid-gestation, the amniotic fluid accumulated radiolabel from non-volatile metabolites, but chloroform itself did not accumulate in fetal brain or other tissue. Radiolabel attached to non-volatile compounds peaked in the fetus around 1 h after inhalation by the dam (Danielsson *et al.*, 1986).

4.2 Toxic effects

4.2.1 *Humans*

Extensive exposure to chloroform is fatal to humans, rapid death being attributed to cardiac arrest and delayed death to liver and kidney damage (Challen *et al.*, 1958;

Matsuki & Zsigmond, 1974). The symptoms of exposure to chloroform include respiratory depression, coma, renal damage and liver damage as measured by elevated serum enzyme levels (Storms, 1973). According to Royston (1925), chloroform was not toxic to the fetus or newborn when administered to women during prolonged labour. Chloroform anaesthesia, under normal conditions, was found to induce minimal or no toxic side-effects, even in young children (Whitaker & Jones, 1965).

4.2.2 *Experimental systems*

The acute toxicity of chloroform is species-, strain-, sex- and age-dependent. Thus, the acute oral LD_{50} in young and older adult male Sprague-Dawley rats was 1300 and 1200 mg/kg bw, respectively whereas it was 440 mg/kg bw in 14-day-old animals (Kimura *et al.*, 1971). The LD_{50} of a single oral dose in male mice varied from 120 mg/kg bw in DBA/2J mice to 490 mg/kg bw in C57BL/6J mice (Hill *et al.*, 1975). The dose that caused a 50% incidence of acute neurological effects (ataxia, loss of coordination and anaesthesia) was 480 mg/kg bw (Balster & Borzelleca, 1982).

Males of many mouse strains are susceptible to renal tubular necrosis, whereas females are not similarly affected. The response to chloroform increased with the age of the mice. Strains C3H, $C3H_f$, A and HR were susceptible, and strains C57BL, C57L, C57BR/cd and ST were resistant to exposure (Deringer *et al.*, 1953).

Renal tubular injury has been observed in mice of a number of strains, including $B6C3F_1$ (Larson *et al.*, 1994a,b, 1996), DBA (Hill *et al.*, 1975), ICR (Smith *et al.*, 1983), C57BL (Hill *et al.*, 1975) and BDF_1 (Templin *et al.*, 1996a, 1998), after oral or inhalational exposure to chloroform. A number of studies indicate that male but not female mice are susceptible to chloroform-induced nephrotoxicity (Eschenbrenner & Miller, 1945; Larson *et al.*, 1996; Templin *et al.*, 1996a, 1998).

Male Sprague-Dawley rats were given 0, 1.2, 2.5, 3.1, 3.7 or 4.4 mmol/kg [0, 140, 300, 370, 440 or 530 mg/kg bw] chloroform in either corn oil or EL 620 emulphor (10 mL/kg) and killed 48 h later. Toxicity to the kidney was evaluated by measuring *para*-aminohippuric acid incorporation into renal cortical slices prepared from treated rats. The nephrotoxicity appeared to be more severe in rats given chloroform in corn oil (Raymond & Plaa, 1997). [The Working Group noted that the large volume of the vehicle used may have influenced these results.]

Liver damage was the cause of death of rats and mice after accidental long-term exposure to and acute administration of chloroform (Doyle *et al.*, 1967; Brown, B.R. *et al.*, 1974). Early dilatation of granular endoplasmic reticulum, with detachment of the ribosomes, was observed in the livers of treated rats (Scholler, 1968). In rats, rabbits and guinea-pigs exposed to 125, 250 or 425 mg/m^3 chloroform in air and in dogs exposed to 125 mg/m^3 for 7 h a day on five days a week for six months, higher mortality rates, changes in organ weights and histopathological alterations in the liver and kidney were observed; centrilobular granular degeneration was seen in rat liver. These effects appeared to be reversible in rats exposed to 125 mg/m^3 (Torkelson *et al.*, 1976).

Chloroform increases ornithine decarboxylase activity in Fischer 344 rats (Savage *et al.*, 1982, 1987) and male B6C3F$_1$ mice (Pereira *et al.*, 1984). Ornithine decarboxylase has been proposed to be a molecular marker for tumour promotion.

Various treatments that affect hepatic drug-metabolizing enzymes alter the hepatotoxicity of chloroform, indicating that a metabolite of chloroform may be responsible for the liver necrosis (McLean, 1970; Scholler, 1970). After administration of [^{14}C]-chloroform, there was extensive, presumably covalent, binding of ^{14}C to liver and kidney proteins in male C57BL/6 mice. The livers of female mice showed similar amounts of covalent binding and a similar degree of hepatic necrosis; the kidneys of female mice appeared to be resistant to chloroform-induced necrosis and showed much less protein binding (Ilett *et al.*, 1973). In similar experiments, binding in the kidneys of mice of two strains was related to their susceptibility to kidney lesions (Vesell *et al.*, 1976). In mice, covalent binding of chloroform to renal proteins correlated with the degree of renal tubular necrosis (Ilett *et al.*, 1973; Smith & Hook, 1983). Other factors, such as the availability of glutathione (Brown, B.R. *et al.*, 1974), the concentration of cytochrome P450 and oxygen tension (Uehleke & Werner, 1975; Sipes *et al.*, 1977), affected the extent of covalent binding and of hepatic centrilobular damage.

Chloroform induced concentration-dependent cytotoxicity in male B6C3F$_1$ mouse and Fischer 344 rat hepatocytes at concentrations greater than 1 mmol/L, which is the threshold concentration for glutathione depletion. Cytochrome P450-dependent metabolism and glutathione depletion, but not reductive metabolism, were found to be involved in the toxicity (Ammann *et al.*, 1998).

Chloroform caused a sustained cytotoxic and regenerative cell proliferative response in the livers of female B6C3F$_1$ mice under conditions of treatment by gavage similar to those that produce cancer (corn oil, 10 mL/kg bw) (Larson *et al.*, 1993, 1994a). Similar total daily doses of chloroform administered in drinking-water at concentrations as high as 1800 ppm [260 mg/kg bw] did not induce hepatocellular damage, cell proliferation or liver tumours (Jorgenson *et al.*, 1985; Larson *et al.*, 1994a). A similar pattern of hepatocellular damage and regeneration was observed in B6C3F$_1$ mice given chloroform by gavage or in the drinking-water (Pereira, 1994).

Male Fischer 344 rats were given oral doses of 0, 10, 34, 90 or 180 mg/kg bw per day chloroform in corn oil for four days, or for five days a week for three weeks. A second group of rats were given chloroform *ad libitum* in the drinking-water at concentrations of 0, 60, 200, 400, 900 or 1800 ppm [0, 6, 17–19, 32–33, 62–68, 57–110 mg/kg bw per day] for four days or three weeks. Bromodeoxyuridine was administered via an osmotic pump 3.5 days before necropsy, and the labelling index was evaluated immunohistochemically. Administration of chloroform by gavage caused more severe hepatic and renal toxicity than exposure in the drinking-water, and regenerative proliferation in the kidney and liver depended on the route of administration (Larson *et al.*, 1995a). Male and female Fischer 344 rats appear to be equally susceptible to chloroform-induced hepatotoxic effects, but the nephrotoxic effects, including the proliferative response, were more severe in females than in males (Larson *et al.*, 1995a,b). Templin *et al.*

(1996b) showed that male Fischer 344 and Osborne-Mendel rats have similar susceptibility to chloroform-induced renal injury.

Female and male B6C3F$_1$ mice were exposed by inhalation to 0, 0.3, 2, 10, 30 or 90 ppm chloroform [0, 1.5, 9.8, 49, 150 or 440 mg/m^3] for 6 h a day on seven days a week for four days or for 3, 6 or 13 consecutive weeks. Additional groups were exposed for five days a week for 13 weeks or exposed for six weeks and then examined at 13 weeks. Bromodeoxyuridine was administered via osmotic pumps implanted 3.5 days before necropsy, and the labelling index was evaluated immunohistochemically. Treatment-induced dose- and time-dependent histological lesions and increased labelling indices were found only in the livers and nasal passages of female and male mice and in the kidneys of male mice. Significant increases in the labelling index (cells in S-phase, a measure of cell proliferation) were sustained in the group exposed to 90 ppm, and no adverse effects were observed in mice exposed to 10 ppm (Larson *et al.*, 1996).

Male and female Fischer 344 rats were exposed to 0, 2, 10, 30, 90 or 300 ppm [0, 9.8, 49, 150, 440 or 1500 mg/m^3] chloroform for 6 h a day on seven days a week for four days or for 3, 6 or 13 weeks. Additional groups were exposed for five days per week for 13 weeks. The primary target in Fischer 344 rats was the kidney, which showed a significantly increased labelling index in the epithelial cells of the proximal tubules of the cortex at concentrations of 30 ppm and above (seven days per week) and 90 ppm and above (five days per week). A concentration-dependent response in the labelling index in the kidney was found in both male and female rats. Hepatocyte alterations were seen mainly in rats exposed to 300 ppm at all times and in those exposed to 90 ppm at later times (Templin *et al.*, 1996c).

4.3 Reproductive and developmental effects

4.3.1 *Humans*

No data were available to the Working Group.

4.3.2 *Experimental systems*

The effects of chloroform on the development of rats, mice and rabbits have been reviewed (Smith *et al.*, 1986). Adverse clinical effects on the dams of each species and some evidence of embryotoxic and fetotoxic effects (predominantly reduced fetal size and weight and retarded skeletal ossification) were reported at the highest doses tested: 300 ppm for 7 h per day by inhalation and up to 400 mg/kg orally on days 6–15 of gestation. Teratogenic effects were reported in rats and mice exposed by inhalation but not in rats or rabbits treated by oral gavage. In one study, abnormal sperm were reported in mice exposed by inhalation to 400 or 800 ppm for 4 h per day for five days (Land *et al.*, 1981).

Sprague-Dawley rats were exposed by inhalation to 0, 30, 100 or 300 ppm chloroform for 7 h per day on days 6–15 of gestation, and their fetuses were examined on day 20 of gestation for viability, growth and morphological appearance. All three doses resulted in significantly reduced maternal body-weight gain, and this effect was marked in females at 300 ppm. Only 3/20 of females at this dose had viable fetuses at term, compared with 88% of the controls. No effects on viability or body weight were noted in the fetuses of dams at the two lower doses, but both viability and body weight were considerably reduced at the high dose, as was crown–rump length. The crown–rump length of fetuses of dams at the low dose was also reduced, and delayed skeletal ossification and an increased incidence of fetuses with wavy ribs were seen. Fetuses of dams at 100 ppm had increased incidences of absent or short tails, imperforate anus, subcutaneous oedema and anomalies of the skull and sternum, with delayed ossification of the sternebrae. The authors concluded that chloroform is not strongly teratogenic but highly embryotoxic (Schwetz *et al.*, 1974).

Groups of 15 Sprague-Dawley rats were exposed to 0, 100, 200 or 400 mg/kg bw chloroform by gavage on days 6–15 of gestation, and their fetuses were examined on day 22. Maternal body-weight gain was decreased in all treated groups, and three females at the high dose died. The relative liver weights were increased at all doses, while the kidney weights were increased only in dams at the high dose. The only fetal effects were a decrease in weight and increased incidences of runts, aberrations of the sternebrae and interparietal malformations at the high dose. The last two effects were considered to be indicative of fetotoxicity (Ruddick *et al.*, 1983).

Male and female mice received 0 or 31 mg/kg bw per day chloroform in an Emulphor-saline vehicle by oral gavage for 21 days before mating, throughout mating (21 days or until a vaginal plug was detected) and throughout gestation and lactation. The offspring in five control and five treated litters received the same doses daily beginning on postnatal day 7 and continuing to the end of the study. No effects were reported on offspring body weights or on a variety of neurobehavioural measures (righting reflex, forelimb placing response, forepaw grasp, rooting reflex, cliff-drop aversion, auditory startle response, bar-holding ability, eye opening, motor activity and passive avoidance learning) (Burkhalter & Balster, 1979).

CF-1 mice were exposed to 0 or 100 ppm chloroform by inhalation for 7 h per day on days 1–7, 6–15 or 8–15 of gestation, and their fetuses were examined on day 18 of gestation for viability, growth and morphological appearance. Reduced body-weight gain during the first few days of exposure was seen in all treated dams. Exposure on days 1–7 or 6–15 significantly reduced the percentage of females that maintained pregnancy. Fetal body weights and crown–rump lengths were reduced in groups treated on days 1–7 or 8–15, and there was a significant increase in the incidence of cleft palate in the latter group (Murray *et al.*, 1979).

The reproductive effects of chloroform were evaluated in CD-1 mice in the continuous breeding protocol of the United States National Toxicology Program (Anon., 1997). As reported in summary form, the mice were exposed to 0, 8, 20 or 50 mg/kg bw per day by gavage, and males and females were maintained in breeding pairs throughout the exposure. There were no reported treatment-related effects on the general health of the parental generation (e.g. body and organ weights, clinical signs) or on their reproductive function (e.g. numbers of litters produced, litter size or pup weight). Mating of control and high-dose offspring to produce an F_2 generation resulted in a higher fertility index and larger litter sizes in the treated groups, while the relative liver weights were increased in treated female offspring (F_1), and the relative weight of the epididymides was increased in treated F_1 males. All treated females showed some degree of hepatocellular degeneration, while individual cases of hepatitis and hepatocellular degeneration were observed in males.

Sprague-Dawley rat embryos (12–15 somites) at day 10.5 of gestation were exposed in whole-embryo culture to chloroform at concentrations of 0.53–3.7 μmol/mL for 40 h. Concentrations of 2 μmol/mL and higher retarded embryonic development. At the highest concentration, yolk sac vascularity was reduced within 4 h of exposure; extensive cell death was seen in the neuroepithelium after 16 h of culture (Brown-Woodman *et al.*, 1998).

4.4 Genetic and related effects

4.4.1 *Humans*

No data were available to the Working Group.

4.4.2 *Experimental systems* (see Table 4 for references)

Chloroform did not induce prophage or SOS DNA repair in *Escherichia coli* in two studies carried out in the presence and absence of exogenous metabolic activation. Weak differential toxicity was observed in *E. coli* in one study with exogenous metabolic activation, but another study gave negative results. A similar assay with *Bacillus subtilis* showed a positive result in the absence of activation, but a second study again gave negative results.

Chloroform did not cause forward mutations in *Salmonella typhimurium* and did not cause reverse mutation in several studies in *S. typhimurium* strains TA100, TA135, TA1537, TA1538 and TA98 and *E. coli* WP2 and WP2 *uvr*A in the presence or absence of exogenous metabolic activation; two exceptions were positive responses in *S. typhimurium* TA1535 transfected with rat glutathione *S*-transferase and in strain TA98 in the presence of metabolic activation from mouse liver.

In lower eukaryotes, chloroform had mixed effects. In one study, it induced mitotic gene conversion, mitotic crossing-over and reversion in the D7 strain of *Saccharomyces cerevisiae* containing cytochrome P450-dependent monooxygenases and, in another study, it induced deletions via intrachromosomal recombination. In contrast, no DNA damage, mitotic gene conversion, mitotic crossing-over, reverse mutation or increase in mitotic aneuploidy were observed in *Saccharomyces cerevisiae* in the presence or absence of exogenous metabolic activation. In *Aspergillus nidulans*, chloroform did not induce mitotic crossing-over, somatic segregation or gene mutation in the absence of metabolic activation; aneuploidy was observed in one of two studies.

In two studies, chloroform did not induce sex-linked recessive lethal mutation in *Drosophila melanogaster*.

Chloroform did not elicit DNA fragmentation in primary rat hepatocytes or DNA repair in either mouse or rat hepatocytes, and it did not induce gene mutation at the *hprt*

Table 4. Genetic and related effects of chloroform

Test system	Result[a]		Dose[b] (LED or HID)	Reference
	Without exogenous metabolic system	With exogenous metabolic system		
Prophage induction, SOS repair, DNA strand breaks, cross-links or related damage	–	–	0.05 μL/mL	Thomson (1981)
Escherichia coli PQ37, SOS repair	–	–	3000	Le Curieux *et al.* (1995)
Escherichia coli pol A/W3110-P3478, differential toxicity (liquid suspension)	–	(+)	250 μg/plate	Rosenkranz *et al.* (1981)
Escherichia coli rec strains, differential toxicity	–	–	NR	Green (1981)
Bacillus subtilis rec strains, differential toxicity	+	NT	NR	San Agustin & Lim-Sylianco (1978)
Bacillus subtilis rec strains, differential toxicity	–	–	20 μL/plate	Kada (1981)
Salmonella typhimurium, forward mutation	–	–	300	Skopek *et al.* (1981)
Salmonella typhimurium Ara forward mutation	–	–	9.6 μmol/plate	Roldán-Arjona *et al.* (1991); Roldán-Arjona & Pueyo (1993)
Salmonella typhimurium TA100, TA98, TA1535, TA1537, TA1538, reverse mutation	–	–	5 mg/plate	Simmon *et al.* (1977)
Salmonella typhimurium TA100, TA98, TA1535, TA1537, TA1538, reverse mutation	NT	–	15 mg/plate	Nestmann *et al.* (1980)
Salmonella typhimurium TA100, TA98, TA1535, TA1537, TA1538, reverse mutation	–	–	3600 μg/plate	Gocke *et al.* (1981)
Salmonella typhimurium TA100, TA98, TA1537, reverse mutation	–	–	5000 μg/plate	MacDonald (1981)
Salmonella typhimurium TA100, TA98, TA1535, TA1537, TA1538, reverse mutation	–	–	1000 μg/plate	Van Abbé *et al.* (1982)
Salmonella typhimurium TA100, reverse mutation (fluctuation test)	–	–	10 000	Le Curieux *et al.* (1995)
Salmonella typhimurium TA1535, reverse mutation	–	NT	0.3% v/v	San Agustin & Lim-Sylianco (1978)

Table 4 (contd)

Test system	Result[a]		Dose[b] (LED or HID)	Reference
	Without exogenous metabolic system	With exogenous metabolic system		
Salmonella typhimurium TA98, TA1535, TA1537, reverse mutation	–	–	10	Gatehouse (1981)
Salmonella typhimurium TA1535, TA1537, TA1538, reverse mutation	–	–	10 000 µg/plate	Richold & Jones (1981)
Salmonella typhimurium TA1535 transfected with human *GST* gene, reverse mutation	(+)	NT	226	Pegram *et al.* (1997)
Salmonella typhimurium TA1537, reverse mutation	–	NT	0.05% v/v	San Agustin & Lim-Sylianco (1978)
Salmonella typhimurium TA98, reverse mutation	–	NT	0.02% v/v	San Agustin & Lim-Sylianco (1978)
Salmonella typhimurium TA98, reverse mutation	NT	+	0.2 mL/2000 cm^3	Norpoth *et al.* (1980)
Escherichia coli WP2 *uvrA*, reverse mutation	–	–	1000	Gatehouse (1981)
Escherichia coli WP2 *uvrA*, reverse mutation	–	–	10 000 µg/plate	Kirkland *et al.* (1981)
Escherichia coli WP2, reverse mutation	–	–	10 000 µg/plate	Kirkland *et al.* (1981)
Saccharomyces cerevisiae, gene conversion	+	NT	6400	Callen *et al.*, (1980)
Saccharomyces cerevisiae, gene conversion	–	–	333 µg/plate	Jagannath *et al.* (1981)
Saccharomyces cerevisiae, gene conversion	–	–	1000	Sharp & Parry (1981)
Saccharomyces cerevisiae, gene conversion	NT	–	3000	Zimmermann & Scheel (1981)
Saccharomyces cerevisiae, homozygosis by mitotic recombination or gene conversion	+	NT	6400	Callen *et al.* (1980)
Saccharomyces cerevisiae, homozygosis by mitotic recombination or gene conversion	–	–	1000	Kassinova *et al.* (1981)
Aspergillus nidulans, genetic crossing-over	–	NT	5 mL/20 L	Crebelli *et al.* (1984)
Aspergillus nidulans, genetic crossing-over	–	NT	0.5%	Gualandi (1984)
Saccharomyces cerevisiae, reverse mutation	+	NT	6400	Callen *et al.* (1980)

Table 4 (contd)

Test system	Result[a]		Dose[b] (LED or HID)	Reference
	Without exogenous metabolic system	With exogenous metabolic system		
Saccharomyces cerevisiae, reverse mutation	–	–	1111	Mehta & von Borstel (1981)
Aspergillus nidulans, forward mutation	–	NT	0.5%	Gualandi (1984)
Saccharomyces cerevisiae, aneuploidy	–	–	100	Parry & Sharp (1981)
Aspergillus nidulans, aneuploidy	–	NT	5 mL/20 L	Crebelli *et al.* (1984)
Aspergillus nidulans, aneuploidy	+	NT	0.16% v/v	Crebelli *et al.* (1988)
Drosophila melanogaster, sex-linked recessive lethal mutations	–		2975	Gocke *et al.* (1981)
Drosophila melanogaster, sex-linked recessive lethal mutations	–		0.2% (adult feeding)	Vogel *et al.* (1981)
DNA strand breaks, cross-links or related damage, rat hepatocytes *in vitro*	–	NT	357	Sina *et al.* (1983)
Unscheduled DNA synthesis, rat hepatocytes *in vitro*	–	NT	1000	Althaus *et al.* (1982)
Unscheduled DNA synthesis, mouse hepatocytes *in vitro*	–	NT	1190	Larson *et al.* (1994c)
Gene mutation, Chinese hamster lung V79 cells, *hprt* locus *in vitro*	–	NT	2.5% gas × 24 h	Sturrock (1977)
Sister cromatid exchange, Chinese hamster cells *in vitro*	–	–	0.71% gas v/v	White *et al.* (1979)
Sister chromatid exchange, Chinese hamster cells *in vitro*	NT	–	10 µg	Perry & Thomson (1981)
Sister chromatid exchange, rat leukemia cells *in vitro*	–	+	119	Fujie *et al.* (1993)
Cell tranformation, SA7/Syrian hamster embryo cells	+	NT	0.25 mL/chamber	Hatch *et al.* (1983)
Unscheduled DNA synthesis, human lymphocytes *in vitro*	–	–	15000	Perocco & Prodi (1981)
Unscheduled DNA synthesis, human hepatocytes *in vitro*	–	NT	119	Butterworth *et al.* (1989)
Sister chromatid exchange, human lymphocytes *in vitro*	NT	–	400	Kirkland *et al.* (1981)
Sister chromatid exchange, human lymphocytes *in vitro*	+	NT	1190	Morimoto & Koizumi (1983)
Chromosomal aberrations, human lymphocytes *in vitro*	NT	–	400	Kirkland *et al.* (1981)

Table 4 (contd)

Test system	Result[a]		Dose[b] (LED or HID)	Reference
	Without exogenous metabolic system	With exogenous metabolic system		
S. typhimurium TA1537, reverse mutation in urine from mice	+		700 × 1	San Agustin & Lim-Sylianco (1978)
Host-mediated assay, *S. typhimurium* TA1535 in mouse peritoneal cavity	–		NG	San Agustin & Lim-Sylianco (1978)
Host-mediated assay, *S. typhimurium* TA1537 in mouse peritoneal cavity	+		NG	San Agustin & Lim-Sylianco (1978)
Host-mediated assay, microbial cells in animal hosts	–		800 ip × 1	Hellmér & Bolcsfoldi (1992)
DNA strand breaks, cross-links or related damage, animal cells *in vivo*	–		400 po	Petzold & Swenberg (1978)
DNA strand breaks, cross-links or related damage, animal cells *in vivo*	–		480 po × 1	Kitchin & Brown (1989)
Unscheduled DNA synthesis, rat hepatocytes *in vivo*	–		400 po	Mirsalis *et al.* (1982)
Unscheduled DNA synthesis, mouse cells *in vivo*	–		477 po × 1	Larson *et al.* (1994c)
Gene mutation, B6C3F1 *lac*I transgenic mice *in vivo*	–		90 ppm 6 h/d × 180 d	Butterworth *et al.* (1998)
Sister chromatid exchange, animal cells *in vivo*	+		50 po × 4	Morimoto & Koizumi (1983)
Micronucleus formation, mice *in vivo*	(+)		700 × 1	San Agustin & Lim-Sylianco (1978)
Micronucleus formation, mice *in vivo*	–		952 ip × 2	Gocke *et al.* (1981)
Micronucleus formation, mice *in vivo*	?		132 ip	Salamone *et al.* (1981)
Micronucleus formation, mice *in vivo*	–		0.06 ml/kg ip × 2	Tsuchimoto & Matter (1981)
Micronucleus formation, rats (kidney) *in vivo*	+		4 mmol/kg po × 1	Robbiano *et al.* (1998)

Table 4 (contd)

Test system	Result[a]		Dose[b] (LED or HID)	Reference
	Without exogenous metabolic system	With exogenous metabolic system		
Micronucleus formation, other animals (newt) *in vivo*	–		50 μg/mL	Le Curieux *et al.* (1995)
Chromosomal aberrations, animal bone-marrow cells *in vivo*	+		10 μmol/kg ip × 1	Fujie *et al.* (1990)
Chromosomal aberrations, animal bone-marrow cells *in vivo*	+		1 mmol/kg po × 5	Fujie *et al.* (1990)
Binding (covalent) to DNA *in vitro*	NT	–	0.8	Diaz Gomez & Castro (1980a)
Binding (covalent) to DNA *in vitro*	–	+	95	Di Renzo *et al.* (1982)
Binding (covalent) to rat liver cell protein *in vitro*	+	NT	0.0008	Diaz Gomez & Castro (1980b)
Binding (covalent) to DNA and RNA, mouse liver cells *in vivo*	–		750 ip × 4	Diaz Gomez & Castro (1980a)
Binding (covalent) to RNA or protein, rat liver cells *in vivo*	+		5 ip × 1	Diaz Gomez & Castro (1980a)

[a] +, positive; (+), weakly positive; –, negative; NT, not tested; ?, inconclusive

[b] LED, lowest effective dose; HID, highest ineffective dose unless otherwise stated; in-vitro test, μg/mL; in-vivo test, mg/kg bw per day; NR, not reported; ip, intraperitoneal; po, oral

locus in Chinese hamster V79 cells in the absence of metabolic activation. No increase in the frequency of sister chromatid exchange was detected, in the presence of a metabolic system from rat liver, in two studies in Chinese hamster ovary cells. A modest but significant increase in sister chromatid exchange frequency was induced by chloroform in cultured rat erythroblastic leukaemia cells, but only in the presence of metabolic activation, and it enhanced transformation of Syrian hamster embryo cells by SA7 adenovirus.

In single studies in cultured human lymphocytes, chloroform increased the frequency of sister chromatid exchange in the absence of metabolic activation, but did not elicit DNA repair with or without activation; it also did not induce chromosomal breakage or sister chromatid exchange in the presence of activation. In cultures of primary human hepatocytes, no DNA repair synthesis was observed after exposure to chloroform.

In a host-mediated assay in mice, chloroform was mutagenic in males but not in females, and the response was weakly positive in *S. typhimurium* strain TA1537 but not in strain TA1535; chloroform was inactive in another host-mediated assay in mice in which the relative survival of *E. coli* k-12 *uvrB/recA* DNA repair-deficient strain was measured in blood, liver, lungs, kidney and testes.

DNA fragmentation was not observed in the livers of rats given a single oral dose of chloroform, and negative responses were obtained in in-vivo–in-vitro assays for DNA repair in rat and mouse hepatocytes. No increase in *lacI* mutant frequency was seen in the livers of female transgenic B6C3F$_1$ mice exposed to chloroform by inhalation for 180 days. Daily oral dosing of mice with chloroform for four successive days caused a significant increase in sister chromatid exchange frequency in bone-marrow cells. Weak induction of micronuclei in polychromatic erythrocytes was observed in chloroform-treated mice in one study, whereas another study of micronucleus formation in mouse bone marrow gave equivocal results and two studies gave negative results. A dose-dependent increase in the frequency of chromosomal aberrations was detected in the bone marrow of rats given a single intraperitoneal dose of chloroform or five successive daily oral doses. A statistically significant increase in the induction of micronucleated cells was observed in the proximal tubules of the kidneys of rats given a single oral dose of chloroform. Micronuclei were not, however, induced in newts.

No covalent binding of reactive metabolites of chloroform to DNA or RNA was observed in the livers of mice and rats injected intraperitoneally with [^{14}C]chloroform or in DNA exposed *in vitro* to [^{14}C]chloroform in the presence of a microsomal suspension containing an NADPH-generating system or liver tissue slices. In contrast, [^{14}C]chloroform bound covalently to calf thymus DNA after activation by hepatic microsomes from phenobarbital-induced rats.

4.5 Mechanistic considerations

There is strong evidence that cytotoxicity is a critical component of the induction of tumours in rodents by chloroform, since it has been shown that oxidative metabolism is necessary for activation of this compound and correlates with cytotoxicity, regenerative cell proliferation and tumour response in the target cell population. The concordance between these responses is strongest for hepatic and renal tumours in mice.

Chloroform-induced liver tumours have been observed in mice only after prolonged exposure to cytotoxic bolus doses given by oral gavage and not after administration of the same total daily dose in drinking-water. The incidence and severity of toxicity in the liver and kidney have been related to the degree of covalent binding of oxidative metabolites of chloroform to tissue proteins. The relationship between metabolism and toxicity is exemplified by localization of covalent binding to protein in both liver and kidney and the increases and decreases in toxic responses that result from pretreatment with inducers and inhibitors of cytochrome P450 activity, respectively. There is a consistent association between oxidative metabolism of chloroform, the pattern of covalent tissue binding and toxic injury (Davidson *et al.*, 1982). A strong dose-related correlation is also seen between induction of hepatic cytotoxicity, a sustained increase in regenerative cell proliferation and induction of liver tumours.

In the kidney of male mice, a strong correlation is also seen between the degree of oxidative metabolism, renal cytotoxicity, compensatory cell regeneration and renal tubular tumours. This correlation includes a strong concordance of these end-points with the sex of the mice and genetic variability. For example, male DBA mice, a parental strain of BDF_1 mice in which chloroform induces renal tumours, developed much more severe renal injury than C57BL mice, in which chloroform does not induce renal tumours.

The evidence for a correlation between cytotoxicity, a sustained increase in regenerative cell proliferation and tumours is weakest in rat kidney and in the tumour-susceptible Osborne-Mendel strain, which has not been investigated in depth; however, the observation of sustained renal cell injury in a two-year bioassay with Osborne-Mendel rats that correlated with tumour-inducing doses is consistent with induction of renal tumours via cytotoxicity induced by high doses and compensatory cell proliferation.

Thus, with the high-dose regimens used in cancer bioassays, chloroform has been shown to induce cytolethality and regenerative cell proliferation in the target organs for cancer.

5. Summary of Data Reported and Evaluation

5.1 Exposure data

Occupational exposure to chloroform may occur during its production and use as a solvent and chemical intermediate. The general population may be exposed as a result of its presence in chlorinated drinking-water, ambient air and some foods.

5.2 Human carcinogenicity data

Two cohort studies of cancer and drinking-water quality were carried out in the United States. One conducted in Maryland showed excess mortality from cancers of the liver and breast in association with water chlorination, while that conducted in Iowa showed increased risks for cancers of the colon and lung and skin melanoma associated with chloroform concentrations in drinking-water.

Eight case–control studies have been reported on bladder cancer in relation to chlorinated drinking-water in the United States. Significant results were obtained in five studies, but there was little consistency in the risk pattern in subgroups defined by sex or surrogate measures of chloroform intake. Significant increasing trends in the risk for bladder cancer were seen in two studies. The study in Colorado showed increasing risk with years of exposure to chlorinated water; the study in Iowa showed increasing risk with lifetime intake of trihalomethanes (from drinking-water), but only in men and not in women.

Seven case–control studies addressed the risk for cancers of the large bowel in association with consumption of chlorinated water. In two of these studies, lifetime exposure to trihalomethanes was assessed. Two studies showed significant associations with rectal cancer. Overall, however, the results were inconsistent with regard to the subsite of the large bowel and sex, and the quality of the studies varied widely.

Exposure to chloroform in the workplace was addressed in two case–control studies, both of which had limited statistical power. The study on brain cancer gave negative results. The other included a number of sites (but not the brain) and showed associations with cancers of the prostate and lung, but no association was seen with bladder cancer.

The presence of various water chlorination by-products, including trihalomethanes, is likely to be highly correlated. Although chloroform is the most ubiquitous, the other by-products therefore may act as confounders in studies of water-mediated exposure. In addition, important sources of chloroform other than drinking-water were ignored in the majority of the studies.

Although the epidemiological evidence for an association between consumption of chlorinated drinking-water and the risk for some cancers, particularly those of the urinary bladder and rectum and possibly of the colon, seems to favour an interpretation of mild excess, a causal inference cannot be made with regard to chloroform because of incomplete control for confounding by other water impurities and other factors and lack of concordance in the results for men and women. Use of surrogate indicators for exposure to chloroform adds to the uncertainty.

5.3 Animal carcinogenicity data

Chloroform was tested for carcinogenicity in several experiments in mice, rats and dogs. In three studies by oral administration and in one study by inhalation exposure in mice, it produced renal tubular tumours and, in one study, hepatocellular tumours. In three studies by oral administration in Osborne-Mendel rats, chloroform produced renal tubule tumours. No increased incidence of tumours was observed in one study in dogs.

5.4 Other relevant data

Chloroform is metabolized by oxidative and reductive pathways. Under normal conditions, oxidative metabolism is the major pathway, and reductive metabolism does not play a significant role. Oxidative metabolism of chloroform results in the generation of phosgene, which either reacts with water to give carbon dioxide and hydrogen chloride or binds covalently to tissue macromolecules. The formation of carbon dioxide as a metabolite of chloroform has been shown in a number of studies in both rodents and humans *in vivo*.

The metabolism of chloroform is more rapid in mice than in rats, and human tissues (liver and kidney) have the lowest activity. CYP2E1 is the predominant enzyme involved in the metabolism of chloroform in both rodent and human tissues.

There is a consistent, tissue-, species-, strain- and sex-specific pattern in the rate of metabolism, cytotoxicity and cell proliferation produced by chloroform in rodent liver and kidney. Under the conditions of the high-dose regimens used in cancer bioassays in which tumours are produced, chloroform induced cytotoxicity and regenerative cell proliferation in the target organs for cancer. These findings are consistent with a mode of action for tumorigenesis in the liver and kidney of rodents that involves cytotoxicity.

Chloroform has been tested for developmental toxicity in mice and rats by gavage and inhalation. Fetal toxicity in the form of growth retardation has been observed in several studies, concurrent with evidence of maternal toxicity. Malformations were observed in one study in rats exposed by inhalation. In a continuous breeding study, no reproductive effects were noted.

No data were available on the genetic and related effects of chloroform in humans. There is weak evidence for the genotoxicity of chloroform in experimental systems *in vivo* and in mammalian cells, fungi and yeast *in vitro*. It was not mutagenic to bacteria.

5.5 Evaluation

There is *inadequate evidence* in humans for the carcinogenicity of chloroform.

There is *sufficient evidence* in experimental animals for the carcinogenicity of chloroform.

Overall evaluation

Chloroform is *possibly carcinogenic to humans (Group 2B)*.

6. References

Alavanja, M., Goldstein, I. & Susser, M. (1980) A case control study of gastrointestinal and urinary tract cancer mortality and drinking water chlorination. In: Jolley, R., Brungs, W.A. & Cumming, R.B., eds, *Water Chlorination. Environmental Impact and Health Effects*, Vol. 3, Ann Arbor, Ann Arbor Science Publishers, pp. 395–409

Althaus, F.R., Lawrence, S.D., Sattler, G.L., Longfellow, D.G. & Pitot, H.C. (1982) Chemical quantification of unscheduled DNA synthesis in cultured hepatocytes as an assay for the rapid screening of potential chemical carcinogens. *Cancer Res.*, **42**, 3010–3015

American Conference of Governmental Industrial Hygienists (1997) *1997 TLVs® and BEIs®*, Cincinnati, OH, p. 19

Amet, Y., Berthou, F., Fournier, G., Dréano, Y., Bardou, L., Clèdes, J. & Ménez, J.-F. (1997) Cytochrome P450 4A and 2E1 expression in human kidney microsomes. *Biochem. Pharmacol.*, **53**, 765–771

Ammann, P., Laethem, C.L., & Kedderis, G.L. (1998) Chloroform-induced cytolethality in freshly isolated male B6C3F$_1$ mouse and Fischer 344 rat hepatocytes. *Toxicol. appl. Pharmacol.*, **149**, 217–225

Anon. (1997) Chloroform. *Environ. Health Perspectives*, **105** (Suppl. 1), 285–286

Balster, R.L. & Borzelleca, J.F. (1982) Behavioral toxicity of trihalomethane contaminants of drinking water in mice. *Environ. Health Perspectives*, **46**, 127–136

Brady, J.F., Li, D., Ishizaki, H., Lee, M., Ning, S.M., Xiao, F., & Yang, C.S. (1989) Induction of cytochromes P450IIE1 and P450IIB1 by secondary ketones and the role of P450IIE1 in chloroform metabolism. *Toxicol. appl. Pharmacol.*, **100**, 342–349

Branchflower, R.V., Nunn, D.S., Highet, R.J., Smith, J.H., Hook, J.B. & Pohl, L.R. (1984) Nephrotoxicity of chloroform: Metabolism to phosgene by the mouse kidney. *Toxicol. appl. Pharmacol.*, **72**, 159–168

Brenniman, G.R., Vasilomanolakis-Lagos, J., Amsel, J., Namekata, T. & Wolff, A.H. (1980) Case–control study of cancer deaths in Illinois communities served by chlorinated or nonchlorinated water. In: Jolley, R., Brungs, W.A. & Cumming, R.B., eds, *Water Chlorination. Environmental Impact and Health Effects*, Vol. 3, Ann Arbor, Ann Arbor Science Publishers, pp. 1043–1057

Brown, B.R., Jr, Sipes, I.G. & Sagalyn, A.M. (1974) Mechanisms of acute hepatic toxicity: Chloroform, halothane and glutathione. *Anesthesiology*, **41**, 554–561

Brown, D.M., Langley, P.F., Smith, D. & Taylor, D.C. (1974) Metabolism of chloroform. I. The metabolism of [^{14}C] chloroform by different species. *Xenobiotica*, **4**, 151–163

Brown-Woodman, P.D.C., Hayes, L.C., Huq, F., Herlihy, C., Picker, K. & Webster, W.S. (1998) In vitro assessment of the effect of halogenated hydrocarbons: Chloroform, dichloromethane, and dibromoethane on embryonic development of the rat. *Teratology*, **57**, 321–333

Budavari, S., ed. (1996) *The Merck Index*, 12th Ed., Whitehouse Station, NJ, Merck & Co., p. 357

Burkhalter, J.E. & Balster, R.L. (1979) Behavioral teratology evaluation of trichloromethane in mice. *Neurobehav. Toxicol.*, **1**, 199–205

Butterworth, B.E., Smith-Oliver, T., Earle, L., Loury, D.J., White, R.D., Doolittle, D.J., Working, P.K., Cattley, R.C., Jirtle, R., Michalopoulos, G. & Strom, S. (1989) Use of primary cultures of human hepatocytes in toxicology studies. *Cancer Res.*, **49**, 1075–1084

Butterworth, B.E., Templin, M.V., Constan, A.A., Sprankle, C.S., Wong, B.A., Pluta, L.J., Everitt, J.I. & Recio, L. (1998) Long-term mutagenicity studies with chloroform and dimethylnitrosamine in female *lacI* transgenic B6C3F$_1$ mice. *Environ. mol. Mutag.*, **31**, 248–256

Callen, D.F., Wolff, C.R. & Philpot, R.M. (1980) Cytochrome P-450 mediated genetic activity and cytotoxicity of seven halogenated aliphatic hydrocarbons in *Saccharomyces cerevisiae*. *Mutat Res.*, **77**, 55–63

Cantor, K.P., Hoover, R., Hartge, P., Mason, T.J., Silverman, D.T., Altman, R., Austin, D.F., Child, M.A., Key, C.R., Marrett, L.D., Myers, M.H., Narayana, A.S., Levin, L.I., Sullivan, J.W., Swanson, G.M., Thomas, D.B. & West, D.W. (1987) Bladder cancer, drinking water source, and tap water consumption: A case–control study. *J. natl Cancer Inst.*, **79**, 1269–1279

Cantor, K.P., Lynch, C.F., Hildesheim, M.E., Dosemeci, M., Lubin, J., Alavanja, M. & Craun, G. (1998) Drinking water source and chlorination byproducts. I. Risk of bladder cancer. *Epidemiology*, **9**, 21–28

Challen, P.J.R., Hickish, D.E. & Bedford, J. (1958) Chronic chloroform intoxication. *Br. J. ind. Med.*, **15**, 243–249

Charlesworth, F.A. (1976) Patterns of chloroform metabolism. *Food Cosmet. Toxicol.*, **14**, 59–60

Chemical Information Services (1995) *Directory of World Chemical Producers 1995/96 Standard Edition*, Dallas, TX, p. 174

Clemens, T.L., Hill, R.N., Bullock, L.P., Johnson, W.D., Sultatos, L.G. & Vesell, E.S. (1979) Chloroform toxicity in the mouse: Role of genetic factors and steroids. *Toxicol. appl. Pharmacol.*, **48**, 117–130

Conkle, J.P., Camp, B.J. & Welch, B.E. (1975) Trace composition of human respiratory gas. *Arch. environ. Health*, **30**, 290–295

Corley, R.A., Mendrala, A.L., Smith, F.A., Staats, D.A., Gargas, M.D., Conolly, R.B., Andersen, M.E. & Reitz, R.H. (1990) Development of a physiologically-based pharmacokinetic model for chloroform. *Toxicol. appl. Pharmacol.*, **103**, 512–527

Crebelli, R. Conti, G., Conti, L. & Carere, A. (1984) Induction of somatic segregation by halogenated aliphatic hydrocarbons in *Aspergillus nidulans*. *Mutat. Res.*, **138**, 33–38

Crebelli, R., Benigni, R., Franekic, J., Conti, G., Conti, L. & Carere, A. (1988) Induction of chromosome malsegregation by halogenated organic solvents in *Aspergillus nidulans*: Unspecific or specific mechanism? *Mutat. Res.*, **201**, 401–411

Cresteil, T., Beaune, P., Leroux, J.P., Lange, M. & Mansuy, D. (1979) Biotransformation of chloroform by rat and human liver microsomes; *in vitro* effect on some enzyme activities and mechanism of irreversible binding to macromolecules. *Chem.-biol. Interactions*, **24**, 153–165

Daniel, F.B., DeAngelo, A.B., Stober, J.A., Pereira, M.A. & Olson, G.R. (1989) Chloroform inhibition of 1,2-dimethylhydrazine-induced gastrointestinal tract tumors in the Fisher 344 rat. *Fundam. appl. Toxicol.*, **13**, 40–45

Danielsson, B.R.G., Ghantous, H. & Dencker, L. (1986) Distribution of chloroform and methyl chloroform and their metabolites in pregnant mice. *Biol. Res. Pregnancy*, **7**, 77–83

Davidson, I.W.F., Sumner, D.D. & Parker, J.C. (1982) Chloroform: A review of its metabolism, teratogenic, mutagenic, and carcinogenic potential. *Drug chem. Toxicol.*, **5**, 1–87

De Curtis, V., Gemma, S., Sbraccia, M., Testai, E. & Vittozzi, L. (1994) The contribution of electrophilic and radicalic intermediates to phospholipid adducts formed by halomethanes *in vivo*. *J. biochem. Toxicol.*, **9**, 305–310

Deml, E. & Oesterle, D. (1985) Dose-dependent promoting activity of chloroform in rat liver foci bioassay. *Cancer Lett.*, **29**, 59–63

Deml, E. & Oesterle, D. (1987) Dose–response of promotion by polychlorinated biphenyls and chloroform in rat liver foci bioassay. *Arch. Toxicol.*, **60**, 209–211

Deringer, M.K., Dunn, T.B. & Heston, W.E. (1953) Results of exposure of strain C3H mice to chloroform. *Proc. Soc. exp. Biol. NY*, **83**, 474–478

Diaz Gomez, M.I. & Castro, J.A. (1980a) Covalent binding of chloroform metabolites to nuclear protein—No evidence for binding to nucleic acids. *Cancer Lett.*, **9**, 213–218

Diaz Gomez, M.I. & Castro, J.A. (1980b) Nuclear activation of carbon tetrachloride and chloroform. *Res. Comm. Chem. Pathol. Pharmacol.*, **2**, 191–194

Dick, D., Ng, K.M.E., Sauder, D.N. & Chu, I. (1995) *In vitro* and *in vivo* percutaneous absorption of ^{14}C-chloroform in humans. *Hum. exp. Toxicol.*, **14**, 260–255

Di Renzo, A.B., Gandolfi, A.J. & Sipes, I.G. (1982) Microsomal bioactivation and covalent binding of aliphatic halides to DNA. *Toxicol. Lett.*, **11**, 243–252

Dix, K.J., Kedderis, G.L. & Borghoff, S.J. (1997) Vehicle-dependent oral absorption and target tissue dosimetry of chloroform in male rats and female mice. *Toxicol. Lett.*, **91**, 197–209

Docks, E.L. & Krishna, G. (1976) The role of glutathione in chloroform-induced hepatotoxicity. *Exp. mol. Pathol.*, **24,** 13–22

Doyle, R.E., Woodard, J.C., Lewis, A.L. & Moreland, A.F. (1967) Mortality in Swiss mice exposed to chloroform. *J. Am. vet. Med. Assoc.*, **141**, 930–934

Doyle, T.J., Zheng, W., Cerhan, J.R., Hong, C.-P., Sellers, T.A., Kushi, L.H. & Folsom, A.R. (1997) The association of drinking water source and chlorination by-products with cancer incidence among postmenopausal women in Iowa: a prospective cohort study. *Am. J. public Health*, **87**, 1168–1172

Eschenbrenner, A.B. & Miller, E. (1945) Induction of hepatomas in mice by repeated oral administration of chloroform, with observations on sex differences. *J. natl Cancer Inst.,* **5**, 251–255

Fry, B.J., Taylor, T. & Hathway, D.E. (1972) Pulmonary elimination of chloroform and its metabolite in man. *Arch. int. Pharmacodyn.*, **196**, 98–111

Fujie, K., Aoki, T. & Wada, M. (1990) Acute and subacute cytogenetic effects of the trihalomethanes on rat bone marrow cells in vivo. *Mutat. Res.*, **242**, 111–119

Fujie, K., Aoki, T., Ito, Y. & Maeda, S. (1993) Sister-chromatid exchanges induced by trihalomethanes in rat erythroblastic cells and their suppression by crude catechin extracted from green tea. *Mutat. Res.*, **300**, 241–246

Gatehouse, D. (1981) Mutagenic activity of 42 coded compounds in the 'microtiter' fluctuation test. In: de Serres, F.J. & Ashby, J., eds, *Progress in Mutation Research*, Vol. 1, *Evaluation of Short-term Tests for Carcinogens. Report of the International Collaborative Program*, New York, Elsevier/North-Holland, pp. 376–386

Gemma, S., Faccioli, S., Chieco, P., Sbraccia, M., Testai, E. & Vittozzi, L. (1996). *In vivo* $CHCl_3$ bioactivation, toxicokinetics, toxicity and induced compensatory cell proliferation in B6C3F1 male mice. *Toxicol. appl. Pharmacol.*, **141**, 394–402

Gocke, E., King, M.T., Eckhardt, K. & Wild, D. (1981) Mutagenicity of cosmetics ingredients licensed by the European Communities. *Mutat. Res.*, **90**, 91–109

Gottlieb, M.S. & Carr, J.K. (1982) Case–control cancer mortality study and chlorination of drinking water in Louisiana. *Environ. Health Perspectives*, **46**, 169–177

Gottlieb, M., Carr, J.K. & Morris, D.T. (1981) Cancer and drinking water in Louisiana: Colon and rectum. *Int. J. Epidemiol.*, **10**, 117–125

Gottlieb, M.S., Carr, J.K. & Clarkson, J.R. (1982) Drinking water and cancer in Louisiana. A retrospective mortality study. *Am. J. Epidemiol.*, **116**, 652–667

Green, M.H.L. (1981) A differential killing test using an improved repair-deficient strain of *Escherichia coli*. In: de Serres, F.J. & Ashby, J., eds, *Progress in Mutation Research*, Vol. 1, *Evaluation of Short-term Tests for Carcinogens. Report of the International Collaborative Program*, New York, Elsevier/North-Holland, pp. 183–194

Gualandi, G. (1984) Genotoxicity of the free-radical producers CCl_4 and lipoperoxide in *Aspergillus nidulans*. *Mutat. Res.*, **136**, 109–114

Guengerich, F.P., Kim, D.-H. & Iwasaki, M. (1991) Role of human cytochrome P-450 II E1 in the oxidation of many low molecular weight cancer suspects. *Chem. Res. Toxicol.*, **4**, 168–179

Hatch, G.G., Mamay, P.D., Ayer, M.L., Casto, B.C. & Nesnow, S. (1983) Chemical enhancement of viral transformation in Syrian hamster embryo cells by gaseous and volatile chlorinated methanes and ethanes. *Cancer Res.*, **43**, 1945–1950

Hathway, D.E. (1974) Chemical, biochemical and toxicological differences between carbon tetrachloride and chloroform. A critical review of recent investigations of these compounds in mammals. *Arzneim.-Forsch.*, **24**, 173–176

Heineman, E.F., Cocco, P., Gomez, M.R., Dosemeci, M., Stewart, P.A., Hayes, R.B., Zahm, S.H., Thomas, T.L. & Blair, A. (1994) Occupational exposure to chlorinated aliphatic hydrocarbons and risk of astrocytic brain cancer. *Am. J. ind. Med.*, **26**, 155–169

Hellmér, L. & Bolcsfoldi, G. (1992) An evaluation of the *E. coli* K-12 *uvrB/recA* DNA repair host-mediated assay. II. In vivo results for 36 compounds tested in the mouse. *Mutat. Res.*, **272**, 161–173

Heywood, R., Sortwell, R.J., Noel, P.R.B., Street, A.E., Prentice, D.E., Roe, F.J.C., Wadsworth, P.F., Worden A.N. & Van Abbé, N.J. (1979) Safety evaluation of toothpaste containing chloroform. III. Long-term study in beagle dogs. *J. environ. Pathol. Toxicol.*, **2**, 835–851

Hildesheim, M.E., Cantor, K.P., Lynch, C.F., Dosemeci, M., Lubin, J., Alavanja, M. & Craun, G. (1998) Drinking water source and chlorination byproducts. II. Risk of colon and rectal cancers. *Epidemiology*, **9**, 29–35

Hill, R.N., Clemens, T.L., Liu, D.K., Vesell, E.S. & Johnson, W.D. (1975) Genetic control of chloroform toxicity in mice. *Science*, **190**, 159–161

IARC (1972) *IARC Monographs on the Evaluation of Carcinogenic Risk of Chemicals to Man*, Vol. 1, *Some Inorganic Substances, Chlorinated Hydrocarbons, Aromatic Amines,* N-*Nitroso Compounds, and Natural Products*, Lyon, pp. 61–65

IARC (1979) *IARC Monographs on the Evaluation of the Carcinogenic Risks of Chemicals to Humans*, Vol. 20, *Some Halogenated Hydrocarbons*, Lyon, pp. 401–427

IARC (1987) *IARC Monographs on the Evaluation of Carcinogenic Risks to Humans*, Suppl. 7, *Overall Evaluations of Carcinogenicity: An Updating of* IARC Monographs *Volumes 1 to 42*, Lyon, pp. 152–154

Ilett, K.F., Reid, W.D., Sipes, I.G. & Krishna, D. (1973) Chloroform toxicity in mice: correlation of renal and hepatic necrosis with covalent binding of metabolities to tissue macromolecules. *Exp. mol. Pathol.*, **19**, 215–229

International Labour Office (1991) *Occupational Exposure Limits for Airborne Toxic Substances*, 3rd. Ed. (Occupational Safety and Health Series No. 37), Geneva, pp. 90–91

International Trade Commission (1991) *Synthetic Organic Chemicals, US Production and Sales*, 75th Ed., Washington DC, US Government Printing Office, p. 15-9

International Trade Commission (1993) *Synthetic Organic Chemicals, US Production and Sales*, 77th Ed., Washington DC, US Government Printing Office, p. 3-18

Jagannath, D.R., Vultaggio, D.M. & Brusick, D.J. (1981) Genetic activity of 42 coded compounds in the mitotic gene conversion assay using *Saccharomyces cerevisiae* strain D4. In: de Serres, F.J. & Ashby, J., eds, *Progress in Mutation Research*, Vol. 1, *Evaluation of Short-term Tests for Carcinogens. Report of the International Collaborative Program*, New York, Elsevier/North-Holland, pp. 456–467

Jorgenson, T.A., Meierhenry, E.F., Rushbrook, C.J., Bull, R.J. & Robinson, M. (1985) Carcinogenicity of chloroform in drinking water to male Osborne-Mendel rats and female $B6C3F_1$ mice. *Fundam. appl. Toxicol.*, **5**, 760–769

Kada, T. (1981) The DNA-damaging activity of 42 coded compounds in the rec-assay. In: de Serres, F.J. & Ashby, J., eds, *Progress in Mutation Research*, Vol. 1, *Evaluation of Short-term Tests for Carcinogens. Report of the International Collaborative Program*, New York, Elsevier/North-Holland, pp. 175-182

Kanarek, M.S. & Young, T.B. (1982) Drinking water treatment and risk of cancer death in Wisconsin. *Environ. Health Perspectives*, **46**, 179–186

Kassinova, G.V., Kovaltsova, S.V., Marfin, S.V. & Zakharov, I.A. (1981) Activity of 40 coded compounds in differential inhibition and mitotic crossing-over assays in yeast. In: de Serres, F.J. & Ashby, J., eds, *Progress in Mutation Research*, Vol. 1, *Evaluation of Short-term Tests for Carcinogens. Report of the International Collaborative Program*, New York, Elsevier/North-Holland, pp. 434–455

Kimura, E.T., Ebert, D.M. & Dodge, P.W. (1971) Acute toxicity and limits of solvent residue for sixteen organic solvents. *Toxicol. appl. Pharmacol.*, **19**, 699–704

Kirkland, D.J., Smith, K.L. & Van Abbé, N.J. (1981) Failure of chloroform to induce chromosome damage or sister-chromatid exchanges in cultured human lymphocytes and failure to induce reversion in *Escherichia coli*. *Food Cosmet. Toxicol.*, **19**, 651–656

Kitchin, K.T. & Brown, J.L. (1989) Biochemical effects of three carcinogenic chlorinated methanes in rat liver. *Teratog. Carcinog. Mutag.*, **9**, 61–69

Klaunig, J.E., Ruch, R.J. & Pereira, M.A. (1986) Carcinogenicity of chlorinated methane and ethane compounds administered in drinking water to mice. *Environ. Health Perspectives*, **69**, 89–95

Land, P.C., Owen, E.L. & Linde, H.W. (1981) Morphologic changes in mouse spermatozoa after exposure to inhalational anesthetics during early spermatogenesis. *Anesthesiology*, **54**, 53–56

Larson, J.L., Wolf, D.C. & Butterworth, B.E. (1993) Acute hepatotoxic and nephrotoxic effects of chloroform in male Fischer 344 rats and female B6C3F1 mice. *Fundam. appl. Toxicol.*, **20**, 302–315

Larson, J.L., Wolf, D.C. & Butterworth, B.E. (1994a) Induced cytotoxicity and cell proliferation in the hepatocarcinogenicity of chloroform in female B6C3F1 mice: Comparison of administration by gavage in corn oil vs *ad libitum* in drinking water. *Fundam. appl. Toxicol.*, **22**, 90–102

Larson, J.L., Wolf, D.C., Morgan, K.T, Méry, S. & Butterworth, B.E. (1994b) The toxicity of 1-week exposures to inhaled chloroform in female B6C3F1 mice and male Fischer 344 rats. *Fundam. appl. Toxicol.*, **22**, 431–446

Larson, J.L., Sprankle, C.S. & Butterworth, B.E. (1994c) Lack of chloroform-induced DNA repair in vitro and in vivo in hepatocytes of female B6C3F_1 mice. *Environ. mol. Mutag.*, **23**, 132–136

Larson, J.L., Wolf, D.C. & Butterworth, B.E. (1995a) Induced regenerative cell proliferation in livers and kidneys of male Fischer 344 rats given chloroform in corn oil by gavage or ad libitum in drinking water. *Toxicology*, **95**, 73–86

Larson, J.L., Wolf, D.C., Méry, S., Morgan, K.T. & Butterworth, B.E. (1995b) Toxicity and cell proliferation in the liver, kidneys and nasal passages of female Fischer 344 rats, induced by chloroform administered by gavage. *Food chem. Toxicol.*, **33**, 443–456

Larson, J.L., Templin, M.V., Wolf, D.C., Jamison, K.C., Leininger, J.R., Méry, S., Morgan, K.T., Wong, B.A., Conolly, R.B. & Butterworth, B.E. (1996) A 90-day chloroform inhalation study in female and male B6C3F_1 mice: Implications for cancer risk assessment. *Fundam. appl. Toxicol.*, **30**, 118–137

Lawrence, C.E., Taylor, P.R., Trock, B.J. & Reilly, A.A. (1984) Trihalomethanes in drinking water and human colorectal cancer. *J. natl Cancer Inst.*, **72**, 563–568

Le Curieux, F., Gauthier, L., Erb, F., & Marzin, D. (1995) Use of the SOS chromotest, the Ames-fluctuation test and the newt micronucleus test to study the genotoxicity of four trihalomethanes. *Mutagenesis*, **10**, 333–341

Lide, D.R., ed. (1997) *CRC Handbook of Chemistry and Physics*, 78th Ed., Boca Raton, FL, CRC Press, p. 3-207

Luke, B.T., Loew, G.H. & McLean, A.D. (1988) Theoretical investigation of the anaerobic reduction of halogenated alkanes by cytochrome P-450. 2. Vertical electron affinities of chlorofluoromethanes as a measure of their activity. *J. Am. chem. Soc.*, **110**, 3396–3400

Lykins, B.W., Jr & Koffskey, W. (1986) Products identified at an alternative disinfection pilot plant. *Environ. Health Perspectives*, **69**, 119–127

MacDonald, D.J. (1981) *Salmonella*/microsome tests on 42 coded chemicals. In: de Serres, F.J. & Ashby, J., eds, *Progress in Mutation Research*, Vol. 1, *Evaluation of Short-term Tests for Carcinogens. Report of the International Collaborative Program*, New York, Elsevier/North-Holland, pp. 285–297

Mansuy, D., Beaune, P., Cresteil, T., Lange, M. & Leroux, J.-P. (1977) Evidence for phosgene formation during liver microsomal oxidation of chloroform. *Biochem. biophys. Res. Comm.*, **79**, 513–517

Matsuki, A. & Zsigmond, E.K. (1974) The first fatal case of chloroform anesthesia in the United States. *Anesth. Analg.*, **53**, 152–154

McConnell, G., Ferguson, D.M. & Pearson, C.R. (1975) Chlorinated hydrocarbons and the environment. *Endeavor*, **34**, 13–18

McGeehin, M.A., Reif, J.S., Becher, J.C. & Mangione, E.J. (1993) Case–control study of bladder cancer and water disinfection methods in Colorado. *Am. J. Epidemiol.*, **138**, 492–501

McLean, A.E.M. (1970) The effects of protein deficiency and microsomal enzyme induction by DDT and phenobarbitone on the acute toxicity of chloroform and a pyrrolizidine alkaloid, retrorsine. *Br. J. exp. Pathol.*, **51**, 317–321

Mehta, R.D. & von Borstel, R.C. (1981) Mutagenic activity of 42 encoded compounds in the haploid yeast reversion assay, strain XV185-14C. In: de Serres, F.J. & Ashby, J., eds, *Progress in Mutation Research*, Vol. 1, *Evaluation of Short-term Tests for Carcinogens. Report of the International Collaborative Program*, New York, Elsevier/North-Holland, pp. 414–423

Mink, F.L., Brown, T.J. & Rickabaugh, J. (1986) Absorption, distribution, and excretion of ^{14}C-trihalomethanes in mice and rats. *Bull. environ. Contam. Toxicol.*, **37**, 752–758

Mirsalis, J.C., Tyson, C.K. & Butterworth, B.E. (1982) Detection of genotoxic carcinogens in the in vivo-in vitro hepatocyte DNA repair assay. *Environ. Mutag.*, **4**, 553–562

Morgan, A., Black, A. & Belcher, D.R. (1970) The excretion in breath of some aliphatic halogenated hydrocarbons following administration by inhalation. *Ann. occup. Hyg.*, **13**, 219–233

Morgan, D.L., Cooper, S.W., Carlock, D.L., Sykora, J.J., Sutton, B., Mattie, D.R. & McDougal, J.N. (1991) Dermal absorption of neat and aqueous volatile organic chemicals in the Fisher-344 rat. *Environ. Res.*, **55**, 51–63

Morimoto, K. & Koizumi, A. (1983) Trihalomethanes induce sister chromatid exchanges in human lymphocytes *in vitro* and mouse bone marrow cells *in vivo*. *Environ. Res.*, **32**, 72–79

Murray, F.J., Schwetz, B.A., McBride, J.G. & Staples, R.E. (1979) Toxicity of inhaled chloroform in pregnant mice and their offspring. *Toxicol. appl. Pharmacol.*, **50**, 515–522

Nagano, K., Nishizawa, T., Yamamoto, S. & Matsushima, T. (1998) Inhalation carcinogenesis studies of six halogenated hydrocarbons in rats and mice. In: Chiyotani K., Hosoda, Y. & Aizawa, Y., eds, *Advances in the Prevention of Occupational Respiratory Diseases*, Amsterdam, Elsevier, pp. 741–746

National Institute for Occupational Safety and Health (1998) *National Occupational Exposure Survey (1981–1983)*, Cincinnati, OH

National Library of Medicine (1998a) *Hazardous Substances Data Bank (HSDB)*, Bethesda, MD [Record No. 56]

National Library of Medicine (1998b) *Toxic Chemical Release Inventory 1987 & 1996* (TRI87 & TRI96), Bethesda, MD

National Toxicology Program (1991) *NTP Chemical Repository Data Sheet: Chloroform*, Research Triangle Park, NC

Nestmann, E.R., Lee, E.G.-H., Matula, T.I., Douglas, G.R. & Mueller, J.C. (1980) Mutagenicity of constituents identified in pulp and paper mill effluents using the Salmonella/mammalian-microsome assay. *Mutat. Res.*, **79**, 203–212

Norpoth, K., Reisch, A. & Heinecke, A. (1980) Biostatistics of Ames-test data. In: Norpoth, K.H. & Garner, R.C., eds, *Short-term Test Systems for Detecting Carcinogens*, New York, Springer-Verlag, pp. 312–322

Palmer A.K., Street, A.E., Roe, F.J.C., Worden, A.N. & Van Abbé, N.J. (1979) Safety evaluation of toothpaste containing chloroform II. Long term studies in rats. *J. environ. Pathol. Toxicol.*, **2**, 821–833

Parry, J.M. & Sharp, D.C. (1981) Induction of mitotic aneuploidy in the yeast strain D6 by 42 coded compounds. In: de Serres, F.J. & Ashby, J., eds, *Progress in Mutation Research*, Vol. 1, *Evaluation of Short-term Tests for Carcinogens. Report of the International Collaborative Program*, New York, Elsevier/North-Holland, pp. 468–480

Paul, B.B. & Rubinstein, D. (1963) Metabolism of carbon tetrachloride and chloroform by the rat. *J. Pharmacol. exp. Ther.*, **141**, 141–148

Pegram, R.A., Andersen, M.E., Warren, S.H., Ross, T.M. & Claxton, L.D. (1997) Glutathione S-transferase-mediated mutagenicity of trihalomethanes in *Salmonella typhimurium*: Contrasting results with bromodichloromethane and chloroform. *Toxicol. appl. Pharmacol.*, **144**, 183–188

Pereira, M.A. (1994) Route of administration determines whether chloroform enhances or inhibits cell proliferation in the liver of B6C3F1 mice. *Fundam. appl. Toxicol.*, **23**, 87–92

Pereira, M.A., Lin, L-H.C., Lippitt, J.M. & Herren, S.L. (1982) Trihalomethanes as initiators and promoters of carcinogenesis. *Environ. Health Perspectives*, **46**, 151–156

Pereira, M.A., Savage, R.E., Jr, Guion, C.W. & Wernsing, P.A. (1984) Effect of chloroform on hepatic and renal DNA synthesis and ornithine decarboxylase activity in mice and rats. *Toxicol. Lett.*, **21**, 357–364

Pereira, M.A., Knutsen G.L. & Herren-Freund, S.L. (1985) Effect of subsequent treatment of chloroform or phenobarbital on the incidence of liver and lung tumors initiated by ethylnitrosourea in 15 day old mice. *Carcinogenesis*, **6**, 203–207

Perocco, P. & Prodi, G. (1981) DNA damage by haloalkanes in human lymphocytes cultured in vitro. *Cancer Lett.*, **13**, 213–218

Perry, P.E. & Thomson, E.J. (1981) Evaluation of the sister chromatid exchange method in mammalian cells as a screening system for carcinogens. In: de Serres, F.J. & Ashby, J., eds, *Progress in Mutation Research*, Vol. 1, *Evaluation of Short-term Tests for Carcinogens. Report of the International Collaborative Program*, New York, Elsevier/North-Holland, pp. 560–569

Petzold, G.L. & Swenberg, J.A. (1978) Detection of DNA damage induced *in vivo* following exposure of rats to carcinogens. *Cancer Res.*, **38**, 1589–1594

Pohl, L.R. (1979) Biochemical toxicology of chloroform. In: Bend, J., Philpot, R.M. & Hodgson, E., eds, *Reviews of Biochemical Toxicology*, Amsterdam, Elsevier North Holland, pp. 79–107

Pohl, L.R., Bhooshan, B., Whittaker, N.F. & Krishna, G. (1977) Phosgene: A metabolite of chloroform. *Biochem. biophys. Res. Comm.*, **79**, 684–691

Pohl, L.R., George, J.W., Martin, J.L. & Krishna, G. (1979) Deuterium isotope effect in *in vivo* bioactivation of chloroform to phosgene. *Biochem. Pharmacol.*, **289**, 561–563

Pohl, L.R., Martin, J.L., & George, J.W. (1980) Mechanism of metabolic activation of chloroform by rat liver microsomes. *Biochem. Pharmacol.*, **29**, 3271–3276

Pohl, L.R., Branchflower, R.V., Highet, R.J., Martin, J.L., Nunn, D.S., Monks, T.J., George, J.W. & Hinson, J.A. (1981) The formation of diglutathionyl dithiocarbonate as a metabolite of chloroform, bromotrichloromethane and carbon tetrachloride. *Drug Metab. Disposition*, **9**, 334–339

Pohl, L.R., George, J.W. & Satoh, H. (1984) Strain and sex differences in chloroform-induced nephrotoxicity *Drug. Metab. Disposition*, **12**, 304–308

Poobalasingham, N. & Payne, J.P. (1978) The uptake and elimination of chloroform in man. *Br. J. Anaesth.*, **50**, 325–329

Raymond, P. & Plaa, G.L. (1997) Effect of dosing vehicle on the hepatotoxicity of CCl_4 and nephrotoxicity of $CHCl_3$ in rats. *J. Toxicol. environ. Health*, **51**, 463–476

Reddy, T.V, Daniel, F.B., Lin, E.L., Stober, J.A. & Olson, G.R. (1992) Chloroform inhibits the development of diethylnitrosamine-initiated, phenobarbital-promoted γ-glutamyltrans-peptidase and placental form glutathione S-transferase-positive foci in rat liver. *Carcinogenesis*, **13**, 1325–1330

Richold, M. & Jones, E. (1981) Mutagenic activity of 42 coded compounds in the *Salmonella/* microsome assay. In: de Serres, F.J. & Ashby, J., eds, *Progress in Mutation Research*, Vol. 1, *Evaluation of Short-term Tests for Carcinogens. Report of the International Collaborative Program*, New York, Elsevier/North-Holland, pp. 314–322

Robbiano, L., Mereto, E., Migliazzi Morando, A., Pastore, P. & Brambilla, G. (1998) Increased frequency of micronucleated kidney cells in rats exposed to halogenated anaesthetics. *Mutat. Res.*, **413**, 1–6

Roe, F.J.C., Palmer, A.K., Worden A.N. & Van Abbé, N.J. (1979) Safety evaluation of toothpaste containing chloroform I. Long-term studies in mice. *J. environ. Pathol. Toxicol.*, **2**, 799–819

Roldán-Arjona, T. & Pueyo, C. (1993) Mutagenic and lethal effects of halogenated methanes in the Ara test of *Salmonella typhimurium*: Quantitative relationship with chemical reactivity. *Mutagenesis*, **8**, 127–131

Roldán-Arjona, T., García-Pedrajas, M.D., Luque-Romero, F.L., Hera, C. & Pueyo, C. (1991) An association between mutagenicity of the Ara test of *Salmonella typhimurium* and carcinogenicity in rodents for 16 halogenated aliphatic hydrocarbons. *Mutagenesis*, **6**, 199–205

Rosenkranz, H.S., Hyman, J. & Leifer, Z. (1981) DNA polymerase deficient assay. In: de Serres, F.J. & Ashby, J., eds, *Progress in Mutation Research*, Vol. 1, *Evaluation of Short-term Tests for Carcinogens. Report of the International Collaborative Program*, New York, Elsevier/ North-Holland, pp. 210–218

Royston, G.D. (1925) Delayed chloroform poisoning following delivery. *Am. J. Obstet. Gynecol.*, **10**, 808–814

Ruddick, J.A., Villeneuve, D.C. & Chu, I. (1983) A teratological assessment of four trihalomethanes in the rat. *J. environ. Sci. Health*, **B18**, 333–349

Salamone, M.F., Heddle, J.A. & Katz, M. (1981) Mutagenic activity of 41 compounds in the in vivo micronucleus assay. In: de Serres, F.J. & Ashby, J., eds, *Progress in Mutation Research*, Vol. 1, *Evaluation of Short-term Tests for Carcinogens. Report of the International Collaborative Program*, New York, Elsevier/North-Holland, pp. 686–697

San Agustin, J. & Lim-Sylianco, C.Y. (1978) Mutagenic and clastogenic effects of chloroform. *Bull. Phil. Biochem. Soc.*, **1**, 17–23

Savage, R.E., Jr, Westrich, C., Guion, C. & Pereira, M.A. (1982) Chloroform induction of ornithine decarboxylase activity in rats. *Environ. Health Perspectives*, **46**, 157–162

Savage, R.E., Jr, DeAngelo, A.B., Guion, C. & Pereira, M.A. (1987) Studies on the mechanism of action of chloroform stimulation of rat hepatic ornithine decarboxylase (ODC). *Res. Comm. chem. Pathol. Pharmacol.*, **58**, 97–113

Scholler, K.L. (1968) Electron-microscopic and autoradiographic studies on the effect of halothane and chloroform on liver cells. *Acta. anaesthesiol. scand.*, **32** (Suppl.), 1–62

Scholler, K.L. (1970) Modification of the effects of chloroform on the rat liver. *Br. J. Anaesth.*, **42**, 603–605

Schwetz, B.A., Leong, B.K.J. & Gehring, P.J. (1974) Embryo- and fetotoxicity of inhaled chloroform in rats. *Toxicol. appl. Pharmacol.*, **28**, 442–451

Sharp, D.C. & Parry, J.M. (1981) Induction of mitotic gene conversion by 41 coded compounds using the yeast culture *JD1*. In: de Serres, F.J. & Ashby, J., eds, *Progress in Mutation Research*, Vol. 1, *Evaluation of Short-term Tests for Carcinogens. Report of the International Collaborative Program*, New York, Elsevier/North-Holland, pp. 491–501

Siemiatycki, J., ed. (1991) *Risk Factors for Cancers in the Workplace*, Boca Raton, FL, CRC Press

Simmon, V.F., Kauhanen, K. & Tardiff, R.C. (1977) Mutagenic activity of chemicals identified in drinking water. In: Scott, D., Bridges, B.A. & Sobels, F.H., eds, *Developments in Toxicology and Environmental Science, Progress in Genetic Toxicology*, Vol. 2, Amsterdam, Elsevier/North-Holland, pp. 249–258

Sina, J.F., Bean, C.L., Dysart, G.R., Taylor, V.I. & Bradley, M.O. (1983) Evaluation of the alkaline elution/rat hepatocyte assay as a predictor of carcinogenic/mutagenic potential. *Mutat. Res.*, **113**, 357–391

Sipes, I.G., Krishna, G. & Gillette, J.R. (1977) Bioactivation of carbon tetrachloride, chloroform and bromotrichloromethane: Role of cytochrome P-450. *Life Sci.*, **20**, 1541–1548

Skopek, T.R., Andon, B.M., Kaden., D.A. & Thilly, W.G. (1981) Mutagenic activity of 42 coded compounds using 8-azaguanine resistance as a genetic marker in *Salmonella typhimurium*. In: de Serres, F.J. & Ashby, J., eds, *Progress in Mutation Research*, Vol. 1, *Evaluation of Short-term Tests for Carcinogens. Report of the International Collaborative Program*, New York, Elsevier/North-Holland, pp. 371–375

Smith, J.H. & Hook, J.B. (1983) Mechanism of chloroform nephrotoxicity. II. *In vitro* evidence for renal metabolism of chloroform in mice. *Toxicol. appl. Pharmacol.*, **70**, 480–485

Smith, J.H., & Hook, J.B. (1984) Mechanism of chloroform nephrotoxicity. III. Renal and hepatic microsomal metabolism of chloroform in mice. *Toxicol. appl. Pharmacol.*, **73**, 511–524

Smith, A.A., Volpitto, P.P., Gramling, Z.W., DeVore, M.B. & Glassman, A.B. (1973) Chloroform, halothane, and regional anesthesia: A comparative study. *Anesth. Analg.*, **52**, 1–11

Smith, J.H., Maita, K., Sleight, S.D. & Hook, J.B. (1983) Mechanism of chloroform nephrotoxicity. I. Time course of chloroform toxicity in male and female mice *Toxicol. appl. Pharmacol.*, **70**, 467–479

Smith, M.K., Zenick, H. & George, E.L. (1986) Reproductive toxicology of disinfection by-products. *Environ. Health Perspectives*, **69**, 177–182

Storms, W.W. (1973) Chloroform parties. *J. Am. med. Assoc.*, **225**, 160

Sturrock, J. (1977) Lack of mutagenic effect of halothane or chloroform on cultured cells using the azaguanine test system. *Br. J. Anaesth.*, **49**, 207–210

Taylor, D.C., Brown, D.M., Keeble, R. & Langley, P.F. (1974) Metabolism of chloroform. II. A sex difference in the metabolism of [^{14}C] chloroform in mice. *Xenobiotica*, **4**, 165–174

Templin, M.V., Jamison, K.C., Sprankle, C.S., Wolf, D.C., Wong, B.A. & Butterworth, B.E. (1996a) Chloroform-induced cytotoxicity and regenerative cell proliferation in the kidneys and liver of BDF1 mice. *Cancer Lett.*, **108**, 225–231

Templin, M.V., Jamison, K.C., Wolf, D.C., Morgan, K.T. & Butterworth, B.E. (1996b) Comparison of chloroform-induced toxicity in the kidneys, liver, and nasal passages of male Osborne-Mendel and Fischer 344 rats. *Cancer Lett.*, **104**, 71–78

Templin, M.V., Larson, J.L., Butterworth, B.E., Jamison, K.C., Leininger, J.R., Méry, S., Morgan, K.T., Wong, B.A. & Wolf, D.C. (1996c) A 90-day chloroform inhalation study in Fischer 344 rats: Profile of toxicity and relevance to cancer studies. *Fundam. appl. Toxicol.*, **32**, 109–125

Templin, M.V., Constan, A.A., Wolf, D.C., Wong, B.A. & Butterworth, B.E. (1998) Patterns of chloroform-induced regenerative cell proliferation in BDF1 mice correlate with organ specificity and dose-response of tumor formation. *Carcinogenesis*, **19**, 187–193

Testai, E. & Vittozzi, L. (1986) Biochemical alterations elicited in rat liver microsomes by oxidation and reduction products of chloroform metabolism. *Chem.-biol. Interactions*, **59**, 157–171

Thomson, J.A. (1981) Mutagenic activity of 42 coded compounds in the lambda induction assay. In: de Serres, F.J. & Ashby, J., eds, *Progress in Mutation Research*, Vol. 1, *Evaluation of Short-term Tests for Carcinogens. Report of the International Collaborative Program*, New York, Elsevier/North-Holland, pp. 224–235

Torkelson, T.R., Oyen, F. & Rowe, V.K. (1976) The toxicity of chloroform as determined by single and repeated exposure of laboratory animals. *Am. ind. Hyg. Assoc. J.*, **37**, 697–705

Tsuchimoto, T. & Matter, B.E. (1981) Activity of coded compounds in the micronucleus test. In: de Serres, F.J. & Ashby, J., eds, *Progress in Mutation Research*, Vol. 1, *Evaluation of Short-term Tests for Carcinogens. Report of the International Collaborative Program*, New York, Elsevier/North-Holland, pp. 705–711

Tumasonis, C.F., McMartin, D.N. & Bush, B. (1987) Toxicity of chloroform and bromodichloromethane when administered over a lifetime in rats. *J. environ. Pathol. Toxicol. Oncol.*, **7**, 55–64

Uehleke, H. & Werner, T. (1975) A comparative study on the irreversible binding of labeled halothane trichlorofluoromethane, chloroform, and carbon tetrachloride to hepatic protein and lipids *in vitro* and *in vivo*. *Arch. Toxicol.*, **34**, 289–308

Van Abbé, N.J., Green, T.J., Jones, E., Richold, M. & Roe, F.J.C. (1982) Bacterial mutagenicity studies on chloroform *in vitro*. *Food chem. Toxicol.*, **20**, 557–561

Verschueren, K. (1996) *Handbook of Environmental Data on Organic Chemicals*, 3rd Ed., New York, Van Nostrand Reinhold Co., pp. 476–482

Vesell, E.S., Lang, C.M., White, W.J., Passananti, G.T., Hill, R.N., Clemens, T.L., Liu, D.K. & Johnson, W.D. (1976) Environmental and genetic factors affecting the response of laboratory animals to drugs. *Fed. Proc.*, **35**, 1125–1132

Vogel, E., Blijleven, W.G.H., Kortselius, M.J.H. & Zijlstra, J.A. (1981) Mutagenic activity of 17 coded compounds in the sex-linked recessive lethal test in *Drosophila melanogaster*. In: de Serres, F.J. & Ashby, J., eds, *Progress in Mutation Research*, Vol. 1, *Evaluation of Short-term Tests for Carcinogens. Report of the International Collaborative Program*, New York, Elsevier/North-Holland, pp. 660–665

Von Oettingen, W.E. (1964) *The Halogenated Hydrocarbons of Industrial and Toxicological Importance*, New York, Elsevier, pp. 77–81, 95–101

Whitaker, A. M. & Jones, C.S. (1965) Report of 1500 chloroform anesthetics administered with a precision vaporizer. *Anesth. Analg.*, **44**, 60–65

White, A.E., Takehisa, S., Eger, E.I., Wolff, S. & Stevens, W.C. (1979) Sister chromatid exchanges induced by inhaled anesthetics. *Anesthesiology*, **50**, 426–430

WHO (1993) *Guidelines for Drinking Water Quality*, 2nd Ed., Vol. 1, *Recommendations*, Geneva, p. 101

WHO (1994) *Chloroform* (Environmental Health Criteria 163), Geneva, International Programme on Chemical Safety

Wilkins, J.R., III & Comstock, G.W. (1981) Source of drinking water at home and site-specific cancer incidence in Washington County, Maryland. *Am. J. Epidemiol.*, **114**, 178–190

Withey, J.R., Collins, B.T. & Collins, P.G. (1983) Effect of vehicle on the pharmacokinetics and uptake of four halogenated hydrocarbons from the gastrointestinal tract of the rat. *J. appl. Toxicol.*, **3**, 249–253

Young, T.B., Kanarek, M.S. & Tsiatis, A.A. (1981) Epidemiologic study of drinking water chlorination and Wisconsin female cancer mortality. *J. natl Cancer Inst.*, **67**, 1191–1198

Young, T.B., Wolf, D.A. & Kanarek, M.Y. (1987) Case–control study of colon cancer and drinking water trihalomethanes in Wisconsin. *Int. J. Epidemiol.*, **16**, 190–197

Zierler, S., Feingold, L., Danley, R.A. & Craun, G. (1988) Bladder cancer in Massachusetts related to chlorinated and chloraminated drinking water: A case–control study. *Arch. environ. Health*, **43**, 195–200

Zimmermann, F.K. & Scheel, I. (1981) Induction of mitotic gene conversion in strain D7 of *Saccharomyces cerevisiae* by 42 coded chemicals. In: de Serres, F.J. & Ashby, J., eds, *Progress in Mutation Research*, Vol. 1, *Evaluation of Short-term Tests for Carcinogens. Report of the International Collaborative Program*, New York, Elsevier/North-Holland, pp. 481–490

CHLOROTHALONIL

This substance was considered by previous working groups, in 1982 (IARC, 1983) and 1987 (IARC, 1987). Since that time, new data have become available, and these have been incorporated into the monograph and taken into consideration in the present evaluation.

1. Exposure Data

1.1 Chemical and physical data

1.1.1 *Nomenclature*

Chem. Abstr. Serv. Reg. No.: 1897-45-6
Deleted CAS Reg. Nos: 37223-69-1; 101963-73-9
Chem. Abstr. Name: 2,4,5,6-Tetrachloro-1,3-benzenedicarbonitrile
IUPAC Systematic Name: Tetrachloroisophthalonitrile
Synonyms: 1,3-Dicyanotetrachlorobenzene; tetrachlorobenzene-1,3-dicarbonitrile; 2,4,5,6-tetrachloro-1,3-dicyanobenzene; 2,4,5,6-tetrachloroisophthalonitrile; 2,4,5,6-tetrachloro-1,3-isophthalonitrile

1.1.2 *Structural and molecular formulae and relative molecular mass*

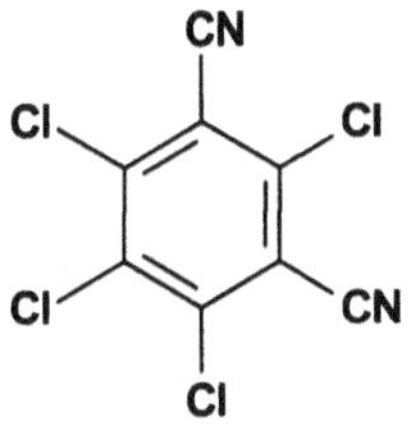

$C_8Cl_4N_2$ Relative molecular mass: 265.91

1.1.3 *Chemical and physical properties of the pure substance*

(*a*) *Description*: White, crystalline solid (National Library of Medicine, 1998a)
(*b*) *Boiling-point*: 350°C (Lide, 1997)
(*c*) *Melting-point*: 250°C (Lide, 1997)
(*d*) *Density*: 1.7 g/cm^3 at 25°C (Lide, 1997)
(*e*) *Solubility*: Insoluble in water; slightly soluble in acetone and cyclohexane (Lide, 1997)
(*f*) *Volatility*: Vapour pressure, < 1 Pa at 40°C (National Toxicology Program, 1991)

(*g*) *Octanol/water partition coefficient (P)*: log P, 2.90 (Hansch *et al.*, 1995)
(*h*) *Conversion factor*: mg/m³ = 10.88 × ppm

1.2 Production and use

Chlorothalonil has been produced commercially since 1969 (WHO, 1996). Information available in 1995 indicated that chlorothalonil was produced in China and Italy (Chemical Information Services, 1995).

Chlorothalonil is used as an agricultural and horticultural fungicide, bactericide and nematocide (Budavari, 1996). It is also used as a preservative in paints and adhesives (National Toxicology Program, 1991).

1.3 Occurrence

1.3.1 *Natural occurrence*

Chlorothalonil is not known to occur naturally.

1.3.2 *Occupational exposure*

According to the 1981–83 National Occupational Exposure Survey (National Institute for Occupational Safety and Health, 1998), approximately 63 000 workers in the United States were potentially exposed to chlorothalonil. Occupational exposure to chlorothalonil may occur during its production and during its use as a pesticide or preservative. Crop workers may be exposed to chlorothalonil by dermal contact and inhalation of dust during application and as a result of contact with treated foliage (National Library of Medicine, 1998a).

1.3.3 *Environmental occurrence*

Chlorothalonil has been detected in some raw agricultural commodities and foods in several countries at concentrations of 0.001–7.5 mg/kg (WHO, 1996; National Library of Medicine, 1998a).

Chlorothalonil has been found in surface water, groundwater and seawater (WHO, 1996; Cox, 1997; National Library of Medicine, 1998a).

The mean concentrations of chlorothalonil in indoor air samples have been reported to range from 0.1 to 6.7 ng/m³ and those in outdoor air samples at the same locations from 0.2 to 0.8 ng/m³ (National Library of Medicine, 1998a).

According to the Environmental Protection Agency Toxic Chemical Release Inventory for 1987, 9600 kg chlorothalonil were released into the air and 110 kg were discharged into water from manufacturing and processing facilities in the United States. By 1996, 7100 kg were released into the air, 10 kg were discharged into water, and 760 kg were released onto the land (National Library of Medicine, 1998b).

1.4 Regulations and guidelines

No occupational exposure limits have been proposed for chlorothalonil in workplace air in the United States, and no international guidelines for chlorothalonil in drinking-water have been established (WHO, 1993).

2. Studies of Cancer in Humans

No data were available to the Working Group.

3. Studies of Cancer in Experimental Animals

Previous evaluation

Chlorothalonil was tested in one experiment in both rats and mice by oral administration. It produced adenomas and adenocarcinomas of the renal tubular epithelium at low incidence in male and female rats. No carcinogenic effect was found in mice (IARC, 1983).

New studies

Oral administration

Mouse: Groups of 60 male and 60 female CD-1 mice [age unspecified] were given diets containing chlorothalonil at doses of 0, 125, 250 or 550 mg/kg bw per day for 24 months. Survival was unaffected by treatment. Chlorothalonil increased the incidence of renal tubular tumours in male mice, but without a clear dose–response relationship, the incidences being: control, 0/60; low dose, 6/60, intermediate dose, 4/60; and high-dose, 5/60. No renal tumours were seen in females. There was a close association between renal tubular hyperplasia and renal tumour incidence in males, and a much lower incidence of tubular hyperplasia in females. Animals of each sex showed increased incidences of forestomach tumours, again with no clear dose–response relationship, the incidences being: males—control, 0/60; low dose, 2/60; intermediate dose, 5/60; and high dose, 2/60; females—control, 0/60; low dose, 2/60; intermediate dose, 4/60; and high dose, 5/59. Forestomach tumours were associated with squamous-cell hyperplasia and hyperkeratosis in all treated groups (Wilkinson & Killeen, 1996).

In a second study, male CD-1 mice were fed diets containing chlorothalonil at 1.6, 4.5, 21.3 and 91.3 mg/kg bw per day for two years. No renal tumours were observed, but there was a slight increase in the incidence of forestomach tumours at the high dose. Dose-related increases in the incidence of associated hyperplasia were seen, commencing at 21.3 mg/kg bw for the renal tubules and at 4.5 mg/kg bw for the forestomach lining (Wilkinson & Killeen, 1996).

Rat: Groups of 60 male and 60 female Fischer 344 rats were given diets containing chlorothalonil at 0, 40, 80 or 175 mg/kg bw per day for 27 months for males and for 30 months for females. Survival was unaffected by treatment. Chlorothalonil increased the incidence of renal tubular tumours (adenomas and carcinomas) in a dose-related manner at all doses in animals of each sex. The incidence of forestomach tumours (squamous-cell papillomas and carcinomas) was also increased in males and females (Table 1). A close association was seen between renal tubular hyperplasia and renal tumorigenicity

Table 1. Incidences of primary tumours in Fischer 344 rats exposed orally to chlorothalonil

Treatment (mg/kg bw per day)	Sex	Animals with tumours	
		Kidney[a]	Forestomach[b]
None	M	0/60	0/60
40		7/60	1/60
80		7/60	1/60
175		19/60	3/60
None	F	0/60	0/60
40		3/60	1/60
80		6/60	2/60
175		23/60	7/60
None	M	1/55	0/55
1.8		1/54	0/54
3.8		1/54	3/54
15		4/54	2/54
175		23/55	5/55
None	F	0/55	1/55
1.8		0/54	1/54
3.8		0/55	2/55
15		0/53	5/53
175		32/55	9/55

From Wilkinson & Killeen (1996); no statistical analysis provided
[a] Renal tubular adenoma or carcinoma
[b] Squamous-cell papilloma or carcinoma

and between squamous-cell hyperplasia and forestomach tumorigenicity (Wilkinson & Killeen, 1996).

In a second study, groups of 55 male and 55 female Fischer 344 rats received diets containing chlorothalonil at doses of 0, 1.8, 3.8, 15 or 175 mg/kg bw for either 23–26 months (males) or 29 months (females). The incidence of renal tubular tumours and forestomach tumours was increased at the high dose in animals of each sex (Table 1; Wilkinson & Killeen, 1996).

4. Other Data Relevant to an Evaluation of Carcinogenicity and its Mechanisms

4.1 Absorption, distribution, metabolism and excretion

4.1.1 *Humans*

No data were available to the Working Group.

4.1.2 *Experimental systems*

The toxicokinetics of chlorothalonil in rats has been reviewed (Wilkinson & Killeen, 1996). After oral administration, the amount of chlorothalonil absorbed is dose-related. Thus, while approximately 30% of an administered dose of up to 50 mg/kg bw was absorbed, absorption at higher doses decreased, being only 15% at 200 mg/kg bw. Chlorothalonil reacts readily with glutathione, and glutathione conjugation is the primary route of metabolism. The liver is the major organ for the conjugation of chlorothalonil with glutathione: 9 and 18 h after oral administration of 5000 mg/kg bw chlorothalonil to rats, hepatic glutathione was depleted by 20 and 40%, respectively. The major urinary metabolites are trithiomonochloroisophthalonitrile and dithiomonochloroisophthalonitrile and the corresponding methylthio derivatives. The di- and tri-glutathione conjugates of chlorothalonil formed in the liver may be secreted into the bile, undergo enterohepatic circulation as intact glutathione conjugates or cysteine conjugates, return to the liver for further processing and be transported directly to the kidney, as demonstrated by their presence in blood. The chlorothalonil metabolites arriving in the kidney consist of a mixture of di-and tri-glutathione conjugates, cysteine *S*-conjugates and possibly some mercapturic acids. The glutathione conjugates are completely cleaved in the proximal tubules by γ-glutamyl transpeptidase and dipeptidases to the cysteine *S*-conjugates, which are subsequently cleaved by β-lyases to the corresponding thiol derivatives. Since mercapturic acids have not been identified in the urine, these compounds are probably deacetylated to the corresponding cysteine *S*-conjugates, which may undergo bioactivation to a reactive thiol by β-lyase (Wilkinson & Killeen, 1996).

A comparative study in rats, dogs and rhesus monkeys demonstrated that rats excrete the largest amount of thiol-derived materials in the urine. During the first 24 h after oral administration of chlorothalonil to rats, about 1.6% of the administered dose (50 mg/kg bw) was excreted in the urine as di- and trithiol-derived metabolites. In contrast, rhesus monkeys excreted less than 0.06% of the applied dose in the form of thiol derivatives during the same time, and no thiol-derived metabolites were identified in the urine of dogs (Savides *et al.*, 1991).

4.2 Toxic effects

4.2.1 *Humans*

Contact dermatitis due to exposure to chlorothalonil was diagnosed over a period of two years in three workers in greenhouses in which chlorothalonil was used (Bruynzeel & van Ketel, 1986).

Contact urticaria was reported after diagnostic application of diluted chlorothalonil (0.01% aqueous solution) to intact skin (Dannaker *et al.*, 1993). The patient had experienced immediate respiratory reactions (tight chest and throat) after entering a nursery greenhouse in which chlorothalonil and other pesticides had been applied. Chlorothalonil was present at 300 ppm in the air, while the other pesticides were not detectable. Since the patient showed skin reactions after direct application of chlorothalonil, but not after that of the other pesticides used in the nursery, chlorothalonil can be considered the cause of the allergic reaction.

Patch tests for chlorothalonil were performed in two groups of field workers in banana plantations in Panama: 39 workers with erythema-dyschromicum-perstans-like dermatitis (ashy dermatitis) and 41 control workers without skin symptoms (Penagos *et al.*, 1996). Thirty-four (87%) of the 39 workers with dermatitis and none of the controls showed positive reactions to chlorothalonil; the difference was highly significant. The group with dermatitis did not have positive reactions to 16 additional pesticides used in the banana plantations.

4.2.2 *Experimental systems*

Daily oral administration of approximately equimolar doses of chlorothalonil (75 mg/kg bw per day) or the monoglutathione conjugate of chlorothalonil (150 mg/kg bw per day) to male Fischer 344 rats over 90 days resulted in significantly increased kidney weights and histopathological signs of nephrotoxicity: proximal tubular hyperplasia, tubular dilatation, vacuolar degeneration and interstitial fibrosis. The parent compound also induced gross and microscopic changes in the forestomach, which were not seen with the glutathione conjugate (Wilson *et al.*, 1990).

Fischer 344 rats fed diets containing chlorothalonil at 175 mg/kg bw per day for up to 91 days showed multifocal ulceration and erosion of the stomach mucosa, which subsequently progressed to hyperplasia and hyperkeratosis. The first evidence of kidney damage was seen on day 4, as marked vacuolization of the proximal tubular epithelial cells; this was followed on day 14 by tubular hyperplasia (Wilkinson & Killeen, 1996).

Chlorothalonil administered in the diet of dogs at daily doses of up to 500 mg/kg bw for 12 months did not induce proliferative or degenerative changes in the kidney (Wilkinson & Killeen, 1996).

Incubation of hepatocytes from male Sprague-Dawley rats for up to 90 min with 0.1 mmol/L chlorothalonil reduced the non-protein sulfhydryl content to 13% that of controls and stimulated lipid peroxidation, as evidenced by malondialdehyde production, while cell viability was reduced to only 84% that of the controls. Chlorothalonil at 1 mmol/L reduced the non-protein sulfhydryl content of hepatocytes to 4.8% that of controls and the cell viability to 14% that of controls. The cytotoxic effects on isolated hepatocytes were probably directly associated with a reduction in non-protein sulfhydryls, since addition of dithiothreitol prevented the cytotoxicity of chlorothalonil (Yamano & Morita, 1995).

A comparative investigation in isolated Wistar rat hepatocytes of cytotoxicity and induction of lipid peroxidation, as assessed by measuring the content of hydroperoxide in phospholipid, showed chlorothalonil to be one of the most potent of 10 pesticides. At 1 mmol/L, chlorothalonil reduced survival to practically zero and increased the phosphatidylcholine hydroperoxide concentration by 23-fold when compared with controls, indicating oxidative damage (Suzuki *et al.*, 1997).

Feeding diets containing chlorothalonil at doses of 125, 250 or 550 mg/kg bw per day to CD1 mice for 24 months resulted in renal tubular tumours, cortical tubular degeneration and proximal tubular hyperplasia in males at all doses and a low incidence of the non-neoplastic changes in female mice (Wilkinson & Killeen, 1996).

Male CD1 mice fed diets containing chlorothalonil at doses of 1.6, 4.5, 21.3 or 91.3 mg/kg bw per day for 24 months showed no renal tumours, but the incidence of tubular hyperplasia was slightly increased at doses ≥ 21.3 mg/kg bw per day. Forestomach tumours were found at the highest dose, and dose-related increases in hyperplasia and hyperkeratosis of the forestomach epithelium were observed at doses ≥ 4.5 mg/kg bw per day (Wilkinson & Killeen, 1996).

4.3 Reproductive and developmental effects

No data were available to the Working Group.

4.4 Genetic and related effects

4.4.1 *Humans*

No data were available to the Working Group.

4.4.2 *Experimental systems* (see Table 2 for references)

Chlorothalonil was not mutagenic to *Salmonella typhimurium* or *Escherichia coli* WP2 *hcr*. It induced point mutations in strains *biA1, meth G1* and 118 of *Aspergillus nidulans* in the absence of metabolic activation. Chlorothalonil did not induce sex-linked recessive lethal mutations in *Drosophila melanogaster*. It weakly induced forward mutation in L5178Y $tk^{+/-}$ mouse lymphoma cells in the absence of metabolic activation in two of three independent experiments. It increased the frequency of sister chromatid exchange in Chinese hamster ovary cells in the presence but not in the absence of a liver microsomal preparation from Aroclor 1254-induced rats. Chlorothalonil induced chromosomal aberrations in Chinese hamster ovary cells.

A statistically significant, dose-dependent increase in DNA damage, as evaluated in the comet assay, was observed in peripheral blood lymphocytes of humans exposed to chlorothalonil.

Chlorothalonil did not form adducts in calf thymus DNA when incubated with rat liver microsomes, as tested by ^{32}P-postlabelling.

A dose-dependent increase in the 8-hydroxy-2-deoxyguanosine concentration in liver DNA, indicative of oxidative damage, was observed in rats treated *in vivo*.

5. Summary of Data Reported and Evaluation

5.1 Exposure data

Exposure to chlorothalonil may occur during its production and during its application as a fungicide, bactericide and nematocide. It has been detected in some foods.

Table 2. Genetic and related effects of chlorothalonil

Test system	Results[a]		Dose[b] (LED or HID)	Reference
	Without metabolic activation	With metabolic activation		
Salmonella typhimurium TA100, TA98, TA1535, TA1537, TA1538, reverse mutation	–	–	7.64 μg/plate	Wei (1982)
Salmonella typhimurium TA100, TA98, TA1535, TA1537, TA1538, reverse mutation	–	–	5000 μg/plate	Moriya *et al.* (1983)
Salmonella typhimurium TA100, TA98, TA1535, TA1537, reverse mutation	–	–	10 μg/plate	Mortelmans *et al.* (1986)
Escherichia coli WP2, reverse mutation	–	–	5000 μg/plate	Moriya *et al.* (1983)
Aspergillus nidulans (strains biA1, methG1 and 118), forward mutation	+	NT	0.4	Martinez-Rossi & Azevedo (1987)
Drosophila melanogaster, sex-linked recessive lethal mutations	–		10 000	Yoon *et al.* (1985)
Gene mutation, mouse lymphoma L5178Y cells, *tk* locus *in vitro*	(+)	NT	0.12	McGregor *et al.* (1988)
Sister chromatid exchange, Chinese hamster ovary cells *in vitro*	–	+	2.50	Galloway *et al.* (1987)
Chromosomal aberrations, Chinese hamster ovary cells *in vitro*	+	+	0.5	Galloway *et al.* (1987)
DNA strand breaks, cross-links or related damage (comet assay), human lymphocytes *in vitro*	+	NT	2.7	Lebailly *et al.* (1997)
DNA damage, rat liver *in vivo*	+		0.13 po × 10	Lodovici *et al.* (1997)
Binding (covalent) to DNA *in vitro*	NT	–	266	Shah *et al.* (1997)

[a] +, positive; (+), weak positive; –, negative; NT, not tested
[b] LED, lowest effective dose; HID, highest ineffective dose; in-vitro tests, μg/mL; in-vivo tests, mg/kg bw per day; po, oral

5.2 Human carcinogenicity data

No data were available to the Working Group.

5.3 Animal carcinogenicity data

Chlorothalonil was tested by oral administration in the diet in three experiments in mice and three experiments in rats. It produced renal tubular tumours (adenomas and carcinomas) in males of each species and in female rats. The incidences of forestomach papillomas and carcinomas were increased in males and females of each species.

5.4 Other relevant data

Chlorothalonil is metabolized in rats by conjugation to glutathione in the gastrointestinal tract and liver. After biliary excretion, uptake and metabolism of these conjugates in the kidney by the action of γ-glutamyl transpeptidase and cysteine–conjugate β-lyase results in the production of di- and tri-thiols, which are thought to be responsible for the toxicity seen in the kidney. Sustained cytotoxicity and the resultant regenerative response in the kidney are found in conjunction with tumour formation after long-term exposure.

There may be less activity of γ-glutamyl transpeptidase and cysteine–conjugate β-lyase in humans than in rats.

Forestomach tumours produced by chlorothalonil were associated with squamous hyperplasia and local irritation.

No data were available on reproductive or developmental effects.

No data were available on the genetic and related effects of chlorothalonil in humans or in rodents *in vivo*. In one study, 8-oxydeoxyguanosine products were observed in the livers of mice exposed *in vivo*. There is some evidence for genotoxicity in mammalian cells *in vitro*. Chlorothalonil was not mutagenic to bacteria.

5.5 Evaluation

There is *inadequate evidence* in humans for the carcinogenicity of chlorothalonil.

There is *sufficient evidence* in experimental animals for the carcinogenicity of chlorothalonil.

Overall evaluation

Chlorothalonil is *possibly carcinogenic to humans (Group 2B)*.

6. References

Bruynzeel, D.P. & van Ketel, W.G. (1986) Contact dermatitis due to chlorothalonil in floriculture. *Contact Derm.*, **14**, 67–68

Budavari, S., ed. (1996) *The Merck Index*, 12th Ed., Whitehouse Station, NJ, Merck & Co., p. 361

Chemical Information Services (1995) *Directory of World Chemical Producers 1995/96 Standard Edition*, Dallas, TX, p. 186

Cox, C. (1997) Fungicide factsheet: Chlorothalonil. *J. Pestic. Reform*, **17**, 14–20

Dannaker, C.J., Maibach, H.I. & O'Malley, M. (1993) Contact urticaria and anaphylaxis to the fungicide chlorothalonil. *Cutis*, **52**, 312–315

Galloway, S.M., Armstrong, M.J., Reuben, C., Colman, S., Brown, B., Cannon, C., Bloom, A.D., Nakamura, F., Ahmed, M., Duk, S., Rimpo, J., Margolin, B.H., Resnick, M.A., Anderson, B. & Zeiger E. (1987) Chromosome aberrations and sister chromatid exchanges in Chinese hamster ovary cells: Evaluations of 108 chemicals. *Environ. mol. Mutag.*, **10** (Suppl. 10), 1–175

Hansch, C., Leo, A. & Hoekman, D. (1995) *Exploring QSAR: Hydrophobic, Electronic, and Steric Constants*, Washington DC, American Chemical Society, p. 27

IARC (1983) *IARC Monographs on the Evaluation of the Carcinogenic Risk of Chemicals to Humans*, Vol. 30, *Miscellaneous Pesticides*, Lyon, pp. 319–328

IARC (1987) *IARC Monographs on the Evaluation of Carcinogenic Risks to Humans,* Suppl. 7, *Overall Evaluations of Carcinogenicity: An Updating of* IARC Monographs *Volumes 1 to 42*, Lyon, p. 60

Lebailly, P., Vigreux, C., Godard, T., Sichel, F., Bar, E., Le Talaër, Y.F., Henry-Amar, M. & Gauduchon, P. (1997) Assessment of DNA damage induced in vitro by etoposide and two fungicides (carbendazim and chlorothalonil) in human lymphocytes with the comet assay. *Mutat. Res.*, **375**, 205–217

Lide, D.R., ed. (1997) *CRC Handbook of Chemistry and Physics*, 78th Ed., Boca Raton, FL, CRC Press, p. 3-38

Lodovici, M., Casalini, C., Briani, C. & Dolara, P. (1997) Oxidative liver DNA damage in rats treated with pesticide mixtures. *Toxicology*, **117**, 55–60

Martinez-Rossi, N.M. & Azevedo, J.L. (1987) Detection of point-mutation mutagens in *Aspergillus nidulans*: comparison of methionine suppressors and arginine resistance induction by fungicides. *Mutat. Res.*, **176**, 29–35

McGregor, D.B., Brown, A., Cattanach, P., Edwards, I., Mc Bride, D., Riach, C. & Caspary, W.J. (1988) Responses of the L5178Y tk^+/tk^- mouse lymphoma cell forward mutation assay: III. 72 coded chemicals. *Environ. mol. Mutag.*, **12**, 85–154

Moriya, M., Ohta, T., Watanabe, K., Miyazawa, T., Kato, K. & Shirasu, Y. (1983) Further mutagenicity studies on pesticides in bacterial reversion assay systems. *Mutat. Res.*, **116**, 185–216

Mortelmans, K., Haworth, S., Lawlor, T., Speck, W., Tainer, B. & Zeiger, E. (1986) *Salmonella* mutagenicity tests: II. Results from the testing of 270 chemicals. *Environ. Mutag.*, **8** (Suppl. 7), 1–119

National Institute for Occupational Safety and Health (1998) *National Occupational Exposure Survey (1981-1983)*, Cincinnati, OH

National Library of Medicine (1998a) *Hazardous Substances Data Bank (HSDB)*, Bethesda, MD [Record No. 1546]

National Library of Medicine (1998b) *Toxic Chemical Release Inventory 1987 & 1996* (TRI87 & TRI96), Bethesda, MD

National Toxicology Program (1991) *NTP Chemical Repository Data Sheet: Chlorothalonil*, Research Triangle Park, NC

Penagos, H., Jimenez, V., Fallas, V., O'Malley, M. & Maibach, H.I. (1996) Chlorothalonil, a possible cause of erythema dyschromicum perstans (ashy dermatitis). *Contact Derm.*, **35**, 214–218

Savides, M.C., Marciniszyn, J.P., Medvedeff, E.D., Killeen, J.C., Jr & Eilrich, G.L. (1991) Comparative studies on the metabolism of chlorothalonil via the gluthathione pathway (Abstract). *Toxicologist*, **11**, 60

Shah, R.G., Lagueux, J., Kapur, S., Levallois, P., Ayotte, P., Tremblay, M., Zee, J. & Poirier, G.G. (1997) Determination of genotoxicity of the metabolites of the pesticides Gluthion, Sencor, Lorox, Reglone, Daconil and Admire by ^{32}P-postlabeling. *Mol. cell. Biochem.*, **169**, 177–184

Suzuki, T., Komatsu, M. & Isono, H. (1997) Cytotoxicity of organochlorine pesticides and lipid peroxidation in isolated rat hepatocytes. *Biol. pharm. Bull.*, **20**, 271–274

Wei, C. (1982) Lack of mutagenicity of the fungicide 2,4,5,6-tetrachloroisophthalonitrile in the Ames *Salmonella*/microsome test. *Appl. environ. Microbiol.*, **43**, 252–254

WHO (1993) *Guidelines for Drinking Water Quality*, 2nd Ed., Vol. 1, *Recommendations*, Geneva

WHO (1996) *Chlorothalonil* (Environmental Health Criteria 183), Geneva, International Programme on Chemical Safety

Wilkinson, C.F. & Killeen, J.C. (1996) A mechanistic interpretation of the oncogenicity of chlorothalonil in rodents and an assessment of human relevance. *Regul. Toxicol. Pharmacol.*, **24**, 69–84

Wilson, N.H., Killeen, J.C., Jr, Ford, W.H., Siou, G., Busey, W.M. & Eilrich, G.L. (1990) A 90-day study in rats with the monoglutathione conjugate of chlorothalonil. *Toxicol. Lett.*, **53**, 155–156

Yamano, T. & Morita, S. (1995) Effects of pesticides on isolated rat hepatocytes, mitochondria, and microsomes II. *Arch. environ. Contam. Toxicol.*, **28**, 1–7

Yoon, J.S., Mason, J.M., Valencia, R., Woodruff, R.C. & Zimmering, S. (1985) Chemical mutagenesis testing in *Drosophila*. IV. Results of 45 coded compounds tested for the National Toxicology Program. *Environ. Mutag.*, **7**, 349–367

CYCLAMATES

These substances were considered by previous working groups, in 1979 (IARC, 1980) and 1987 (IARC, 1987). Since that time, new data have become available, and these have been incorporated into the monograph and taken into consideration in the present evaluation.

1. Exposure Data

1.1 Chemical and physical data

1.1.1 *Nomenclature*

Cyclamic acid

Chem. Abstr. Serv. Reg. No.: 100-88-9
Deleted CAS Reg. No.: 45951-45-9
Chem. Abstr. Name: Cyclohexylsulfamic acid
IUPAC Systematic Name: Cyclohexanesulfamic acid
Synonyms: Cyclamate; cyclohexylamidosulfuric acid; cyclohexylaminesulfonic acid; *N*-cyclohexylsulfamic acid; hexamic acid; sucaryl; sucaryl acid

Sodium cyclamate

Chem. Abstr. Serv. Reg. No.: 139-05-9
Deleted CAS Reg. No.: 53170-91-5
Chem. Abstr. Name: Cyclohexylsulfamic acid, monosodium salt
IUPAC Systematic Name: Cyclohexanesulfamic acid, monosodium salt
Synonyms: Cyclamate sodium; cyclohexylsulfamate sodium; *N*-cyclohexylsulfamic acid sodium salt; sodium cyclohexanesulfamate; sodium cyclohexylaminesulfonate; sodium cyclohexylsulfamate; sodium sucaryl; sucaryl sodium

Calcium cyclamate

Chem. Abstr. Serv. Reg. No.: 139-06-0
Deleted CAS Reg. No.: 201280-50-4
Chem. Abstr. Name: Cyclohexylsulfamic acid, calcium salt (2:1)
IUPAC Systematic Name: Cyclohexanesulfamic acid, calcium salt (2:1)
Synonyms: Calcium cyclohexanesulfamate; calcium sucaryl

1.1.2 *Structural and molecular formulae and relative molecular mass*

Cyclamic acid

$C_6H_{13}NO_3S$ Relative molecular mass: 179.2

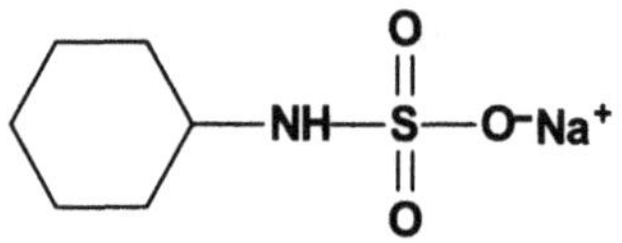

Sodium cyclamate

$C_6H_{12}NO_3S.Na$ Relative molecular mass: 201.2

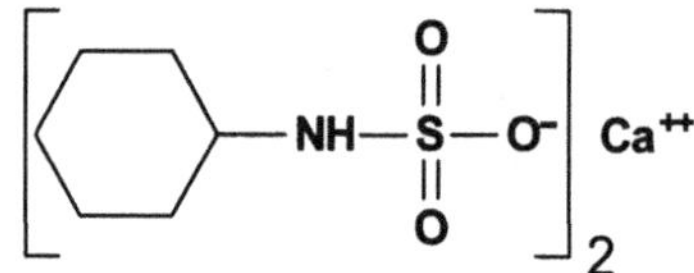

Calcium cyclamate

$(C_6H_{12}NO_3S)_2Ca$ Relative molecular mass: 396.5

1.1.3 *Chemical and physical properties of the pure substances*

From Lewis (1993) and Budavari (1996) unless otherwise noted

Cyclamic acid

(*a*) *Description*: White odourless, crystalline powder with a sweet taste

(*b*) *Melting-point*: 169–170°C

(*c*) *Solubility*: Soluble in water (130 g/L) and ethanol (Bopp & Price, 1991); insoluble in oils

(*c*) *pH of a 10% aqueous solution*: 0.8–1.6 (Bopp & Price, 1991)

(*d*) *Conversion factor*: $mg/m^3 = 7.33 \times ppm$

Sodium cyclamate

(*a*) *Description*: White, odourless, crystalline powder with a sweet taste (about 30 times as sweet as refined cane sugar)

(*b*) *Solubility*: Freely soluble in water; practically insoluble in benzene, chloroform, ethanol and diethyl ether

(*c*) *pH of a 10% aqueous solution*: 5.5–7.5

(*d*) *Conversion factor*: $mg/m^3 = 8.23 \times ppm$

(*e*) Stability: Cyclamate solutions are stable to heat, light and air throughout a wide range of pH.

Calcium cyclamate

(*a*) *Description*: White odourless, crystalline powder with a sweet taste, somewhat less than that of sodium cyclamate

(*b*) *Solubility*: Freely soluble in water; practically insoluble in benzene, chloroform ethanol and diethyl ether

(*c*) *pH of a 10% aqueous solution*: Neutral to litmus (5.5–7.5)

(*d*) *Conversion factor*: mg/m^3 = 16.22 × ppm

(*e*) *Stability*: More resistant to cooking temperatures than saccharin

1.2 Production and use

Cyclamates are produced from cyclohexylamine (obtained by the reduction of aniline) by sulfonation (Bizzari *et al.*, 1996).

Production of sodium and calcium cyclamates in western Europe (annual capacity, 4200 tonnes) in 1995 was estimated to be 4000 tonnes. Brazil (annual capacities of 4000 and 2000 tonnes of sodium and calcium cyclamate, respectively) produced over 2300 and 300 tonnes of sodium and calcium cyclamate, respectively, in 1993. There is no commercial production of cyclamates in Japan or the United States (Bizzari *et al.*, 1996).

Information available in 1995 indicated that cyclamic acid was produced in Japan, Spain, Taiwan and the United States, that sodium cyclamate was produced in Argentina, Brazil, Germany, Indonesia, Japan, the Netherlands, Romania, South Africa, Spain, Taiwan, Thailand and the United States and that calcium cyclamate was produced in Argentina, Brazil, Japan, South Africa, Taiwan and the United States (Chemical Information Services, 1995).

Sodium and calcium cyclamates are used as non-nutritive sweeteners (Lewis, 1993; Budavari, 1996); sodium cyclamate, simply known as 'cyclamate', is the more common salt. Calcium cyclamate is used in low-sodium and sodium-free products. World consumption of cyclamates in 1995 was estimated to be 15 000 tonnes. Western European consumption of cyclamates was estimated to be 4000 tonnes. Canadian consumption of cyclamates in 1995 was estimated to be 60 tonnes. Consumption of sodium cyclamate in China in 1995 was estimated to be 4400 tonnes (Bizzari *et al.*, 1996).

1.3 Occurrence

1.3.1 *Natural occurrence*

Cyclamates are not known to occur naturally.

1.3.2 *Occupational exposure*

According to the 1981–83 National Occupational Exposure Survey (National Institute for Occupational Safety and Health, 1998), approximately 5300 workers in the United States were potentially exposed to sodium cyclamate. Occupational exposure to sodium cyclamate may occur during its production.

1.3.3 *Dietary intake*

The dietary intake of cyclamate in Spain was evaluated in 1992. The average daily intake of cyclamate was 0.44 mg/kg bw for the whole population and 2.44 mg/kg bw among consumers of cyclamates. Subjects following a diet, such as diabetic patients, reported the highest intakes, and only 0.16% of the sample studied consumed more than the acceptable daily intake (ADI) of 11 mg/kg bw (Serra-Majem *et al.*, 1996).

A survey of intense sweetener consumption in Australia was conducted in 1994, which consisted of a seven-day survey of high consumers of the main sources of sweeteners (i.e. carbonated drinks, cordials and table-top sweeteners), with allowance for body weight. The mean intake (expressed as percentage of the ADI of 11 mg/kg bw) of cyclamates was 23% by all consumers 12–39 years of age (men, 27%; women, 21%), 34% by all consumers 12–17 years of age, 20% by all consumers 18–24 years of age and 20% by all consumers 25–39 years of age (National Food Authority, 1995).

In a study of the potential intake of intense sweeteners in Brazil in 1990–91, 67% of the studied population was found to consume cyclamate. Table-top sweeteners were the major source, followed by soft drinks. The median daily intake of cyclamate was approximately 16% of the ADI (11 mg/kg bw) (Toledo & Ioshi, 1995).

The use of table-top sweeteners and diet soft-drinks and intake of cyclamate were assessed from the second Dutch National Food Consumption Survey, conducted in 1992. Users of intense sweeteners assessed from two-day records had a median daily intake of cyclamate of 0.8 mg/kg bw; those assessed from a food frequency questionnaire had a median daily intake of 1.1 mg/kg bw. Less than 0.5% of the total population had an intake above the ADI (11 mg/kg bw) (Hulshof *et al.*, 1995).

The dietary intake of intense sweeteners was evaluated in Germany in 1988–89. Complete 24-h records of the amounts and types of all foods and drinks consumed were obtained from 2291 individuals. The mean intake of cyclamate by users of intense sweeteners was 2.62 mg/kg bw per day. Sweetener intake was further evaluated during a seven-day period in those subjects who in the one-day study had a consumption of any of the sweeteners in excess of 75% of the ADI (11 mg/kg bw). The mean intake of cyclamate for this group was 4.53 mg/kg bw per day, corresponding to 41% of the ADI (Bär & Biermann, 1992).

A survey of general food additive intakes in Finland in 1980 included an assessment of the intake of cyclamate (Penttilä *et al.*, 1988). The paper gave few details of the study design or method and reported only that the average daily intake of sodium cyclamate (calculated from data on the consumption of various foods and drinks) was 12.3 mg/person.

1.4 Regulations and guidelines

No national or international occupational exposure limits have been proposed for cyclamic acid, sodium cyclamate, or calcium cyclamate in workplace air, and no international guidelines for cyclamates in drinking-water have been established (WHO, 1993).

Cyclamate is approved for use in over 55 countries, including Canada (for table-top use only), Australia, and the European Union (Bizzari *et al.*, 1996). An ADI of 11 mg/kg bw for cyclamate was established by the WHO/FAO Joint Expert Committee on Food Additives and the Scientific Committee for Food of the European Union (Renwick, 1995). Cyclamate was banned in the United States in 1970 (Bopp & Price, 1991).

2. Studies of Cancer in Humans

Studies on artificial sweeteners in which the actual compound used was not specified are summarized in the monograph on saccharin; however, four of the studies included specific analyses of the risk for urinary bladder cancer associated with exposure to cyclamates (Simon *et al.*, 1975; Kessler & Clark, 1978; Møller Jensen *et al.*, 1983; Risch *et al.*, 1988).

In the study of Simon *et al.* (1975; see the monograph on saccharin), cyclamate use was evaluated in coffee-drinkers and tea-drinkers separately. Among the coffee-drinkers (122 cases and 349 controls), nine patients with bladder cancer and 22 controls reported use of cyclamate, yielding a crude odds ratio of 1.2 (95% confidence interval [CI], 0.5–2.6). Among the tea-drinkers (98 cases and 281 controls), eight patients and 20 controls reported use of cyclamate, yielding a crude odds ratio of 1.2 (95% CI, 0.5–2.7). The groups of tea-drinkers and coffee-drinkers were mutually exclusive.

In the study of Kessler and Clark (1978), 130 of the 519 patients (25%) and 135 of the 519 controls (26%) had ever used cyclamate, yielding an odds ratio of 1.0 (95% CI, 0.7–1.3). The risk did not differ substantially between men (odds ratio, 1.1; 95% CI, 0.8–1.6) and women (odds ratio, 0.7; 95% CI, 0.5–1.2), and the results did not change when the odds ratios were adjusted in a multivariate analysis for several potential confounders (smoking, occupation, age, race, sex, diabetes mellitus, marital status, education, overweight, dieting and memory) or when the odds ratios for different types of artificial sweeteners were estimated simultaneously.

In the study of Risch *et al.* (1988), odds ratios of 1.1 (95% CI, 0.60–2.0) for men and 0.9 (95% CI, 0.6–1.4) for women were reported when 'total lifetime intake' was included in a continuous regression model and after adjustment for lifetime cigarette consumption and history of diabetes, but not for other use of artificial sweeteners.

In the study of Møller Jensen *et al.* (1983), 11% of the subjects reported having used cyclamate only. There was no indication that cyclamate users had an elevated risk. The odds ratio was 0.72 (95% CI, 0.3–2.0) for men and 1.3 (95% CI, 0.22–8.3) for women.

3. Studies of Cancer in Experimental Animals

Previous evaluation

Sodium cyclamate was tested by oral administration in two experiments in mice, one of which was a multigeneration study, and in three experiments in rats. A few benign and malignant bladder tumours were observed in rats, but the incidences were not statistically greater than those in controls in any single experiment. An increased incidence of lymphosarcomas was seen in female but not in male mice in one experiment. Sodium cyclamate was also tested by oral administration in other experiments in mice, rats, hamsters and monkeys, but these experiments could not be evaluated because of various inadequacies or incomplete reporting.

Pellets of sodium cyclamate in cholesterol have been tested in mice by implantation into the bladder in one experiment: exposure by this route increased the incidence of bladder carcinomas.

When sodium cyclamate was administered to rats in one experiment by subcutaneous injection, no tumours were seen at the site of injection.

Calcium cyclamate has been tested by oral administration in one two-generation experiment in rats; no difference in tumour incidence was seen between treated and control animals. Two further experiments in rats showing a few bladder tumours and one in hamsters were considered to be inadequate for evaluation. When calcium cyclamate was administered to rats by subcutaneous injection, tumours were produced at the site of injection.

In one study in rats fed sodium cyclamate after receiving a single instillation into the bladder of a low dose of *N*-nitroso-*N*-methylurea, transitional-cell neoplasms of the bladder were produced. No such tumours were observed in animals that received *N*-nitroso-*N*-methylurea alone. [The present Working Group noted inadequacies in this study and noted that these results were not repeated in a second study.]

Cyclohexylamine, an intestinal biotransformation product of cyclamates, has been tested by oral administration in two experiments in mice, one of which was a multi-generation study, and in four experiments in rats; there were no differences in tumour incidence between treated and control animals. A further experiment in rats was considered to be inadequate for evaluation (IARC, 1980).

[The present Working Group noted, in relation to the study of Bryan and Ertürk (1970) summarized in the previous monograph, that it is difficult to interpret the results of studies involving bladder implantation, since the pellet itself has significant carcinogenic effects (Clayson, 1974; Jull, 1979; De Sesso, 1989). Furthermore, virtually all of the sodium cyclamate was reported to have leached out of the pellets within 7 h of implantation (Bryan & Ertürk, 1970), which would have left the pellet with a roughened surface, unlike the control pellets (De Sesso, 1989). The low incidence of bladder tumours in the groups receiving control pellets in the study of Bryan and Ertürk, which was not seen in subsequent studies involving implantation of pellets in the bladder, was also noted. The Working Group also noted, in relation to the study of Brantom *et al.* (1973) in which an increased incidence of lymphosarcomas was reported in female mice, that the study included only limited sampling of tissues for histopathological examination.]

For summaries of studies of combined administration of saccharin and cyclamates, see the monograph on saccharin and its salts.

New studies

No new data were available to the Working Group.

4. Other Data Relevant to an Evaluation of Carcinogenicity and its Mechanisms

4.1 Absorption, distribution, metabolism and excretion

4.1.1 *Humans*

Absorption of cyclamate from the gut is incomplete, and absorbed cyclamate is excreted in the urine. When three men received 1 g calcium [^{14}C]cyclamate orally, 87–90% was recovered in the urine and faeces in about equal amounts within four days (Renwick & Williams, 1972a). When the subjects had received a cyclamate-containing diet for 17–30 days before the radioactive dose, 96–99% of the dose was recovered within four to five days, and urinary excretion was greater than before the cyclamate diet. Most humans convert only small amounts of cyclamate to cyclohexylamine, and the majority converted < 0.1–8%; however, there is wide interindividual variation in the daily urinary excretion of cyclohexylamine, which can amount to 60% of a dose of cyclamate (IARC, 1980; Buss *et al.*, 1992). Gastrointestinal microflora are the source of the conversion of unabsorbed cyclamate to cyclohexylamine (Drasar *et al.*, 1972). Other aspects of the conversion of cyclamate to cyclohexylamine have been reviewed extensively (National Research Council, 1985; Ahmed & Thomas, 1992).

Two metabolites were definitely identified in the urine of volunteers who received an oral dose of [^{14}C]cyclohexylamine, namely cyclohexanol and *trans*-cyclohexane-1,2-diol. No *N*-hydroxycyclohexylamine was found in human urine (Renwick & Williams, 1972b).

4.1.2 *Experimental systems*

In guinea-pigs, rats and rabbits, 30, 50 and 5% of orally administered cyclamate was excreted in the faeces and 65, 40 and 95% in the urine, respectively, over two to three days. Cyclamate thus appears to be readily absorbed by rabbits but less readily by guinea-pigs and rats (Renwick & Williams, 1972a).

When given to lactating dogs and rats, calcium cyclamate reached higher concentrations in the milk than in the blood (Sonders & Wiegand, 1968; Ward & Zeman, 1971). In pregnant rats, significant amounts of sodium cyclamate were distributed to fetal tissues (Schechter & Roth, 1971). In rhesus monkeys, cyclamate crossed the placenta (Pitkin *et al.*, 1969).

Cyclohexylamine can be formed to a variable extent by microbial biotransformation of cyclamate in the gastrointestinal tract of all species studied; after absorption, it is further metabolized to several compounds that are excreted in the urine (Golberg *et al.*, 1969; Parekh *et al.*, 1970; Asahina *et al.*, 1971; Ichibagase *et al.*, 1972; Coulston *et al.*, 1977).

Administration to rats of 0.1% calcium cyclamate in the diet for eight months, followed by a single dose of [^{14}C]cyclamate, resulted in traces of dicyclohexylamine in the urine, but no *N*-hydroxycyclohexylamine was detected. Rats that had received a control diet did not convert [^{14}C]cyclamate to additional products (Prosky & O'Dell, 1971).

Most of the cyclohexylamine given by gavage or intraperitoneal injection to rats and guinea-pigs was excreted unchanged, and only 4–5% was metabolized within 24 h. In rabbits, 30% was metabolized. Cyclohexylamine has been reported to be metabolized further to cyclohexanone and then to cyclohexanol in guinea-pigs, rabbits and rats. A number of hydroxylated products of cyclohexylamine have been reported in these species, which were excreted in part as glucuronides (Renwick & Williams, 1972b).

In rhesus monkeys receiving 200 mg/kg bw cyclamate orally for several years, more than 99.5% was excreted unchanged. The principal metabolites found were cyclohexylamine, cyclohexanone and cyclohexanol (Coulston *et al.*, 1977).

Comparison of the integrated area under the concentration–time curve (AUC) in the testis of rats and mice showed that the lower clearance of cyclohexylamine in rats resulted in greater exposure of the target organ for toxicity. In rat plasma and testes, the cyclohexylamine concentration was non-linearly related to intake, and elevated concentrations were found in these tissues after administration of doses above 200 mg/kg per day because of decreased urinary output. At a dose of 400 mg/kg per day, which caused testicular atrophy in rats but not mice, the plasma and testicular levels of cyclohexylamine were lower in mice than in rats (Roberts & Renwick, 1989; Roberts *et al.*, 1989).

4.1.3 *Comparison of humans and rodents*

Orally administered cyclamate appears to be readily absorbed by rabbits but less readily by guinea-pigs, rats and humans. All of these species convert cyclamate to cyclohexylamine, *via* the action of gastrointestinal microflora on unabsorbed cyclamate. The metabolism of cyclohexylamine to other products differs somewhat in humans and other species, although most cyclohexylamine is rapidly excreted unchanged in the urine. In rats, it is metabolized mainly by hydroxylation of the cyclohexane ring; in humans, it is metabolized by deamination; and in guinea-pigs and rabbits, it is metabolized by ring hydroxylation and deamination (Renwick & Williams, 1972b).

4.2 Toxic effects

4.2.1 *Humans*

No data were available to the Working Group.

4.2.2 *Experimental systems*

The oral LD_{50} of sodium cyclamate in mice and rats is 10–12 g/kg bw (Richards *et al.*, 1951); the oral LD_{50} in male and female hamsters—based on eight days' administration in drinking-water and calculated on the basis of mortality up to day 16—was 9.8

and 12 g/kg bw, respectively; for calcium cyclamate, the respective values were 4.5 and 6 g/kg bw (Althoff *et al.*, 1975).

Several studies have shown that cyclohexylamine affects the testis of rats (Oser *et al.*, 1976; Mason & Thompson, 1977). In one study, cyclohexylamine produced testicular atrophy in DA and Wistar rats, but not in mice, at a dietary dose of 400 mg/kg per day for up to 13 weeks. The testicular toxicity was not due to the formation of hydroxylated metabolites but to cyclohexylamine *per se*. The lack of sensitivity of mouse testis is probably due to the lower tissue concentrations of cyclohexylamine in this species in comparison with rats (Roberts *et al.*, 1989).

Sodium cyclamate inhibited binding of ^{125}I-labelled mouse epidermal growth factor to dog kidney, rat hepatoma and rat liver cells, mouse fibroblasts, human foreskin and human skin fibroblasts, human carcinoma and human xeroderma pigmentosum cells *in vitro* (Lee, 1981).

In cultured bladders from young female Fischer 344 rats, 12 or 24 mmol/L sodium cyclamate produced pronounced urethelial hyperplasia and dysplasia, as confirmed by histology (Knowles *et al.*, 1986). Sodium cyclamate alone or after exposure to *N*-methyl-*N*-nitrosourea induced foci of cell proliferation in explanted bladder epithelium cultures derived from young female Fischer 344 rats (Knowles & Jani, 1986; Nicholson & Jani, 1988).

4.3 Reproductive and developmental effects

4.3.1 *Humans*

No data were available to the Working Group.

4.3.2 *Experimental systems*

No adverse effects on fetal viability, growth or morphology as a consequence of exposure to cyclamates were reported in mice, rats, rabbits, hamsters, dogs and rhesus monkeys exposed during some or all periods of prenatal development (Fritz & Hess, 1968; Klotzsche, 1969; Lorke, 1969; Adkins *et al.*, 1972). The chemical form used was usually the sodium salt, which was given either orally or in the diet. The concentrations used in the studies in rodents were up to 5% in the diet; in the study in dogs (Fancher *et al.*, 1968), doses of up to 1 g/kg of a 10:1 combination of sodium cyclamate:saccharin were used; and monkeys received up to 2000 mg/kg on one of several four-day periods during gestation (Wilson, 1972). Adverse effects attributed to cyclamates were noted in two other studies. In one, reduced postnatal growth and altered reproductive capacity were found in the offspring of rats given diets containing 5 or 10% calcium cyclamate; food intake was markedly reduced in both treatment groups (Nees & Derse, 1965, 1967). In the other study, offspring of rats treated with 300 mg/L sodium and calcium cyclamate in the drinking-water during pregnancy had increased motor activity (Stone *et al.*, 1969a).

In their review of the toxicity of cyclamates, Bopp *et al.* (1986) summarized a number of studies on the effects of these compounds on the testis, reproductive function and prenatal development, some of which were unpublished. With regard to male reproductive effects, they concluded that the testicular atrophy observed in cyclamate-treated rats was associated with exposure to dietary concentrations of 5–10% (i.e. about 2.5–5.0 g/kg bw per day), was accompanied by reductions in body weight and was evident only after long-term exposure and hence appeared to be a secondary or indirect effect of exposure. [The Working Group noted that testicular effects are generally not seen in dietary restriction studies until body-weight deficits of more than 80% occur (Chapin & Gulati, 1997).] The authors also noted that the testicular effects were present only in rats (and not mice, dogs or rhesus monkeys). With regard to effects on reproductive function, they concluded that high doses adversely affected the viability and growth of rat pups during lactation, although the pups might also have eaten their mothers' feed, and that mice and dogs are insensitive to such exposure. With regard to developmental toxicity, they noted that numerous investigations in mice, rats and rabbits and isolated studies in dogs and rhesus monkeys have shown no reproducible effect of cyclamate on embryonic viability or on the frequency of malformations after exposure during organogenesis.

Sodium cyclamate did not affect growth or viability or induce malformations in a short-term screening test for teratogenicity at a minimally maternally toxic dose given orally on days 8–12 of gestation to ICR/SIM mice (Seidenberg *et al.*, 1986).

Cyclamate did not affect the development of cultured rat embryos exposed on days 9.5–11.5 of gestation to concentrations of up to 810 μg/mL (Cicurel & Schmid, 1988). As reported in an abstract, exposure of NMRI mouse embryos to sodium cyclamate [dose not given] in culture for 26 h beginning on day 8.5 of gestation was not teratogenic (Delhaise *et al.*, 1989).

The concentration of cyclamic acid that caused 50% inhibition of proliferation of human epithelial palatal mesenchyme cells was reported to be 6500 μg/mL (32 mmol/L). The authors considered that a concentration of less than 1 mmol/L was indicative of teratogenic potential in this assay (Pratt & Willis, 1985). A subsequent interlaboratory comparison provided no evidence that sodium cyclamate is teratogenic in either this cell growth inhibition assay or the mouse ovarian tumour cell attachment inhibition assay, which monitors cell attachment to concanavalin A-coated beads (Steele *et al.*, 1988).

Cyclamate was considered to be ineffective in a test with rat embryonic limb bud micromass in culture. The mean concentrations that affected chondrogenesis and cell proliferation were 6200 and 3100 μg/mL, respectively (Renault *et al.*, 1989).

Exposure of developing *Drosophila* larvae to cyclamate caused a dose-related increase in the number of extra bristles and reduced the whole-body size of adults, but these effects were not considered to be the most predictive of developmental toxicity in mammals (Lynch *et al.*, 1991).

The effects of sodium cyclamate on the development of frog embryos were evaluated in a validation study in seven laboratories. The median lethal concentration, the concentration that induced malformations in 50% of the surviving embryos and the teratogenic index, i.e. the ratio of the two other measures, were 16 mg/mL, 14 mg/mL and 1.1 mg/mL, respectively. These results suggest that sodium cyclamate has low potential selective embryotoxicity (Bantle *et al.*, 1994).

Cyclohexylamine

Studies have been carried out in rats, mice and rhesus monkeys exposed to cyclohexylamine during some or all of gestation and in a one-generation study in mice and a multigeneration study in rats. The exposure included intraperitoneal injection on a single day of gestation (mice; Gibson & Becker, 1971), oral administration for several days during pregnancy (mice, Takano & Suzuki, 1971; rats, Tanaka *et al.*, 1973; and monkeys, Wilson, 1972) and long-term dietary administration (Lorke & Machemer, 1975; Kroes *et al.*, 1977). No treatment-related malformations were seen in these studies, but several found evidence of developmental toxicity in the form of reduced growth or viability of fetuses and/or postnatal offspring (see also IARC, 1980).

Exposure of day-10.5 rat embryos in whole-embryo cultures to 1.0 mmol/L cyclohexylamine reduced growth and increased the incidence of morphologically abnormal embryos. No significant effects were seen at 0.3 mmol/L, and the addition of hepatic microsomes did not alter the dose–response relationship (Kitchin & Ebron, 1983).

In their review of the toxicity of cyclohexylamine, Bopp *et al.* (1986) summarized a number of studies of effects on the testis, reproductive function and prenatal development, some of which were unpublished. They concluded that the testicular effects, which included reduced organ weights, sperm counts, sperm motility and impairment of spermatogenesis, were among the most sensitive effects of cyclohexylamine at the target organ and that rats were more sensitive than other species, but that the mode of action was not discernible; hyperthermia, direct endocrine imbalance and primary Sertoli cell toxicity were dismissed as possible explanations for the testicular effects. With regard to effects on reproductive function, they noted that exposed male rats showed reduced fertility (evidenced by fewer impregnated females and implantation sites) and that mice had reduced litter sizes and pup weights at birth. In studies of prenatal toxicity, no malformations were seen after exposure of mice, rats, rabbits or monkeys to cyclohexylamine during gestation, but a study in mice and another in rats showed potential embryolethality. One study in which rat embryos were exposed *in vitro* showed an effect on growth and morphogenesis from doses of 1 mmol/L (Kitchin & Ebron, 1983). None of the studies of mammals *in vivo* demonstrated teratogenic effects.

4.4 Genetic and related effects

The genetic toxicology and other toxicological aspects of cyclamate and its principal metabolite cyclohexylamine have been reviewed (Bopp *et al.*, 1986).

4.4.1 *Humans*

Chromosomal breaks were observed in lymphocytes from 11 human patients suffering from chronic liver and kidney diseases, who had taken daily doses of cyclamate (2–5 g) for up to three years. The number of chromosomal breaks per cell in this group was significantly higher than that in a similar group of patients who were not taking cyclamate or in healthy controls. The frequency of other types of cytogenetic damage, however, was significantly different only between the two patient groups and the controls

(Bauchinger *et al.*, 1970). The other study involved three groups of healthy volunteers, each comprising two men and two women 20–54 years of age. The first group received no cyclamate and served as the control group. The second group consisted of four subjects who were capable of metabolically converting cyclamate to cyclohexylamine, and the third group comprised four subjects who could not convert cyclamate to cyclohexylamine. The last two groups received sodium cyclamate capsules three times a day for four days, providing an average daily dose of 70 mg/kg bw. Analysis of peripheral blood lymphocytes collected on the first and fifth days of the study showed no increase in the frequency of chromosomal aberrations in the two treated groups over that in the control subjects (Dick *et al.*, 1974). [The Working Group considered that the second study was rather weak because of the limited size of the treated groups and the short exposure.]

4.4.2 *Experimental systems* (see Tables 1–3 for references)

Calcium cyclamate

In one study, calcium cyclamate did not induce gene mutation in *Salmonella typhimurium* strains TA100, TA1537 or TA98 in the presence or absence of exogenous metabolic activation at the highest concentration tested. It did not induce aneuploidy in *Drosophila melanogaster*; but in one of three studies it induced sex-linked recessive lethal mutations, and in one of two studies it induced heritable translocations when males were exposed to calcium cyclamate in the diet.

In separate studies, calcium cyclamate did not induce unscheduled DNA synthesis in rat primary hepatocyte cultures, gene mutation in Chinese hamster ovary cells at the *hprt* locus with or without exogenous metabolic activation, or chromosomal aberrations in a rat-kangaroo kidney cell line. Calcium cyclamate induced chromosomal aberrations in human lymphocytes cultured *in vitro* in the absence of metabolic activation.

Calcium cyclamate did not affect sperm morphology or induce micronuclei in the bone marrow of mice treated on five consecutive days by intraperitoneal injection, bone marrow or sperm samples being collected 4 h or 35 days, respectively, after the last injection. Chromosomal aberrations were induced in the bone marrow of Mongolian gerbils given five daily intraperitoneal injections of calcium cyclamate. Aberrations were not induced in the bone marrow or spermatogonia of rats given calcium cyclamate and casein in a semisynthetic diet for 10 months, nor were dominant lethal mutations observed in these rats. Calcium cyclamate did not induce dominant lethal mutations in mice of two strains given calcium cyclamate by gavage daily for five or 30 days, respectively. In a single study, calcium cyclamate did not induce heritable translocations in mice given the compound by gavage on five days per week for six weeks.

Sodium cyclamate

In one study, the frequency of chromosomal aberrations in the callus and root tips of *Haworthia* exposed to sodium cyclamate *in vitro* was not significantly greater than that in control cultures. Sodium cyclamate did not induce sex-linked recessive lethal mutation or aneuploidy in *D. melanogaster*.

Table 1. Genetic and related effects of calcium cyclamate

Test system	Result [a]		Dose[b] (LED or HID)	Reference
	Without exogenous metabolic activation	With exogenous metabolic activation		
Salmonella typhimurium TA100, TA98, TA1537, reverse mutation	–	–	500 μg/plate	Bruce & Heddle (1979)
Drosophila melanogaster, sex-linked mutation	+		50000 ppm feed	Majumdar & Freedman (1971) [abst]
Drosophila melanogaster, sex-linked mutation	–		50000 ppm feed	Rotter & Mittler (1972) [abst]
Drosophila melanogaster, sex-linked mutation	–		100 mg/mL feed	Brusick *et al.* (1989)
Drosophila melanogaster, heritable translocations	–		50000 ppm feed	Rotter & Mittler (1972) [abst]
Drosophila melanogaster, heritable translocations	+		12500 ppm feed	Wu & Smith (1981) [abst]
Drosophila melanogaster, aneuploidy	–		50000 ppm feed	Rotter & Mittler (1972) [abst]
Drosophila melanogaster, aneuploidy	–		12500 ppm feed	Wu & Smith (1981) [abst]
Unscheduled DNA synthesis, Fischer 344 rat primary hepatocytes *in vitro*	–	NT	5000	Brusick *et al.* (1989)
Gene mutation, Chinese hamster ovary cells, *hprt* locus *in vitro*	–	–	10000	Brusick *et al.* (1989)
Chromosomal aberrations, rat-kangaroo kidney cells *in vitro*	–	NT	200	Green *et al.* (1970)
Chromosomal aberrations, human lymphocytes *in vitro*	+	NT	250	Stone *et al.* (1969b)
Chromosomal aberrations, human lymphocytes *in vitro*	+	NT	4000	Jemison *et al* (1984)
Micronucleus formation, mouse bone marrow *in vivo*	–		2500 × 5 ip	Bruce & Heddle (1979)
Chromosomal aberrations, gerbil bone marrow *in vivo*	+		30 × 5 ip	Majumdar & Solomon (1971)
Chromosomal aberrations, Holzman rat bone marrow *in vivo*	–		500 diet 10 mo	Friedman *et al.* (1972)
Chromosomal aberrations, Holzman rat spermatogonia *in vivo*	–		500 diet 10 mo	Friedman *et al.* (1972)
Dominant lethal mutation, ICR/Ha Swiss mice *in vivo*	–		1000 × 5 po	Epstein *et al.* (1972)
Dominant lethal mutation, (C3H × 101) F_1 mice *in vivo*	–		4000 × 30 po	Cain *et al.* (1988)
Dominant lethal mutation, Osborne-Mendel rats *in vivo*	–		1000 diet 10 mo	Friedman *et al.* (1972)

Table 1 (contd)

Test system	Result [a]		Dose[b] (LED or HID)	Reference
	Without exogenous metabolic activation	With exogenous metabolic activation		
Heritable translocation, mice *in vivo*	–		4000 × 30 po	Cain *et al.* (1988)
Sperm morphology, (C57BL/6 × C3H/He) F_1 mice *in vivo*	–		500 × 5 ip	Wyrobek & Bruce (1975)
Sperm morphology, (C57BL/6 × C3H/He) F_1 mice *in vivo*	–		2500 × 5 ip	Bruce & Heddle (1979)

[a] +, positive; –, negative; NT, not tested

[b] LED, lowest effective dose; HID, highest ineffective dose; unless otherwise stated, in-vitro tests, μg/mL; in-vivo tests, mg/kg bw per day; ip, intraperitoneal; mo, month; po, oral

Table 2. Genetic and related effects of sodium cyclamate

Test system	Result[a]		Dose[b] (LED or HID)	Reference
	Without exogenous metabolic system	With exogenous metabolic system		
Haworthia variegata, chromosomal aberrations	–	NT	20000	Majumdar & Lane (1970)
Drosophila melanogaster, sex-linked mutation	–		2 µg/fly inj	Šrám & Ondrej (1968) [abst]
Drosophila melanogaster, sex-linked mutation	–		5000	Vogel & Chandler (1974)
Drosophila melanogaster, aneuploidy	–		160 mg/mL feed	Félix & de la Rosa (1971)
Chromosomal aberrations, Chinese hamster cells *in vitro*	+	NT	250	Kristoffersson (1972)
Cell transformation, Fischer 344 rat bladder explant *in vitro*	+	NT	240	Nicholson & Jani (1988)
Sister chromatid exchange, human lymphocytes *in vitro*	+	NT	7500	Wolff (1983)
Chromosomal aberrations, human fibroblasts *in vitro*	+	NT	200	Stone *et al.* (1969b)
Chromosomal aberrations, human lymphocytes *in vitro*	+	NT	250	Stone *et al.* (1969b)
Chromosomal aberrations, human lymphocytes *in vitro*	+	NT	200	Stoltz *et al.* (1970)
Chromosomal aberrations, human lymphocytes *in vitro*	+	NT	5000	Collin (1971)
Chromosomal aberrations, human lymphocytes *in vitro*	+	NT	2000	Tokomitsu (1971)
Chromosomal aberrations, human lymphocytes *in vitro*	+	NT	4500	Perez Requejo (1972)
Chromosomal aberrations, human lymphocytes *in vitro*	–	NT	20	Shamberger *et al.* (1973)
Host-mediated assay, *Salmonella typhimurium* in NMRI mice	–		500	Buselmaier *et al.* (1972)
Chromosomal aberrations, BALB/c mice spermatogonia *in vivo*, spermatocytes observed	–		3400 drink 150 d	Leonard & Linden (1972)
Chromosomal aberrations, Chinese hamster spermatogonia *in vivo*	–		2000 × 5 po	Machemer & Lorke (1975a)
Dominant lethal mutation, NMRI mice *in vivo*	–		10000 × 5 po	Lorke (1973)
Dominant lethal mutation, mice *in vivo*	–		2000 diet 70 d	Lorke & Machemer (1975)

Table 2 (contd)

Test system	Result[a]		Dose[b] (LED or HID)	Reference
	Without exogenous metabolic system	With exogenous metabolic system		
Dominant lethal mutation, mice *in vivo*	–		10000 × 1 po	Machemer & Lorke (1975b)
Sperm morphology, (CBA × BALB/c) F_1 mice *in vivo*	–		1000 × 5 ip	Topham (1980)

[a] +, positive; –, negative; NT, not tested

[b] LED, lowest effective dose; HID, highest ineffective dose; in-vitro tests, μg/mL; in-vivo tests, mg/kg bw per day; d, day; inj, injection; po, oral; ip, intraperitoneal

Table 3. Genetic and related effects of cyclohexylamine

Test system	Result[a]		Dose[b] (LED or HID)	Reference
	Without exogenous metabolic activation	With exogenous metabolic activation		
Prophage, induction, SOS repair test, DNA strand breaks, cross-links or related damage	–	NT	NR	Mayer *et al.* (1969)
Salmonella typhimurium TA100, TA98, TA1535 TA1537, reverse mutation	–	–	2500 μg/plate	Herbold (1981)
Salmonella typhimurium TA100,, TA98, TA1535, TA1537, reverse mutation	–	–	10000 μg/plate	Mortelmans *et al.* (1986)
Salmonella typhimurium TA100, TA98, TA1535, TA1538, reverse mutation	NT	–	2500 μg/plate	Anderson & Styles (1978)
Drosophila melanogaster, sex-linked recessive lethal mutation	–		990 μg/mL feed	Vogel & Chandler (1974)
Drosophila melanogaster, sex-linked recessive lethal mutation	–		1720 μg/mL feed	Brusick *et al.* (1989)
Drosophila melanogaster, sex-linked recessive lethal mutation	–		0.2% feed or 1 mg/fly inj	Knaap *et al.* (1973)
Drosophila melanogaster, heritable translocations	–		NR	Knaap *et al.* (1973)
Drosophila melanogaster, aneuploidy	–		6880 ppm feed	Félix & de la Rosa (1971)
Unscheduled DNA synthesis, Fischer 344 rat primary hepatocytes *in vitro*	–	NT	860	Brusick *et al.* (1989)
Gene mutation, Chinese hamster ovary cells, *hprt* locus *in vitro*	–	–	1376	Brusick *et al.* (1989)
Chromosomal aberrations, rat-kangaroo kidney cells *in vitro*	+	NT	50	Green *et al.* (1970)
Cell transformation, SA7/Syrian hamster embryo cells	+	NT	62	Casto (1981)
Sister chromatid exchange, human lymphocytes *in vitro*	+	NT	99	Wolff (1983)
Chromosomal aberrations, human lymphocytes *in vitro*	(+)	NT	99	Stoltz *et al.* (1970)
Chromosomal aberrations, human lymphocytes *in vitro*	–	NT	500	Brewen *et al.* (1971)
Host-mediated assay, *Salmonella typhimurium* G46 and *Serratia marcescns* a21 in mouse peritoneal cavity	–	NT	100	Buselmaier *et al.* (1972)

Table 3 (contd)

Test system	Result[a]		Dose[b] (LED or HID)	Reference
	Without exogenous metabolic activation	With exogenous metabolic activation		
Host-mediated assay, human leukocytes in Chinese hamster peritoneal cavity	–	NT	450 ip × 1	Brewen *et al.* (1971)
Mouse spot test	(+)		200 ip × 1	Fahrig (1982)
Chromosomal aberrations, rat bone-marrow cells *in vivo*	+		50 ip × 5	Legator *et al.* (1969)
Chromosomal aberrations, rat bone-marrow cells *in vivo*	–		50 po/ip × 5	Dick *et al.* (1974)
Chromosomal aberrations, fetal sheep bone-marrow cells *in vivo*	–		250 iv × 1	Turner & Hutchinson (1974)
Chromosomal aberrations, Chinese hamster bone-marrow *in vivo*	–		450 ip × 1	Brewen *et al.* (1971)
Chromosomal aberrations, rat leukocytes *in vivo*	–		50 ip × 35	Mostardi *et al.* (1972)
Chromosomal aberrations, fetal sheep leukocytes *in vivo*	+		50 iv × 1	Turner & Hutchinson (1974)
Chromosomal aberrations, Chinese hamster leukocytes *in vivo*	+		200 po × 3	Van Went-deVries *et al.* (1975)
Chromosomal aberrations, mouse spermatogonia *in vivo*, spermatocytes observed	–		100 ip × 5	Cattanach & Pollard (1971)
Chromosomal aberrations, rat spermatogonia treated *in vivo*, spermatogonia observed	+		50 ip × 1	Legator *et al.* (1969)
Chromosomal aberrations, Chinese hamster spermatogonia treated *in vivo*, spermatogonia observed	–		102 po × 5	Machemer & Lorke (1976)
Dominant lethal mutation, ICR/Ha Swiss mice *in vivo*	–		25 ip × 1	Epstein *et al.* (1972)
Dominant lethal mutation, male mice *in vivo*	–		100 ip × 5	Cattanach & Pollard (1971)
Dominant lethal mutation, mice *in vivo*	+		100 ip × 5	Petersen *et al.* (1972)
Dominant lethal mutation, male NMRI mice *in vivo*	–		102 po × 5	Lorke & Machemer (1975)

Table 3 (contd)

Test system	Result[a]		Dose[b] (LED or HID)	Reference
	Without exogenous metabolic activation	With exogenous metabolic activation		
Dominant lethal mutation, male and female mice *in vivo*	–		0.11% diet equival. to 136 mg/kg/d, 10 wk	Lorke & Machemer (1975)
Dominant lethal mutation, male mice *in vivo*	–		150 po × 1	Machemer & Lorke (1975b)
Dominant lethal mutation, male and female rats *in vivo*	– (dec. fert.)		145 po × 3 wk[c]	Khera & Stoltz (1970)

[a] +, positive; (+), weakly positive; –, negative; NT, not tested; dec. fert., decreased fertility
[b] LED, lowest effective dose; HID, highest ineffective dose; unless otherwise stated, *in-vitro* tests, μg/mL; *in-vivo* tests, mg/kg bw per day: NR, not reported; inj, injection; ip, intraperitoneal; po, oral; iv, intravenous; d, day; wk, week
[c] Male and female rats treated with 2% cyclohexylamine in drinking-water for three weeks. Males were then gavaged daily with 220 mg/kg for four weeks followed by three weeks without treatment then two more weeks of gavage treatment; each male was mated with two females on five days/week throughout the treatment period.

Results from a single study showed a high incidence of epithelial foci in Fischer 344 rat bladder explants exposed to sodium cyclamate. Chromosomal aberrations were induced in Chinese hamster embryonic lung cells cultured with sodium cyclamate in one study, in human skin fibroblasts cultured with sodium cyclamate in another study, and in human lymphocytes treated with sodium cyclamate *in vitro* in five studies. Sister chromatid exchange was induced in human lymphocyte cultures exposed to sodium cyclamate in a single study.

Gene mutation was not induced in a host-mediated assay in which mice were injected intraperitoneally with *S. typhimurium* strain G46 and exposed to sodium cyclamate by subcutaneous injection. Chromosomal aberrations were not induced in the spermatogonia of mice or Chinese hamsters exposed to sodium cyclamate in drinking-water for 150 days or by gavage for five consecutive days, respectively. Dominant lethal mutations were not induced in male and female mice fed a diet containing sodium cyclamate for 10 weeks or in male mice treated orally for five days or female mice dosed once. Sperm morphology was unaffected in mice treated by intraperitoneal injection on five consecutive days with sodium cyclamate.

Cyclohexylamine

Cyclohexylamine did not induce bacterial prophage in *E. coli* or gene mutations in *S. typhimurium*. It did not induce somatic cell mutation or recombination, sex-linked recessive lethal mutation, heritable translocation or aneuploidy in *D. melanogaster*. *In vitro*, it did not induce unscheduled DNA synthesis in rat hepatocytes or gene mutations in Chinese hamster ovary cells, but it did induce chromosomal aberrations in rat-kangaroo kidney cells and transformation of Syrian hamster embryo cells. In human lymphocyte cultures, cyclohexylamine induced sister chromatid exchange, but the frequency of chromosomal aberrations was increased only slightly in one study and not at all in another. After intraperitoneal injection of cyclohexylamine, gene mutations were not induced in host-mediated assays in bacteria in the peritoneal cavity of mice or in human lymphocytes in the peritoneal cavity of Chinese hamsters. *In vivo*, cyclohexylamine was weakly mutagenic in one mouse spot test. While the frequency of chromosomal aberrations was increased in one of two studies in rat bone marrow, no aberrations were seen in the bone marrow of Chinese hamsters or fetal sheep, nor in rat leukocytes. Chromosomal aberrations were induced by cyclohexamine in leukocytes of Chinese hamsters and fetal sheep. The compound also induced chromosomal aberrations in rat spermatogonia when these cells were recovered shortly after exposure *in vivo*, but there was no increase in the frequency of chromosomal aberrations in mouse spermatocytes when their precursors had been exposed to cyclohexylamine during the spermatogonial stage. Dominant lethal effects were enhanced in mice in one study, while there was no effect in five other studies. In a single study in rats, cyclohexylamine did not induce dominant lethal mutations.

5. Summary of Data Reported and Evaluation

5.1 Exposure data

Cyclamates are widely used as non-caloric sweeteners, the average daily dietary intake generally being less than 3 mg/kg bw.

5.2 Human carcinogenicity data

Use of cyclamates was analysed separately in only four of the studies summarized in the monograph on saccharin and its salts. No increase in the risk for urinary bladder cancer was seen.

5.3 Animal carcinogenicity data

Sodium cyclamate was tested by oral administration in two experiments in mice, one of which was a multigeneration study, and in three experiments in rats. No treatment-related increase in tumour incidence was found. Sodium cyclamate was also tested by oral administration in other experiments in mice, rats, hamsters and monkeys, but these experiments could not be evaluated because of various inadequacies or incomplete reporting.

Pellets containing sodium cyclamate induced bladder tumours in mice after implantation into the bladder; however, the protocol was considered to be inadequate for determining carcinogenicity.

Calcium cyclamate was tested by oral administration in a two-generation experiment in rats; no difference in tumour incidence was seen between treated and control animals.

In two studies in rats, sodium cyclamate was administered orally after a known carcinogen. The incidence of urinary bladder tumours was increased in one study, whereas only slight enhancement was found in a second study.

5.4 Other relevant data

Cyclamates are incompletely absorbed from the gastrointestinal tract of humans and other mammals. Most is excreted in the urine unchanged. Cyclamates are partially converted by gastrointestinal microflora to cyclohexylamine, which is absorbed. Cyclamates and cyclohexylamine can produce testicular toxicity in rats.

Cyclamates have not been observed to produce developmental toxicity in mice, rats, rabbits, hamsters, dogs or rhesus monkeys. Negative results were obtained in a number of short-term assays for teratogenicity *in vitro* and *in vivo*. Cyclamates were not teratogenic in mice, rats or rhesus monkeys, but there were some indications of reduced growth and viability of embryos in some studies. Rat embryos exposed *in vitro* showed altered morphological development in one study.

Cyclamates did not produce chromosomal aberrations in peripheral lymphocytes of volunteers. Cyclamates were not genotoxic in rodents *in vivo* but were genotoxic in mammalian cells *in vitro*.

5.5 Evaluation

There is *inadequate evidence* in humans for the carcinogenicity of cyclamates.

There is *inadequate evidence* in experimental animals for the carcinogenicity of cyclamates.

Overall evaluation

Cyclamates are *not classifiable as to their carcinogenicity to humans (Group 3).*

6. References

Adkins, A., Hupp, E.W. & Gerdes, R.A. (1972) Biological activity of saccharins and cyclamates in golden hamsters (Abstract). *Texas J. Sci.*, **23**, 575

Ahmed, F.E. & Thomas, D.B. (1992) Assessment of the carcinogenicity of the nonnutritive sweetener cyclamate. *Crit. Rev. Toxicol.*, **22**, 81–118

Althoff, J., Cardesa, A., Pour, P. & Shubik, P. (1975) A chronic study of artificial sweeteners in Syrian golden hamsters. *Cancer Lett.*, **1**, 21–24

Anderson, D. & Styles, J.A. (1978) The bacterial mutation test. *Br. J. Cancer*, **37**, 924–930

Asahina, M., Yamaka, T., Watanabe, K. & Sarrazin, G. (1971) Excretion of cyclohexylamine, a metabolite of cyclamate, in human urine. *Chem. pharm. Bull.*, **19**, 628–632

Bantle, J.A., Burton, D.T., Dawson, D.A., Dumont, J.N., Finch, R.A., Fort, D.J., Linder, G., Rayburn, J.R., Buchwalter, D., Gaudet-Hull, A.M., Maurice, M.A. & Turley, S.D. (1994) FETAX interlaboratory validation study: Phase II testing. *Environ. Toxicol. Chem.*, **13**, 1629–1637

Bär, A. & Biermann, C. (1992) Intake of intense sweeteners in Germany. *Z. Ernährungswiss*, **31**, 25–29

Bauchinger, M., Schmid, E., Pieper, M. & Zollner, N. (1970) [Cytogenetic effects of cyclamate on human peripheral lymphocytes in vivo.] *Dtsch. med. Wochenschr.*, **95**, 2220–2223 (in German)

Bizzari, S.N., Leder, A.E. & Ishikawa, Y. (1996) High-intensity sweeteners. In: *Chemical Economics Handbook*, Menlo Park, CA, SRI International

Bopp, B.A. & Price, P. (1991) Cyclamate. In: O'Brien Nabors, L. & Gelardi, R.C., eds, *Alternative Sweeteners*, 2nd Ed., New York, Marcel Dekker, pp. 72–95

Bopp, B., Sonders, R.C. & Kesterson, J.W. (1986) Toxicological aspects of cyclamate and cyclohexylamine. *Crit. Rev. Toxicol.*, **16**, 213–306

Brantom, P.G., Gaunt, I.F. & Grasso, P. (1973) Long-term toxicity of sodium cyclamate in mice. *Food Cosmet. Toxicol.*, **11**, 735–746

Brewen, J.G., Pearson, F.G., Jones, K.P. & Luippold, H.E. (1971) Cytogenetic effects of cyclohexylamine and N-OH-cyclohexamine on human leukocytes and Chinese hamster bone marrow. *Nature New Biol.*, **230**, 15–16

Bruce, W.R. & Heddle, J.A. (1979) The mutagenic activity of 61 agents as determined by the micronucleus, Salmonella, and sperm abnormality assays. *Can. J. Genet. Cytol.*, **21**, 319–334

Brusick, D., Cifone, M., Young, R. & Benson, S. (1989) Assessment of the genotoxicity of calcium cyclamate and cyclohexylamine. *Environ. mol. Mutag.*, **14**, 188–199

Bryan, G.T. & Ertürk, E. (1970) Production of mouse urinary bladder carcinomas by sodium cyclamate. *Science*, **167**, 996–998

Budavari, S., ed. (1996) *The Merck Index*, 12th Ed., Whitehouse Station, NJ, Merck & Co., Inc., pp. 272–273, 454–455

Buselmaier, W., Rohrborn, G. & Propping, P. (1972) Mutagenicity investigations with pesticides in the host-mediated assay and the dominant lethal test in mice. *Biol. Zentralbl.*, **91**, 311–325

Buss, N.E., Renwick, A.G., Donaldson, K.M. & George, C.F. (1992) The metabolism of cyclamate to cyclohexylamine and its cardiovascular consequences in human volunteers. *Toxicol. appl. Pharmacol.*, **115**, 199–210

Cain, K.T., Cornett, C.V., Cacheiro, N.L., Hughes, L.A., Owens, J.G. & Generoso, W.M. (1988) No evidence found for induction of dominant lethal mutations and heritable translocations in male mice by calcium cyclamate. *Environ. mol. Mutag.*, **11**, 207–213

Casto, B.C. (1981) Detection of chemical carcinogens and mutagens in hamster cells by enhancement of adenovirus transformation. In: Mishra, N., Dunkel, V. & Mehlman, I., eds, *Advances in Modern Environmental Toxicology*, Vol. 1, Princeton, NJ, Senate Press, pp. 241–271

Cattanach, B.M. & Pollard, C.E. (1971) Mutagenicity tests with cyclohexylamine in the mouse. *Mutat. Res.*, **12**, 472–474

Chapin, R.E. & Gulati, D.K. (1997) Feed restriction in rats. *Environ. Health Perspectives*, **105** (Suppl. 1), 381–382

Chemical Information Services (1995) *Directory of World Chemical Producers 1995/96 Standard Edition*, Dallas, TX, pp. 143, 213, 625

Cicurel, L. & Schmid, B.P. (1988) Post-implantation embryo culture: Validation with selected compounds for teratogenicity testing. *Xenobiotica*, **18**, 617–624

Clayson, D.B. (1974) Bladder carcinogenesis in rats and mice: Possibility of artifacts. *J. natl Cancer Inst.*, **52**, 1685–1689

Collin, J.P. (1971) [Cytogenetic effect of sodium cyclamate, cyclohexanone and cyclohexanol.] *Diabete*, **19**, 215–221 (in French)

Coulston, F., McChesney, E.W. & Benitz, K.-F. (1977) Eight-year study of cyclamate in rhesus monkeys (Abstract No. 80). *Toxicol. appl. Pharmacol.*, **41**, 164–165

Delhaise, F., van Cutsem, P., van Maele-Fabry, G., Roba, J. & Picard, J.J. (1989) Assessment of the validity of an in vitro teratogenicity test using post-implantation mouse embryos. *Teratology*, **40**, 279–280

De Sesso, I.M. (1989) Confounding factors in direct bladder exposure studies. *Comments Toxicol.*, **3**, 317–334

Dick, C.E., Schniepp, M., Sonders, R.C. & Wiegand, R.G. (1974) Cyclamate and cyclohexylamine: Lack of effect on the chromosomes of man and rats *in vivo*. *Mutat. Res.*, **26**, 199–203

Drasar, B.S., Renwick, A.G. & Williams, R.T. (1972) The role of the gut flora in the metabolism of cyclamate. *Biochem. J.*, **129**, 881–890

Epstein, S.S., Arnold, E., Andrea, J., Bass, W. & Bishop, Y. (1972) Detection of chemical mutagens by the dominant lethal assay in the mouse. *Toxicol. appl. Pharmacol.*, **23**, 288–325

Fahrig, R. (1982) Effects in the mammalian spot test: Cyclamate versus saccharin. *Mutat. Res.*, **103**, 43–47

Fancher, O.E., Palazzolo, R.J., Blockhus, L., Weinberg, M.S. & Calandra, J.C. (1968) Chronic studies with sodium saccharin and sodium cyclamate in dogs (Abstract No. 15). *Toxicol. appl. Pharmacol.*, **12**, 291

Félix, R. & de la Rosa, M.E. (1971) Cytogenetic studies with sodium cyclamate in D. melanogaster females. *Drosophila Info. Serv.*, **47**, 102–104

Friedman, L., Richardson, H.L., Richardson, M.E., Lethco, E.J., Wallace, W.C. & Saura, F.M. (1972) Toxic response of rats to cyclamates in chow and semisynthetic diets. *J. natl Cancer Inst.*, **49**, 751–764

Fritz, H. & Hess, R. (1968) Prenatal development in the rat following the administration of cyclamate, saccharin and sucrose. *Experientia*, **24**, 1140–1141

Gibson, J.E. & Becker, B.A. (1971) Teratogenicity of structural truncates of cyclophosphamide in mice. *Teratology*, **4**, 141–150

Golberg, L., Parekh, C., Patti, A. & Soike, K. (1969) Cyclamate degradation in mammals and *in vitro* (Abstract No. 107). *Toxicol. appl. Pharmacol.*, **14**, 654

Green, S., Palmer, K.A. & Legator, M.S. (1970) In vitro cytogenetic investigation of calcium cyclamate, cyclohexylamine and triflupromazine. *Food Cosmet. Toxicol.*, **8**, 617–623

Herbold, B.A. (1981) Studies to evaluate artificial sweeteners, especially Remsen-Fahlberg saccharin, and their possible impurities, for potential mutagenicity by the Salmonella/ mammalian liver microsome test. *Mutat. Res.*, **90**, 365–372

Hulshof, K.F.A.M., Kistemaker, C., Bouman, M. & Löwik, M.R.H. (1995) *Use of Various Types of Sweeteners in Different Population Groups: 1992 Dutch National Food Consumption Survey* (TNO Report V-95.301), Zeist, TNO Nutrition and Food Research Institute

IARC (1980) *IARC Monographs on the Evaluation of the Carcinogenic Risk of Chemicals to Humans*, Vol. 22, *Some Non-nutritive Sweetening Agents*, Lyon, pp. 55–109, 171–185

IARC (1987) *IARC Monographs on the Evaluation of Carcinogenic Risks to Humans*, Suppl. 7, *Overall Evaluations of Carcinogenicity: An Updating of* IARC Monographs *Volumes 1 to 42*, Lyon, pp. 178–182

Ichibagase, H., Kojima, S., Suenaga, A. & Inoue, K. (1972) Studies on synthetic sweetening agents. XVI. Metabolism of sodium cyclamate. 5. The metabolism of sodium cyclamate in rabbits and rats after prolonged administration of sodium cyclamate. *Chem. pharm. Bull.*, **20**, 1093–1101

Jemison, E.W., Brown, K., Rivers, B. & Knight, R. (1984) Cytogenetic effects of cyclamates. *Adv. exp. Med. Biol.*, **172**, 91–117

Jull, J.W. (1979) The effect of time on the incidence of carcinomas obtained by the implantation of paraffin wax pellets into mouse bladder. *Cancer Lett.*, **6**, 21–25

Kessler, I.I. & Clark, J.P. (1978) Saccharin, cyclamate and human bladder cancer. *J. Am. med. Assoc.*, **240**, 349–355

Khera, K.S. & Stoltz, D.R. (1970) Effects of cyclohexylamine on rat fertility. *Experientia*, **26**, 761–762

Kitchin, K.T. & Ebron, M.T. (1983) Studies of saccharin and cyclohexylamine in a coupled microsomal activating/embryo culture system. *Food chem. Toxicol.*, **21**, 537–541

Klotzsche, C. (1969) [On the teratogenic and embryotoxic effect of cyclamate, saccharin and sucrose.] *Arzneimitt. Forsch.*, **19**, 925–928 (in German)

Knaap, A.G.A.C., Kramers, P.G.N. & Sobels, F.H. (1973) Lack of mutagenicity of the cyclamate metabolites in Drosophila. *Mutat. Res.*, **21**, 341–344

Knowles, M.A. & Jani, H. (1986) Multistage transformation of cultured rat urothelium: The effects of *N*-methyl-*N*-nitrosourea, sodium saccharin, sodium cyclamate and 12-*O*-tetradecanoylphorbol-13-acetate. *Carcinogenesis*, **7**, 2059–2065

Knowles, M.A., Jani, H. & Hicks, R.M. (1986) Induction of morphological changes in the urothelium of cultured adult rat bladder by sodium saccharin and sodium cyclamate. *Carcinogenesis*, **7**, 767–774

Kristoffersson, U. (1972) Effect of cyclamate and saccharin on the chromosomes of a Chinese hamster cell line. *Hereditas*, **70**, 271–282

Kroes, R., Peters, P.W.J., Berkvens, J.M., Verschuuren, H.G., De Vries, T. & van Esch, G.J. (1977) Long-term toxicity and reproduction study (including a teratogenicity study) with cyclamate, saccharin and cyclohexylamine. *Toxicology*, **8**, 285–300

Lee, L.S. (1981) Saccharin and cyclamate inhibit binding of epidermal growth factor. *Proc. natl Acad. Sci. USA*, **78**, 1042–1046

Legator, M.S., Palmer, K.A., Green, S. & Petersen, K.W. (1969) Cytogenetic studies in rats of cyclohexylamine, a metabolite of cyclamate. *Science*, **165**, 1139–1140

Leonard, A. & Linden, G. (1972) Mutagenic properties of cyclamates in mammals. *C.R. Soc. Biol.*, **166**, 468–470

Lewis, R.J., Jr (1993) *Hawley's Condensed Chemical Dictionary*, 12th Ed., New York, Van Nostrand Reinhold, pp. 202, 335, 1054

Lorke, D. (1969) [Studies on the embryotoxic and teratogenic effects of cyclamate and saccharin in the mouse.] *Arzneimitt. Forsch.*, **19**, 920–922 (in German)

Lorke, D. (1973) Investigation of cyclamate for mutagenic effects by use of the dominant lethal assay in the mouse. *Humangenetik*, **18**, 165–170

Lorke, D. & Machemer, L. (1975) [The effect of several weeks' treatment of male and female mice with saccharin, cyclamate or cyclohexylamine sulfate on fertility and dominant lethal effects.] *Humangenetik*, **26**, 199–205 (in German)

Lynch, D.W., Schuler, R.L., Hood, R.D. & Davis, D.G. (1991) Evaluation of *Drosophila* for screening developmental toxicants: Test results with eighteen chemicals and presentation of a new *Drosophila* bioassay. *Teratog. Carcinog. Mutag.*, **11**, 147–173

Machemer, L. & Lorke, D. (1975a) Method for testing mutagenic effects of chemicals on spermatogonia of the Chinese hamster. *Arzneimitt. Forsch.*, **25**, 1889–1896

Machemer, L. & Lorke, D. (1975b) Experiences with the dominant lethal test in female mice: Effects of alkylating agents and artificial sweeteners on pre-ovulatory oocyte stages. *Mutat. Res.*, **29**, 209–214

Machemer, L. & Lorke, D. (1976) Evaluation of the mutagenic potential of cyclohexylamine on spermatogonia of the Chinese hamster. *Mutat. Res.*, **40**, 243–250

Majumdar, S.K. & Freedman, C. (1971) Mutation test of calcium cyclamate in Drosophila melanogaster (Abstract). *Drosophila Info. Serv.*, **46**, 114

Majumdar, S.K. & Lane, D.J. (1970) Effects of sodium cyclamate on Haworthia callus cultured in vitro: Development, differentiation, and the chromosomes. *J. Hered.*, **61**, 193–195

Majumdar, S.K. & Solomon, M. (1971) Chromosome changes in Mongolian gerbil following calcium cyclamate administration. *Nucleus*, **14**, 168–170

Mason, P.L. & Thompson, G.R. (1977) Testicular effects of cyclohexylamine hydrochloride in the rat. *Toxicology*, **8**, 143–156

Mayer, V.W., Gabridge, M.G. & Oswald, E.J. (1969) Rapid plate test for evaluating phage induction capacity. *Appl. Microbiol.*, **18**, 697–698

Møller Jensen, O., Knudsen, J.R., Sorensen, R.L. & Clemmesen, J. (1983) Artificial sweeteners and absence of bladder cancer risk in Copenhagen. *Int. J. Cancer*, **32**, 577–582

Mortelmans, K., Haworth, S., Lawlor, T., Speck, W., Tainer, B. & Zeiger, E. (1986) Salmonella mutagenicity tests: II. Results from the testing of 270 chemicals. *Environ. Mol. Mutag.*, **8** (Suppl. 7), 1–119

Mostardi, R.A., Keller, R. & Koo, R. (1972) Cytogenetic studies of cyclohexylamine, a metabolite of cyclamate. *Ohio J. Sci.*, **72**, 313–318

National Food Authority (1995) *Survey of Intense Sweetener Consumption in Australia. Final Report*, Canberra

National Institute for Occupational Safety and Health (1998) *National Occupational Exposure Survey 1981–83*, Cincinnati, OH

National Research Council (1985) *Evaluation of Cyclamate for Carcinogenicity*, Washington DC, National Academy Press

Nees, P.O. & Derse, P.H. (1965) Feeding and reproduction of rats fed calcium cyclamate. *Nature*, **208**, 81–82

Nees, P.O. & Derse, P.H. (1967) Effect of feeding calcium cyclamate to rats. *Nature*, **211**, 1191–1195

Nicholson, L.J. & Jani, H. (1988) Effects of sodium cyclamate and sodium saccharin on focus induction in explant cultures of rat bladder. *Int. J. Cancer*, **42**, 295–298

Oser, B.L., Carson, S., Cox, G.E., Vogin, E.E. & Sternberg, S.S. (1976) Long-term and multigeneration toxicity studies with cyclohexylamine hydrochloride. *Toxicology*, **6**, 47–65

Parekh, C., Goldberg, E.K. & Goldberg, L. (1970) Fate of sodium cyclamate-^{14}C in the rhesus monkey (*M. mulatta*) (Abstract No. 26). *Toxicol. appl. Pharmacol.*, **17**, 282

Penttilä, P.-L., Salminen, S. & Niemi, E. (1988) Estimates on the intake of food additives in Finland. *Z. Lebensm. Unters. Forsch.*, **186**, 11–15

Perez Requejo, J.L. (1972) In vitro effect of sodium cyclamate on human chromosomes. *Sangre*, **17**, 386–394

Petersen, K.W., Legator, M.S. & Figge, F.H.J. (1972) Dominant-lethal effects of cyclohexylamine in C57BL/FE mice. *Mutat. Res.*, **14**, 126–129

Pitkin, R.M., Reynolds, W.A. & Filer, L.J. (1969) Cyclamate and cyclohexylamine: Transfer across the hemocharial placenta. *Proc. Soc. exp. Biol.*, **132**, 993–995

Pratt, R.M. & Willis, W.D. (1985). In vitro screening assay for teratogens using growth inhibition of human embryonic cells. *Proc. natl Acad. Sci. USA*, **82**, 5791–5794

Prosky, L. & O'Dell, R.G. (1971) *In vivo* conversion of ^{14}C-labeled cyclamate to cyclohexylamine. *J. pharm. Sci.*, **60**, 1341–1343

Renault, J.-Y., Melcion, C. & Cordier, A. (1989) Limb bud cell culture for in vitro teratogen screening: Validation of an improved assessment method using 51 compounds. *Teratog. Carcinog. Mutag.*, **9**, 83–96

Renwick, A.G. (1995) Intense sweeteners intake surveys: Methods, results and comparisons. In: *Intake Studies—Lessons Learnt, ISA Symposium, Brussels, November 27, 1995*, Brussels, International Sweeteners Association, pp. 79–97

Renwick, A.G. & Williams, R.T. (1972a) The fate of cyclamate in man and other species. *Biochem. J.*, **129**, 869–879

Renwick, A.G. & Williams, R.T. (1972b) The metabolites of cyclohexylamine in man and certain animals. *Biochem. J.*, **129**, 857–867

Richards, R.K., Taylor, J.D., O'Brien, J.L. & Duescher, H.O. (1951) Studies on cyclamate sodium (sucaryl sodium), a new noncaloric sweetening agent. *J. Am. Pharmacol. Assoc.*, **40**, 1–6

Risch, J.A., Burch, J.D., Miller, A.B., Hill, G.B., Steel, R. & Howe, G.R. (1988) Dietary factors and the incidence of cancer of the urinary bladder. *Am. J. Epidemiol.*, **127**, 1179–1191

Roberts, A. & Renwick, A.G. (1989) The pharmacokinetics and tissue concentrations of cyclohexylamine in rats and mice. *Toxicol. appl. Pharmacol.*, **98**, 230–242

Roberts, A., Renwick, A.G., Ford, G., Creasy, D.M. & Gaunt, I. (1989) The metabolism and testicular toxicity of cyclohexylamine in rats and mice during chronic dietary administration. *Toxicol. appl. Pharmacol.*, **98**, 216–229

Rotter, D. & Mittler, S. (1972) Failure of mono sodium glutamate and calcium cyclamate to induce chromosomal aberrations in Drosophila (Abstract). *Mutat. Res.*, **21**, 12

Schechter, P.J. & Roth, L.J. (1971) Whole-body autoradiography of ^{14}C sodium cyclamate in pregnant and fetal rats. *Toxicol. appl. Pharmacol.*, **20**, 130–133

Seidenberg, J.M., Anderson, D.G. & Becker, R.A. (1986) Validation of an in vivo developmental toxicity screen in the mouse. *Teratog. Carcinog. Mutag.*, **6**, 361–374

Serra-Majem, L., Ribas, L., Inglès, C., Fuentes, M.., Lloveras, G. & Salleras, L. (1996) Cyclamate consumption in Catalonia, Spain (1992): Relationship with the body mass index. *Food Addit. Contam.*, **13**, 695–703

Shamberger, R.J., Baughman, F.F., Kalchert, S.L.,Willis, C.E. & Hoffman, G.C. (1973) Carcinogen-induced chromosomal breakage decreased by antioxidants. *Proc. natl Acad. Sci. USA*, **70**, 1461–1463

Simon, D., Yen, S. & Cole, P. (1975) Coffee drinking and cancer of the lower urinary tract. *J. natl Cancer Inst.*, **54**, 587–591

Sonders, R.C. & Wiegand, R.G. (1968) Absorption and excretion of cyclamate in animals and man (Abstract No. 16). *Toxicol. appl. Pharmacol.*, **12**, 291

Šrám, R. & Ondrej, M. (1968) Mutagenic activity of some drugs and pesticides (Abstract). *Drosophila Info. Serv.*, **43**, 164

Steele, V.E., Morrissey, R.E., Elmore, E.L., Gurganus-Rocha, D., Wilkinson, B.P., Curren, R.D., Schmetter, B.S., Louie, A.T., Lamb, J.C., IV & Yang, L.L. (1988) Evaluation of two in vitro assays to screen for potential developmental toxicants. *Fundam. appl. Toxicol.*, **11**, 673–684

Stoltz, D.R., Khera, K.S., Bendall, R. & Gunner, S.W. (1970) Cytogenetic studies with cyclamate and related compounds. *Science*, **167**, 1501–1502

Stone, D., Matalka, E. & Riordan, J. (1969a) Hyperactivity in rats bred and raised on relatively low amounts of cyclamates. *Nature*, **224**, 1326–1328

Stone, D., Lamson, E., Chang, Y.S. & Pickering, K.W. (1969b) Cytogenetic effects of cyclamates on human cells in vitro. *Science*, **164**, 568–569

Takano, K. & Suzuki, M. (1971) [Cyclohexylamine, a chromosome-aberration inducing substance: No teratogenicity in mice.] *Congen. Anomalies*, **11**, 51–57 (in Japanese)

Tanaka, S., Nakaura, S., Kawashima, K., Nagao, S., Kuwamura, T. & Omori, T. (1973) Studies on the teratogenicity of food additives. 2. Effects of cyclohexylamine and cyclohexylamine sulfate on the fetal development in rats. *J. Food Hyg. Soc.*, **14**, 542–548

Tokomitsu, T. (1971) Some aspects of cytogenetic effects of sodium cyclamate on human leukocytes in vitro. *Proc. Jpn. Acad.*, **47**, 635–639

Toledo, M.C.F. & Ioshi, S.H. (1995) Potential intake of intense sweeteners in Brazil. *Food Add. Contam.*, **12**, 799–808

Topham, J.C. (1980) Do induced sperm-head abnormalities in mice specifically identify mammalian mutagens rather than carcinogens? *Mutat. Res.*, **74**, 379–387

Turner, J.H. & Hutchinson, D.L. (1974) Cyclohexylamine mutagenicity: An in vivo evaluation utilizing fetal lambs. *Mutat. Res.*, **26**, 407–412

Van Went-de Vries, G.F., Freudenthal, J., Hogendoorn, A.M., Kragten, M.G.T. & Gramberg, L.G. (1975) In vivo chromosome damaging effect of cyclohexylamine in the Chinese hamster. *Food. Cosmet. Toxicol.*, **13**, 415–418

Vogel, E. & Chandler, J.L.R. (1974) Mutagenicity testing of cyclamate and some pesticides in Drosophila melanogaster. *Experientia*, **30**, 621–623

Ward, V.L. & Zeman, F.J. (1971) Distribution of ^{14}C-cyclamate in the lactating rat. *J. Nutr.*, **101**, 1635–1646

WHO (1993) *Guidelines for Drinking Water Quality*, 2nd Ed., Vol. 1, *Recommendations*, Geneva

Wilson, J.G. (1972) Use of primates in teratological investigations. In: Goldsmith, E.I. & Moor-Jankowski, J., eds, *Medical Primatology*, Basel, Karger, pp. 286–295

Wolff, S. (1983) Sister chromatid exchange as a test for mutagenic carcinogens. *Ann. N.Y. Acad. Sci.*, **407**, 142–153

Wu, C.K. & Smith, P. (1981) Calcium cyclamate induced lethal effect and genetic damage in spermatocytes of Drosophila. *Drosophila Info. Serv.*, **56**, 161–162

Wyrobek, A.J. & Bruce, W.R. (1975) Chemical induction of sperm abnormalities in mice. *Proc. natl Acad. Sci. USA*, **72**, 4425–4429

DICHLOROBENZENES

ortho- and *para*-Dichlorobenzenes were considered by previous working groups, in 1981 (IARC, 1982) and 1987 (IARC, 1987). Since that time, new data have become available, and these have been incorporated into the monograph and taken into consideration in the present evaluation.

1. Exposure Data

1.1 Chemical and physical data

1.1.1 *Nomenclature*

***ortho*-Dichlorobenzene**

Chem. Abstr. Serv. Reg. No.: 95-50-1
Chem. Abstr. Name: 1,2-Dichlorobenzene
IUPAC Systematic Name: *o*-Dichlorobenzene
Synonyms: *o*-Dichlorobenzol

***meta*-Dichlorobenzene**

Chem. Abstr. Serv. Reg. No.: 541-73-1
Chem. Abstr. Name: 1,3-Dichlorobenzene
IUPAC Systematic Name: *m*-Dichlorobenzene
Synonyms: *m*-Dichlorobenzol; *m*-phenylene dichloride

***para*-Dichlorobenzene**

Chem. Abstr. Serv. Reg. No.: 106-46-7
Chem. Abstr. Name: 1,4-Dichlorobenzene
IUPAC Systematic Name: *p*-Dichlorobenzene
Synonyms: *p*-Chlorophenyl chloride; paradichlorobenzene; PDB

1.1.2 *Structural and molecular formulae and relative molecular mass*

Cl Cl Cl Cl Cl Cl

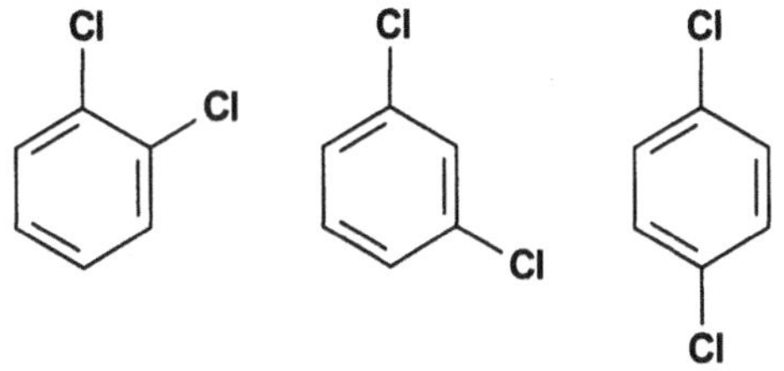

ortho *meta* *para*

$C_6H_4Cl_2$ Relative molecular mass: 147.01

1.1.3 *Chemical and physical properties of the pure substance*

***ortho*-Dichlorobenzene**

(*a*) *Description*: Colourless liquid (Verschueren, 1996)
(*b*) *Boiling-point*: 180°C (Lide, 1997)
(*c*) *Melting-point*: –16.7°C (Lide, 1997)
(*d*) *Density*: 1.3059 g/cm^3 at 20°C (Lide, 1997)
(*e*) *Spectroscopy data*: Infrared (prism [1003], grating [201]), ultraviolet [303] and nuclear magnetic resonance (proton [746], C-13 [1844]) spectral data have been reported (Sadtler Research Laboratories, 1980).
(*f*) *Solubility*: Insoluble in water; soluble in ethanol and diethyl ether; miscible in acetone (Lide, 1997)
(*g*) *Volatility*: Vapour pressure, 200 Pa at 25°C; relative vapour density (air = 1), 5.07 (Verschueren, 1996)
(*h*) *Octanol/water partition coefficient (P)*: log P, 3.43 (Hansch *et al*., 1995)
(*i*) *Conversion factor*: mg/m^3 = 6.01 × ppm

***meta*-Dichlorobenzene**

(*a*) *Description*: Colourless liquid (National Toxicology Program, 1991a)
(*b*) *Boiling-point*: 173°C (Lide, 1997)
(*c*) *Melting-point*: –24.8°C (Lide, 1997)
(*d*) *Density*: 1.2884 g/cm^3 at 20°C (Lide, 1997)
(*e*) *Spectroscopy data*: Infrared (prism [5934], grating [18109]), ultraviolet [1671] and nuclear magnetic resonance (proton [8596], C-13 [6235]) spectral data have been reported (Sadtler Research Laboratories, 1980).
(*f*) *Solubility*: Insoluble in water; soluble in ethanol and diethyl ether; miscible in acetone (Lide, 1997)
(*g*) *Volatility*: Vapour pressure, 665 Pa at 39°C; relative vapour density (air = 1), 5.08 (National Toxicology Program, 1991a)
(*h*) *Octanol/water partition coefficient (P)*: log P, 3.53 (Hansch *et al*., 1995)
(*i*) *Conversion factor*: mg/m^3 = 6.01 × ppm

***para*-Dichlorobenzene**

(*a*) *Description*: Volatile crystals with a characteristic penetrating odour (Budavari, 1996)
(*b*) *Boiling-point*: 174°C (Lide, 1997)
(*c*) *Melting-point*: 52.7°C (Lide, 1997)
(*d*) *Density*: 1.2475 g/cm^3 at 55°C (Lide, 1997)
(*e*) *Spectroscopy data*: Infrared (prism [146], grating [44]), ultraviolet [55] and nuclear magnetic resonance (proton [715], C-13 [37]) spectral data have been reported (Sadtler Research Laboratories, 1980).
(*f*) *Solubility*: Insoluble in water; soluble in diethyl ether; miscible in ethanol and acetone (Lide, 1997)

(*g*) *Volatility*: Vapour pressure, 80 Pa at 20°C; relative vapour density (air = 1), 5.07 (Verschueren, 1996)
(*h*) *Octanol/water partition coefficient (P)*: log P, 3.44 (Hansch *et al.*, 1995)
(*i*) *Conversion factor*: mg/m³ = 6.01 × ppm

1.1.4 *Technical products and impurities*

Industrial processes for the production of dichlorobenzenes give the *ortho*, *meta* and *para* isomers with varying amounts of the other isomers and of mono- and trichlorobenzenes. Technical-grade *ortho*-dichlorobenzene typically consists of 70–85% *ortho*-dichlorobenzene, < 0.05% chlorobenzene and < 0.5% trichlorobenzene, with the remainder as *meta*- and *para*-dichlorobenzene. Pure-grade *ortho*-dichlorobenzene consists of > 99.8% *ortho*-dichlorobenzene, < 0.05% chlorobenzene, < 0.1% trichlorobenzene and < 0.1% *para*-dichlorobenzene. Commercial-grade *meta*-dichlorobenzene typically consists of 85–99% *meta*-dichlorobenzene, < 0.01% chlorobenzene and < 0.1% *ortho*-dichlorobenzene, with the remainder as *para*-dichlorobenzene. Pure-grade *para*-dichlorobenzene consists of > 99.8% *para*-dichlorobenzene, < 0.05% chlorobenzene and trichlorobenzene and < 0.1% *ortho*- and *meta*-dichlorobenzene (Beck, 1986).

Trade names for *ortho*-dichlorobenzene include Cloroben, Dilatin DB and Dowtherm E. Trade names for *para*-dichlorobenzene include Di-chloricide, Dichlorocide, Evola, Paradi, Paradow, Paramoth, Persia-Perazol and Santochlor.

1.1.5 *Analysis*

Selected methods of analysis for dichlorobenzenes in various matrices are presented in Table 1.

1.2 Production and use

1.2.1 *Production*

Chlorobenzenes are prepared industrially by reaction of liquid benzene with gaseous chlorine in the presence of a catalyst at moderate temperature and atmospheric pressure. Hydrogen chloride is formed as a by-product. Generally, mixtures of isomers and compounds with varying degrees of chlorination are obtained. Lewis acids ($FeCl_3$, $AlCl_3$, $SbCl_3$, $MnCl_2$, $MoCl_3$, $SnCl_4$, $TiCl_4$) are the main catalysts used (Beck, 1986).

Dichlorobenzenes are formed in this process as isomeric mixtures with a low content of the 1,3-isomer. A maximum dichlorobenzene yield of 98% is obtainable in a batch process in which 2 mol of chlorine per mol of benzene are reacted in the presence of ferric chloride and sulfur monochloride at mild temperatures. The remainder of the product consists of mono- and trichlorobenzene. About 75% *para*-dichlorobenzene, 25% *ortho*-dichlorobenzene and only 0.2% *meta*-dichlorobenzene are obtained (Beck, 1986).

Only three chlorinated benzenes are currently produced in large volumes: monochlorobenzene, *ortho*-dichlorobenzene and *para*-dichlorobenzene. Total combined production of chlorobenzenes amounted to approximately 400 thousand tonnes in 1988, with 46% in the

Table 1. Selected methods for the analysis of dichlorobenzenes

Sample matrix	Sample preparation	Assay procedure	Limit of detection	Reference
Air	Adsorb on charcoal; desorb with carbon disulfide	GC/FID	0.01 mg/sample	Occupational Safety and Health Administration (1990) [Method 07]; Eller (1994) [Method 1003]
Air, water, soil, solid waste	Adsorb on particulate matter; filter; extract with dichloromethane; dry; concentrate (air); liquid–liquid or solid-phase extraction (water); Soxhlet, pressurized fluid, ultrasonic or supercritical fluid extraction (soil/sediment/waste)	GC/MS	10 μg/L (groundwater); 660 μg/kg (soil/sediment) [EQL]	Environmental Protection Agency (1996a) [Method 8270C]
Water	Extract (purge) with inert gas; trap on suitable sorbent; thermally desorb	GC/PID/ELCD GC/PID	0.01–0.02 μg/L (PID); 0.01–0.05 μg/L (ELCD) 0.006–0.02 μg/L (PID)	Environmental Protection Agency (1991, 1995a) [Methods 502.2 & 503.1]
	Extract (purge) with inert gas; trap on suitable sorbent; thermally desorb on capillary column	GC/MS	0.03–0.12 μg/L	Environmental Protection Agency (1995b) [Method 524.2]
Waste water, municipal, industrial	Extract (purge) with inert gas; trap on suitable sorbent; thermally desorb	GC/HSD GC/PID	0.15–0.32 μg/L 0.3–0.4 μg/L	Environmental Protection Agency (1997a,b) [Methods 601 & 602]
	Extract with dichloromethane; dry; exchange to hexane; concentrate	GC/ECD	1.14–1.34 μg/L	Environmental Protection Agency (1997c) [Method 612]
	Extract with dichloromethane; dry; concentrate	GC/MS	1.9–4.4 μg/L	Environmental Protection Agency (1997d) [Method 625]

Table 1 (contd)

Sample matrix	Sample preparation	Assay procedure	Limit of detection	Reference
Waste water, municipal, industrial (contd)	Add isotope-labelled analogue; extract with dichloromethane; dry over sodium sulfate; concentrate	GC/MS	10 μg/L	Environmental Protection Agency (1997e) [Method 1625B]
Solid waste matrices[a]	Extract (purge) with inert gas; trap on suitable sorbent; thermally desorb, sample headspace or inject directly	GC/PID/ELCD GC/MS	0.007–0.05 μg/L (PID); 0.01–0.02 μg/L (ELCD) 0.03–0.12 μg/L	Environmental Protection Agency (1996b,c) [Methods 8021B & 8260B]
Water, soil, waste	Extract with dichloromethane or dichloromethane:acetone (1:1); exchange to hexane	GC/ECD	0.27–0.89 μg/L	Environmental Protection Agency (1994a) [Method 8121]
Waste water, soil, sediment, solid waste	Liquid–liquid extraction (water); Soxhlet or ultrasonic extraction (soil/ sediment/ waste)	GC/FT-IR	25 μg/L	Environmental Protection Agency (1994b) [Method 8410]

Abbreviations: GC, gas chromatography; FID, flame ionization detection; MS, mass spectrometry; PID; photoionization detection; ELCD, electrolytic conductivity detection; HSD, halide-specific detection; ECD, electron capture detection; FT-IR, Fourier transform-infrared detection

[a] Samples include groundwater, aqueous sludges, caustic liquors, acid liquors, waste solvents, oily wastes, mousses, tars, fibrous wastes, polymeric emulsions, filter cakes, spent carbons, spent catalysts, soils and sediments.

United States, 34% in western Europe and 20% in Japan; monochlorobenzene accounted for over 50% of the total production of chlorinated benzenes (Bryant, 1993).

Production of *ortho*-dichlorobenzene in the United States has decreased since the 1970s, from approximately 24 700 tonnes in 1975 to approximately 15 800 tonnes in 1993 (International Trade Commission, 1993; Environmental Protection Agency, 1998a). Production of *meta*-dichlorobenzene in the Federal Republic of Germany in 1987 was 3000–4000 tonnes (German Chemical Society, 1987), while that in the United States in 1983 was less than 500 tonnes. Production of *para*-dichlorobenzene in the United States has increased since the 1980s, from approximately 6800 tonnes in 1981 to approximately 32 600 tonnes in 1993 (International Trade Commission, 1993; Environmental Protection Agency, 1998b).

Information available in 1995 indicated that *ortho*-dichlorobenzene was produced in 19 countries, that *meta*-dichlorobenzene was produced in four countries and that *para*-dichlorobenzene was produced in 17 countries (Chemical Information Services, 1995).

1.2.2 *Use*

In western Europe and the United States, *ortho*-dichlorobenzene is used mainly in the production of 3,4-dichloroaniline, the base material for several herbicides; in Japan it is used for garbage treatment (Bryant, 1993). The estimated pattern of use of *ortho*-dichlorobenzene in the United States in 1987 was: organic synthesis (mainly for herbicides), 90%; toluene diisocyanate processing solvent, 5%; and miscellaneous uses, 5% (Environmental Protection Agency, 1998a). *ortho*-Dichlorobenzene is also used as a solvent for waxes, gums, resins, tars, rubbers, oils and asphalts; as an insecticide for termites and locust borers; as a degreasing agent for metals, leather, paper, dry-cleaning, bricks, upholstery and wool; as an ingredient of metal polishes; in motor oil additive formulations; and in paints (National Toxicology Program, 1991b; Budavari, 1996; Environmental Protection Agency, 1998b).

meta-Dichlorobenzene has been used in the production of various herbicides and insecticides; it has also been used in the production of pharmaceuticals and dyes (Beck, 1986; German Chemical Society, 1987; National Toxicology Program, 1991a).

In the United States and Canada, *para*-dichlorobenzene is used mainly as an air freshener and a moth repellent (e.g. as 'moth balls' or 'moth crystals') and in a range of pesticidal applications. It is also used in the manufacture of 2,5-dichloroaniline and pharmaceuticals; in the manufacture of polyphenylene sulfide resins used for surface coatings and moulding resins; and to control mildew. In Japan, the pattern of use of *para*-dichlorobenzene is about 81% for moth control, 11% for polyphenylene sulfide resins and 8% for dyestuffs (Beck, 1986; National Toxicology Program, 1991c; Bryant, 1993; Budavari, 1996; Government of Canada, 1993a; Environmental Protection Agency, 1998b).

1.3 Occurrence

1.3.1 *Natural occurrence*

Dichlorobenzenes are not known to occur naturally.

1.3.2 *Occupational exposure*

***ortho*-Dichlorobenzene**

According to the 1981–83 United States National Occupational Exposure Survey (National Institute for Occupational Safety and Health, 1988), approximately 92 000 workers in the United States were potentially exposed to *ortho*-dichlorobenzene. Mechanics and persons working in textiles and dry-cleaning or laundering accounted for a large number of those potentially exposed. Occupational exposure to *ortho*-dichlorobenzene may occur by inhalation and eye or skin contact during its manufacture and its use as a chemical intermediate, as a deodorizing agent, as a fumigant, as a cleaner and degreaser, as a solvent for the application and removal of surface coatings, as a heat-transfer medium and in textile dyeing (National Institute for Occupational Safety and Health, 1978a).

In a study of three plants for the manufacture of chlorobenzene in the United States, personal concentrations of *ortho*-dichlorobenzene, a by-product, ranged from below the limit of detection to 13.7 mg/m^3 (Cohen *et al.*, 1981). Concentrations in a dye manufacture factory in Germany in which *ortho*-dichlorobenzene was used as a solvent ranged from 0.3 to 14 mg/m^3 (German Chemical Society, 1990). Kumagai and Matsunaga (1997a,b) measured 8-h time-weighted personal exposure concentrations of 0.1–2.3 ppm for 10 workers employed in a plant synthesizing intermediate products for dyes. The concentrations of 2,3- and 3,4-dichlorophenols and 3,4- and 4,5-dichlorocatechol in urine samples collected at the end of a shift correlated with the level of exposure to *ortho*-dichlorobenzene (correlation coefficient, 0.8–0.9). According to Zenser *et al.* (1997), *N*-acetyl-*S*-(dichlorophenyl)cysteines (also known as dichlorophenylmercapturic acids) are also suitable biomarkers for monitoring occupational exposure to *ortho*-dichlorobenzene (study on volunteers). The determination of 2,3- and 2,4-dichlorophenylmercapturic acids in urine was considered to be more suitable for monitoring exposure to *ortho*-dichorobenzene than 2,3- and 3,4-dichlorophenols or 3,4- and 4,5-dichlorocathecols, which are excreted as glucurono and sulfo conjugates and may thus not be hydrolysed efficiently during the analytical procedure.

***meta*-Dichlorobenzene**

No data were available to the Working Group.

***para*-Dichlorobenzene**

According to the 1981–83 United States National Occupational Exposure Survey (National Institute for Occupational Safety and Health, 1998), approximately 34 000 workers in the United States were potentially exposed to *para*-dichlorobenzene; most of these were janitors and cleaners, mortuary employees and workers in pest control. Occupational exposure to *para*-dichlorobenzene may occur by inhalation and ocular or dermal contact during its manufacture, formulation and use as an insecticide, a moth control agent, a fumigant, a deodorant and in organic syntheses for preparation of dye intermediates (National Institute for Occupational Safety and Health, 1978b).

Few data are available, especially on recent occupational exposure (Table 2). Unmodified *para*-dichlorobenzene and its metabolite 2,5-dichlorophenol have been found in the urine of exposed workers at the end of their shift and have been suggested for use as biological indicators of exposure (Pagnotto & Walkley, 1965; Ghittori *et al.*, 1985).

1.3.3 *Environmental occurrence*

Both *ortho*- and *para*-dichlorobenzenes are considered priority and/or hazardous pollutants in the United States by the Environmental Protection Agency (1979), in Canada (Meek *et al.*, 1994a,b,c) and in the European Communities (1976a,b; Bro-Rasmussen, 1994) and have been reported, generally at low parts per thousand million levels, in air, surface, ground-, drinking- and seawater, sediments, sludges, fish, birds' eggs, foods and human tissues (Environmental Protection Agency, 1980, 1985, 1988; German Chemical Society, 1990; WHO, 1991; Government of Canada, 1993a,b; Agency for Toxic Substances and Disease Registry, 1997). The level of human exposure to *ortho*- and *para*-dichlorobenzenes has been estimated from daily intake via multiple pathways (WHO, 1991; Meek *et al.*, 1994b,c).

The production and use of *ortho*-dichlorobenzene, primarily as a solvent and as an intermediate in organic synthesis, and the production and use of *para*-dichlorobenzene, primarily in a variety of consumer products (space deodorants, room fresheners, toilet deodorizer, general insecticide) and as an agricultural fumigant, are the main sources of their release to the environment from various waste streams. The *para* isomer is generally found at higher concentrations than the *ortho* isomer (Environmental Protection Agency, 1980, 1985, 1988; WHO, 1991; Agency for Toxic Substances Disease Registry, 1997).

(*a*) *Air*

According to the Toxic Release Inventory of the Environmental Protection Agency (1996d), emissions of *ortho*-dichlorobenzene to the air from 33 industrial facilities in the United States were 111 000 kg in 1994, and the estimated emissions of *para*-dichlorobenzene from 23 facilities were 117 000 kg.

The major sources of *ortho*-dichlorobenzene in the atmosphere have been reported to be solvent applications, which may account for 25% of annual releases to the atmosphere (Singh *et al.*, 1981; Oliver & Nicol, 1982; Harkov *et al.*, 1983; WHO, 1991; Agency for Toxic Subtances Disease Registry, 1997). *ortho*-Dichlorobenzene exists primarily in the vapour phase in the atmosphere.

The mean concentration of *ortho*-dichlorobenzene detected in air in Newark, NJ (United States), was 0.18 μg/m^3 in 29 of 38 samples; that in Elizabeth, NJ, was 0.12 μg/m^3 in 24 of 37 samples; and that in Camden, NJ, was 0.06 μg/m^3 in 27 of 35 samples during July–August 1981 (Harkov *et al.*, 1983). Ambient mean air concentrations of 0.24–5.2 μg/m^3 *ortho*-dichlorobenzene were detected above six abandoned hazardous waste sites in New Jersey (Harkov *et al.*, 1985). *ortho*-Dichlorobenzene was detected at concentrations of 0.09–0.66 μg/m^3 in ambient air in Bound Brook, NJ, during a one-day period in September 1978 (Krost *et al.*, 1982). Mean concentrations of 75, 136 and 24 μg/m^3

Table 2. Occupational exposure to *para*-dichlorobenzene

Activity	Air concentration (mg/m^3)		Type and duration of sampling	No. of samples	Reference
	Mean	Range			
Manufacturing plant			NR	NR	Pagnotto & Walkley (1965)
Washing	204	42–288			
Shovelling and centrifuging	198	60–294			
Crushing and sizing	144	48–276			
Household product packaging plant					
Pulverizing					
Moth cake line	150	108–204			
Dumping crystals	55	48–72			
Crystal line	54	42–60			
Abrasive wheel manufacturing plant	66	48–108			
Mixing					
Wheel-forming	69	48–87			
	48	42–54			
Monochlorobenzene manufacturing plant		30.7–52.1	Area and personal	3	Albrecht (1980)
Drumming *para*-dichlorobenzene					
Chemical factory	44.7[a]	25–78	Personal, 8-h[b]	20	Ghittori *et al.* (1985)
Toilet-block manufacturing plants		30–487	Personal, 1–3.5-h	13	Fairhurst *et al.* (1994)
Hardwood bleaching plant	0.15×10^{-3} median[c]	$(0.06–0.8) \times 10^{-3}$	Area	34	Rosenberg *et al.* (1991)

NR, not reported
[a] Geometric mean
[b] Time-weighted average
[c] 24 samples below detection limit

ortho-dichlorobenzene were detected in the ambient air of Los Angeles, CA, Phoenix, AZ, and Oakland, CA (United States), respectively, during July–August 1981 (Singh *et al.*, 1981).

The average 1-h concentrations of total isomeric dichlorobenzenes in 1980 were 0.36 μg/m³ (maximum, 7.3 μg/m³) in polluted parts of the Netherlands (Delft, Vlaardingen) and 0.18 μg/m³ (maximum, 2.0 μg/m³) on the island of Terschelling (Guicherit & Schulting, 1985).

The major sources of *para*-dichlorobenzene in the atmosphere are due to volatilization during its consumer or commercial use and from waste sites and emissions from waste incinerator facilities (Agency for Toxic Substances Disease Registry, 1997). In 1981, the mean ambient air concentrations of *para*-dichlorobenzene in three cities in New Jersey (United States) were 0.30 μg/m³ (detected in 32 of 38 samples) in Newark, 0.42 μg/m³ (30 of 37 samples) in Elizabeth and 0.24 μg/m³ (34 of 35 samples) in Camden during July–August (Harkov *et al.*, 1983).

Isomeric dichlorobenzenes have been found in emissions from municipal waste incinerator plants in Germany at concentrations of 0.02 μg/m³ *ortho*-dichlorobenzene, 0.51 μg/m³ *para*-dichlorobenzene and 0.21 μg/m³ *meta*-dichlorobenzene (Jay & Stieglitz, 1995).

Because of its extensive indoor use (i.e. room deodorants, air fresheners, moth repellants), *para*-dichlorobenzene is often found at higher concentrations in indoor than ambient outdoor air (Barkley *et al.*, 1980; Wallace *et al.*, 1984; Pellizzari *et al.*, 1986; Wallace *et al.*, 1987; Wallace, 1991a; Fellin & Otson, 1994; Kostianinen, 1995). In a comparison of indoor and outdoor residential air concentrations of volatile organic chemicals in five areas in the United States (Greensboro, NC; Baton Rouge/Geismar, LA; Deer Park/Pasadena, TX; Elizabeth/Bayonne, NJ; Antioch/W. Pittsburg, CA), the medians and maximum indoor levels were generally higher than the corresponding outdoor concentrations for mixtures of *meta*- and *para*-dichlorobenzenes and *para*-dichlorobenzene alone and to a much lesser extent for *ortho*-dichlorobenzene. In some cases, the median indoor:outdoor ratios were greater than 10 (Pellizzari *et al.*, 1986).

Moth crystals and room deodorizers are important sources of *para*-dichlorobenzene in homes. In the Total Exposure Assessment Methodology (TEAM) Study carried out by the Environmental Protection Agency between 1979 and 1985, personal exposures to toxic substances were estimated for 400 residents of the states of New Jersey, North Carolina and North Dakota (United States). The mean 24-h personal air and breath concentrations were consistently higher than the outdoor air concentrations for 10 compounds including *para*-dichlorobenzene (Wallace *et al.*, 1987). In another comparison, the outdoor air concentration of 0.6 μg/m³ found in the backyards of 175 homes in six urban areas in the United States was much lower than the mean 24-h average exposure (22 μg/m³) of 750 persons living in these homes. In about one-third of the homes, *para*-dichlorobenzene was used for moth control or as a deodorizer (Wallace, 1991a).

Three large studies of volatile organic compounds, involving more than 100 homes each have been carried out in Germany, the Netherlands and the United States. The arithmetic mean concentrations of *para*-dichlorobenzene in indoor air were 14 μg/m³ in Germany and 25 μg/m³ in the United States, and the median found in the Netherlands was 1 μg/m³; the maximum levels found were 1260 μg/m³ in Germany, 299 μg/m³ in the Netherlands and 1600 μg/m³ in the United States (Wallace, 1991b).

In a nationwide study of the indoor air concentrations of 26 volatile compounds in Canada in 1991, the mean *para*-dichlorobenzene concentrations were 36 μg/m³ in winter, 15 μg/m³ in spring, 11 μg/m³ in summer and 15 μg/m³ in autumn; the concentrations declined with increasing ambient air temperature. Indoor sources of *para*-dichlorobenzene (household products and moth-repellant crystal) were judged to have a greater influence on indoor air concentration than climatic variables (Fellin & Otson, 1994).

The concentration of total dichlorobenzenes in the ambient air of household basements near industrial and chemical waste disposal sites in the Love Canal area of New York State (United States) were 2.3–190 μg/m³ (Pellizzari, 1982). The concentrations of dichlorobenzenes in ambient air outside this area ranged from traces to 0.44 μg/m³ (Barkley *et al.*, 1980).

(*b*) *Water and sediments*

(i) *Surface water*

The isomeric dichlorobenzenes are generally considered to persist in the aquatic environment, since they are not readily biodegraded, hydrolysed or photodegraded (WHO, 1991; Agency for Toxic Substances Disease Registry, 1997). According to the National Library of Medicine (1998) Toxic Chemicals Release Inventory, in 1994 1277 kg of *ortho*-dichlorobenzene were released to surface waters from 33 facilities in the United States and 723 kg of *para*-dichlorobenzene were released from 23 facilities.

ortho-Dichlorobenzene was detected in 15 of 463 bodies of surface water in New Jersey, United States, during 1977–79, 8.2 μg/L being the highest concentration found (Page, 1981). In 1980, mean concentrations of 5 ng/L (range, 2–7 ng/L) and 45 ng/L (range, 33–64 ng/L) *ortho*- and *para*-dichlorobenzenes, respectively, were found in open waters at five locations in Lake Ontario, Canada. Mean concentrations of 4 ng/L (range, 3–6 ng/L) *para*-dichlorobenzene were found at five open water locations in Lake Huron. Ten monitoring stations on Grand River, Canada (the largest tributary of the Canadian Great Lakes), registered mean concentrations of 6 ng/L (range, not detected–31 ng/L) *ortho*-dichlorobenzene and 10 ng/L (range, not detected–42 ng/L) *para*-dichlorobenzene. These concentrations were highest below cities from which treated sewage was discharged into the River, and dissipated further downstream (Oliver & Nicol, 1982).

The concentrations of dichlorobenzene in the Niagara River at four sites near Niagara Falls, New York (United States), ranged from not detected to 56 ng/L for *ortho*-dichlorobenzene and from 1 to 94 ng/L for *para*-dichlorobenzene. The effluents and raw sewage of four activated sludge waste-water treatment plants in Canada, two discharging into Lake Ontario and two into the Grand River, contained mean concentrations of 13 ng/L (range, 6–22 ng/L) *ortho*-dichlorobenzene and 600 ng/L (range, 484–920 ng/L) *para*-dichlorobenzene (Oliver & Nicol, 1982).

The approximate input from the Niagara River to Lake Ontario (North America) was estimated to be 2000 kg each of *ortho*- and *para*-dichlorobenzenes on the basis of measurements between September 1981 and September 1983 (Oliver & Nicol, 1984).

ortho-Dichlorobenzene was detected in industrial effluents from 2.5% of 1311 sites and in 0.6% of ambient water samples at 1077 sites in the United States, in both cases at a median concentration < 10 g/L. *para*-Dichlorobenzene was found in industrial effluents from 1.7% of 1306 sites and in 3% of ambient water samples from 8575 sites, at a median concentration < 0.1 μg/L (Staples et al., 1985).

Sewage effluents are believed to be the most important source of *para*-dichlorobenzene in Lake Zurich, Switzerland, and the total annual amount discharged to the central basin from treatment plants was estimated to be 62 kg (Schwarzenbach *et al.*, 1979). Volatilization was found to be the predominant mechanism of elimination of *para*-dichlorobenzene from Lake Zurich in one-year monitoring studies, and the average residence time for this isomer was approximately five months.

(ii) *Drinking-water*

para-Dichlorobenzene is the main dichlorobenzene found in drinking-water, probably resulting from its release into surface waters after its extensive use in urinal deodorant blocks (Oliver & Nicol, 1982; WHO, 1991).

In a survey of the groundwater supply in the United States in 1980, *ortho*-dichlorobenzene was found at concentrations of 2.2 and 2.7 μg/L in two of 945 finished water supplies (Westrick *et al.*, 1984), and *para*-dichlorobenzene was found at mean concentrations of 0.60–0.74 μg/L in nine of these supplies (Westrick, 1990).

para-Dichlorobenzene was detected in five of 29 raw and treated (day 1) potable water supplies of Canadian municipalities at concentrations < 1 μg/L but was not detected after the second day of treatment during August-September 1979 and was not detected in raw or treated potable water during November–December 1979 (Otson *et al.*, 1982a,b).

Drinking-water samples collected from three cities in the Lake Ontario, Canada, area in 1980 contained mean concentrations of 3 μg/L (range, not detected–7 μg/L) *ortho*-dichlorobenzene and 13 μg/L (range, 8–20 μg/L) *para*-dichlorobenzene (Oliver & Nicol, 1982).

(iii) *Leachates and sediments*

The isomeric dichlorobenzenes were monitored in wetland-treated leachate water at a municipal solid-waste landfill site in central Florida (United States) in 1989–90 and 1992–93. During the first sampling period, *para*-dichlorobenzene was detected in surface water samples at 0.04–0.13 μg/L and in groundwater samples at 0.08–11 μg/L. During the second sampling period, *para*-dichlorobenzene was not detected in surface water and was found at concentrations of 0.45 and 3.7 μg/L in two of the four groundwater samples (Chen & Zoltek, 1995).

In Canada, the mean *ortho*-dichlorobenzene concentrations found in surface sediments in 1980 were 1 μg/mL from 13 sites at Lake Superior, 8 μg/L from 42 sites at Lake Huron,

2 µg/L from five sites at Lake Erie and 11 µg/L from 11 sites at Lake Ontario. The mean *para*-dichlorobenzene concentrations at these sites were 5 µg/L at Lake Superior, 16 µg/L at Lake Huron, 9 µg/L at Lake Erie and 94 µg/L at Lake Ontario. The major source of the chlorobenzenes appeared to be leachates from chemical waste dumps and direct chemical manufacturing effluents. *ortho*- and *para*-Dichlorobenzene were found at mean concentrations of 2–19 µg/kg and 17–230 µg/kg, respectively, in seven Lake Ontario sediment cores (0–7 cm in depth) from the Niagara Basin between 1932–41 and 1976–80, indicating that contamination of the Lake had begun over 40 years earlier (Oliver & Nicol, 1982).

(*c*) *Soil and sludges*

The concentrations of dichlorobenzenes in contemporary sewage sludges vary significantly according to waste-water source, sludge type and treatment technique as well as temporally and spatially (Rogers *et al.*, 1989; Wang *et al.*, 1992). Municipal sludge is often applied to agricultural land in Canada, the United Kingdom and the United States (Jacobs & Zabik, 1983; Webber & Lesage, 1989; Wang *et al.*, 1992; Rogers, 1996). In an analysis of 12 industrial sludges in the United Kingdom, *ortho*-dichlorobenzene was found at concentrations (dry weight) of not detected to 14 mg/kg (median, 7.9 mg/kg) and *para*-dichlorobenzene at not detected to 34 mg/kg (median, 9.8 mg/kg) (Rogers *et al.*, 1989).

In a survey of 215 sewage sludges in the United States, the concentration ranges (dry weight) were 0.02–810 mg/kg *ortho*-dichlorobenzene and 0.04–630 mg/kg *para*-dichlorobenzene (Jacobs & Zabik, 1983; Rogers, 1996).

ortho-Dichlorobenzene was found in nine Canadian municipal sludges and sludge composts at levels ranging from 0.03 to 0.32 mg/kg between September 1993 and February 1994. During the same period, *para*-dichlorobenzene was found in 11 Canadian sludge samples at levels ranging from 0.26 to 2.6 mg/kg dry weight (Webber *et al.*, 1996).

The principal sources of *para*-dichlorobenzene on land are disposal of industrial waste in landfills, application of sewage sludge containing *para*-dichlorobenzene to agricultural land and atmospheric deposition (Webber & Lesage, 1989; Wang *et al.*, 1992, 1995; Webber *et al.*, 1996). In the United Kingdom, *para*-dichlorobenzene was found at increasing concentrations in sewage sludge samples stored from 1942 to 1961. It was detected in 100% of the sludge samples at concentrations of 7.8–72 µg/kg (median, 26 µg/kg; mean, 30 µg/kg) (Wang *et al.*, 1995).

In 1994, industrial releases of *ortho*-dichlorobenzene to the land from 33 facilities in the United States amounted to 11 000 kg, and those of *para*-dichlorobenzene were 500 kg (National Library of Medicine, 1998).

(*d*) *Food*

Dichlorobenzenes may be present as contaminants in foods, although little information is available. *para*-Dichlorobenzene has been found in a variety of Canadian foods, including some samples of soft drinks (0.1 µg/kg), butter (1.3–2.7 µg/kg), margarine (12.2–14.5 µg/kg), peanut butter (1.2–8.8 µg/kg), flour (7.3 µg/kg) and pastry mix (22 µg/kg) (Page & Lacroix, 1995).

para-Dichlorobenzene was detected at a concentration of 0.55 ng/kg in cows' milk from Ontario, Canada, but not in four other composites analysed, i.e. leafy vegetables, fruits, root vegetables and eggs/meat. *ortho*-Dichlorobenzene was detected at a level of 1.8 ng/kg in food composites containing eggs or meat but was not found (limit of detection, 0.1 ng/kg) in leafy vegetables, fruits, root vegetables (including potatoes) or milk (Davies, 1988).

ortho-Dichlorobenzene was found at concentrations of 0.3, 1, 1 and 1 µg/kg in trout taken from Lakes Superior, Huron, Erie and Ontario (Canada), respectively, during 1980 (Oliver & Nicol, 1982).

The mean concentrations of *ortho*-dichlorobenzene found in samples of cows' milk and beef from markets in Yugoslavia were 2.6 and 1.0 µg/kg, respectively, and the mean concentrations of *para*-dichlorobenzene were 5.3 and 5.0 µg/kg, respectively (Jan, 1983a).

In an isolated incident in England, tainted pork (lean and fat meat) contained 5–20 mg/kg *para*-dichlorobenzene. This isomer was also present in other batches of pork from the same source. Other meat products from various commercial sources contained concentrations of < 10 µg/kg during the period 1979–81 (Watson & Patterson, 1982).

para-Dichlorobenzene was detected in Yugoslavia in the oils of seeds from corn, soya bean, rape, sunflower, peanut, sesame, walnut, hazelnut and poppy, the highest level (0.90 µg/kg) being found in corn (Jan, 1980).

(*e*) *Human tissues and secretions*

In a national Canadian survey, *ortho*-dichlorobenzene was found at a maximum concentration of 29 µg/kg (mean, 3 µg/kg) in breast milk (three to four weeks after parturition) and 890 µg/kg in milk fat (mean, 84 µg/kg). The mean concentration of *meta*- and *para*-dichlorobenzenes (combined) in whole breast milk was 6.0 µg/kg, and that in milk fat was 160 µg/kg (Mes *et al.*, 1986).

ortho-Dichlorobenzene was found at an average concentration of 9 µg/kg (range, 5–12 µg/kg) in 12 samples of human whole milk in Yugoslavia. The corresponding average concentration of *para*-dichlorobenzene was 25 µg/kg (range, 5–35 µg/kg). Mean concentrations of 13 µg/kg *ortho*-dichlorobenzene and 140 µg/kg *para*-dichlorobenzene were found in 15 samples of human adipose tissue in Yugoslavia (Jan, 1983b).

ortho-Dichlorobenzene (1–4 µg/L), *meta*-dichlorobenzene (3–8 µg/L) and *para*-dichlorobenzene (26 µg/L) were found in samples of blood from residents of the Love Canal area in Niagara Falls, New York (United States) (Bristol *et al.*, 1982).

Median *para*-dichlorobenzene concentrations of 1.3, 1.3 and 1.2 µg/m^3 were found in the autumn of 1981, the summer of 1982 and the winter of 1983, respectively, in 344 breath samples from individuals in New Jersey (United States) who were participating in the United States Environmental Protection Agency TEAM Study in 1979–85. Median *para*-dichlorobenzene levels of 1.2 µg/m^3 and 0.82 µg/m^3 were found in 33 and 23 breath samples from individuals from Greensboro, NC, and Devils Lake, ND, respectively (Wallace *et al.*, 1987).

In a study of 1000 adults in the United States, 96% had detectable concentrations of *para*-dichlorobenzene in their blood (≤ 49 μg/L; median, 0.33 μg/L; mean, 2.1 μg/L). Additionally, 98% of these adults had detectable levels of 2,5-dichlorophenol, a metabolite of *para*-dichlorobenzene, in their urine (Hill *et al.*, 1995).

1.4 Regulations and guidelines

Occupational exposure limits and guidelines for dichlorobenzenes in a number of countries are presented in Table 3.

WHO (1993) has established international drinking-water guidelines of 1 mg/L for *ortho*-dichlorobenzene and 300 mg/L for *para*-dichlorobenzene. Canada has recommended a maximum acceptable concentration (MAC) for *ortho*-dichlorobenzene in drinking-water of 0.2 mg/L (0.005 mg/L for *para*-dichlorobenzene) and an odour/taste threshold concentration of ≤ 0.003 mg/L (0.001 mg/L for *para*-dichlorobenzene). The Czech Republic has set MACs for dichlorobenzenes combined of 300 ng/L in drinking-water and 0.001 mg/L in surface water. Germany has set an air emission standard maximum for *ortho*-dichlorobenzene of 20 mg/m³ at a mass flow ≥ 0.1 kg/h (100 mg/m³ at a mass flow ≥ 2 kg/h for *para*-dichlorobenzene). The maximum residue limit of *para*-dichlorobenzene in all food products in Germany is 0.01 mg/kg. The Russian Federation has set a preliminary exposure standard for *ortho*-dichlorobenzene in ambient air of 0.03 mg/m³ (0.035 mg/m³ for *meta*- and *para*-dichlorobenzene) and a MAC in surface water of 0.002 mg/L [all isomers] (United Nations Environment Programme, 1998). The Environmental Protection Agency (1998a,b) in the United States has set maximum contaminant levels of 0.6 mg/L for *ortho*-dichlorobenzene and 0.075 mg/L for *para*-dichlorobenzene in primary drinking-water. The European Union has set a standard of 12 mg/kg for the concentration of *para*-dichlorobenzene that can migrate from plastics and articles intended to come in contact with foodstuffs. Sweden has banned the use and handling of *para*-dichlorobenzene as a pesticide on the basis of its suspected carcinogenicity (United Nations Environment Programme, 1998).

Separate regulations and guidelines have not been established for *meta*-dichlorobenzene (WHO, 1993; United Nations Environment Programme, 1998).

2. Studies of Cancer in Humans

2.1 Case reports

One report of a series of five cases suggested an association between leukaemia and exposure to dichlorobenzenes (IARC, 1982).

2.2 Cohort study

Mortality from cancer was studied among 14 457 workers exposed to a large number of organic solvents and other chemicals, including *ortho*-dichlorobenzene, during employment in one aircraft maintenance facility in the United States (Spirtas *et al.*, 1991). In

Table 3. Occupational exposure limits for dichlorobenzenes

Country	Year	Concentration (mg/m^3)		Interpretation
		ortho isomer	*para* isomer	
Argentina	1991	300	450	TWA
Australia	1993	300	450	TWA
			675	STEL
Austria	1993	300		TWA
Belgium	1993		451	TWA
		301 (skin)	661	STEL
Canada	1994	300 (ceiling)	450	TWA
			675	STEL
Denmark	1993		450	TWA
		300		STEL
Finland	1998	300 (skin)	450 (skin)	TWA
		450	690	STEL
France	1993		450	TWA
		300	675	STEL
Germany	1997	300 (skin)	300 (skin)	TWA
Hungary	1993	50 (skin)		TWA
		100		STEL
Ireland	1997		150	TWA
		300	300	STEL
Japan	1996	150	300 (Ca)	TWA
Netherlands	1997	150	150	TWA
		300	300	STEL
Philippines	1993	300	450	TWA
Poland	1993	20	20	TWA
Russian Federation	1993		300	TWA
		50		STEL
Sweden	1993		450	TWA
		300	700	STEL
Switzerland	1993	300	450	TWA
		600	900	STEL
Thailand	1993	300		TWA
Turkey	1993	300	450	TWA
United Kingdom	1997		153	TWA
		300	306	STEL

Table 3 (contd)

Country	Year	Concentration (mg/m^3)		Interpretation
		ortho isomer	*para* isomer	
United States				
OSHA (PEL)	1997	300	450	Ceiling
NIOSH (REL)	1994	300	lfc	Ceiling
ACGIH (TLV)[a]	1997	150 (A4)	60 (A3)	TWA
		301 (A4)		STEL

From International Labour Office (1991); American Conference of Governmental Industrial Hygienists (1997, 1998); National Library of Medicine (1998); United Nations Environment Programme (1998)
TWA, time-weighted average; STEL, short-term exposure limit; A3, animal carcinogen; A4, not classifiable as a human carcinogen; Ca, carcinogen designation; lfc, lowest feasible concentration; PEL, permissible exposure limit; REL, recommended exposure limit; skin, potential dermal absorption; TLV, threshold limit value
[a] The following countries follow the exposure limits suggested by the ACGIH: Bulgaria, Colombia, Jordan, Republic of Korea, New Zealand, Singapore and Viet Nam.

comparison with the general male population, the rate of mortality from any cancer in the cohort was slightly reduced (standardized mortality ratio, 0.90; 95% confidence interval, 0.8–1.0). The only cancers evaluated in a subgroup of workers with estimated exposure to *ortho*-dichlorobenzene [size of the subgroup not given] were multiple myeloma, from which no deaths occurred, and non-Hodgkin lymphoma, from which one death occurred among men and one among women with 1.4 and 0.5 expected, respectively.

3. Studies of Cancer in Experimental Animals

3.1 Oral administration

3.1.1 ortho-*Dichlorobenzene*

Mouse: Groups of 50 male and 50 female B6C3F$_1$ mice, seven weeks of age, were given *ortho*-dichlorobenzene (purity, > 99%) by oral gavage in corn oil at doses of 0, 60 or 120 mg/kg bw on five days per week for 103 weeks. The body-weight gain of treated mice was not decreased when compared with controls. No significant difference in survival was observed between groups or between sexes; the rates ranged from 52% in control males to 70% in those at the high dose and from 66% in control females to 80% in those at the low dose. *ortho*-Dichlorobenzene did not increase the incidence of tumours in mice of either sex (National Toxicology Program, 1985).

Rat: Groups of 50 male and 50 female Fischer 344/N rats, seven weeks of age, were given *ortho*-dichlorobenzene by oral gavage in corn oil at doses of 0, 60 or 120 mg/kg bw on five days per week for 103 weeks. The body-weight gain of treated males was reduced in comparison with controls. The survival of males at the high dose (38%) was significantly reduced when compared with controls (84%; $p < 0.001$) and those at the low dose (72%; $p = 0.014$). The survival rates of female rats ranged from 62% in controls to 66% at the low dose. *ortho*-Dichlorobenzene did not increase the incidence of tumours in either male or female rats (National Toxicology Program, 1985).

3.1.2 meta-*Dichlorobenzene*

No data were available to the Working Group.

3.1.3 para-*Dichlorobenzene*

Mouse: Groups of 50 male and 50 female B6C3F$_1$ mice, eight weeks of age, were given *para*-dichlorobenzene (purity, > 99%) by oral gavage in corn oil at doses of 0, 300 or 600 mg/kg bw on five days per week for 103 weeks. There was no significant difference in survival between groups or sexes; the survival rates at termination ranged from 56 to 64% in male groups and 70 to 72% in female groups. As shown in Table 4, *para*-dichlorobenzene increased the incidences of hepatocellular tumours (adenomas and carcinomas) in both male and female mice. The incidence rates of liver tumours, adjusted for survival, were 43% in controls, 58% at 300 mg/kg bw and 100% at 600 mg/kg bw in males and 39, 26 and 90% in females, respectively. A marginal increase in the incidence of phaeochromocytomas of the adrenal gland was seen in male mice, but the incidence was within the historical control range for that laboratory (National Toxicology Program, 1987).

Rat: Groups of 50 male and 50 female Fischer 344/N rats, seven weeks of age, were given *para*-dichlorobenzene (purity, > 99%) by oral gavage in corn oil at doses of 0, 150 or 300 mg/kg bw for male rats and 0, 300 or 600 mg/kg bw for female rats on five days per week for 103 weeks. The survival rate of the high-dose males was significantly lower

Table 4. Incidences of primary hepatocellular tumours in B6C3F$_1$ mice exposed by oral administration to *para*-dichlorobenzene

Tumour	Animals with tumours					
	Males			Females		
	Control	300 mg/kg bw	600 mg/kg bw	Control	300 mg/kg bw	600 mg/kg bw
Adenoma	5/50	13/49 ($p = 0.035$)	16/50 ($p = 0.015$)	10/50	6/48	21/50 ($p = 0.012$)
Carcinoma	14/50	11/49	32/50 ($p < 0.001$)	5/50	5/48	19/50 ($p < 0.001$)

From National Toxicology Program (1987)

(40%) than that of the control males (64%) at study termination, but no significant difference in survival was observed between female groups, the rates ranging from 58% at the high dose to 70% in controls and 78% at the low dose. *para*-Dichlorobenzene increased the incidence of renal tubular carcinoma in males at the high dose (control, 1/50; low-dose, 3/50; high-dose, 7/50; $p = 0.03$, Fisher's exact test) but not in females. The incidence rates of kidney carcinomas in male rats (adjusted for survival) were 3.1% in controls, 9.2% at 150 mg/kg bw and 26% at 300 mg/kg bw (National Toxicology Program, 1987).

3.2 Inhalation

Mouse: Groups of 75 male and 75 female Alderley Park SPF mice [age unspecified] were exposed by inhalation to *para*-dichlorobenzene vapour at concentrations of 0, 75 or 500 ppm [0, 45 and 3000 mg/m^3] in air for 57 weeks. The male mice were killed after week 57 since their mortality rate due to fighting and respiratory infection approached 80%. The surviving females were killed at weeks 75–76, i.e. 18–19 weeks after cessation of exposure. The tumour incidence was thus based on 64, 63 and 67% surviving females at 0, 75 and 500 ppm, respectively. Under these conditions, *para*-dichlorobenzene did not increase the tumour incidence (Loeser & Litchfield, 1983). [The Working Group noted the inadequacy of the study due to the short duration and the poor survival.]

Rat: Groups of 76–79 male and female Alderley Park Wistar-derived SPF rats [age unspecified] were exposed by inhalation to *para*-dichlorobenzene vapour at concentrations of 0, 75 or 500 ppm [0, 45 and 3000 mg/m^3] in air for 5 h per day, on five days per week for 76 weeks. Surviving rats were given control air for up to 36 weeks after cessation of exposure. Under these conditions *para*-dichlorobenzene did not increase the tumour incidence (Loeser & Litchfield, 1983). [The Working Group noted the inadequacy of the study due to the short duration of exposure.]

3.3 Administration with known carcinogens

Rat: In a model of liver carcinogenesis, groups of 12 (vehicle control) or 18 male Fischer 344 rats, 10 weeks of age, received a single intraperitoneal injection of either 200 mg/kg bw *N*-nitrosodiethylamine (NDEA) dissolved in 0.9% saline or saline alone. Two weeks after the NDEA or saline injection, *para*-dichlorobenzene [purity unspecified] was administered by gavage at doses of 0.1 or 0.4 mmol/kg bw per day in corn oil for six weeks; control groups received only corn oil or NDEA in corn oil. One week after the start of *para*-dichlorobenzene treatment (i.e. week 3), all animals underwent a partial hepatectomy. The study was terminated at the end of week 8. Hepatic foci were identified by immunohistochemical staining for the placental form of glutathione *S*-transferase. The incidence of hepatic foci was not increased, and the authors concluded that *para*-dichlorobenzene is not a liver tumour promoter (Gustafson *et al.*, 1998).

4. Other Data Relevant to an Evaluation of Carcinogenicity and its Mechanisms

4.1 Absorption, distribution, metabolism and excretion

4.1.1 *Humans*

2,5-Dichlorophenol has been detected in the urine of persons exposed to *para*-dichlorobenzene (Hill *et al.*, 1995). Studies of the occurrence of dichlorobenzenes in human tissues and secretions are described on pp. 236–237.

4.1.2 *Experimental systems*

(*a*) ortho-*Dichlorobenzene*

After oral administration to rabbits (500 mg/kg bw), *ortho*-dichlorobenzene is metabolized mainly to 3,4-dichlorophenol, but 2,3-dichlorophenol, 3,4-dichlorophenylmercapturic acid and 3,4- and 4,5-dichlorocatechol are also formed (Azouz *et al.*, 1955).

The relationship between the metabolism and the toxicity of *ortho*-dichlorobenzene was investigated by evaluating its biotransformation, tissue distribution, blood kinetics and excretion after oral administration of 5, 50 or 250 mg/kg bw to male Wistar rats. The dose of 250 mg/kg bw had been demonstrated to be toxic in previous studies. The major route of elimination of *ortho*-dichlorobenzene (75–85%) was via the kidneys; excretion in the faeces represented 19% of the low dose and 7% of the high dose. Excretion was nearly complete within 24 h after the low and intermediate doses and within 48 h after the high dose. Pretreatment with phenobarbital accelerated excretion of the high dose and resulted in an overall higher proportion of urinary excretion. Biliary excretion constituted 50–60% of the dose, indicating significant enterohepatic recirculation. The highest concentrations of radiolabel after a low dose were found in fat, liver and kidney 6 h after administration; these then declined rapidly. The maximal concentration in blood was reached 6–8 h after administration of the low and intermediate doses and 24 h after the high dose. *ortho*-Dichlorobenzene was detected in blood only during the first 2 h after administration of 5 mg/kg bw. The major route of biotransformation was via the glutathione pathway, 60% of the urinary metabolites being mercapturic acids; the major metabolites in bile were also conjugates of glutathione. Other major metabolites in urine were the sulfate conjugates of 2,3- and 3,4-dichlorophenol. No significant differences in metabolic profiles were observed with dose. Induction with phenobarbital increased excretion of sulfate conjugates (30% in induced rats, 20% in control rats), the main one being the conjugate of 3,4-dichlorophenol. The mercapturic acids in urine and the glutathione conjugates in bile were epoxide-derived metabolites, and no quinone- or hydroquinone-derived metabolites were observed. A high dose of *ortho*-dichlorobenzene results in depletion of glutathione, followed by oxidative stress and possibly binding to macromolecules (Hissink *et al.*, 1996a).

The oxidative biotransformation of *ortho*-dichlorobenzene was investigated in hepatic microsomes from male Wistar, Fischer 344 and Sprague-Dawley rats, phenobarbital- and isoniazid-treated male Wistar rats and humans; in addition, microsomes from cell lines that selectively express cytochrome P450 (CYP) 2E1, 1A1, 1A2, 2B6, 2C9, 2D6, 2A6 or 3A4 were used. The rate of conversion was 0.09 nmol/min per mg protein in both Wistar and Fischer 344 rat microsomes, 0.04 in Sprague-Dawley microsomes and 0.14 in human microsomes. Induction of Wistar rats with isoniazid, a CYP 2E1 inducer, or phenobarbital, a CYP 2B1/2 inducer, resulted in increased conversion rates of 0.20 and 0.42 nmol/min per mg protein, respectively. Covalent binding of radiolabel to microsomal proteins was similar in Wistar, Fischer and isoniazid-treated Wistar rats (16–17% of total metabolites), whereas induction with phenobarbital resulted in a slightly increased covalent binding rate of 23% of total metabolites. The covalent binding rate was 31% in Sprague-Dawley microsomes but only 4.6% in human microsomes. Ascorbic acid reduced covalent binding only in Sprague-Dawley microsomes, indicating that quinones are probably major contributors to macromolecular binding in these microsomes. Conjugation of epoxides with glutathione inhibited most covalent binding in all microsomes. In the absence of glutathione, the epoxides were hydrolysed by epoxide hydrolase to dihydrodiols, and inhibition of epoxide hydrolase increased the covalent binding for all microsomes tested, indicating a role of epoxides in the covalent binding. The finding that Fischer 344 rat liver microsomes had less epoxide hydrolase activity than microsomes from Wistar and Sprague-Dawley rats may explain the greater sensitivity of rats of this strain to the hepatotoxicity of *ortho*-dichlorobenzene *in vivo*. Conjugation of the epoxides with glutathione was predominantly non-enzymatic in rats, whereas in humans conjugation was catalysed almost exclusively by glutathione *S*-transferases. This difference may be due to formation of a 'non-reactive' 3,4-epoxide by CYP 2E1 in human microsomes: incubation with microsomes that selectively express human CYP 2E1 or with human liver microsomes resulted in the formation of similar amounts of 2,3- and 3,4-dichlorophenol and two glutathione–epoxides in equal amounts. In rat microsomes, one major glutathione–epoxide conjugate was found, with a much higher covalent binding index, particularly for the phenobarbital-induced microsomes. The authors suggested that rat CYP 2B1/2 preferentially oxidizes the 4,5 site of *ortho*-dichlorobenzene, while human CYP 2E1 forms predominantly the 'non-reactive' 3,4-epoxide. They concluded that the risk for liver toxicity due to exposure to 1,2-dichlorobenzene will be overestimated when it is based solely on toxicity in rats (Hissink *et al.*, 1996b).

2,3- and 3,4-Dichlorophenyl methyl sulfoxides (2,3- and 3,4-sulfoxides) and 2,3- and 3,4-dichlorophenyl methyl sulfones (2,3- and 3,4-sulfones) were detected in the urine of rats given *ortho*-dichlorobenzene. After administration, swift decreases were observed in the concentrations of *ortho*-dichlorobenzene in blood, liver and kidneys, whereas 3,4-sulfone appeared in blood, liver, kidneys and adipose tissue. The concentrations of 3,4-sulfone in the blood and three tissues reached maxima at 24 h. The activities of aminopyrine *N*-demethylase and aniline hydroxylase and the cytochrome P450 content of hepatic microsomes decreased 24 h after administration of *ortho*-dichlorobenzene. In contrast, the 3,4-sulfone increased the activities of these enzymes and the cytochrome P450 and b_5 contents of rat liver microsomes. The concentrations of 2,3- and 3,4-sulfones in blood, liver, kidneys and adipose tissue were dramatically reduced in both antibiotic-pretreated and bile duct-cannulated rats dosed with *ortho*-dichlorobenzene, suggesting that the process of formation of methylsulfonyl metabolites of *ortho*-dichlorobenzene involves biliary secretion of the sulfones and/or their precursors, which are subjected to metabolism by intestinal microflora. In antibiotic-pretreated rats, the inhibitory effects of administration of *ortho*-dichlorobenzene on the activities of aminopyrine- and aniline-metabolizing enzymes and the contents of cytochromes P450 and b_5 in hepatic microsomes were greater than those observed in the intact rats. In bile duct-cannulated rats, the decrease in aminopyrine *N*-demethylase activity after administration of *ortho*-dichlorobenzene was greater than that observed in the intact rats. Hence, metabolites other than the sulfones dominate the effects of the parent compound on liver enzymes (Kato & Kimura, 1997).

(*b*) meta-*Dichlorobenzene*

No data were available to the Working Group.

(*c*) para-*Dichlorobenzene*

Following repeated whole-body exposure of female CFY (Sprague-Dawley-derived strain) rats to atmospheres containing [^{14}C]*para*-dichlorobenzene (1000 ppm) for 3 h per day for up to 10 days or administration of oral or subcutaneous doses of 250 mg/kg bw per day for up to 10 days, ^{14}C was measured in tissues 24 h after the last dose. After the atmospheric or oral doses, the highest concentrations of radiolabel were measured in fat, followed by kidneys, liver and lungs. The concentration declined rapidly in plasma and tissues five days after the last dose. During the five days after repeated dosing, 91–97% of the excreted radiolabel was found in the urine, indicating biotransformation to polar metabolites. Excretion was more prolonged after subcutaneous administration. After single doses to bile duct-cannulated animals, 46–63% of the excreted radiolabel was found in the bile over 24 h, indicating extensive enterohepatic circulation. The pattern of metabolites in urine and bile was similar after each type of administration, although there were quantitative differences. Urine extracts contained two major ^{14}C components, namely a sulfate and a glucuronide of 2,5-dichlorophenol, representing 46–54% and 31–34% of the urinary radiolabel, respectively. Two minor components were identified by mass spectrometry as a dihydroxydichlorobenzene and the mercapturic acid of *para*-dichlorobenzene. The glucuronide of 2,5-dichlorophenol was the major (30–42%) component of radiolabel in bile (Hawkins *et al.*, 1980).

Male and female Fischer 344 rats were given 900 mg/kg bw [^{14}C]*para*-dichlorobenzene by gavage, housed for 72 h in metabolic cages for collection of urine and then killed. Selected organs were excised to determine total and protein-bound radiolabel. In liver, kidney, lung and spleen, the radiolabel bound to proteins was below the limit of detection. Approximately 38–42% of the dose was recovered in urine, where both sulfate and glucuronide conjugates of 2,5-dichlorophenol were identified. These results confirm those of other studies that 2,5-dichlorophenol is a major metabolite of *para*-dichlorobenzene. 2,5-Dichlorohydroquinone was identified in urine as a minor metabolite only after acid hydrolysis. The authors note that hydroquinones are relatively inert chemically and may be conjugated to glucuronides and excreted without resulting in covalent binding or toxicity (Klos & Dekant, 1994).

The distribution of *para*-dichlorobenzene in organs was compared in male and female Fischer 344/DuCrj rats after they had inhaled 500 ppm for 24 h in a whole-body chamber. The concentrations of *para*-dichlorobenzene in serum, liver, kidney and fatty tissues were measured by gas chromatography at intervals up to 24 h after treatment. Although no significant differences in serum concentrations were observed between male and female rats, those in the livers of female rats were significantly higher than in male rats. Conversely, significantly higher levels of *para*-dichlorobenzene were found in the kidneys of male than female rats. The authors concluded that the distribution correlates with the finding of nephrotoxic changes only in male rats and of minor hepatotoxic changes only in females (Umemura *et al.*, 1990).

The biotransformation and kinetics of *para*-dichlorobenzene were studied in male Wistar rats given doses of 10, 50 or 250 mg/kg bw orally. At all doses, excretion was predominantly via the urine (78–85%) with only a small amount via the faeces (2–5%); excretion in the bile represented < 5% of the low dose and 30% of the high dose. The major biliary metabolite was the glucuronide of 2,5-dichlorophenol. The time at which the plasma concentrations of the parent compound and the metabolites were maximal and the maximal concentrations increased with dose. Induction of CYP 2E1 by isoniazid resulted in faster urinary elimination, whereas the time at which the plasma concentrations of the parent compound and the metabolites were maximal and the maximal concentrations were lower. At 50 mg/kg bw, the integrated area under the curve of time–concentration in blood was smaller (148 versus 244 μmol × h/L) and total clearance was higher (33 versus 24 mL/min per kg bw) in induced rats. At this dose, the plasma half-life was approximately 7 h in uninduced rats and 4.5 h in induced rats; these values were similar at the high dose. *para*-Dichlorobenzene was metabolized mainly to 2,5-dichlorophenol (~90%), which was detected in urine as its sulfate (50–60%), glucuronide (20–30%) and the free form (5–10%). Minor metabolites were *N*-acetyl-cysteine-*S*-dihydro-hydroxy-1,4-dichlorobenzene and the corresponding dehydrated *N*-acetyl-cysteine-*S*-1,4-dichlorobenzene, which comprised about 10% of total metabolites. No hydroquinones were observed, even under conditions of induced oxidative metabolism (Hissink *et al.*, 1997a).

Conversion of *para*-dichlorobenzene to oxidized metabolites, glutathione conjugates and covalently bound metabolites was investigated in hepatic microsomes from humans, male B6C3F$_1$ mice and male Fischer 344, Sprague-Dawley and Wistar rats to determine possible species and strain differences. *para*-Dichlorobenzene is hepatocarcinogenic in B6C3F$_1$ mice but not in Wistar or Fischer rats, and is nephrotoxic and nephrocarcinogenic in male Fischer rats. The species rank order for total conversion of *para*-dichlorobenzene *in vitro* was mouse > rat >> human. Microsomes from Fischer and Wistar rats showed similar conversion, whereas those from Sprague-Dawley rats converted less of the compound. Liver microsomes prepared from mice produced most of the reactive metabolites, as indicated by covalent binding to macromolecules: > 20% of total metabolites were formed, whereas the amounts formed by rat and human microsomes were not detectable to 13%. Covalent binding by mouse microsomes was extensively inhibited by ascorbic acid, with a concomitant increase in hydroquinone formation, suggesting that benzoquinones are the reactive metabolites. Phenobarbital pretreatment of rats enhanced the conversion of *para*-dichlorobenzene *in vitro* and the amount of covalent binding. Covalent binding by all rat microsomes was partly (33–79%) inhibited by ascorbic acid. Addition of glutathione and ascorbic acid further diminished the covalent binding, with a concomitant increase in the formation of the glutathione-conjugated epoxide. Human microsomes produced the least reactive metabolites, > 70% of the covalent binding being prevented by the addition of glutathione (Hissink *et al.*, 1997b).

(*d*) *Comparative studies of* ortho-, para- *and* meta-*dichlorobenzenes*

The oxidation of [^{14}C]*ortho*- and *para*-dichlorobenzene was investigated in liver microsomes from male Wistar rats. The major metabolites of both isomers were dichlorophenols (2,5-dichlorophenol for *para*-dichlorobenzene and 2,3- and 3,4-dichlorophenol for *ortho*-dichlorobenzene) and dichlorohydroquinones. Formation of polar dihydrodiols appeared to be a major route for *ortho*- but not for *para*-dichlorobenzene. Both the hepatotoxic *ortho*-dichlorobenzene and the non-hepatotoxic *para*-dichlorobenzene were oxidized to metabolites that interacted covalently with protein and to only a small extent with DNA. Protein binding could be inhibited by the addition of ascorbic acid, with a concomitant increase in the formation of hydroquinones and catechols, indicating involvement of reactive benzoquinone metabolites in protein binding. In the presence of ascorbic acid, a substantial amount of protein-bound metabolites of *ortho*-dichlorobenzene was still observed, while protein binding of *para*-dichlorobenzene metabolites was nearly completely inhibited. This effect was ascribed to the direct formation of reactive benzoquinone metabolites in a single cytochrome P450-mediated oxidation of the primary oxidation product, a dichlorophenol. The presence of a chlorine *para* to the phenolic group (such as in 3,4-dichlorophenol, which is produced from *ortho*-dichlorobenzene) results in direct formation of a reactive benzoquinone and elimination of the chlorine as an anion. In contrast, 2,5-dichlorophenol, the major phenol isomer derived from *para*-dichlorobenzene is oxidized to its hydroquinone derivative, which requires prior oxidation in order to generate the reactive benzoquinone species. Reactive intermediates in the secondary metabolism of *ortho*-dichlorobenzene lead to more covalent binding than those derived from *para*-dichlorobenzene, and this finding correlates very well with their reported hepatotoxic potency (den Besten *et al.*, 1992). [The Working Group noted that after administration of *ortho*-dichlorobenzene to rats *in vivo*, the glutathione conjugates in bile and the mercapturic acids in urine were epoxide-derived and quinone- or hydroquinone-derived *S*-conjugates were not observed.]

4.2 Toxic effects

4.2.1 *Humans*

(*a*) ortho-*Dichlorobenzene*

Occupational exposure to *ortho*-dichlorobenzene at a concentration of 100 ppm caused some irritation of the eyes and upper respiratory tract (American Conference of Governmental Industrial Hygienists, 1991).

(*b*) meta-*Dichlorobenzene*

No data were available to the Working Group.

(*c*) para-*Dichlorobenzene*

A case of acute haemolytic anaemia was described in a three-year-old boy whose mother had seen him playing with moth crystals containing *para*-dichlorobenzene. Traces of 2,5-dichloroquinol and two other phenols where identified in urine collected six days later, but 2,5-dichlorophenol, the major metabolite of *para*-dichlorobenzene, could not be identified (Hallowell, 1959).

A case of aplastic anaemia was reported in a 68-year-old female employee of a clothing resale store who had handled a total of 5.5 kg *para*-dichlorobenzene and 7 kg naphthalene over a period of one month in a poorly ventilated storage area (Harden & Baetjer, 1978).

[The Working Group noted that neither report provides proof of a causal involvement of *para*-dichlorobenzene in the observed anaemia.]

4.2.2 *Experimental systems*

(*a*) ortho-*Dichlorobenzene*

Rats treated by gavage on five days a week with 188 or 376 mg/kg bw *ortho*-dichlorobenzene for 27 weeks had increased liver and kidney weights. Exposure by inhalation to 539 ppm (3200 mg/m^3) *ortho*-dichlorobenzene for one to three days for 3–6.5 h per day resulted in marked centrilobular necrosis of the liver and swelling of the kidney tubular epithelium (Hollingsworth *et al.*, 1958).

Liver damage resulting from acute 4-h exposure to 246, 369, 610 or 739 ppm (1500, 2200, 3700 or 4400 mg/m^3) *ortho*-dichlorobenzene was found in male Sprague-Dawley rats. An inverse linear relationship was established between the logarithmic values of serum glutamate dehydrogenase and sorbitol dehydrogenase activities and decreased centrilobular liver-cell glucose-6-phosphatase staining intensity; the levels of exposure were linearly related to the same two parameters (Brondeau *et al.*, 1986).

The ability of acetone and three other ketone vapours to affect the hepatotoxicity of inhaled *ortho*-dichlorobenzene was examined in male Sprague-Dawley rats and OF1 mice. Methylethylketone, methylisobutylketone or cyclohexanone increased liver cytochrome P-450 content and glutathione *S*-transferase activity but did not affect serum glutamate dehydrogenase activity in rats. Pre-exposure to these ketones enhanced the *ortho*-dichlorobenzene-induced increase in serum glutamate dehydrogenase activity by

8–63-fold, while the increases in cytochrome P450 content (33–86%) and glutathione *S*-transferase activity (42–64%) were identical to those resulting from exposure to the ketones alone. Acetone elicited cytochrome P450 and glutathione *S*-transferase responses comparable to those caused by the other ketones; however, pre-exposure to acetone potentiated (at 4785 ppm), reduced (at 10 670 ppm) or suppressed (at 14 790 ppm) *ortho*-dichlorobenzene-induced liver toxicity. The authors suggested that the concentration-dependent effects of acetone were due to induction of different microsomal enzymes: a toxifying isozyme at the lower concentration and a detoxifying isozyme at the higher concentration, as has been observed with 1,1-dichloroethylene (Brondeau *et al.*, 1989).

ortho-Dichlorobenzene was administered to male and female Sprague-Dawley rats at doses of 37.5, 75, 150 or 300 mg/kg bw per day for 10 days or at 25, 100 or 400 mg/kg bw per day for 90 days in corn oil by gavage; control animals received corn oil. In the 10-day study, male rats treated with 300 mg/kg bw had significantly decreased final body weights; heart, kidney, spleen, testis and thymus weights; and relative spleen and thymus weights. These animals also had significantly increased absolute and relative liver weights. Males also displayed significant increases in water consumption (at 300 mg/kg bw), alanine aminotransferase activity (at 300 mg/kg bw) and number of leukocytes (at 150 and 300 mg/kg bw). A significant increase in the incidence of hepatocellular necrosis was seen in males at 300 mg/kg bw when compared with controls. In the 90-day study, male rats exposed to 400 mg/kg bw *ortho*-dichlorobenzene had significantly decreased body weights and absolute and relative spleen weights and significantly increased absolute weights of kidney and liver and relative weights of heart, kidney, liver, lung, brain and testis. Females at this dose had increased absolute and relative weights of both kidney and liver. The only effects on clinical chemical parameters were increased alanine aminotransferase activity at 100 and 400 mg/kg bw, increased blood urea nitrogen and total bilirubin concentrations in males at 400 mg/kg bw and increased total bilirubin content in females at this dose. Histopathological evaluation showed hepatocellular lesions associated with treatment, which included centrilobular degeneration and hypertrophy and single-cell necrosis in males and females receiving 400 mg/kg bw *ortho*-dichlorobenzene. No adverse effect was observed at 25 mg/kg bw per day (Robinson *et al.*, 1991).

The hepatic toxicity of *ortho*-dichlorobenzene was studied in Fischer 344 rats given methyl palmitate in order to inhibit Kupffer-cell function or superoxide dismutase (conjugated to polyethylene glycol) to scavenge superoxide anions. Administration of either compound dramatically reduced the severity of *ortho*-dichlorobenzene-induced liver injury, and both agents reduced the increase in plasma alanine aminotransferase activity by 80%; light microscopic examination confirmed that the reductions in enzyme activity reflected protection from hepatocellular injury. Interestingly, methyl palmitate did not protect against *ortho*-dichlorobenzene-induced hepatotoxicity in phenobarbital-pretreated rats, and the degree of inhibition of hepatotoxicity by polyethylene glycol–superoxide dismutase was not significantly different from that in normal rats. The lack of significant inhibition of phenobarbital-potentiated hepatotoxicity by both polyethylene glycol–

superoxide dismutase and methyl palmitate suggests that reactive oxygen species released from a non-parenchymal source are not as crucial to the hepatotoxicity of *ortho*-dichlorobenzene in phenobarbital-pretreated as in the normal rats. The results suggest that reactive oxygen species released from Kupffer cells play a major role in the progression of *ortho*-dichlorobenzene hepatotoxicity (Gunawardhana *et al.*, 1993).

Twenty-two hours after intraperitoneal injection of [^{14}C]*ortho*-dichlorobenzene (127 μCi/kg bw, 42 μCi/μmol) to male Wistar rats and BALB/c mice, covalent binding of radiolabel was detected in the DNA, RNA and proteins of liver, kidney, lung and stomach. The authors stated that the covalent binding index to liver DNA (17 in rats, 50 in mice) was typical of that of carcinogens classified as weak initiators. The enzyme-mediated interaction of *ortho*-dichlorobenzene with calf thymus DNA of synthetic polyribonucleotides *in vitro* was mediated by a microsomal mixed-function oxidase system and microsomal glutathione transferases, which seemed to be effective only in liver and lung of rats and mice. Cytosolic glutathione transferases played a minor role in the bioactivation of *ortho*-dichlorobenzene (Colacci *et al.*, 1990). [The Working Group noted that DNA adducts were not identified.]

(*b*) meta-*Dichlorobenzene*

See the section on comparative studies of the toxicity of *ortho*-, *para*- and *meta*-dichlorobenzene, below.

(*c*) para-*Dichlorobenzene*

Daily oral administration of 0–200 mg/kg bw *para*-dichlorobenzene to female rats [strain unspecified] did not increase their liver weights or the concentrations of liver or urinary porphyrins (Carlson, 1977).

Groups of male and female Wistar rats and female Alderley Park mice were exposed for 5 h per day on five days a week to *para*-dichlorobenzene at concentrations of 0, 75 or 500 ppm (0, 450 or 3000 mg/m^3) for 76 weeks (rats) or 57 weeks (female mice), followed by 36 weeks (rats) or 19 weeks (female mice) without exposure. No clinical signs of toxicity were apparent at 75 ppm, nor were there any treatment-related effects on blood or urinary clinical chemistry. Slightly elevated urinary coproporphyrin excretion and increased liver and kidney weights were considered to be treatment-related effects in rats exposed to 500 ppm *para*-dichlorobenzene. [The Working Group noted that no quantitative data were included in the report]. Histopathological evaluation of non-neoplastic lesions did not indicate any treatment-related effects in either species (Loeser & Litchfield, 1983).

Fischer 344 rats were given 37.5–1500 mg/kg bw *para*-dichlorobenzene by gavage on five days per week for 13 weeks. Body-weight gain was decreased at doses ≥ 600 mg/kg bw, and the mortality rate was increased at doses ≥ 900 mg/kg bw. At doses ≥ 300 mg/kg bw, male rats developed kidney damage characterized by tubular degeneration and necrosis, while females had no adverse renal effects at doses ≤ 1500 mg/kg bw. Hepatotoxicity was observed in rats at doses ≥ 600 mg/kg bw, and the urinary concentration of coproporhyrins was increased at 1200 mg/kg bw. In the animals treated with 1200 or 1500 mg/kg bw, additional adverse effects were seen, consisting of bone-marrow hypoplasia, lymphoid depletion of the spleen and thymus and necrosis in the nasal turbinates and intestinal mucosa. In the same study, B6C3F$_1$ mice were treated with daily oral doses of 84–1800 mg/kg bw. Body-weight gain was affected at doses > 1000 mg/kg bw; deaths were seen only at 1800 mg/kg bw. Histological and clinical hepatotoxicity was induced at 600 mg/kg bw but not at 338 mg/kg bw. Mice treated with 1500 mg/kg bw or 1800 mg/kg bw developed lymphoid necrosis in the thymus, lymphoid depletion in the spleen and haematopoietic hypoplasia of the spleen and bone marrow. No effect on the kidney was observed (National Toxicology Program, 1987).

Groups of 10 male and 10 female Fischer 344 rats were dosed by gavage with 0, 75, 150, 300 or 600 mg/kg bw per day of *para*-dichlorobenzene in corn oil. Half of the animals were killed after four weeks and the remainder after 13 weeks. Increased urinary lactate dehydrogenase activity, increased epithelial cell excretion and exacerbation of hyaline droplet accumulation in the cytoplasm of renal cortical cells were observed in male rats over the entire dose range investigated. Tubular single-cell necrosis and dilated tubules with granular cast formation in the outer zone of the medulla were evident in male rats after 4 and 13 weeks of treatment with doses of 150–600 mg/kg bw per day. Female rats showed no indication of nephrotoxicity. The authors concluded that the morphological characteristics of the sex-specific effects on the kidney corresponded to the light hydrocarbon nephropathy observed after short-term treatment with a number of aliphatic and cyclic hydrocarbons (Bomhard *et al.*, 1988).

Male Fischer 344 rats were given a single dose of 300 or 500 mg/kg bw [^{14}C]*para*-dichlorobenzene or [^{14}C]*ortho*-dichlorobenzene by gavage, placed in metabolism cages for collection of urine and killed 24 h later. Gel filtration chromatography of soluble renal proteins from *para*-dichlorobenzene-treated rats showed that the radiolabel co-eluted with α_{2u}-globulin in a single sharp peak, and *para*-dichlorobenzene and its metabolite, 2,5-dichlorophenol, were found to be reversibly bound to this globulin. *ortho*-Dichlorobenzene-derived radiolabel, but not that from *para*-dichlorobenzene, was found to bind covalently to liver and high-molecular-mass plasma proteins. *para*-Dichlorobenzene increased protein droplet formation in male rat kidneys, whereas equimolar doses of *ortho*-dichlorobenzene had no effect. Renal-cell proliferation, measured by [^{3}H]thymidine incorporation into renal DNA, was increased after treatment with *para*- but not *ortho*-dichlorobenzene (Charbonneau *et al.*, 1989).

Male NCI-Black-Reiter rats are the only animals known not to synthesize α_{2u}-globulin in the liver. Under conditions of exposure that clearly induced α_{2u}-globulin nephropathy in male Fischer 344 rats (500 mg/kg bw per day on four consecutive days), *para*-dichlorobenzene did not induce α_{2u}-globulin accumulation, hyaline (protein) droplet formation or renal lesions in these animals (Dietrich & Swenberg, 1991).

Increases in the amount of kidney-type α_{2u}-globulin (16 kDa), which result from renal processing of the 19 kDa native-type α_{2u}-globulin produced in the liver, were detected in the urine of male rats treated with 220 mg/kg bw per day *para*-dichlorobenzene for seven consecutive days. The increase correlated directly with increased concentrations of kidney-type α_{2u}-globulin in renal tissue and with accumulation of hyaline droplets in the proximal convoluted tubules. Similar changes were not observed with the nephrotoxic chemicals puromycin aminonucleoside and hexachlorobutadiene, but a marked increase in kidney-type α_{2u}-globulin was detected after administration of 2,2,4-trimethylpentane, *d*-limonene, decalin or isophorone (Saito *et al.*, 1996).

B6C3F$_1$ mice were exposed to *para*-dichlorobenzene in corn oil by gavage for up to five days at a dose of 600 mg/kg bw per day, and male Fischer 344 rats were exposed to 300 mg/kg bw per day on five days per week for up to three weeks. The percentage of cells in S-phase (labelling index) was compared in tissues of animals given either 5-bromo-2′-deoxyuridine (BrDU) or [^{3}H]thymidine as a single intraperitoneal injection 2 h before being killed or continuously via a subcutaneously implanted osmotic pump for three or six days. Cell proliferation was increased in the livers of animals of both species treated with *para*-dichlorobenzene when compared with controls. After four days of treatment with the chemical and continuous administration of a DNA precursor label during the last three days of treatment, the labelling indices in control and *para*-dichlorobenzene-treated mouse livers were 0.7 and 19% for BrDU and 0.9 and 15% for [^{3}H]thymidine, respectively. The labelling indices for BrDU- and [^{3}H]thymidine-labelled renal proximal tubular cells were 7.7 and 8.0%, respectively, in male rats receiving *para*-dichlorobenzene for four days, while those in controls were 4.3 and 3.7%, respectively. The renal proximal tubular cell labelling index increased to 11% in male BrDU-labelled rats treated with *para*-dichlorobenzene for three weeks (Eldridge *et al.*, 1990).

A sharp increase in labelling index was seen in female B6C3F$_1$ mice and Fischer 344 rats 24 h after a single treatment with 600 mg/kg bw *para*-dichlorobenzene, and after 48 h in male mice. No increase in the activity of liver-associated plasma enzymes was seen at doses up to 1200 mg/kg bw. In mice treated for 13 weeks with *para*-dichlorobenzene by gavage at 300 or 600 mg/kg bw per day, a statistically significant, transient peak of hepatocellular proliferation was observed during week 1 at 600 mg/kg bw per day. Hepatocellular proliferation was also observed in female rats, which had no increase in liver tumour incidence when compared with controls. The relative liver weights (percentage of body weight) in comparison with controls were increased in male and female mice and female rats at the high dose, but not in male rats. No significant increases in the activities of liver-associated plasma enzymes were found at any time, indicating a lack of overt hepatotoxicity. Histopathological evaluation revealed no evidence of hepatocellular necrosis in any group. The authors considered that their data indicated early mitogenic stimulation of cell proliferation rather than regeneration secondary to cytotoxicity in the livers of *para*-dichlorobenzene-treated mice, which correlates with the observed tumour formation in a dose-dependent manner. The induction of cell proliferation by *para*-dichlorobenzene in rat liver in the absence of a tumorigenic response was suggested by the authors to imply important species differences in the relationship between cell proliferation and carcinogenesis (Eldridge *et al.*, 1992).

Cell proliferation in the kidneys and livers of Fischer 344 rats and B6C3F$_1$ mice treated by gavage with *para*-dichlorobenzene at 0, 150, 300 or 600 mg/kg bw per day for four days was evaluated by measuring BrDU incorporation into nuclei of DNA-synthesizing cells. The cumulative fraction of proliferating cells was increased in the proximal tubular epithelial cells of male rats at the high dose but not at the lower doses or in females at either dose, when the γ-glutamyl transferase reaction was used to identify tubular cells. No increase in cell proliferation was found in mouse kidney. The fractions of proliferating cells in the livers of rats and mice of each sex were also increased at the two higher doses. Although the increased cell proliferation in male rat kidney and in the livers of mice of each sex correlates with the reported carcinogenic effects of *para*-dichlorobenzene in those tissues, cell proliferation was also induced in the livers of rats of each sex and in female mice at the low dose in the absence of an increased incidence of liver tumours, indicating that acute induction of cell proliferation is not sufficient to lead to or explain tumour formation (Umemura *et al.*, 1992).

A single administration of 300 mg/kg bw *para*-dichlorobenzene or 950 mg/kg bw diethylhexyl phthalate to male Fischer 344 rats by gavage induced an increase in the hepatic labelling index and in the expression of the immediate early genes c-*fos*, c-*myc* and c-*jun* in the liver similar to that in untreated controls (Hasmall *et al.*, 1997). The authors concluded that neither the labelling index nor the expression of immediate early genes can distinguish between hepatocarcinogenic (diethylhexyl phthalate) and non-hepatocarcinogenic (*para*-dichlorobenzene) liver mitogens. [The Working Group noted that the experimental design, involving a single administration, is not suitable for evaluating mechanisms of carcinogenicity and that *para*-dichlorobenzene is hepato-carcinogenic at doses that concomitantly induce liver injury.]

B6C3F$_1$ mice and Fischer 344 rats were treated by gavage for four weeks with *para*-dichlorobenzene in corn oil. The doses for mice were 150, 300 or 600 mg/kg bw (the maximal tolerated dose, which also increased liver tumour formation), and those for rats were 75, 150 or 300 mg/kg bw. In mice at the high dose, the incidence of hepatic cell proliferation was increased by 16-fold at one week and by fourfold at four weeks; at 300 mg/kg bw, the increase was seen only at one week and had subsided by four weeks. In rats at doses of 150 and 300 mg/kg bw, the incidence of hepatic cell proliferation was increased after one week but had returned to normal after four weeks. The authors concluded that sustained cell proliferation occurs only in susceptible species at a carcino-genic dose (Umemura *et al.*, 1998).

Male Fischer 344 rats and male B6C3F$_1$ mice were given 0, 25, 75, 150, 300 or 600 mg/kg bw per day *para*-dichlorobenzene by gavage on five days a week for 1, 4 or 13 weeks. *para*-Dichlorobenzene produced significant, dose-related increases in relative liver weights in both rats and mice, which was associated with mild and marked centri-lobular hypertrophy, respectively. Dose-related increases in cytochrome P450 content and 7-pentoxyresorufin-*O*-depentylase activity were observed throughout the 13-week treatment period in animals of each sex. CYP 2B isoenzymes were induced by *para*-dichlorobenzene in both rat and mouse liver microsomes. The hepatic labelling index was increased in rats treated for one week with 300 mg/kg bw *para*-dichlorobenzene, whereas in mice the hepatic labelling index was increased by treatment with 300 or 600 mg/kg bw *para*-dichlorobenzene for one and four weeks. The labelling index in the kidney proximal tubular cells of rats was increased at 1, 4 and 13 weeks of *para*-dichlorobenzene administration, while little effect was seen in mouse kidney (Lake *et al.*, 1997).

(*d*) *Comparative studies of the toxicity of* ortho-, para- *and* meta-*dichlorobenzenes*

The flow of bile duct and pancreatic fluid was increased and the protein concentration of the fluid was decreased 24 h after intraperitoneal administration of 5 mmol/kg bw *ortho*-dichlorobenzene to male Holtzman rats, while *para*-dichlorobenzene had no such action. This effect did not involve secretin or cholinergic stimulation of the pancreas and was not associated with hepatotoxicity, as shown by the absence of an increase in serum glutamate pyruvate transaminase activity (Yang *et al.*, 1979).

Tenfold more covalent binding was observed in the livers of male C57BL/6J mice treated with 0.5 mmol/kg bw *ortho*- compared with *para*-dichlorobenzene. The amount of covalent binding was increased by pretreatment with phenobarbital, and this increase was prevented by concomitant pretreatment with SKF 525-A (Reid & Krishina, 1973).

The acute hepatotoxicity of the three isomers of dichlorobenzene was evaluated in male Fischer 344 rats at various times after intraperitoneal administration. Plasma alanine aminotransferase activity, measured 24 h after treatment with 1.8–5.4 mmol/kg bw *ortho*-dichlorobenzene, was dramatically elevated. In contrast, equimolar doses of *para*-dichlorobenzene had no effect, and *meta*-dichlorobenzene had a clearly weaker effect on enzyme activity at doses ≥ 2.7 mmol/kg bw. Histopathological changes in the livers of treated animals correlated with the alterations in enzyme activities. Phenobarbital pretreatment potentiated the acute hepatotoxicity of *ortho*- and *meta*-dichlorobenzene but did not affect the toxicity of *para*-dichlorobenzene. Similarly, SKF-525A pretreatment inhibited the hepatotoxicity of *ortho*-dichlorobenzene. Equimolar doses of *ortho*- and *meta*-dichlorobenzene produced approximately equivalent depletion of intrahepatic glutathione, while *para*-dichlorobenzene had no effect on this parameter. Prior depletion of hepatic glutathione by pretreatment with phorone markedly potentiated the hepatotoxicity of *ortho*- and *meta*-dichlorobenzene but only slightly increased the toxicity of *para*-dichlorobenzene. These quantitative and qualitative differences could not be explained by differences in hepatic distribution or covalent binding to hepatic proteins. Interestingly, male Fischer rats are 75 times more sensitive than Sprague-Dawley rats to the acute hepatotoxicity of *ortho*-dichlorobenzene, and this is one of the most dramatic strain differences in toxicity (Gunawardhana & Sipes, 1991; Stine *et al.*, 1991).

Toxic effects on the liver, kidneys and thyroid were monitored after a single intraperitoneal administration of 1, 2 or 4 mmol/kg bw *ortho*- or *para*-dichlorobenzene to male Wistar rats. *ortho*-Dichlorobenzene was the most potent hepatotoxicant, as determined by plasma alanine aminotransferase activity and histopathological appearance after 72 h. Protein droplets were observed in tubular epithelial cells 72 h after administration of *para*-

dichlorobenzene, but not after administration of *ortho*-dichlorobenzene. Both chlorinated benzenes reduced the plasma thyroxine concentration (den Besten *et al.*, 1991).

Male Fischer 344 rats were injected intraperitoneally with 2, 3 or 4 mmol/kg bw *ortho*-, *meta*- or *para*-dichlorobenzene, and pair-fed control animals were injected intraperitoneally with corn oil (1 mL/kg bw). After 24 h, plasma alanine aminotransferase activity was found to be increased by *ortho*-dichlorobenzene in a dose-dependent manner. Centrilobular necrosis was observed in rats treated with *ortho*-dichlorobenzene, while the morphological appearance was relatively normal in rats treated with *meta*- or *para*-dichlorobenzene. Kidney weights and blood urea nitrogen concentration were not altered by treatment with *meta*- or *para*-dichlorobenzene. Accumulation of *para*-aminohippurate in renal cortical slices was decreased by *meta*- (2 and 4 mmol/kg bw) and *ortho*-dichlorobenzene (3 and 4 mmol/kg bw), while accumulation of the cation tetraethylammonium was decreased by 4 mmol/kg bw *para*-dichlorobenzene. The results demonstrate that *ortho* substitution enhances hepatic toxicity and that the liver is more sensitive than the kidney to the toxic effects of dichlorobenzenes (Valentovic *et al.*, 1993).

Although Fischer 344 rats are many times more sensitive to the hepatotoxic effect of *ortho*-dichlorobenzene than Sprague-Dawley rats, the LD_{50} values (1.7 mL/kg bw in male Fischer 344 and 1.8 mL/kg bw in Sprague-Dawley rats) were similar. In age-matched male Sprague-Dawley and Fischer 344 rats given *ortho*-dichlorobenzene intraperitoneally (0.2, 0.6 or 1.2 mL/kg bw), liver injury over time was assessed by measuring plasma alanine aminotransferase and sorbitol dehydrogenase activities and histopathology. Fischer 344 rats showed larger increases in plasma alanine aminotransferase activity after administration of 0.2 or 0.6 mL/kg bw *ortho*-dichlorobenzene than Sprague-Dawley rats. When sorbitol dehydrogenase was used as a marker of liver injury, the strain difference was seen only at 0.2 mL/kg bw. Liver regeneration was estimated from [^{3}H]thymidine incorporation into liver DNA and an assay for proliferating cell nuclear antigen. These markers indicated that Fischer 344 rats had up to fourfold more hepatocellular regeneration than Sprague-Dawley rats. The significantly greater depletion of hepatic glycogen observed in Fischer 344 rats after administration of 0.2 or 0.6 mL/kg bw *ortho*-dichlorobenzene was not accompanied by significant changes in plasma glucose concentration and was consistent with the stimulated tissue repair seen in these rats at the corresponding doses (Kulkarni *et al.*, 1996).

The acute hepatotoxicity of the dichlorobenzene isomers was compared in the livers of male B6C3F$_1$ mice at different times after a single intragastric administration of *ortho*-, *meta*- or *para*-dichlorobenzene at 300, 300 or 1800 mg/kg bw, respectively. Acute hepatic injury was assessed from serum alanine aminotransferase activity, histopathological appearance and hepatocyte replication (BrDU labelling). Both *ortho*- and *meta*-dichlorobenzene significantly increased liver weights and serum alanine aminotransferase activity and caused extensive liver-cell necrosis. In contrast, *para*-dichlorobenzene induced slight hepatocyte injury only at the sixfold higher dose of 1800 mg/kg bw; however, it induced hepatocyte proliferation at 1000 mg/kg bw, in the absence of any signs of hepatotoxicity while increased cell proliferation due to *ortho*- or *meta*-dichlorobenzene occurred only at doses that caused hepatic injury. These data suggest that the hepatocyte proliferation induced by *ortho*- or *meta*-dichlorobenzene is compensatory regeneration, while that induced by *para*-dichlorobenzene is a response to mitogenic stimulation (Umemura *et al.*, 1996).

4.3 Reproductive and developmental effects

4.3.1 *Humans*

No data were available to the Working Group.

4.3.2 *Experimental systems*

The developmental effects of *para*-dichlorobenzene in experimental systems have been reviewed (Loeser & Litchfield, 1983). In rats exposed by inhalation to 0, 75, 200 or 500 ppm (0, 450, 1200 or 3000 mg/m^3) for 6 h per day on days 6–15 of gestation, isolated malformations were seen at all doses, but the authors concluded that these did not constitute evidence of embryo- or fetotoxicity or teratogenicity.

Groups of 30–32 Fischer 344 rats were exposed to *ortho*-dichlorobenzene (purity, 98.81%) by inhalation on days 6–15 of gestation, and groups of 28–30 New Zealand rabbits were exposed on days 6–18 of gestation to 0, 100, 200 or 400 ppm (0, 600, 1200 or 2400 mg/m^3). Further groups of rabbits were exposed to 0, 100, 300 or 800 ppm (0, 600, 1800 or 4800 mg/m^3) *para*-dichlorobenzene (purity, 99.9%) on days 6–18 of gestation. In rats, maternal toxicity, evident as decreased weight gain and increased relative liver weights, was seen in all treated groups, but there was no indication of an effect on the developing organism. In rabbits, decreased maternal body weights were noted in all exposed groups, but the effect was largely limited to changes manifest within the first three days of exposure; again, there were no effects on the developing offspring attributable to *ortho*-dichlorobenzene. With *para*-dichlorobenzene, maternal body-weight gain was reduced at the high dose at several periods during gestation, but no other dose-related effects were seen in the does or fetuses (Hayes *et al.*, 1985).

The developmental effects of *para*-dichlorobenzene (99% pure) in groups of 13–17 CD rats were evaluated after exposure to 0, 250, 500, 750 or 1000 mg/kg bw per day by oral gavage in corn oil. Decreased food consumption was seen in all treated groups, and females at the highest dose had decreased body-weight gain during treatment. There were no effects on fetal viability, but fetal body weights were decreased at the highest dose, and the incidence of extra ribs was increased at all doses above 250 mg/kg bw per day (Giavini *et al.*, 1986).

4.4 Genetic and related effects

4.4.1 *Humans*

A study of 26 individuals accidentally exposed to *ortho*-dichlorobenzene (presumably > 100 ppm) for four days revealed a statistically significant (4.4-fold) increase in the frequency of chromosomal aberrations in peripheral blood lymphocytes as compared with a control group; six months later, chromosomal aberrations were still more frequent than in the control group (Zapata-Gayon *et al.*, 1982).

4.4.2 *Experimental systems* (see Table 5 for references)

ortho-Dichlorobenzene did not induce point mutations in eight histidine-requiring mutants of *Salmonella typhimurium*, which involve the *C*, *D* and *G* genes of the *histidine* operon, and was not mutagenic to *S. typhimurium* strains TA100, TA1535, TA1537, TA1538 or TA98 with and without metabolic activation. It induced mitotic gene conversion and reverse mutation in the D7 strain of *Saccharomyces cerevisiae* in the presence of an exogenous metabolic system from the livers of induced mice and was very weakly mutagenic in a methionine-requiring auxotroph of *Aspergillus nidulans*. A dose-dependent increase in the frequency of micronucleated polychromatic erythrocytes was detected in the bone marrow of male mice after intraperitoneal injection of two equal doses of *ortho*-dichlorobenzene. DNA damage was not induced in the livers of female rats given two oral doses of *ortho*-dichlorobenzene. Covalent binding of [^{14}C]*ortho*-dichlorobenzene to calf thymus DNA was detected *in vitro* after incubation with various subcellular preparations of liver from induced mice. Weak covalent binding of *ortho*-dichlorobenzene to the DNA of various organs in male rats and mice was also reported *in vivo* after a single intraperitoneal treatment.

meta-Dichlorobenzene did not induce mutation in *S. typhimurium* strains TA100, TA1535, TA1537, TA1538 or TA98 or in *Escherichia coli* WP2 *uvr*A with and without metabolic activation; it had contrasting effects in differential toxicity assays with *E. coli* and *Bacillus subtilis* and caused gene conversion in *Saccharomyces cerevisiae*. A dose-dependent increase in the frequency of micronucleated polychromatic erythrocytes was detected in the bone marrow of male mice after intraperitoneal injection of two equal doses of *meta*-dichlorobenzene.

para-Dichlorobenzene was not mutagenic to *S. typhimurium* strains TA100, TA1535, TA1537, TA1538 or TA98 with and without metabolic activation; in only one study, a more than twofold increase in the number of revertant colonies was observed in the presence of metabolic activation in one of two experiments carried out in strain TA1535. *para*-Dichlorobenzene induced mitotic gene conversion and reverse mutation in the D7 strain of *Saccharomyces cerevisiae* in the presence of a metabolic activation system from liver of induced mice. It was reported to induce reverse mutations of a methionine-requiring auxotroph of *Aspergillus nidulans* and to induce chromosomal abnormalities and breakage in the root tips of two *Vicia* species. *para*-Dichlorobenzene did not induce DNA fragmentation in primary cultures of either rat or human hepatocytes. It did not significantly increase the frequency of mutants in mouse lymphoma L5178Y $tk^{+/-}$ cells and did not induce sister chromatid exchange in Chinese hamster ovary cells either in the absence or in the presence of liver preparations from Aroclor 1254-induced rats. *para*-Dichlorobenzene significantly increased the frequency of micronucleated cells in primary cultures of rat hepatocytes, but not in primary cultures of human hepatocytes under the same experimental conditions. It did not increase the frequency of chromosomal aberrations in Chinese hamster ovary cells in the absence or in the presence of a metabolic system from the liver of Aroclor 1254-induced rats. *para*-Dichlorobenzene increased the frequency of sister chromatid exchange in human

Table 5. Genetic and related effects of dichlorobenzenes

Test system	Results[a]		Dose[b] (LED or HID)	Reference
	Without exogenous metabolic activation	With exogenous metabolic activation		
***ortho*-Dichlorobenzene**				
Salmonella typhimurium TA100, TA98, TA1535, TA1537, reverse mutation	–	–	100 µg/plate	Haworth *et al.* (1983)
Salmonella typhimurium TA100, TA98, TA1535, TA1537, TA1538, reverse mutation	–	–	832 µg/plate	Shimizu *et al.* (1983)
Salmonella typhimurium (eight unidentified strains), reverse mutation	–	NT	NR	Andersen *et al.* (1972)
Aspergillus nidulans, reverse mutation	(+)	NT	200	Prasad (1970)
Saccharomyces cerevisiae, homozygosis by mitotic recombination or gene conversion	–	+	74	Paolini *et al.* (1998)
Saccharomyces cerevisiae, reverse mutation	–	+	74	Paolini *et al.* (1998)
DNA strand breaks, cross-links or related damage, female rat liver cells *in vivo*	–		300 po × 2	Kitchin *et al.* (1993)
Micronucleus formation, male mouse bone-marrow cells *in vivo*	+		93.5 ip × 2	Mohtashamipur *et al.* (1987)
Binding (covalent) to calf thymus DNA *in vitro*	–	+	15	Paolini *et al.* (1998)
Binding (covalent) to DNA, male rat liver, lung, kidney and stomach *in vivo*	+		0.4 ip × 1	Colacci *et al.* (1990)
Binding (covalent) to DNA, male mouse liver, lung, kidney and stomach *in vivo*	+		0.4 ip × 1	Colacci *et al.* (1990)
***meta*-Dichlorobenzene**				
Escherichia coli pol A/W3110-P3478, differential toxicity (spot test)	+	NT	13000	Environmental Protection Agency (1984)
Bacillus subtilis rec strains, differential toxicity	–	NT	13000	Environmental Protection Agency (1984)
Salmonella typhimurium TA100, TA98, TA1535, TA1537, TA1538, reverse mutation	–	–	820 µg/plate	Shimizu *et al.* (1983)

Table 5 (contd)

Test system	Results[a]		Dose[b] (LED or HID)	Reference
	Without exogenous metabolic activation	With exogenous metabolic activation		
***meta*-Dichlorobenzene (contd)**				
Salmonella typhimurium TA100, TA98, TA1535, TA1537, TA1538, reverse mutation	–	–	325	Environmental Protection Agency (1984)
Escherichia coli WP2 *uvr*A, reverse mutation	–	–	325	Environmental Protection Agency (1984)
Saccharomyces cerevisiae, gene conversion	+	+	30	Environmental Protection Agency (1984)
Micronucleus formation, male mouse bone-marrow cells *in vivo*	+		87.5 ip × 2	Mohtashamipur *et al.* (1987)
***para*-Dichlorobenzene**				
Salmonella typhimurium TA100, TA98, TA1535, TA1537, reverse mutation	–	–	100 μg/plate	Haworth *et al.* (1983)
Salmonella typhimurium TA100, TA98, TA1538, reverse mutation	–	–	2500 μg/plate	Loeser & Litchfield (1983)
Salmonella typhimurium TA1535, reverse mutation	–	?	500 μg/plate	Loeser & Litchfield (1983)
Salmonella typhimurium TA100, TA98, TA1535, TA1537, TA1538, reverse mutation	–	–	6552 μg/plate	Shimizu *et al.* (1983)
Saccharomyces cerevisiae, homozygosis by mitotic recombination or gene conversion	–	+	74	Paolini *et al.* (1998)
Saccharomyces cerevisiae, reverse mutation	–	+	147	Paolini *et al.* (1998)
Aspergillus nidulans, reverse mutation	(+)	NT	200	Prasad (1970)
Vicia sativa, chromosomal aberrations	+	NT	NR	Sharma & Bhattacharyya (1956)
Vicia faba, chromosomal aberrations	+	NT	NR	Srivastava (1966)

Table 5 (contd)

Test system	Results[a]		Dose[b] (LED or HID)	Reference
	Without exogenous metabolic activation	With exogenous metabolic activation		
***para*-Dichlorobenzene (contd)**				
DNA strand breaks, cross-links or related damage, rat hepatocytes *in vitro*	–	NT	470	Canonero *et al.* (1997)
Gene mutation, mouse lymphoma L5178Y cells, *tk* locus *in vitro*	–	–	100	US National Toxicology Program (1987)
Sister chromatid exchange, Chinese hamster ovary cells *in vitro*	–	–	150	Galloway *et al.* (1987)
Micronucleus formation, rat hepatocytes *in vitro*	+	NT	150	Canonero *et al.* (1997)
Chromosomal aberrations, Chinese hamster ovary cells *in vitro*	–	–	150	Galloway *et al.* (1987)
DNA strand breaks, cross-links or related damage, human hepatocytes *in vitro*	–	NT	470	Canonero *et al.* (1997)
Micronucleus formation, human hepatocytes *in vitro*	–	NT	470	Canonero *et al.* (1997)
Sister chromatid exchange, human lymphocytes *in vitro*	(+)	NT	0.1000	Carbonell *et al.* (1991)
DNA strand breaks, cross-links or related damage, mouse liver and spleen cells *in vivo*	+		2000 ip × 1	Sasaki *et al.* (1997)
DNA strand breaks, cross-links or related damage, mouse kidney, lung and bone-marrow cells *in vivo*	–		2000 ip × 1	Sasaki *et al.* (1997)
Unscheduled DNA synthesis, male and female mouse hepatocytes *in vivo*	–		1000 po × 1	Sherman *et al.* (1998)
Unscheduled DNA synthesis, male and female rat kidney *in vivo*	–		1000 po × 1	Sherman *et al.* (1998)
Micronucleus formation, male mouse bone-marrow cells *in vivo*	+		177.5 ip × 2	Mohtashamipur *et al.* (1987)
Micronucleus formation, male mouse erythrocytes in *vivo*	–		1800 po × 13 wk	National Toxicology Program (1987)
Micronucleus formation, male and female mouse bone-marrow cells *in vivo*	–		1600 ip × 2	Morita *et al.* (1997)
Micronucleus formation, mouse bone-marrow cells *in vivo*	–		2000 po × 2	Morita *et al.* (1997)
Chromosomal aberrations, rat bone-marrow cells *in vivo*	–		682 ppm in air 2 h × 1	Loeser & Litchfield (1983)

Table 5 (contd)

Test system	Results[a]		Dose[b] (LED or HID)	Reference
	Without exogenous metabolic activation	With exogenous metabolic activation		
***para*-Dichlorobenzene (contd)**				
Chromosomal aberrations, rat bone-marrow cells *in vivo*	–		500 ppm in air 5 h/d × 3 mo	Loeser & Litchfield (1983)
Dominant lethal mutation, mice	–		450 ppm in air 6 h/d × 5	Loeser & Litchfield (1983)
Binding (covalent) to calf thymus DNA *in vitro*	–	+	0.003	Lattanzi *et al.* (1989)
Binding (covalent) to calf thymus DNA *in vitro*	–	+	15	Paolini *et al.* (1998)
Binding (covalent) to DNA, male mouse liver, lung, kidney and stomach *in vivo*	+		0.4 ip × 1	Lattanzi *et al.* (1989)
Binding (covalent) to DNA, male rat liver, lung, kidney and stomach *in vivo*	–		0.4 ip × 1	Lattanzi *et al.* (1989)
Binding (covalent) to RNA or protein, male mouse liver, lung, kidney and stomach *in vivo*	+		0.4 ip × 1	Lattanzi *et al.* (1989)
Binding (covalent) to RNA or protein, male rat liver, lung, kidney and stomach *in vivo*	–		0.4 ip × 1	Lattanzi *et al.* (1989)

[a] +, positive; (+), weak positive; –, negative; NT, not tested; ?, inconclusive

[b] LED, lowest effective dose; HID, highest ineffective dose; unless otherwise stated, in-vitro tests, μg/mL; in-vivo tests, mg/kg bw per day; NR, not reported; po, oral; ip, intraperitoneal; wk, week; mo, month; d, day

peripheral blood lymphocytes to a modest but significant extent in the absence of metabolic activation.

A significant increase in the frequency of alkali-labile DNA lesions was detected by means of the comet assay in liver and spleen, but not in kidney, lung or bone marrow, of mice given a single intraperitoneal dose of *para*-dichlorobenzene. A dose-dependent increase in the frequency of micronucleated polychromatic erythrocytes was detected in the bone marrow of male mice after intraperitoneal injection of two equal doses of *para*-dichlorobenzene, but no response was found in another study in mice of each sex; moreover, no significant increase in the frequency of micronucleated peripheral blood reticulocytes was seen in male mice given oral or intraperitoneal doses, and no increase in the frequency of chromosomal abnormalities was detected in bone-marrow cells of rats after single or multiple exposures to *para*-dichlorobenzene by inhalation.

para-Dichlorobenzene did not induce unscheduled DNA synthesis in mouse hepatocytes or rat kidney cells after single oral doses comparable to the daily doses given in carcinogenicity assays conducted with this chemical (see section 3).

para-Dichlorobenzene did not induce dominant lethal mutations at any maturation stage of the eight-week spermatogenic cycle of mice.

Covalent binding of [^{14}C]*para*-dichlorobenzene to calf thymus DNA was detected *in vitro* after incubation with various subcellular fractions of liver from induced mice. After intraperitoneal injection of [^{14}C]*para*-dichlorobenzene, DNA, RNA and protein adducts were detected in liver, lung, kidney and stomach of male mice but not male rats. Studies of the interaction of *para*-dichlorobenzene with calf thymus DNA *in vitro* indicated that microsomal mixed-function oxidases and microsomal glutathione tranferases are involved in its metabolic activation.

4.5 Mechanistic considerations

4.5.1 *Renal tumours in male rats*

The criteria for establishing that an agent causes renal tumours in male rats through a response associated with α_{2u}-globulin (Capen *et al.*, 1999) are as follows:

- lack of genotoxic activity (the agent and/or a metabolite) on the basis of an overall evaluation of results obtained *in vitro* and *in vivo*;
- nephropathy and renal tumorigenicity seen only in male rats;
- induction in shorter studies of the characteristic sequence of histopathological changes, of which protein droplet accumulation is obligatory;
- identification of the protein that accumulates in tubular cells as α_{2u}-globulin;
- reversible binding of the chemical metabolite to α_{2u}-globulin;
- induction of a sustained increase in cell proliferation in the renal cortex; and
- similarities between the dose–response relationship for tumour outcome with those for histopathological end-points (protein droplets, α_{2u}-globulin accumulation, cell proliferation).

The results of several 13-week studies in male and female rats showed that *para*-dichlorobenzene causes renal damage characterized by tubular degeneration and necrosis in male rats but no adverse effects in female rats. Necrosis in single tubular cells and dilated tubules with granular cast formation were seen in the outer zone of the medulla in male rats. In male Fischer 344 rats, *para*-dichlorobenzene increased the number of protein droplets that stained for α_{2u}-globulin. In contrast, in NCI-Black Reiter rats, which do not synthesize α_{2u}-globulin, *para*-dichlorobenzene did not increase the number of protein droplets.

para-Dichlorobenzene and its metabolite 2,5-dichlorophenol bound to α_{2u}-globulin isolated from *para*-dichlorobenzene-treated male rats; the binding was found to be reversible. *In vitro*, *para*-dichlorobenzene and 2,5-dichlorophenol competed with 2,4,4-trimethyl-2-pentanol for binding to α_{2u}-globulin (Borghoff *et al.*, 1991). Binding of 2,5-dichlorophenol, but not *para*-dichlorobenzene, to α_{2u}-globulin *in vitro* reduced the rate of lysosomal degradation relative to the native protein (Lehman-McKeeman *et al.*, 1990).

A number of studies showed that *para*-dichlorobenzene increases cell proliferation in the renal cortex of male, but not female, rats. This increased cell proliferation is sustained during up to 13 weeks of administration of the chemical. Increased protein droplet accumulation and renal-cell proliferation were observed at a concentration that causes renal tumours in male rats.

para-Dichlorobenzene, but not *ortho*-dichlorobenzene, induces renal tumours specifically in male rats. There is substantial evidence that *para*-dichlorobenzene induces these tumours through an α_{2u}-globulin-associated response. Although *para*-dichlorobenzene does not bind to DNA in the male rat kidney, there is weak evidence that it binds to DNA in several tissues in treated mice. Both *ortho*- and *para*-dichlorobenzene have been reported to bind to proteins and DNA in the same mouse tissues. No attempt was made to isolate any DNA adducts. The data available on the genotoxicity of *para*-dichlorobenzene and *ortho*-dichlorobenzene also do not allow any distinction to be made between these two compounds, which differ significantly in their tumorigenicity: *ortho*-dichlorobenzene does not cause tumours, whereas *para*-dichlorobenzene causes liver tumours in mice and kidney tumours in male rats. Overall, the data on genotoxicity do not support a mechanism for renal-cell tumour induction in rats involving direct interaction of *para*-dichlorobenzene with DNA. Therefore, the overall data, including those on genotoxicity, indicate that *para*-dichlorobenzene causes renal tumours in male rats through an α_{2u}-globulin associated response.

4.5.2 *Hepatic tumours in mice*

para-Dichlorobenzene produces liver tumours in mice, and there is some evidence that it is genotoxic in mouse liver. *para*-Dichlorobenzene bound to purified calf thymus DNA when microsomal and cytosolic activating enzymes from mouse liver were present. *In vivo*, *para*-dichlorobenzene bound covalently to DNA fractions purified from the livers of mice that had been treated by intraperitoneal injection; however, the amount of binding was low (covalent binding index, 14). DNA adducts were not identified in other tests, such as ^{32}P-postlabelling. DNA damage was seen in mouse liver in two further assays. Overall, the data preclude a determination that a DNA-reactive mechanism is operative in the formation of liver tumours in mice. There is evidence of enhanced cell proliferation in mouse liver, but this proliferative response was also present in rats.

5. Summary of Data Reported and Evaluation

5.1 Exposure data

Dichlorobenzenes are chemical intermediates used widely in the manufacture of dyes, pesticides and various industrial products. *ortho*-Dichlorobenzene is further used as a solvent and an insecticide. *para*-Dichlorobenzene is used widely as a moth repellent and an air deodorizer and also as a pesticide.

Occupational exposure to dichlorobenzenes may occur during their manufacture and use, at levels reaching up to a few hundred milligrams per cubic meter in the case of *para*-dichlorobenzene. *ortho*-Dichlorobenzene and *para*-dichlorobenzene are found in ambient air at levels usually below 1 μg/m^3; in indoor air, *para*-dichlorobenzene is typically found at a level an order of magnitude higher. These two isomers have been detected in some drinking-water supplies at levels usually below 1 μg/L and in some foods at levels up to 10 μg/kg. Concentrations of 5–30 μg/kg *ortho*- and *para*-dichlorobenzene have been reported in human milk.

meta-Dichlorobenzene is produced in smaller quantities than the *ortho* and *para* isomers and is used primarily as a chemical intermediate. The data on exposure to this chemical are limited.

5.2 Human carcinogenicity data

In a cohort study from the United States, no association was observed between occupational exposure to *ortho*-dichlorobenzene and mortality from multiple myeloma or non-Hodgkin lymphoma; however, the risk estimates were based on exceedingly few observations.

5.3 Animal carcinogenicity data

ortho-Dichlorobenzene was tested by oral administration in one well-conducted study in mice and one well-conducted study in rats. No increased incidence of tumours was observed.

meta-Dichlorobenzene has not been adequately tested for potential carcinogenicity in laboratory animals.

para-Dichlorobenzene was tested by oral administration and inhalation in mice and rats. After oral administration, it increased the incidence of adenomas and carcinomas of the liver in male and female mice and of renal tubular carcinomas in male rats. Studies in mice and rats exposed by inhalation were judged to be inadequate. *para*-Dichlorobenzene did not promote hepatic foci in a two-stage model of carcinogenesis in rats.

5.4 Other relevant data

No data were available on the absorption, distribution, metabolism or excretion of *ortho-*, *meta-* or *para-*dichlorobenzene in humans.

The major route of biotransformation of *ortho-*dichlorobenzene in male rats was via the glutathione pathway; most of the urinary metabolites were mercapturic acids. Other metabolites were conjugates of 2,3- and 3,4-dichlorophenol. A high dose of *ortho-*dichlorobenzene results in depletion of glutathione. The major metabolite of *para-*dichlorobenzene is 2,5-dichlorophenol. After administration of a high oral dose of *para-*dichlorobenzene to male rats, dichlorohydroquinone was identified in the urine only after acid hydrolysis.

No data were available to evaluate the toxicity of *meta-*dichlorobenzene in humans. Occupational exposure to *ortho-* and *para-*dichlorobenzene caused ocular irritation; *ortho-*dichlorobenzene also caused irritation in the upper respiratory tract.

*para-*Dichlorobenzene was reported to be hepatotoxic at doses of 600 mg/kg bw and higher in rats. *ortho-*Dichlorobenzene was found to be a more potent hepatotoxicant in rats than *para-*dichlorobenzene. *para-*Dichlorobenzene was reported to cause a mitogenic response in both mouse and rat liver under the dosing conditions used in the cancer bioassay.

*para-*Dichlorobenzene causes male rat-specific nephrotoxicity resulting from accumulation of the male rat-specific protein α_{2u}-globulin. Both *para-*dichlorobenzene and its major metabolite, 2,5-dichlorophenol, bind reversibly to α_{2u}-globulin. *para-*Dichlorobenzene causes sustained cell proliferation in proximal renal tubular cells, and the dose–response relationships for tumour outcome, enhanced cell proliferation and other histopathological end-points typical of α_{2u}-globulin nephropathy are similar. Female rats, male rats of strains that do not express this protein and mice are not susceptible to the nephrotoxic action of *para-*dichlorobenzene.

*ortho-*Dichlorobenzene did not cause developmental toxicity in rats or rabbits exposed by inhalation during gestation. After administration by gavage to rats during gestation, decreased fetal growth and an increased incidence of extra ribs were observed. *para-*Dichlorobenzene did not cause developmental toxicity in rabbits exposed during gestation.

A statistically significant, fourfold increase in the frequency of persistent chromosomal aberrations was observed in peripheral blood lymphocytes of individuals accidentally exposed to *ortho-*dichlorobenzene. No data were available on the genetic and related effects of *meta-*dichlorobenzene or *para-*dichlorobenzene in humans.

*ortho-*Dichlorobenzene induced micronuclei in the bone marrow of mice treated *in vivo*. Radiolabelled *ortho-*dichlorobenzene was found to bind covalently to DNA, RNA and proteins of the liver, kidney, lung and stomach of treated rats and mice. It bound to DNA *in vitro* in the presence but not in the absence of metabolic activation. It was mutagenic to yeast and fungi but not to bacteria.

*meta-*Dichlorobenzene increased the frequency of micronuclei in the bone marrow of mice treated *in vivo*. It caused gene conversion in yeast. It was not mutagenic to bacteria but gave contradictory results with respect to DNA damage.

para-Dichlorobenzene bound to DNA in liver, lung and kidney of mice but not of male rats. It induced DNA damage in liver and spleen but not in kidney, lung or bone marrow of mice. No conclusion can be drawn from the few data on genotoxicity *in vivo*. There is weak evidence for the genotoxicity of *para*-dichlorobenzene in mammalian cells *in vitro*. It was not mutagenic to bacteria. Overall, the results of tests for genotoxicity do not support a mechanism for renal-cell tumour induction in male rats that involves a direct interaction between *para*-dichlorobenzene or its metabolites and DNA.

5.5 Evaluation

There is *inadequate evidence* in humans for the carcinogenicity of dichlorobenzenes.

There is *evidence suggesting lack of carcinogenicity* in experimental animals of *ortho*-dichlorobenzene.

There is *inadequate evidence* in experimental animals for the carcinogenicity of *meta*-dichlorobenzene.

There is *sufficient evidence* in experimental animals for the carcinogenicity of *para*-dichlorobenzene.

Overall evaluation

In making its overall evaluation of the carcinogenicity of *para*-dichlorobenzene to humans, the Working Group concluded that *para*-dichlorobenzene produces renal tubular tumours in male rats by a non-DNA-reactive mechanism, through an α_{2u}-globulin-associated response. Therefore, the mechanism by which *para*-dichlorobenzene increases the incidence of renal tubular tumours in male rats is not relevant to humans.

para-Dichlorobenzene caused a high incidence of liver tumours in male and female mice. Supporting evidence that its mechanism of carcinogenesis may be relevant for humans includes evidence that it causes DNA damage in liver and spleen of mice and weakly binds to DNA in mouse liver.

ortho-Dichlorobenzene is *not classifiable as to its carcinogenicity to humans (Group 3).*

meta-Dichlorobenzene is *not classifiable as to its carcinogenicity to humans (Group 3).*

para-Dichlorobenzene is *possibly carcinogenic to humans (Group 2B).*

6. References

Agency for Toxic Substances and Disease Registry (1997) *Toxicological Profile for 1,4-Dichlorobenzene (Update)* (PB/93/182459/AS), Research Triangle Park, NC

Albrecht, W.N. (1980) *Health Hazard Evaluation Report, PPG Industries/Natrium Plant, New Martinsville, West Virginia* (HE 80-082-773), Cincinnati, OH, Hazard Evaluations and Technical Assistance Branch, National Institute for Occupational Safety and Health

American Conference of Governmental Industrial Hygienists (ACGIH) (1991) *Documentation of the Threshold Limit Values and Biological Exposure Indices*, 6th Ed., Vol. 1, Cincinnati, OH

American Conference of Governmental Industrial Hygienists (ACGIH) (1997) *1997 TLVs® and BEIs®*, Cincinnati, OH, p. 21

American Conference of Governmental Industrial Hygienists (ACGIH) (1998) *TLVs and Other Occupational Exposure Values—1998 CD-ROM*, Cincinnati, OH

Andersen, K.J., Leighty, E.G. & Takahashi, M.T. (1972) Evaluation of herbicides for possible mutagenic properties. *J. agric. Food Chem.*, **20**, 649–656

Azouz, W.M., Parke, D.V. & Williams, R.T. (1955) Studies in detoxication. 62. The metabolism of halogenobenzenes. *ortho-* and *para-*Dichlorobenzenes. *Biochem. J.*, **59**, 410–415

Barkley, J., Bunch, J., Bursey, J.T., Castillo, N., Cooper, S.D., Davis, J.M., Erickson, M.D., Harris, B.S.H., III, Kirkpatrick, M., Michael, L.C., Parks, S.P., Pellizzari, E.D., Ray, M., Smith, D., Tomer, K.B., Wagner, R. & Zweidinger, R.A. (1980) Gas chromatography mass spectrometry computer analysis of volatile halogenated hydrocarbons in man and his environment—A multimedia environmental study. *Biomed. mass Spectrom.*, **7**, 139–147

Beck, U. (1986) Chlorinated hydrocarbons: Chlorinated benzenes. In: Gerhartz, W. & Yamamoto, Y.S., eds, *Ullmann's Encyclopedia of Industrial Chemistry*, 5th Ed., Vol. A6, New York, VCH Publishers, pp. 330–340

den Besten, C., Vet, J.J.R.M., Besselink, H.T., Kiel, G.S., van Berkel, B.J.M, Beems, R. & van Bladeren, P.J. (1991) The liver, kidney, and thyroid toxicity of chlorinated benzenes. *Toxicol. appl. Pharmacol.*, **111**, 69–81

den Besten, C., Ellenbroek, M., van der Ree, M.A.E., Rietjens, I.M. & van Bladeren, P.J. (1992) The involvement of primary and secondary metabolism in the covalent binding of 1,2- and 1,4-dichlorobenzenes. *Chem.-biol. Interactions*, **84**, 259–275

Bomhard, E., Luckhaus, G., Voigt, W.H. & Loeser, E. (1988) Induction of light hydrocarbon nephropathy by *p*-dichlorobenzene. *Arch. Toxicol.*, **61**, 433–439

Borghoff, S.J., Miller, A.B., Bowen, J.P. & Swenberg, J.A. (1991) Characteristics of chemical binding to α_{2u}-globulin in vitro—Evaluating structure–activity relationships. *Toxicol. appl. Pharmacol.*, **107**, 228–238

Bristol, P.W., Crist, H.L., Lewis, R.G., Macleod, K.E. & Sovocool, G.W. (1982) Chemical analysis of human blood for assessment of environmental exposure to semivolatile organochlorine chemical contaminants. *J. anal. Toxicol.*, **6**, 269–275

Brondeau, M.T., Ban, M., Bonnet, P., Guenier, J.P. & de Ceaurriz, J. (1986) Concentration-related changes in blood and tissue parameters of hepatotoxicity and their interdependence in rats exposed to bromobenzene and 1,2-dichlorobenzene. *Toxicol. Lett.*, **31**, 159–166

Brondeau, M.T., Ban, M., Bonnet, P., Guenier, J.P. & de Ceaurriz, J. (1989) Acetone compared to other ketones in modifying the hepatotoxicity of inhaled 1,2-dichlorobenzene in rats and mice. *Toxicol. Lett.*, **49**, 69–78

Bro-Rasmussen, F. (1994) EEC water quality objectives for chemicals dangerous to aquatic environments (List 1). *Rev. environ. Contam. Toxicol.*, **137**, 83–110

Bryant, J.G. (1993) Chlorocarbons and chlorohydrocarbons: Chlorinated benzenes. In: Kroschwitz, J.I. & Howe-Grant, M., eds, *Kirk-Othmer Encyclopedia of Chemical Technology*, 4th Ed., Vol. 6, New York, John Wiley & Sons, pp. 87–100

Budavari, S., ed. (1996) *The Merck Index*, 12th Ed., Whitehouse Station, NJ, Merck & Co., p. 517

Canonero, R., Brambilla Campart, G., Mattioli, F., Robbiano, L. & Martelli, A. (1997) Testing of p-dichlorobenzene and hexachlorobenzene for their ability to induce DNA damage and micronucleus formation in primary cultures of rat and human hepatocytes. *Mutagenesis*, **12**, 35–39

Capen, C.C., Dybing, E., Rice, J.M. & Wilbourn, J.D., eds (1999) *Species Differences in Thyroid, Kidney and Urinary Bladder Carcinogenesis* (IARC Scientific Publications No. 147), Lyon, IARC

Carbonell, E., Puig, M., Xamena, N., Creus, A. & Marcos, R. (1991) Sister-chromatid exchanges (SCE) induced by p-dichlorobenzene in cultured human lymphocytes. *Mutat. Res.*, **263**, 57–59

Carlson, G.P. (1977) Chlorinated benzene induction of hepatic porphyria. *Experientia*, **33**, 1627–1629

Charbonneau, M., Strasser, J., Jr, Lock, E.A., Turner, M.J., Jr & Swenberg, J.A. (1989) Involvement of reversible binding to α_{2u}-globulin in 1,4-dichlorobenzene-induced nephrotoxicity. *Toxicol. appl. Pharmacol.*, **99**, 122–132

Chemical Information Services (1995) *Directory of World Chemical Producers 1995/96 Standard Edition*, Dallas, TX, p. 245

Chen, C.S. & Zoltek, J., Jr (1995) Organic priority pollutants in wetland-treated leachates at a landfill in central Florida. *Chemosphere*, **31**, 3455–3464

Cohen, J.M., Dawson R. & Koketsu, M. (1981) *Extent of Exposure Survey of Monochlorobenzene* (Publication No. 81-105), Cincinnati, OH, National Institute for Occupational Safety and Health

Colacci, A., Bartoli, S., Bonora, B., Niero, A., Silingardi, P. & Grilli, S. (1990) In vivo and in vitro interaction of 1,2-dichlorobenzene with nucleic acids and proteins of mice and rats. *Tumori*, **76**, 339–344

Davies, K. (1988) Concentrations and dietary intake of selected organochlorines, including PCBs, PCDDs and PCDFs in fresh food composites grown in Ontario, Canada. *Chemosphere*, **17**, 263–276

Dietrich, D.R. & Swenberg, J.A. (1991) NCI-Black-Reiter (NBR) male rats fail to develop renal disease following exposure to agents that induce alpha-2u-globulin (α_{2u}) nephropathy. *Fundam. appl. Toxicol.*, **16**, 749–762

Eldridge, S.R., Tilbury, L.F., Goldsworthy, T.L. & Butterworth, B.E. (1990) Measurement of chemically induced cell proliferation in rodent liver and kidney: A comparison of 5-bromo-2′-deoxyuridine and [^{3}H]thymidine administered by injection or osmotic pump. *Carcinogenesis*, **11**, 2245–2251

Eldridge, S.R., Goldsworthy, T.L., Popp, J.A. & Butterworth, B.E. (1992) Mitogenic stimulation of hepatocellular proliferation in rodents following 1,4-dichlorobenzene administration. *Carcinogenesis*, **13**, 409–415

Eller, P.M., ed. (1994) Method 1003: Hydrocarbons, halogenated. In: *NIOSH Manual of Analytical Methods (NMAM)* (DHHS (NIOSH) Publication No. 94-113), 4th Ed., Cincinnati, OH, National Institute for Occupational Safety and Health

Environmental Protection Agency (1979) Guidelines establishing test procedures for the analysis of pollutants; proposed regulations. *Fed. Reg.*, **44**, 69464–69525

Environmental Protection Agency (1980) *Ambient Water Quality Criteria for Dichlorobenzenes* (EPA 440/5-80-039; NTIS PB 81-117509), Washington DC, Office of Water Regulations and Standards

Environmental Protection Agency (1984) *In Vitro and In Vivo Mutagenicity Studies of Environmental Chemicals* (EPA-600/1-84-003; NTIS Report PB84-138973), Washington DC

Environmental Protection Agency (1985) *Health Assessment Document for Chlorinated Benzenes. Final Report* (EPA/600/8-84/015F; NTIS PB 85-150-332), Washington DC, Office of Health and Environment Assessment

Environmental Protection Agency (1988) *National Ambient Volatile Organic Compounds (VOCs). Data Base Update* (EPA /600/3-88/01a; NTIS PB 88-195-631), Research Triangle Park, NC, Office of Research and Development

Environmental Protection Agency (1991) Method 503.1. Volatile aromatic and unsaturated organic compounds in water by purge and trap gas chromatography [Rev. 2.0]. In: *Methods for the Determination of Organic Compounds in Drinking Water* (EPA Report No. EPA-600/4-88/039: US NTIS PB91-231480), Cincinnati, OH, Environmental Monitoring Systems Laboratory, pp. 63–108

Environmental Protection Agency (1994a) Method 8121. Chlorinated hydrocarbons by gas chromatography: Capillary column technique [Rev. 0]. In: *Test Methods for Evaluating Solid Waste—Physical/Chemical Methods* (US EPA No. SW-846), Washington DC, Office of Solid Waste

Environmental Protection Agency (1994b) Method 8410. Gas chromatography/Fourier transform infrared (GC/FT-IR) spectrometry for semivolatile organics: Capillary column. [Rev. 0]. In: *Test Methods for Evaluating Solid Waste—Physical/Chemical Methods* (US EPA No. SW-846), Washington DC, Office of Solid Waste

Environmental Protection Agency (1995a) Method 502.2. Volatile organic compounds in water by purge and trap capillary column gas chromatography with photoionization and electrolytic conductivity detectors in series [Rev. 2.1]. In: *Methods for the Determination of Organic Compounds in Drinking Water, Supplement III* (EPA Report No. EPA-600/R-95/131; US NTIS PB95-261616), Cincinnati, OH, Environmental Monitoring Systems Laboratory

Environmental Protection Agency (1995b) Method 524.2—Measurement of purgeable organic compounds in water by capillary column gas chromatography/mass spectrometry [Rev. 4.1]. In: *Methods for the Determination of Organic Compounds in Drinking Water, Supplement III* (EPA Report No. EPA-600/R-95/131; US NTIS PB95-261616), Cincinnati, OH, Environmental Monitoring Systems Laboratory

Environmental Protection Agency (1996a) Method 8270C. Semivolatile organic compounds by gas chromatography/mass spectrometry (GC/MS) [Rev. 3]. In: *Test Methods for Evaluating Solid Waste—Physical/Chemical Methods*, (US EPA No. SW-846), Washington DC, Office of Solid Waste

Environmental Protection Agency (1996b) Method 8021B. Aromatic and halogenated volatiles by gas chromatography using photoionization and/or electrolytic conductivity detectors [Rev. 2]. In: *Test Methods for Evaluating Solid Waste—Physical/Chemical Method* (US EPA No. SW-846), Washington DC, Office of Solid Waste

Environmental Protection Agency (1996c) Method 8260B. Volatile organic compounds by gas chromatography/mass spectrometry (GC/MS) [Rev. 2]. In: *Test Methods for Evaluating Solid Waste—Physical/Chemical Methods* (US EPA No. SW-846), Washington DC, Office of Solid Waste

Environmental Protection Agency (1996d) *1994 Toxins Release Inventory (EPA/45-R96-002)*, Washington DC, p. 242

Environmental Protection Agency (1997a) Methods for organic chemical analysis of municipal and industrial wastewater. Method 601—Purgeable halocarbons. *US Code fed. Regul.*, **Title 40**, Part 136, App. A, pp. 29–43

Environmental Protection Agency (1997b) Methods for organic chemical analysis of municipal and industrial wastewater. Method 602—Purgeable aromatics. *US Code fed. Regul.*, **Title 40**, Part 136, App. A, pp. 44–55

Environmental Protection Agency (1997c) Methods for organic chemical analysis of municipal and industrial wastewater. Method 612—Chlorinated hydrocarbons. *US Code fed. Regul.*, **Title 40**, Part 136, App. A, pp. 169–179

Environmental Protection Agency (1997d) Methods for organic chemical analysis of municipal and industrial wastewater. Method 625—Base/neutrals and acids. *US Code fed. Regul.*, **Title 40**, Part 136, App. A, pp. 204–231

Environmental Protection Agency (1997e) Methods for organic chemical analysis of municipal and industrial wastewater. Method 1625B—Semivolatile organic compounds by isotope dilution GC/MS. *US Code fed. Regul.*, **Title 40**, Part 136, App. A, pp. 245–264

Environmental Protection Agency (1998a) *Drinking Water and Health, National Primary Drinking Water Regulations, Technical Factsheet on o-Dichlorobenzene*, Washington DC, Office of Ground Water and Drinking Water [http://www.epa.gov/OGWDW/dwh/t-voc/o-dichlo.html]

Environmental Protection Agency (1998b) *Drinking Water and Health, National Primary Drinking Water Regulations, Technical Factsheet on p-Dichlorobenzene*, Washington DC, Office of Ground Water and Drinking Water [http://www.epa.gov/OGWDW/dwh/t-voc/p-dichlo.html]

European Communities (1976a) Council Directive 76/464. *Off. J. Eur. Comm.*, **L 129**, 23

European Communities (1976b) Communication from the Commission to the Council on dangerous substances which might be included in List 1 of Council Directive 76/464. *Off. J. Eur. Comm.*, **C176**, 3

Fairhurst, S., Girling, G. & White, J. (1994) *1,4-Dichlorobenzene. Criteria Document for an Occupational Exposure Limit*, London, Health and Safety Executive

Fellin, P. & Otson, R. (1994) Assessment of the influence of climatic factors on concentration levels of volatile compounds (VOCs) in Canadian homes. *Atmos. Environ.*, **28**, 3581–3586

Galloway, S.M., Armstrong, M.J., Reuben, C., Colman, S., Brown, B., Cannon, C., Bloom, A.D., Nakamura, F., Ahmed, M., Duk, S., Rimpo, J., Margolin, B.H., Resnick, M.A., Anderson, B. & Zeiger, E. (1987) Chromosome aberrations and sister chromatid exchanges in Chinese hamster ovary cells: Evaluations of 108 chemicals. *Environ. mol. Mutag.*, **10**, 1–175

German Chemical Society (1987) *m-Dichlorobenzene* (BUA Report 8), Stuttgart, GDCh-Advisory Committee on Existing Chemicals of Environmental Relevance (BUA), Stuttgart, S. Hirzel-Wissenschaftliche Verlagsgesellschaft

German Chemical Society (1990) *o-Dichlorobenzene* (BUA Report 53), Stuttgart, GDCh-Advisory Committee on Existing Chemicals of Environmental Relevance (BUA), Stuttgart, S. Hirzel-Wissenschaftliche Verlagsgesellschaft

Ghittori, S., Imbriani, M., Pezzagno, G. & Capodaglio, E. (1985) Urinary elimination of p-dichlorobenzene (p-DCB) and weighted exposure concentration. *G. ital. Med. Lav.*, **7**, 59–63

Giavini, E., Broccia, M.L., Prati, M. & Vismara, C. (1986) Teratologic evaluation of *p*-dichlorobenzene in the rat. *Bull. environ. Contam. Toxicol.*, **37**, 164–168

Government of Canada (1993a) *Priority Substances List Assessment Report: 1,4-Dichlorobenzene*, Ottawa, Canada Communication Group

Government of Canada (1993b) *Priority Substances List Assessment Report: 1,2-Dichlorobenzene*, Ottawa, Canada Communication Group

Guicherit, R & Schulting, F.L. (1985) The occurrence of organic chemicals in the atmosphere of the Netherlands. *Sci. total Environ.*, **43**, 193–219

Gunawardhana, L. & Sipes, I.G. (1991) Dichlorobenzene hepatotoxicity strain differences and structure activity relationships. *Adv. exp. Med. Biol.*, **283**, 731–734

Gunawardhana, L., Mobley, S.A. & Sipes, I.G. (1993) Modulation of 1,2-dichlorobenzene hepatotoxicity in the Fischer-344 rat by a scavenger of superoxide anions and an inhibitor of Kupffer cells. *Toxicol. appl. Pharmacol.*, **119**, 205–213

Gustafson, D.L., Coulson, A.L., Feng, L., Pott, W.A., Thomas, R.S., Chubb, L.S., Saghir, S.A., Benjamin, S.A. & Yang, R.S. (1998) Use of a medium-term liver focus bioassay to assess the hepatocarcinogenicity of 1,2,4,5-tetrachlorobenzene and 1,4-dichlorobenzene. *Cancer Lett.*, **129**, 39–44

Hallowell, M. (1959) Acute haemolytic anaemia following the ingestion of para-dichlorobenzene. *Arch. Dis. Child.*, **34**, 74–75

Hansch, C., Leo, A. & Hoekman, D. (1995) *Exploring QSAR: Hydrophobic, Electronic, and Steric Constants*, Washington DC, American Chemical Society, p. 17

Harden, R.A. & Baetjer, A.M. (1978) Aplastic anemia following exposure to paradichlorobenzene and naphthalene. *J. occup. Med.*, **20**, 820–822

Harkov, R., Kebbekus, B., Bozzelli, J.W & Lioy, P.J. (1983) Measurement of selected volatile organic compounds at three locations in New Jersey during the summer season. *J. Air Pollut. Control Assoc.*, **33**, 1177–1183

Harkov, R., Gianti, S.J., Bozzelli, J.W. & La Regina, J.E. (1985) Monitoring volatile organic compounds at hazardous and sanitary landfills in New Jersey. *J. environ. Sci. Health*, **A20**, 491–501

Hasmall, S.C., Pyrah, I.T.G., Soames, A.R. & Roberts, R.A. (1997) Expression of the immediate early genes c-*fos*, c-*jun* and c-*myc*: A comparison in rats of nongenotoxic hepatocarcinogens with noncarcinogenic liver mitogens. *Fundam. appl. Toxicol.*, **40**, 129–137

Hawkins, D.R., Chasseaud, L.F., Woodhouse, R.N. & Cresswell, D.G. (1980) The distribution, excretion and biotransformation of *p*-dichloro[^{14}C]benzene in rats after repeated inhalation, oral and subcutaneous doses. *Xenobiotica*, **10**, 81–95

Haworth, S., Lawlor, T., Mortelmans, K., Speck, W. & Zeiger, E. (1983) Salmonella mutagenicity test results for 250 chemicals. *Environ. Mutag.*, **5** (Suppl. 1), 3–142

Hayes, W.C., Hanley, T.R., Jr, Gushow, T.S., Johnson, K.A. & John, J.A. (1985) Teratogenic potential of inhaled dichlorobenzene in rats and rabbits. *Fundam. appl. Toxicol.*, **5**, 190–202

Hill, R.H., Jr, Ashley, D.L., Head, S.L., Needham, L.L. & Pirkle, J.L. (1995) p-Dichlorobenzene exposure among 1000 adults in the United States. *Arch. environ. Health*, **50**, 277–280

Hissink, A.M., van Ommen, B. & van Bladeren, P.J. (1996a) Dose-dependent kinetics and metabolism of 1,2-dichlorobenzene in rat: Effect of pretreatment with phenobarbital. *Xenobiotica*, **26**, 89–105

Hissink, A.M., Oudshoorn, M.J., van Ommen, B., Haenen, G.R.M.M. & van Bladeren, P.J. (1996b) Differences in cytochrome P450-mediated biotransformation of 1,2- dichlorobenzene by rat and man: Implications for human risk assessment. *Chem. Res. Toxicol.*, **9**, 1249–1256

Hissink, A.M., Dunnewijk, R., van Ommen, B. & van Bladeren, P.J. (1997a) Kinetics and metabolism of 1,4-dichlorobenzene in male Wistar rats: No evidence for quinone metabolites. *Chem.-biol. Interactions*, **103**, 17–33

Hissink, A.M., Oudshoorn, M.J., van Ommen, B. & van Bladeren, P.J. (1997b) Species and strain differences in the hepatic cytochrome P450-mediated biotransformation of 1,4-dichlorobenzene. *Toxicol. appl. Pharmacol.*, **145**, 1–9

Hissink, A.M., van Ommen, B., Krüse, J. & van Bladeren, P.J. (1997c) A physiologically based pharmacokinetic (PB-PK) model for 1,2-dichlorobenzene linked to two possible parameters of toxicity. *Toxicol. appl. Pharmacol.*, **145**, 301–310

Hollingsworth, R.L., Rowe, V.K., Oyen, F., Torkelson, T.R. & Adams, E.M. (1958) Toxicity of *o*-dichlorobenzene. *Arch. ind. Health*, **17**, 180–187

IARC (1982) *IARC Monographs on the Evaluation of the Carcinogenic Risk of Chemicals to Humans,* Vol. 29, *Some Industrial Chemicals and Dyestuffs*, Lyon, pp. 213–238

IARC (1987) *IARC Monographs on the Evaluation of Carcinogenic Risks to Humans*, Suppl. 7, *Overall Evaluations of Carcinogenicity: An Updating of* IARC Monographs *Volumes 1 to 42*, Lyon, pp. 192–193

International Labour Office (1991) *Occupational Exposure Limits for Airborne Toxic Substances*, 3rd. Ed. (Occupational Safety and Health Series No. 37), Geneva, pp. 138–139

International Trade Commission (1993) *Synthetic Organic Chemicals, US Production and Sales*, 77th Ed., Washington DC, United States Government Printing Office, p. 3-22

Jacobs, L.W. & Zabik, M.J. (1983) Importance of sludge-borne organic chemicals for land application programs. In: *Proceedings of the 6th Annual Madison Conference on Application Residue Practices. Municipal and Industrial Wastes*, Madison, WI, University of Wisconsin, pp. 418–426

Jan, J. (1980) Chlorinated benzene residues in some seeds. *Chemosphere*, **9**, 165–167

Jan, J. (1983a) Chlorobenzene residues in market milk and meat. *Mitt. Geb. Lebensm. Hyg.*, **74**, 420–425

Jan, J. (1983b) Chlorobenzene residues in human fat and milk. *Bull. environ. Contam. Toxicol.*, **30**, 595–599

Jay, K. & Stieglitz, l. (1995) Identification and quantification of volatile organic components in emissions of waste incineration plants. *Chemosphere*, **30**, 1249–1260

Kato, Y. & Kimura, R. (1997) Role of 3,4-dichlorophenyl methyl sulfone, a metabolite of o-dichlorobenzene, in the changes in hepatic microsomal drug-metabolizing enzymes caused by o-dichlorobenzene administration in rats. *Toxicol. appl. Pharmacol.*, **145**, 277–284

Kitchin, K.T., Brown, J.L. & Kulkarni, A.P. (1993) Predicting rodent carcinogenicity of halogenated hydrocarbons by in vivo biochemical parameters. *Teratog. Carcinog. Mutag.*, **13**, 167–184

Klos, C. & Dekant, W. (1994) Comparative metabolism of the renal carcinogen 1,4-dichlorobenzene in rat: Identification and quantitation of novel metabolites. *Xenobiotica*, **24**, 965–976

Kostianinen, R. (1995) Volatile organic compounds in the indoor air of normal and sick houses. *Atmos. Environ.*, **29**, 693–702

Krost, K.J., Pellizzari, E.D., Walburn, S.G. & Hubbard, S.A. (1982) Collection and analysis of hazardous organic emissions. *Anal. Chem.*, **54**, 810–817

Kulkarni, S.G., Duong, H., Gomila, R. & Mehendale, H.M. (1996) Strain differences in tissue repair response to 1,2-dichlorobenzene. *Arch. Toxicol.*, **70**, 714–723

Kumagai, S. & Matsunaga, I. (1997a) Relations between exposure to *o*-dichlorobenzene and concentrations of urinary metabolites. *J. occup. Health*, **39**, 124–129

Kumagai, S. & Matsunaga, I. (1997b) Quantitative determination of urinary metabolites of *o*-dichlorobenzene using a gas chromatograph. *Ind. Health*, **35**, 399–403

Lake, B.G., Cunninghame, M.E. & Price, R.J. (1997) Comparison of the hepatic and renal effects of 1,4-dichlorobenzene in the rat and mouse. *Fundam. appl. Toxicol.*, **39**, 67–75

Lattanzi, G., Bartoli, S., Bonora, B., Colacci, A., Grilli, S., Niero, A. & Mazzullo, M. (1989) The different genotoxicity of p-dichlorobenzene in mouse and rat: Measurement of the in vivo and in vitro covalent interaction with nucleic acids. *Tumori*, **75**, 305–310

Lehmann-McKeeman, L.D., Rivera-Torres, M.I. & Caudill, D. (1990) Lysosomal degradation of α_{2u}-globulin and α_{2u}-globulin–xenobiotic conjugates. *Toxicol. appl. Pharmacol.*, **103**, 539–548

Lide, D.R., ed. (1997) *CRC Handbook of Chemistry and Physics*, 78th Ed., Boca Raton, FL, CRC Press, p. 3-39

Loeser, E. & Litchfield, M.H. (1983) Review of recent toxicology studies on *p*-dichlorobenzene. *Food chem. Toxicol.*, **21**, 825–832

Meek, M.E., Newhook, R., Liteplo, R.G. & Armstrong, V.C. (1994a) Approach to assessment of risk to human health for priority substances under the Canadian Environmental Protection Act. *Environ. Carcinog. Ecotoxicol. Rev.*, **C12**, 105–134

Meek, M.E., Giddings, M. & Gomes, R. (1994b) 1,2-Dichlorobenzene: Evaluation of risks to health from environmental exposure in Canada. *Environ. Carcinog. Ecotoxicol. Rev.*, **C12**, 269–275

Meek, M.E., Giddings, M. & Gomes, R. (1994c) 1,4-Dichlorobenzene: Evaluation of risks to health from environmental exposure in Canada. *Environ. Carcinog. Ecotoxicol. Rev.*, **C12**, 277–285

Mes, J., Davies, D.J., Turton, D. & Sun, W.-F. (1986) Levels and trends of chlorinated hydrocarbon contaminants in the breast milk of Canadian women. *Food Addit. Contam.*, **3**, 313–322

Mohtashamipur, E., Triebel, R., Straeter, H. & Norpoth, K. (1987) The bone marrow clastogenicity of eight halogenated benzenes in male NMRI mice. *Mutagenesis*, **2**, 111–113

Morita, T., Asano, N., Awogi, T., Sasaki, Y.F., Sato, S., Shimada, H., Sutou, S., Suzuki, T., Wakata, A., Sofuni, T. & Hayashi, M. (1997) Evaluation of the rodent micronucleus assay in the screening of IARC carcinogens (Groups 1, 2A and 2B). The summary report of the 6th collaborative study by CSGMT/JEMS-MMS. *Mutat. Res.*, **389**, 3–122

National Institute for Occupational Safety and Health (1978a) *Occupational Health Guideline for o-Dichlorobenzene*, Cincinnati, OH

National Institute for Occupational Safety and Health (1978b) *Occupational Health Guideline for p-Dichlorobenzene*, Cincinnati, OH

National Institute for Occupational Safety and Health (1998) *National Occupational Exposure Survey (1981–1983)*, Cincinnati, OH

National Library of Medicine (1998) *Toxic Chemical Release Inventory 1994* (TRI94), Bethesda, MD

National Toxicology Program (1985) *Toxicology and Carcinogenesis Studies of 1,2-Dichlorobenzene (o-Dichlorobenzene) (CAS No. 95-50-1) in F344/N rats and B6C3F$_1$ Mice (Gavage Studies)* (Tech. Rep. Ser. No. 255; NIH Publ. No. 86-2511), Research Triangle Park, NC

National Toxicology Program (1987) *Toxicology and Carcinogenesis Studies of 1,4-Dichlorobenzene (CAS No. 106-46-7) in F344/N Rats and B6C3F$_1$ Mice (Gavage Studies)* (Tech. Rep. Ser. No. 319; NIH Publ. No. 87-2575), Research Triangle Park, NC

National Toxicology Program (1991a) *NTP Chemical Repository Data Sheet:* meta-*Dichlorobenzene*, Research Triangle Park, NC

National Toxicology Program (1991b) *NTP Chemical Repository Data Sheet:* ortho-*Dichlorobenzene*, Research Triangle Park, NC

National Toxicology Program (1991c) *NTP Chemical Repository Data Sheet:* para-*Dichlorobenzene*, Research Triangle Park, NC

Occupational Safety and Health Administration (1990) Method 07: Organic vapors. In: *OSHA Analytical Methods Manual*, 2nd Ed., Part 1, *Organic Substances*, Vol. 1, Salt Lake City, UT, US Department of Labor

Oliver, B.G. & Nicol, K.D. (1982) Chlorobenzenes in sediments, water and selected fish from Lakes Superior, Huron, Erie and Ontario. *Environ. Sci. Technol.*, **16**, 532–536

Oliver, B.G. & Nicol, K.D. (1984) Chlorinated contaminants in the Niagara River. *Sci. total Environ.*, **39**, 57–70

Otson, R., Williams, D.T. & Bothwell, P.D. (1982a) Volatile organic compounds in water at thirty Canadian potable water treatment facilities. *J. Assoc. off. anal. Chem.*, **65**, 1370–1374

Otson, R., Williams, D.T. & Biggs, D.C. (1982b) Relationship between raw water quality, treatment, and occurrence of organics in Canadian potable water. *Bull. environ. Contam. Toxicol.*, **28**, 396–403

Page, G.W. (1981) Comparison of ground water and surface water for patterns and levels of contamination by toxic substances. *Environ. Sci. Technol.*, **15**, 1475–1481

Page, B.D. & Lacroix, G.M. (1995) On-line steam distillation/purge and trap analysis of halogenated, non polar, volatile contaminants in foods. *J. Assoc. off. anal Chem. int.*, **78**, 1416–1428

Pagnotto, L.D. & Walkley, J.E. (1965) Urinary dichlorophenol as an index of para-dichlorobenzene exposure. *Am. ind. Hyg. Assoc. J.*, **26**, 137–142

Paolini, M., Pozzetti, L., Silingardi, P., Della Croce, C., Bronzetti, G. & Cantelli-Forti, G. (1998) Isolation of a novel metabolizing system enriched in phase-II enzymes for short-term genotoxicity bioassays. *Mutat. Res.*, **413**, 205–217

Pellizzarri, E.D. (1982) Analysis for organic vapor emissions near industrial waste disposal sites. *Environ. Sci. Technol.*, **16**, 781–785

Pellizzarri, E.D., Hartwell, T.D., Perritt, R.L., Sparacino, C.M., Sheldon, L.S., Zelon, H.S., Whitmore, R.W., Breen, J.J. & Wallace, L. (1986) Comparison of indoor and outdoor residential levels of volatile organic chemicals in five US geographical locations. *Environ. int.*, **12**, 619–623

Prasad, I. (1970) Mutagenic effecs of the herbicide 3′,4′-dichloropropionanilide and its degradation products. *Can. J. Microbiol.*, **16**, 369–372

Reid, W.D. & Krishina, C. (1973) Centrilobular hepatic necrosis related to covalent binding of metabolites of halogenated aromatic hydrocarbons. *Exp. mol. Pathol.*, **18**, 80–99

Robinson, M., Bercz, J.P., Ringhand, H.P., Condie, L.W. & Parnell, M.J. (1991) Ten- and ninety-day toxicity studies of 1,2-dichlorobenzene administered by oral gavage to Sprague-Dawley rats. *Drug chem. Toxicol.*, **14**, 83–112

Rogers, H.R. (1996) Sources, behavior and fate of organic contaminants during sewage treatment and in sewage sludges. *Sci. total Environ.*, **185**, 3–26

Rogers, H.R., Campbell, J.A., Crathorne, B. & Dobbs, A.J. (1989) The occurrence of chlorobenzenes and permethrins in twelve UK sewage sludges. *Water Res.*, **23**, 913–921

Rosenberg, C., Nylund, L., Aalto, T., Kontsas, H., Norppa, H., Jäppinen, P. & Vainio, H. (1991) Volatile organohalogen compounds from the bleaching of pulp—Occurrence and genotoxic potential in the work environment. *Chemosphere*, **23**, 1617–1628

Sadtler Research Laboratories (1980) *Standard Spectra Collection, 1980 Cumulative Index*, Philadelphia, PA

Saito, K., Uwagawa, S., Kaneko, H., Shiba, K., Tomigahara, Y. & Nakatsuka, I. (1996) α_{2u}-Globulins in the urine of male rats: A reliable indicator for α_{2u}-globulin accumulation in the kidney. *Toxicology*, **106**, 149–157

Sasaki, Y.F., Izumiyama, F., Nishidate, E., Matsusaka, N. & Tsuda, S. (1997) Detection of rodent liver carcinogen genotoxicity by the alkaline single-cell gel electrophoresis (Comet) assay in multiple mouse organs (liver, lung, spleen, kidney, and bone marrow). *Mutat. Res.*, **391**, 201–214

Schwarzenbach, R.P., Molnar-Kubica, E., Giger, W. & Wakeham, S.G. (1979) Distribution, residence time and fluxes of tetrachloroethylene and 1,4-dichlorobenzene in Lake Zurich, Switzerland. *Environ. Sci. Technol.*, **13**, 1367–1373

Sharma, A.K. & Bhattacharyya, N.K. (1956) Chromosome breakage through paradichlorobenzene treatment. *Cytologia*, **21**, 353–360

Sherman, J.H., Nair, R.S., Steinmetz, K.L., Mirsalis, J.C., Nestmann, E.R. & Barter, J.A. (1998) Evaluation of unscheduled DNA synthesis (UDS) and replicative DNA synthesis (RDS) following treatment of rats and mice with p-dichlorobenzene. *Teratog. Carcinog. Mutag.*, **18**, 309–318

Shimizu, M., Yasui, Y. & Matsumoto, N. (1983) Structural specificity of aromatic compounds with special reference to mutagenic activity in *Salmonella typhimurium*—A series of chloro- or fluoro-nitrobenzene derivatives. *Mutat. Res.*, **116**, 217–238

Singh, H.B., Salas, L.J., Smith, A.J. & Shigeishi, H. (1981) Measurements of some potentially hazardous organic chemicals in urban environments. *Atmos. Environ.*, **15**, 601–612

Spirtas, R., Stewart, P.A., Lee, J.S., Marano, D.E., Forbes, C.D., Grauman, D.J., Pettigrew, H.M., Blair, A., Hoover, R.N. & Cohen, J.L. (1991) Retrospective cohort mortality study of workers at an aircraft maintenance facility. I. Epidemiological results. *Br. J. ind. Med.*, **48**, 515–530

Srivastava, L.M. (1966) Induction of mitotic abnormalities in certain genera of *Tribe Viciae* by paradichlorobenzene. *Cytologia*, **31**, 166–171

Staples, C.A., Werner, A.F. & Hoogeheem, T.J. (1985) Assessment of priority pollutant concentrations in the United States using STORET data base. *Environ. Toxicol. Chem.*, **4**, 131–142

Stine, E.R., Gunawardhana, L. & Sipes, I.G. (1991) The acute hepatotoxicity of the isomers of dichlorobenzene in Fischer-344 and Sprague-Dawley rats: Isomer-specific and strain-specific differential toxicity. *Toxicol. appl. Pharmacol.*, **109**, 472–481

Umemura, T., Takada, K., Ogawa, Y., Kamata, E., Saito, M. & Kurokawa, Y. (1990) Sex difference in inhalation toxicity of *p*-dichlorobenzene (*p*-DCB) in rats. *Toxicol. Lett.*, **52**, 209–214

Umemura, T., Tokumo, K. & Williams, G.M. (1992) Cell proliferation induced in the kidneys and livers of rats and mice by short term exposure to the carcinogen *p*-dichlorobenzene. *Arch. Toxicol.*, **66**, 503–507

Umemura, T., Saito, M., Takagi, A. & Kurokawa, Y. (1996) Isomer-specific acute toxicity and cell proliferation in livers of B6C3F1 mice exposed to dichlorobenzene. *Toxicol. appl. Pharmacol.*, **137**, 268–274

Umemura, T., Takada, K., Schulz, C., Gebhardt, R., Kurokawa, Y. & Williams, G.M. (1998) Cell proliferation in the livers of male mice and rats exposed to the carcinogen *p*-dichlorobenzene: Evidence for thresholds. *Drug chem. Toxicol.*, **21**, 57–66

United Nations Environment Programme (1998) *UNEP Chemicals (IRPTC) Data Bank Legal File, Recommendations and Legal Mechanisms*, Geneva, World Health Organization [http:/irptc.unep.ch/irptc]

Valentovic, M.A., Ball, J.G., Anestis, D. & Madan, E. (1993) Acute hepatic and renal toxicity of dichlorobenzene isomers in Fischer 344 rats. *J. appl. Toxicol.*, **13**, 1–7

Verschueren, K. (1996) *Handbook of Environmental Data on Organic Chemicals*, 3rd Ed., New York, Van Nostrand Reinhold Co., pp. 661–670

Wallace, L.A. (1991a) Comparison of risks from outdoor and indoor exposure to toxic chemicals. *Environ. Health Perspectives*, **95**, 7–13

Wallace, L.A. (1991b) Volatile organic compounds. In: Samet, J.M. & Spengler, J.P., eds, *Indoor Air Pollution—A Health Perspective,* Baltimore, MD, Johns Hopkins Press, pp. 252–272

Wallace, L.A., Pellizzarri, E.D., Hartwell, T., Rosenzweig, M., Erikson, M., Sparacino, C. & Zelon, H.I. (1984) Personal exposure to volatile compounds. I. Direct measurements in breathing-zone air, drinking water, food, and exhaled breath. *Environ. Res.*, **33**, 293–319

Wallace, L.A., Pellizzarri, E.D., Hartwell, T.D., Sparacino, C., Whitmore, R., Sheldon, L., Zelon, H. & Perritt, R. (1987) The TEAM Study: Personal exposures to toxic substances in air, drinking water, and breath of 400 residents of New Jersey, North Carolina and North Dakota. *Environ. Res.*, **43**, 290–307

Wang, M.J., McGrath, S.P. & Jones, K.C. (1992) The chlorobenzene content of archived sewage sludges. *Sci. total Environ.*, **121**, 159–175

Wang, M.J., McGrath, S.P. & Jones, K.C. (1995) Chlorobenzenes in field soil with a history of multiple sewage sludge applications. *Environ. Sci. Technol.*, **29**, 356–362

Watson, A. & Patterson, R.L.S. (1982) Tainting of pork meat by 1,4-dichlorobenzene. *J. Sci. Food Agric.*, **33**, 103–105

Webber, M.D. & Lesage, S. (1989) Organic contaminants in Canadian municipal sludges. *Waste Manage. Res.*, **7**, 63–82

Webber, M.D., Rogers, H.R., Watts, C.D., Boxall, A.B.A., Davis, R.D. & Scoffin, R. (1996) Monitoring and prioritisation of organic contaminants in sewage sludges using specific chemical analyses and predictive, non-analytical methods. *Sci. total Environ.*, **185**, 27–44

Westrick, J.J. (1990) National surveys of volatile organic compounds in ground and surface waters. In: Ram, N.M., Christman, R.R. & Cantor, K.P., eds, *Significance and Treatment of Volatile Organic Compounds in Water Supplies*, Chelsea, MI, Lewis Publishers, pp. 103–128

Westrick, J.J., Mello, J.W. & Thomas, R.F. (1984) The groundwater supply survey. *J Am. Water Works Assoc.*, **76**, 52–59

WHO (1991) *Chlorobenzenes other than Hexachlorobenzene* (Environmental Health Criteria 128), Geneva

WHO (1993) *Guidelines for Drinking Water Quality*, 2nd Ed., Vol. 1, *Recommendations*, Geneva, pp. 69–70

Yang, K.H., Peterson, R.E. & Fujimoto, J.M. (1979) Increased bile duct-pancreatic fluid flow in benzene and halogenated benzene-treated rats. *Toxicol. appl. Pharmacol.*, **47**, 505–514

Zapata-Gayon, C., Zapata-Gayon, N. & Gonzáles-Angulo, A. (1982) Clastogenic chromosomal aberrations in 26 individuals accidentally exposed to ortho dichlorobenzene vapors in the National Medical Center in Mexico City. *Arch. environ. Health*, **37**, 231–235

Zenser, L.-P., Lang, A. & Knecht, U. (1997) *N*-Acetyl-*S*-(dichlorophenyl)cysteines as suitable biomarkers for the monitoring of occupational exposure to 1,2-dichlorobenzene. *Int. Arch. occup. environ. Health*, **69**, 252–254

HEXACHLOROBUTADIENE

This substance was considered by previous working groups, in 1978 (IARC, 1979) and 1987 (IARC, 1987). Since that time, new data have become available, and these have been incorporated into the monograph and taken into consideration in the present evaluation.

1. Exposure Data

1.1 Chemical and physical data

1.1.1 *Nomenclature*

Chem. Abstr. Serv. Reg. No.: 87-68-3

Chem. Abstr. Name: 1,1,2,3,4,4-Hexachloro-1,3-butadiene

IUPAC Systematic Name: Hexachlorobutadiene

Synonyms: HCB; hexachloro-1,3-butadiene; perchloro-1,3-butadiene; perchlorobutadiene

1.1.2 *Structural and molecular formulae and relative molecular mass*

```
Cl     Cl        Cl
  \    |        /
   C=C—C=C
  /        |    \
Cl        Cl     Cl
```

C_4Cl_6 Relative molecular mass: 260.76

1.1.3 *Chemical and physical properties of the pure substance*

(*a*) *Description*: Clear, colourless liquid with mild odour (Lewis, 1993)

(*b*) *Boiling-point*: 215°C (Lide, 1997)

(*c*) *Melting-point*: –21°C (Lide, 1997)

(*d*) *Density*: 1.556 g/cm^3 at 25°C (Lide, 1997)

(*e*) *Solubility*: Insoluble in water; soluble in ethanol and diethyl ether (Lide, 1997)

(*f*) *Volatility*: Vapour pressure: 2926 Pa at 100°C (Verschueren, 1996)

(*g*) *Octanol/water partition coefficient (P)*: log P, 4.78 (Verschueren, 1996)

(*h*) *Conversion factor*: mg/m^3 = 10.66 × ppm

1.2 Production and use

Hexachlorobutadiene is produced chiefly as a by-product in the manufacture of chlorinated solvents and related products, in which it occurs in the heavy fractions (WHO, 1994).

Information available in 1994 indicated that hexachlorobutadiene was produced only in Austria (Chemical Information Services, 1995).

Hexachlorobutadiene is used as a solvent for natural rubber, synthetic rubber and other polymers. It is used as a heat-transfer liquid, a transformer liquid, a hydraulic fluid and as a washing liquor for removing hydrocarbons (Verschueren, 1996). It is also used as a pesticide, insecticide, herbicide, algicide and chemical intermediate (National Toxicology Program, 1991).

1.3 Occurrence

1.3.1 *Natural occurrence*

Hexachlorobutadiene is not known to occur naturally.

1.3.2 *Occupational exposure*

According to the 1981–83 National Occupational Exposure Survey (National Institute for Occupational Safety and Health, 1998), approximately 1000 workers in the United States were potentially exposed to hexachlorobutadiene. Occupational exposure to hexachlorobutadiene may occur during its production and during its use as a solvent, heat-transfer liquid, transformer liquid, hydraulic fluid, washing liquor, pesticide or chemical intermediate (National Toxicology Program, 1991).

1.3.3 *Environmental occurrence*

Hexachlorobutadiene has been measured in urban air at concentrations < 0.5 μg/m³; the concentrations in remote areas were < 1 pg/m³. Hexachlorobutadiene is frequently detected in ambient water and has been detected in drinking-water at 2–3 ng/L. In lake and river water in Europe, concentrations up to 2 μg/L have been recorded, but the mean level is usually < 0.1 μg/L. In the Great Lakes area of Canada, much lower concentrations (around 1 ng/L) were measured; however, the concentrations in bottom sediment can be as high as 120 μg/kg of dry weight. Sediment layers from around 1960 contained up to 550 μg/kg of wet weight (Agency for Toxic Substances and Disease Registry, 1994; WHO, 1994).

The concentrations of hexachlorobutadiene detected in aquatic organisms, birds and mammals indicate bioaccumulation but not biomagnification. In several species in polluted waters, concentrations > 1000 μg/kg of wet weight have been measured, and 120 mg/kg (lipid base) were found in one species. The concentrations in organisms distant from industrial outflows are generally < 100 μg/kg of wet weight. Hexachlorobutadiene has been detected in human urine, blood and tissues. Certain food items with a high lipid fraction, such as fish, have been found to contain up to 40 μg/kg and, in one case, over 1000 μg/kg (WHO, 1994).

According to the Environmental Protection Agency Toxic Chemical Release Inventory for 1987, 1600 kg hexachlorobutadiene were released into the air, 86 kg were discharged into water, and 32 kg were disposed of by underground injection from manufacturing and processing facilities in the United States. By 1996, the concentrations were 1100 kg released into air, 120 kg discharged into water and 430 kg disposed of by underground injection (National Library of Medicine, 1998).

1.4 Regulations and guidelines

The American Conference of Governmental Industrial Hygienists (1997) recommended 0.21 mg/m^3 as the 8-h time-weighted average threshold limit value, with a skin notation for potential dermal absorption, for exposure to hexachlorobutadiene in workplace air. Values of 0.21–0.25 mg/m^3 have been used as standards or guidelines in other countries (International Labour Office, 1991).

WHO (1993) has established an international drinking-water guideline for hexachlorobutadiene of 0.6 μg/L.

2. Studies of Cancer in Humans

No data were available to the Working Group.

3. Studies of Cancer in Experimental Animals

Previous evaluation

Hexachlorobutadiene was tested in one experiment in rats by oral administration, producing renal tubule adenomas and carcinomas in animals of each sex. It was tested inadequately in one experiment in mice by intraperitoneal injection (IARC, 1979).

New studies

3.1 Skin application

Mouse: Groups of 30 female non-inbred Ha:ICR Swiss mice, six to eight weeks of age, each received applications of 2 or 6 mg hexachlorobutadiene (purity confirmed) in 0.2 mL acetone on the dorsal skin three times per week for 440–594 days. Their rate of survival was described as 'excellent'. The treatment produced no squamous-cell papillomas or carcinomas of the skin (Van Duuren *et al.*, 1979).

3.2 Administration with known carcinogens or modifying factors

Mouse: Groups of 30 female non-inbred Ha:ICR Swiss mice received a single application of 15 mg hexachlorobutadiene (purity 'confirmed') in 0.2 mL acetone on the dorsal skin, followed 14 days later by 5 μg phorbol myristate acetate in 0.2 mL acetone three times a week as a promoting agent for 428–576 days. The rate of survival was described as 'excellent'. The compound did not initiate skin tumours (Van Duuren *et al.*, 1979).

Rat: Groups of 21 male Wistar rats, six weeks of age, were given 0.1% *N*-nitroso-ethylhydroxyethylamine (NEHEA) in the drinking-water for two weeks and then 0.1%

hexachlorobutadiene (purity, > 99%) in the diet for 30 weeks. Three other groups received either hexachlorobutadiene or NEHEA according to the same regimen or basal diet for 32 weeks. The rate of survival was 100%. The incidence of renal tubular tumours in the group given NEHEA plus hexachlorobutadiene (15/21) was greater than that in rats given NEHEA alone (5/10), and the incidence of preneoplastic renal tubular hyperplasia was also increased (21/21 versus 4/10) (Nakagawa *et al.*, 1998).

4. Other Data Relevant to an Evaluation of Carcinogenicity and its Mechanisms

4.1 Absorption, distribution, metabolism and excretion

4.1.1 *Humans*

The sulfoxidation of the mercapturic acid *N*-acetyl-*S*-(1,2,3,4,4-pentachlorobuta-1,3-dienyl)-L-cysteine (*N*-ac-PCBC), a urinary metabolite of the glutathione-dependent bioactivation of hexachlorobutadiene, was studied in liver microsomes from male and female donors with use of reconstituted recombinant cytochrome P450 enzymes (Werner *et al.*, 1995). *N*-ac-PCBC sulfoxide is a major urinary metabolite of hexachlorobutadiene in male rats dosed orally, and only liver microsomes from male rats catalyse the sulfoxidation of *N*-ac-PCBC (Birner *et al.*, 1995; see section 4.1.2). In contrast, liver microsomes from both male and female donors are capable of oxidizing *N*-ac-PCBC to the corresponding sulfoxide diastereomers. The correlation of *N*-ac-PCBC sulfoxidation with the rates of oxidation of P450 enzyme-specific substrates suggests that only cytochrome P450 3A enzymes oxidize *N*-ac-PCBC. Moreover, only gestodene and troleandomycin, two selective inhibitors for P450 3A isozymes, significantly reduced the rates of *N*-ac-PCBC sulfoxidation. No reduction in sulfoxidation rates was observed with inhibitors for other P450 enzymes. Incubation of *N*-ac-PCBC with purified and reconstituted recombinant P450s 1A2, 2E1, 3A4 and 3A5 resulted in sulfoxide formation only with P450s 3A4 and 3A5. In summary, these results indicate that P450 from the 3A family may sulfoxidize *N*-ac-PCBC (Werner *et al.*, 1995).

4.1.2 *Experimental systems*

Hexachlorobutadiene caused a marked reduction in glutathione concentration when incubated with male or female rat hepatic microsomal or cytosolic fractions fortified with glutathione. The depletion of glutathione in the microsomal fraction was not related to the formation of metabolites via cytochrome P450 but appeared to be due to a direct reaction catalysed by a microsomal glutathione *S*-transferase. Mass spectral analysis of a glutathione adduct of hexachlorobutadiene showed that the structure was *S*-(pentachlorobutadienyl)glutathione, confirming a direct substitution reaction without prior oxidation. This conjugate was formed faster by the hepatic microsomal fraction than by the cytosolic fraction. Glutathione adducts were also formed by male and female kidney cytosol and microsomal fractions but at a slower rate than in the liver fractions. It was suggested that the glutathione conjugate of hexachlorobutadiene is converted to the cysteine derivative, the structure of which is similar to that of *S*-dichlorovinyl-L-cysteine, and may therefore be nephrotoxic by a similar mechanism (Wolf *et al.*, 1984).

The hepatic metabolism of hexachlorobutadiene was investigated in isolated rat hepatocytes and after administration *in vivo*. Exposure of isolated hepatocytes to hexachlorobutadiene resulted in dose-dependent depletion of glutathione, and formation of both a mono- and a bis-substituted glutathione conjugate of hexachlorobutadiene was observed. The identity of the mono- and bis-glutathione conjugates was confirmed by high-performance liquid chromatography in which synthetic standards had identical retention times. The production of total and individual glutathione conjugates was both dose- and time-dependent. The production of total conjugates and the ratio of mono- to bis-conjugate was found to depend on the availability of glutathione. After exposure of isolated hepatocytes to a low concentration of hexachlorobutadiene, the bis-substituted conjugate accounted for more than 20% of the total conjugate produced, while this value decreased at higher concentrations. Analysis of bile collected from rats given hexachlorobutadiene intraportally revealed the presence of both the mono- and bis-substituted glutathione conjugates and additional ^{14}C-containing metabolites (Jones *et al.*, 1985).

The glutathione conjugate of hexachlorobutadiene formed in the liver, *S*-(pentachlorobutadienyl)glutathione, is secreted into bile (because of its high molecular mass and the presence of an effective transporter at the canalicular membrane of the hepatocyte), reabsorbed in the gut, intact or after hydrolysis to *S*-(pentachlorobutadienyl)-L-cysteine, and undergoes enterohepatic circulation or translocation to the kidney. Hepatic uptake and metabolism of *S*-(pentachlorobutadienyl)glutathione and *S*-(pentachlorobutadienyl)-L-cysteine may thus influence their renal disposition. In isolated perfused rat liver, dose-dependent uptake of both the glutathione and the cysteine conjugate from the perfusion medium was demonstrated, the cysteine conjugate being cleared from the perfusion medium to a much greater extent than the glutathione conjugate. Both conjugates were extensively biotransformed by further conjugation with glutathione and subsequent hydrolysis of the glutathione moieties. Hepatic biosynthesis of *N*-ac-PCBC from the cysteine conjugate was a minor pathway in both cysteine and glutathione conjugate metabolism in liver. These results indicate that hepatic biosynthesis of mercapturic acids may not contribute to the disposition of *S*-conjugates formed from hexachlorobutadiene *in vivo* and that *S*-(pentachlorobutadienyl)glutathione is, at least in part, delivered intact to the kidney (Koob & Dekant, 1992).

After administration of [^{14}C]-hexachlorobutadiene to male and female Wistar rats at 200 mg/kg bw by gavage, no significant difference was observed between males and females in the disposition or rate of excretion of radiolabel. Of the dose, 16% (± 4.2%) was excreted in the faeces and 3.1% (± 0.7%) in the urine of male rats and 11% (± 3.8%) in the faeces and 4.5% (± 1.5%) in the urine of female rats. The major metabolite excreted by female rats was *N*-ac-PCBC; small amounts of *S*-(pentachlorobutadienyl)-L-cysteine were detected. The urine of male rats contained these two compounds and also *N*-ac-PCBC sulfoxide and unmetabolized hexachlorobutadiene (Birner *et al.*, 1995).

Birner *et al.* (1995) reported the excretion of unmetabolized hexachlorobutadiene in the urine of male but not female rats. In order to investigate the basis for the excretion of highly lipophilic hexachlorobutadiene in the urine, [^{14}C]hexachlorobutadiene (200 mg/kg bw) was administered orally to male and female rats of the Sprague-Dawley strain and to NCI Black-Reiter (NBR) rats which are deficient in α_{2u}-globulin. No significant difference in the disposition or rate of excretion of radiolabel was observed between male and female animals of either strain. The previously observed sex-specific differences in the formation of urinary metabolites in Wistar rats were confirmed in Sprague-Dawley rats and were also found in NBR rats. In contrast to male Sprague-Dawley rats, however, NBR rats did not excrete unmetabolized hexachlorobutadiene in the urine. [^{14}C]Hexachlorobutadiene (10% of total urinary metabolites) was present only in the urine of male Sprague-Dawley rats and was associated with the α_{2u}-globulin fraction in urine and renal cytosol; the radiolabelled compound was identified as hexachlorobutadiene bound to the protein. The results indicate that male-specific urinary excretion of hexachlorobutadiene is associated with its binding to α_{2u}-globulin (Pähler *et al.*, 1997).

4.2 Toxic effects

4.2.1 *Humans*

No data were available to the Working Group.

4.2.2 *Experimental systems*

A single intraperitoneal dose of 100 mg/kg bw hexachlorobutadiene given to male Sprague-Dawley rats caused reductions in body weight and urine osmolality throughout the 96-h observation period. The rate of urine flow increased slightly, and marked increases in urinary protein, glucose and ketones content were observed. Renal slices taken after the same dose showed reduced accumulation of polycyclic aromatic hydrocarbons, whereas the transport of other organic compounds was affected only slightly. After daily administration on four successive days of 25–100 mg/kg bw hexachlorobutadiene, a dose-dependent response was observed for both transport and overall renal function. Glutathione administered in a 2.5-fold molar excess did not prevent the nephrotoxic effects of hexachlorobutadiene (Berndt & Mehendale, 1979).

Intraperitoneal administration of 300 mg/kg bw hexachlorobutadiene to male Sprague-Dawley rats decreased the urine osmolality and glomerular filtration rate and increased urinary excretion of proteins and ketones within 4 h. At 24 h, an elevated blood urea nitrogen concentration was found; however, no definite signs of hepatotoxicity were observed up to 48 h after treatment. Control rats excreted 40% of an intraperitoneal tracer dose (0.1 mg/kg bw) of [^{14}C]hexachlorobutadiene in the faeces and 30% in the urine over 48 h, whereas rats with hexachlorobutadiene-induced nephrotoxicity excreted only 7% in faeces and 6% in urine. Extraction of urine and bile samples with hexane revealed that all of the radiolabel in bile and 87% of that in urine was water-soluble, indicating that the insoluble hexachlorobutadiene was extensively biotransformed into polar metabolites (Davis *et al.*, 1980).

Two-month-old male Wistar rats given a single intraperitoneal injection of 100 mg/kg bw hexachlorobutadiene showed necrosis of the S_3 portion of the proximal convoluted tubule 24 h after administration. Significant increases in the activity of glutamine transaminase K (β-lyase) were detected in the urine as early as 10 h after dosing (Trevisan *et al.*, 1998).

The renal and hepatic glutathione concentrations were measured after treatment of male Sprague-Dawley rats with hexachlorobutadiene or citrinin (a nephrotoxic mycotoxin), alone or in combination, and after pretreatment with the glutathione-depleting agent diethylmaleate. Both renal and hepatic glutathione depletion was increased significantly when either citrinin (35 mg/kg bw) or hexachlorobutadiene (300 mg/kg bw) was given after diethylmaleate, while no difference in glutathione concentration was observed in the absence of pretreatment. When hexachlorobutadiene and citrinin were given in combination, the effect on the glutathione concentration was approximately additive. Renal tubular organic ion transport in kidney slices was also compromised significantly when either citrinin or hexachlorobutadiene was given after pretreatment with diethylmaleate. Hexachlorobutadiene depressed tetraethylammonium transport after diethylmaleate treatment; when given alone, hexachlorobutadiene had no effect on tetraethylammonium transport (Baggett & Berndt, 1984).

In isolated rat renal tubular cells, *N*-ac-PCBC sulfoxide was more cytotoxic than *N*-ac-PCBC. After identical doses of hexachlorobutadiene, the extent of necrosis of the pars recta of the proximal tubules was greater in male than in female rats. While the livers of female animals appeared normal histologically, those of male rats had slight toxic centrilobular changes. *In vitro*, only liver microsomes from male rats catalysed the formation of *N*-ac-PCBC sulfoxide from *N*-ac-PCBC. The authors concluded that formation of this mercapturic acid sulfoxide from hexachlorobutadiene in male rats might contribute to the sex difference in nephrotoxicity (Birner *et al.*, 1995).

Administration of a single intraperitoneal dose of 50 mg/kg bw hexachlorobutadiene caused necrosis of the renal proximal tubules of male Alderly Park albino mice. The earliest morphological changes observed by light microscopy were seen after 4 h; by 16 h, extensive proximal tubular necrosis was seen throughout the cortex. Active tubular regeneration was apparent by day 5, and substantial recovery had occurred by day 14. Electron microscopy showed mitochondrial swelling in the S_1 and S_2 segments of the proximal tubule 1 and 2 h after dosing, whereas by 4 and 8 h the major pathological changes were confined to the lower S_2 and S_3 segments and consisted of mitochondrial swelling and cellular necrosis. The extent of renal injury and regeneration correlated well with measurements of renal function, i.e. plasma urea, renal water and non-protein sulfhydryl content (Ishmael *et al.*, 1984).

Hexachlorobutadiene (50 mg/kg bw intraperitoneally) produced a time- and dose-related increase in hepatic water content in male Alderley Park mice. The increase in liver water was maximal one to two days after a treatment, but the content had returned to normal by day 5. The increased water was accompanied by a parallel increase in Na^+ and K^+ ion concentrations, with no overall change in the intracellular cation concentration. The liver non-protein sulfhydryl content was not decreased after administration of 50 mg/kg bw hexachlorobutadiene. Histopathological examination of the liver showed fine cytoplasmic vacuolation of periportal hepatocytes, which was more marked after a dose of 100 or 200 mg/kg bw than after 50 mg/kg bw hexachlorobutadiene. Ultrastructural changes were evident 4 h after administration of 50 mg/kg bw and consisted of mitochondrial swelling in periportal hepatocytes; in contrast, the pericentral hepatocytes appeared to be normal. By 16 h, marked mitochondrial swelling and some proliferation of the smooth endoplasmic reticulum were evident in periportal hepatocytes. Male mice of the C57BL/10J and C3H strains appeared to be more sensitive to hexachlorobutadiene-induced hepatic hydropic change than male or female Alderley Park strain or male BALB/c and DBA/2J strains. The authors concluded that hexachlorobutadiene or a metabolite may disrupt mitochondria in periportal hepatocytes, resulting in an influx of water and ions into the cell without compromising the Na^+ pump (Lock *et al.*, 1985).

Male and female Alderley Park rats, six to eight weeks of age, were given a single intraperitoneal injection of 0–200 mg/kg bw hexachlorobutadiene or its glutathione conjugate, its cysteine conjugate or its *N*-acetylcysteine conjugate (0–100 mg/kg bw) and killed 24 h later. Nephrotoxicity was assessed by histological examination and plasma urea concentration. All three glutathione-derived conjugates increased the amount of necrosis in the pars recta of the renal proximal tubules, with corresponding increases in plasma urea, as did hexachlorobutadiene. The *S*-conjugates were stronger nephrotoxins than hexachlorobutadiene itself. Hexachlorobutadiene was about four times more toxic to female rats than males, and females were also more susceptible to the metabolites (Ishmael & Lock, 1986).

Renal damage was assessed by histopathological examination and urine analysis in male Wistar rats treated with either hexachlorobutadiene (a single intraperitoneal dose of 170 mg/kg bw, which caused proximal tubule necrosis), adriamycin (a single intraperitoneal dose of 5 mg/kg bw, which caused minimal glomerular changes up to 35 days) or hexachlorobutadiene given two weeks after adriamycin; the animals were then compared with age-matched control rats for 21 days. Analysis of the urine of adriamycin-treated rats showed minimal renal changes. Hexachlorobutadiene significantly increased the urine volume (10-fold), protein (5-fold), glucose (175-fold) and brush border enzyme activities (10–600-fold), indicating severe proximal tubular damage, but most of these parameters had returned to pretreatment levels six days after treatment. In adriamycin-pretreated rats subsequently given hexachlorobutadiene, both urinary alkaline phosphatase activity and the ratio of kidney:body weight were significantly higher for longer periods. Histopathological examination showed that the hexachlorobutadiene-induced proximal tubular lesions were confined to the outer stripe of the outer medulla. Advanced regeneration and repair were evident 21 days after treatment. In the adriamycin-pretreated rats, the hexachlorobutadiene-induced lesions were more severe, affected the entire cortex and were characterized by marked tubular epithelial calcification, with little evidence of repair 21 days after treatment. Enzyme histochemistry showed that γ-glutamyl transpeptidase was localized to the proximal tubules. The enzyme staining was lost after hexachlorobutadiene treatment, but returned in parallel with histological recovery up to 21 days. The distribution and intensity of γ-glutamyl transpeptidase was unchanged in adriamycin-treated rats, but the distribution and intensity of this enzyme in kidneys of adriamycin-pretreated rats given hexachlorobutadiene had not returned to normal by day 21. The results indicate that pretreatment with adriamycin increases hexachlorobutadiene-induced nephrotoxic damage and decreases renal cortical repair capacity (Kirby & Bach, 1995).

Light microscopic examination of the kidneys from the study of Pähler *et al.* (1997) described in section 4.1 revealed the formation of hyaline droplets, indicative of the accumulation of α_{2u}-globulin, in the kidneys of male Sprague-Dawley rats. Haematoxylin- and-eosin staining demonstrated more pronounced necrotic changes in the renal tubules of male Sprague-Dawley rats than in those of females, as previously described for Wistar rats. [The Working Group noted that the changes in α_{2u}-globulin took place against a background of severe renal toxicity.]

The intranephron distribution of two major cysteine *S*-conjugate β-lyases was determined in order to clarify the role of these enzymes in promoting the nephrotoxicity associated with certain halogenated xenobiotics. Collagenase-treated rat kidneys were microdissected in order to isolate various nephron segments: glomeruli, early, middle and terminal portions of the proximal tubules (S_1, S_2 and S_3, respectively), thick ascending limbs, distal tubules and collecting tubules. Each segment was dissected in Hanks' solution, solubilized with Triton X-100 and applied to a micropolyacrylamide gel constructed with a continuous gradient. The gels were subjected to electrophoresis and then incubated in the dark in a solution containing dichlorovinylcysteine, sodium α-keto-γ-methiolbutyrate, phenazine methosulfate and nitroblue tetrazolium. The positions of the cysteine *S*-conjugate β-lyase and L-amino acid oxidase activities in the gels were revealed by the presence of blue formazan dye bands, and the relative intensities of the bands were determined by optical scanning with a microdensitometer. Three bands were detected: band I (M_r approximately 330 000), corresponding to a recently described high-molecular-mass cysteine *S*-conjugate β-lyase; band III (M_r approximately 90 000), corresponding to a lower M_r cysteine *S*-conjugate β-lyase identical to cytosolic glutamine transaminase K; and band II (M_r approximately 240 000), corresponding to L-amino acid oxidase, a unique activity of the B isoform of rat kidney L-hydroxy acid oxidase (Kim *et al.*, 1997).

4.3 Reproductive and developmental effects

4.3.1 *Humans*

No data were available to the Working Group.

4.3.2 *Experimental systems*

No deleterious effects on fertility or on the health of chicks were noted when adult male and female Japanese quail were maintained on a diet that contained up to 30 ppm (320 mg/m³) per day hexachlorobutadiene for 90 days prior to mating (Schwetz *et al.*, 1974).

Groups of six female Wistar-derived rats were fed a diet containing 0, 150 or 1500 ppm hexachlorobutadiene (purity, > 95%; coresponding to 0, 1600 and 16 000 mg/m^3) for four weeks prior to mating with untreated males. Exposure continued until the offspring were 18 weeks of age, when they were necropsied. Females at the high dose lost weight progressively during exposure and produced no litters. The pups of dams at the low dose had significantly reduced birth weights and subsequent growth but no grossly observable malformation. At necropsy, the kidneys of pups of dams at the low dose were heavier and displayed hypercellularity of the epithelial lining and hydropic degeneration and necrosis of cells in the straight limbs of the proximal tubules (Harleman & Seinen, 1979).

Hexachlorobutadiene was administered at 0 or 10 mg/kg bw by intraperitoneal injection to groups of 10–15 Sprague Dawley rats on days 1–15 of gestation, and the fetuses were examined for viability, growth and morphology on gestation day 21. Maternal toxicity [nature not specified] and fetal toxicity (delayed development of the heart and urogenital tract) but no teratogenic effects were reported (Hardin *et al.*, 1981). [The Working Group noted the limited reporting of the experimental results.]

Groups of 24 female Sprague Dawley rats were exposed via inhalation to hexachlorobutadiene (purity, 99%) at concentrations of 0, 2, 5 or 15 ppm (corresponding to 0, 21, 53, 110 and 160 mg/m^3) for 6 h per day on days 6–20 of gestation. Fetuses were examined on gestation day 21 by standard teratological techniques. Maternal weight gain during gestation was significantly reduced at the two highest doses. There was no effect on fetal viability, but the body weights of fetuses of dams at 15 ppm were reduced. No significant effects were observed on fetal morphology (Saillenfait *et al.*, 1989).

4.4 Genetic and related effects

4.4.1 *Humans*

No data were available to the Working Group.

4.4.2 *Experimental systems* (see Table 1 for references)

Hexachlorobutadiene produced a dose-dependent increase in Ara^r forward mutation frequency in *Salmonella typhimurium* that was more marked in the absence than in presence of an exogenous metabolic system. Hexachlorobutadiene was not mutagenic to *S. typhimurium* strains TA98 and TA100 either in the presence or the absence of the usual metabolic activation systems; however, it was mutagenic to the TA100 strain when a fortified system was used and when glutathione was added during preincubation. Furthermore, the mutagenic effect was enhanced by a longer preincubation time and by the inclusion of rat kidney microsomes. In the presence of metabolic activation, the mutagenic response induced by the mercapturic acid derivative of hexachlorobutadiene was 80 times greater than that of the parent compound (Wild *et al.*, 1986). Perchloro-3-butenoic acid and perchloro-3-butenoic acid chloride, two possible oxidative metabolites of hexachlorobutadiene, were mutagenic in the absence of metabolic activation and exerted a mutagenic effect two- to threefold higher than that of hexachlorobutadiene in

Table 1. Genetic and related effects of hexachlorobutadiene

Test system	Result[a]		Dose[b] (LED or HID)	Reference
	Without exogenous metabolic activation	With exogenous metabolic activation		
Salmonella typhimurium BA13/BAL13, L-arabinose resistance (Ara[r]) forward mutation	+	+	26100 μg/plate	Roldán-Arjona *et al.* (1991)
Salmonella typhimurium TA100, reverse mutation	–	NT	1000 μg/plate	Rapson *et al.* (1980)
Salmonella typhimurium TA100, reverse mutation	–	–	5000 μg/plate	Stott *et al.* (1981)
Salmonella typhimurium TA100, TA98, TA1535, TA1537, reverse mutation	–	–	33 μg/plate	Haworth *et al.* (1983)
Salmonella typhimurium TA100, reverse mutation	–	–	16700 μg/plate	Reichert *et al.* (1983)
Salmonella typhimurium TA100, reverse mutation	–	+[c]	167 μg/plate	Reichert *et al.* (1984)
Salmonella typhimurium TA100, reverse mutation	–	+[d]	1.3 μg/plate	Vamvakas *et al.* (1988a)
Salmonella typhimurium TA100, reverse mutation	NT	+[c]	320 μg/plate	Wild *et al.* (1986)
Drosophila melanogaster, sex-linked recessive lethal mutations	–		15 feed or inj	Woodruff *et al.* (1985)
Unscheduled DNA synthesis, Sprague-Dawley rat primary hepatocytes *in vitro*	–	NT	7800	Stott *et al.* (1981)
Sister chromatid exchange, Chinese hamster ovary cells *in vitro*	+	+	1.4	Galloway *et al.* (1987)
Chromosomal aberrations, Chinese hamster ovary cells *in vitro*	–	–	35	Galloway *et al.* (1987)
Cell transformation, Syrian hamster embryo cells, clonal assay	+	NT	10	Schiffmann *et al.* (1984)
Binding (covalent) to DNA, Sprague-Dawley rat kidney *in vivo*	+		20 po × 1	Stott *et al.* (1981)
Binding (covalent) to mitochondrial DNA, female NMRI mouse liver and kidney cells *in vivo*	+		30 po × 1	Schrenk & Dekant (1989)

[a] +, positive; –, negative; NT, not tested

[b] LED, lowest effective dose; HID, highest ineffective dose; unless otherwise stated, in-*vitro* tests, μg/mL; in-*vivo* tests, mg/kg bw per day; inj, injection; po, oral

[c] Containing 30% of a 9000 × *g* supernatant of rat liver

[d] Rat liver microsomes and reduced glutathione

the presence of activation (Reichert *et al.*, 1984). Hexachlorobutadiene did not induce sex-linked recessive lethal mutations in *Drosophila melanogaster*.

Unscheduled DNA synthesis, as measured by liquid scintillation counting, was not induced in rat primary hepatocytes but was elicited by hexachlorobutadiene and its putative metabolite pentachlorobutanoic acid in Syrian hamster embryo fibroblasts, the responses being approximately three times greater in the presence than in the absence of exogenous metabolization. Morphological transformation was induced in Syrian hamster embryo fibroblasts by hexachlorobutadiene and its putative metabolite pentachlorobutenoic acid. Hexachlorobutadiene increased the frequency of sister chromatid exchange in Chinese hamster ovary cells in both the absence and presence of an exogenous metabolic system from liver, but did not induce chromosomal aberrations under the same experimental conditions.

Covalent binding of [^{14}C]hexachlorobutadiene metabolites to rat kidney DNA and to renal and hepatic mitochondrial DNA was detected in mice given a single oral dose of 30 mg/kg bw of the parent compound, binding being 15-fold higher in kidneys. The metabolites bound to a much greater extent to mitochondrial DNA than to nuclear DNA in the kidneys, probably because of greater β-lyase activity in the mitochondrial membrane and the absence of histones (Schrenk & Dekant, 1989).

Further information on the reactive metabolites of hexachlorobutadiene is provided by the results of the following studies. The cysteine and glutathione conjugates of hexachlorobutadiene were mutagenic to *S. typhimurium* TA100 in the absence and to a greater extent in the presence of a metabolic activation system from rat kidney. The cysteine conjugate was found to be metabolized by rat kidney slices and rat kidney β-lyase to pyruvate, ammonia and an unidentified reactive metabolite, and this effect is consistent with the known renal carcinogenicity of hexachlorobutadiene (Green & Odum, 1985). *S*-(Pentachlorobutadienyl)-L-cysteine, which is regarded as the penultimate metabolite of hexachlorobutadiene, was mutagenic to *S. typhimurium* strains TA100, TA2638 and TA98 without the addition of a metabolic activation system. In the presence of a 100 000 × *g* supernatant from these bacteria, which contain significantly higher concentrations of β-lyase than rat subcellular fractions, the cleavage of *S*-(pentachlorobutadienyl)-L-cysteine resulted in a time-dependent, linear formation of pyruvate, ammonia and a thiol which is regarded as the ultimate genotoxic metabolite (Dekant *et al.*, 1986). *S*-(Pentachlorobutadienyl)-L-cysteine was shown to be activated by β-lyase to thioacylating reactive intermediates which bind covalently to DNA of *S. typhimurium* TA100 and of isolated rat renal proximal tubular cells (Vamvakas *et al.*, 1988b). No DNA single-strand breaks but some evidence of DNA cross-links was observed in isolated rabbit renal tubules after exposure to 1 mmol/L *S*-(pentachlorobutadienyl)cysteine (Jaffe *et al.*, 1983).

4.5 Mechanistic considerations

The cysteine *S*-conjugate of hexachlorobutadiene is concentrated in the renal proximal tubules and cleaved by β-lyases, which are very active in this part of the nephron, and the reactive thioketene formed can acylate proteins and DNA. This toxification pathway is responsible for the renal-specific toxicity and carcinogenicity of hexachlorobutadiene in rodents (Anders *et al.*, 1992; Koob & Dekant, 1992). The metabolism of hexachlorobutadiene has not been investigated in humans; however, the demonstrated glutathione pathway of the structurally related haloalkenes tri- and tetrachloroethene in humans indicates that hexachlorobutadiene is metabolized similarly in humans and rodents and has similar renal-specific toxicity.

Hexachlorobutadiene is a selective nephrotoxin in experimental animals, causing damage primarily to the proximal tubules. Renal toxicity is presumed to be due to bioactivation by glutathione *S*-conjugate formation. Hexachlorobutadiene is conjugated with glutathione to *S*-(pentachlorobutadienyl)glutathione and further transformed to *S*-(pentachlorobutadienyl)-L-cysteine, which is *N*-acetylated in the liver to form *N*-ac-PCBC. This metabolite accumulates in the kidney, where renal acylases cleave it to *S*-(pentachlorobutadienyl)-L-cysteine, which is a substrate for renal cysteine conjugate β-lyase and is transformed into a reactive thioketene. Binding of this intermediate to renal macromolecules is probably responsible for the nephrotoxicity of hexachlorobutadiene.

Studies in rats given kidney-specific toxins as single intraperitoneal or subcutaneous injections were conducted to determine the distribution of β-lyase within the nephron. When potassium dichromate was given as a single subcutaneous injection of 25 mg/kg bw, vacuolar degeneration and focal necrosis of the S_1–S_2 segment of the proximal convoluted tubule were accompanied by significant increases in the activity of β-lyase in the urine. When mercuric chloride was given as a single intraperitoneal dose of 1 mg/kg bw and separate groups of rats were given a single intraperitoneal dose of 100 mg/kg bw hexachlorobutadiene, both chemicals resulted in diffuse necrosis of the S_3 portion of the proximal tubule 24 h later. These changes were accompanied by increased urinary β-lyase activity, which also peaked 24 h after administration of either compound. These results show that necrosis in the S_1–S_2 or S_3 portion of the proximal tubules is accompanied by the release of β-lyase into the urine and support the conclusion that β-lyase is distributed throughout the proximal tubules. Although the distribution of necrosis in the rat kidney is more limited than that of β-lyase, the relative contribution of additional factors such as specific uptake systems and the differing concentrations of the second enzyme involved, γ-glutamyl transpeptidase, suggest that the proposed mechanism is consistent with the data (Trevisan *et al.*, 1998).

The activity of γ-glutamyl transpeptidase in human kidney is reported to be approximately 10-fold lower than that in Fischer rat kidney (Lau *et al.*, 1990). In addition, the activity of β-lyase in human kidney has been reported to be a further 10-fold lower than that in rat kidney (Lash *et al.*, 1990). These two factors have important implications with respect to the relative hazard of hexachlorobutadiene to human kidney.

The molecular mechanism of the bioactivation of hexachlorobutadiene that accounts for the kidney-selective tumour induction has been elucidated. The conjugation of hexachlorobutadiene with glutathione, catalysed by hepatic glutathione *S*-transferase, results in the formation of *S*-(pentachlorobutadienyl)glutathione, which is eliminated from rat liver with the bile and translocated to the kidney either intact or after metabolism to the corresponding cysteine-*S*-conjugate. These conjugates are metabolized by renal tubular cysteine conjugate β-lyase to a reactive intermediate, which is most likely a thioacyl-chloride or a thioketene.

5. Summary of Data Reported and Evaluation

5.1 Exposure data

Exposure to hexachlorobutadiene has occurred principally as a result of its production and release as a by-product from the manufacture of chlorinated solvents and related products. It has been widely detected in ambient air, water, foods and human tissues.

5.2 Human carcinogenicity data

No data were available to the Working Group.

5.3 Animal carcinogenicity data

Hexachlorobutadiene was tested by oral administration in one study in rats, by skin application in mice and inadequately in one experiment in mice by intraperitoneal injection. After oral administration in rats, it produced benign and malignant tumours in the kidneys of animals of each sex. It did not produce skin tumours after repeated application or show initiating activity in a two-stage initiation–promotion study in mice. It enhanced the incidence of renal tubular tumours induced by *N*-nitrosoethylhydroxy-ethylamine in a two-stage model of renal carcinogenesis.

5.4 Other relevant data

Hexachlorobutadiene is metabolized exclusively by glutathione conjugation and γ-glutamyl transpeptidase to its corresponding cysteine *S*-conjugate, *S*-(1,2,3,4,4-penta-chloro-1,3-butadienyl)-L-cysteine, which is concentrated in the renal proximal tubules. This conjugate is partly acetylated to the corresponding mercapturic acid and excreted in urine. It is also a substrate for β-lyases, which have high activity in this part of the nephron and cleave the *S*-conjugate to produce a reactive thioketene, which can acylate proteins and DNA. This toxification pathway is responsible for the kidney-specific toxicity and carcino-genicity of hexachlorobutadiene in rodents. The metabolism of hexachlorobutadiene has not been investigated in humans; however, the demonstrated formation of mercapturic acids from the structurally related haloalkenes tri- and tetrachloroethylene in humans indi-cates that hexachlorobutadiene would be metabolized in humans in a manner similar to that in rodents.

In rats exposed during development, fetal growth retardation has been observed, usually at maternally toxic doses. Malformations have not been reported. Negative results were obtained in a short-term assay to screen for teratogenicity in mice exposed by gavage.

No data were available on the genetic and related effects of hexachlorobutadiene in humans or in rodents *in vivo*. There is weak evidence for its genotoxicity in mammalian cells *in vitro*. The findings for mutagenicity in bacteria are equivocal.

5.5 Evaluation

There is *inadequate evidence* in humans for the carcinogenicity of hexachlorobutadiene.

There is *limited evidence* in experimental animals for the carcinogenicity of hexachlorobutadiene.

Overall evaluation

Hexachlorobutadiene is *not classifiable as to its carcinogenicity to humans (Group 3)*.

6. References

Agency for Toxic Substances and Disease Registry (1994) *ATSDR Toxicological Profiles: Hexachlorobutadiene*, Department of Health and Human Services, Public Health Service (CD ROM)

American Conference of Governmental Industrial Hygienists (1997) *1997 TLVs® and BEIs®*, Cincinnati, OH, p. 26

Anders, M.W., Dekant, W. & Vamvakas, S. (1992) Glutathione dependent toxicity. *Xenobiotica*, **22**, 1135–1145

Baggett, J.M. & Berndt, W.O. (1984) Renal and hepatic glutathione concentrations in rats after treatment with hexachloro-1,3-butadiene and citrinin. *Arch. Toxicol.*, **56**, 46–49

Berndt, W.O. & Mehendale, H.M. (1979) Effects of hexachlorobutadiene (HCBD) on renal function and renal organic ion transport in the rat. *Toxicology*, **14**, 55–65

Birner, G., Werner, M., Ott, M.M. & Dekant, W. (1995) Sex differences in hexachlorobutadiene biotransformation and nephrotoxicity. *Toxicol. appl. Pharmacol.*, **132**, 203–212

Chemical Information Services (1995) *Directory of World Chemical Producers 1995/96 Standard Edition*, Dallas, TX, p. 556

Davis, M.E., Berndt, W.O. & Mehendale, H.M. (1980) Disposition and nephrotoxicity of hexachloro-1,3-butadiene. *Toxicology*, **16**, 179–191

Dekant, W., Vamvakas, S., Berthold, K., Schmidt, S., Wild, D. & Henschler, D. (1986) Bacterial β-lyase mediated cleavage and mutagenicity of cysteine conjugates derived from the nephrocarcinogenic alkenes trichloroethylene, tetrachloroethylene and hexachlorobutadiene. *Chem.-biol. Interactions*, **60**, 31–45

Galloway, S.M., Armstrong, M.J., Reuben, C., Colman, S., Brown, B., Cannon, C., Bloom, A.D., Nakamura, F., Ahmed, M., Duk, S., Rimpo, J., Margolin, B.H., Resnick, M.A., Anderson, B. & Zeiger, E. (1987) Chromosome aberrations and sister chromatid exchanges in Chinese hamster ovary cells: Evaluations of 108 chemicals. *Environ. mol. Mutag.*, **10** (Suppl. 10), 1–175

Green, T. & Odum, J. (1985) Structure/activity studies of the nephrotoxic and mutagenic action of cysteine conjugates of chloro-and fluoroalkenes. *Chem.-biol. Interactions,* **54**, 15–31

Hardin, B.D., Bond, G.P., Sikov, M.R., Andrew, F.D., Beliles, R.P. & Niemeier, R.W. (1981) Testing of selected workplace chemicals for teratogenic potential. *Scand. J. Work Environ. Health*, **7**, 66–75

Harleman, J.H. & Seinen, W. (1979) Short-term toxicity and reproduction studies in rats with hexachloro-(1,3)-butadiene. *Toxicol. appl. Pharmacol.*, **47**, 1–14

Haworth, S., Lawlor, T., Mortelmans, K., Speck, W. & Zeiger, E. (1983) Salmonella mutagenicity test results for 250 chemicals. *Environ. Mutag.*, **5** (Suppl. 1), 3–142

IARC (1979) *IARC Monographs on the Evaluation of the Carcinogenic Risk of Chemicals to Humans,* Vol. 20, *Some Halogenated Hydrocarbons*, Lyon, pp. 179–193

IARC (1987) *IARC Monographs on the Evaluation of Carcinogenic Risks to Humans*, Suppl. 7, *Overall Evaluations of Carcinogenicity: An Updating of* IARC Monographs *Volumes 1 to 42*, Lyon, p. 64

International Labour Office (1991) *Occupational Exposure Limits for Airborne Toxic Substances*, 3rd Ed. (Occupational Safety and Health Series No. 37), Geneva, pp. 216–217

Ishmael, J. & Lock, E.A. (1986) Nephrotoxicity of hexachlorobutadiene and its glutathione-derived conjugates. *Toxicol. Pathol.*, **14**, 258–262

Ishmael, J., Pratt, I. & Lock, E.A. (1984) Hexachloro-1:3-butadiene-induced renal tubular necrosis in the mouse. *J. Pathol.*, **142**, 195–203

Jaffe, D.R., Hassal, C.D., Brendel, K. & Gandolfi, A.J. (1983) *In vivo* and *in vitro* nephrotoxicity of the cysteine conjugate of hexachlorobutadiene. I. *Toxicol. environ. Health*, **11**, 857–867

Jones, T.W., Gerdes, R.G., Ormstad, K. & Orrenius, S. (1985) The formation of both a mono- and a bis-substituted glutathione conjugate of hexachlorobutadiene by isolated hepatocytes and following in vivo administration to the rat. *Chem.-biol. Interactions*, **56**, 251–267

Kim, H.S., Cha, S.H., Abraham, D.G., Cooper, A.J.L. & Endou, H. (1997) Intranephron distribution of cysteine S-conjugate β-lyase activity and its implication for hexachloro 1,3 butadiene induced nephrotoxicity in rats. *Arch. Toxicol.*, **71**, 131–141

Kirby, G.M. & Bach, P.H. (1995) Enhanced hexachloro-1:3-butadiene nephrotoxicity in rats with a preexisting adriamycin-induced nephrotic syndrome. *Toxicol. Pathol.*, **23**, 303–312

Koob, M. & Dekant, W. (1992) Biotransformation of the hexachlorobutadiene metabolites 1-(glutathion-*S*-yl)-pentachlorobutadiene and 1-(cystein-*S*-yl)-pentachlorobutadiene in the isolated perfused rat liver. *Xenobiotica*, **22**, 125–138

Lash, L.H., Nelson, R.M., Van Dyke, R.A. & Anders, M.W. (1990) Purification and characterization of human kidney cytosolic cysteine conjugate β-lyase activity. *Drug Metab. Disposition*, **18**, 50–54

Lau, S.S., Jones, T.W., Sioco, R., Hill, B.A., Pinon, R.K. & Monks, T.J. (1990) Species differences in renal γ-glutamyltranspeptidase activity do not correlate with susceptibillity to 2-bromo-(diglutathion-S-yl)-hydroquinone nephrotoxicity. *Toxicology*, **64**, 291–311

Lewis, R.J., Jr (1993) *Hawley's Condensed Chemical Dictionary*, 12th Ed., New York, Van Nostrand Reinhold Co., p. 595

Lide, D.R., ed. (1997) *CRC Handbook of Chemistry and Physics*, 78th Ed., Boca Raton, FL, CRC Press, p. 3-88

Lock, E.A., Pratt, I.S. & Ishmael, J. (1985) Hexachloro-1,3-butadiene-induced hydropic change in mouse liver. *J. appl. Toxicol.*, **5**, 74–79

Nakagawa, Y., Kitahori, Y., Cho, M., Konishi, N., Tsumatani, K-I, Ozono, S., Okajima, E., Hirao, Y. & Hiasa, Y. (1998) Effect of hexachloro-1,3-butadiene on renal carcinogenesis in male rats pretreated with *N*-ethyl-*N*-hydroxyethylnitrosamine. *Toxicol. Pathol.*, **26**, 361–366

National Institute for Occupational Safety and Health (1998) *National Occupational Exposure Survey (1981–83)*, Cincinnati, OH

National Library of Medicine (1998) *Toxic Chemical Release Inventory 1987 and 1996* (TRI87 and TRI96), Bethesda, MD

National Toxicology Program (1991) *NTP Chemical Repository Data Sheet: Hexachloro-1,3-butadiene*, Research Triangle Park, NC

Pähler, A., Birner, G., Ott, M.M. & Dekant, W. (1997) Binding of hexachlorobutadiene to α_{2u}-globulin and its role in nephrotoxicity in rats. *Toxicol. appl. Pharmacol.*, **147**, 372–380

Rapson, W.H., Nazar, M.A. & Butsky, V.V. (1980) Mutagenicity produced by aqueous chlorination of organic compounds. *Bull. environ. Contam. Toxicol.*, **24**, 590–596

Reichert, D., Neudecker, T., Spengler, U. & Henschler, D. (1983) Mutagenicity of dichloroacetylene and its degradation products trichloroacetyl chloride, trichloroacryloyl chloride and hexachlorobutadiene. *Mutat Res.*, **117**, 21–29

Reichert, D., Neudecker, T. & Schütz, S. (1984) Mutagenicity of hexachlorobutadiene, perchlorobutenoic acid and perchlorobutenoic acid chloride. *Mutat. Res.*, **137**, 89–93

Roldán-Arjona, T., Garciá-Pedrajas, M.D., Luque-Romero, F.L., Hera, C. & Pueyo, C. (1991) An association between mutagenicity of the Ara test of *Salmonella typhimurium* and carcinogenicity in rodents for 16 halogenated aliphatic hydrocarbons. *Mutagenesis*, **6**, 199–205

Saillenfait, A.M., Bonnet, P., Guenier, J.P. & de Ceaurriz, J. (1989) Inhalation teratology study on hexachloro-1-3-butadiene in rats. *Toxicol. Lett.*, **47**, 235–240

Schiffmann, D., Reichert, D. & Henschler, D. (1984) Induction of morphological transformation and unscheduled DNA synthesis in Syrian hamster embryo fibroblasts by hexachlorobutadiene and its putative metabolite pentachlorobutenoic acid. *Cancer Lett.*, **23**, 297–305

Schrenk, D. & Dekant, W. (1989) Covalent binding of hexachlorobutadiene metabolites to renal and hepatic mitochondrial DNA. *Carcinogenesis*, **10**, 1139–1141

Schwetz, B.A., Norris, J.M., Kociba, R.J., Keeler, P.A., Cornier, R.F. & Gehring, P.J. (1974) Reproduction study in Japanese quail fed hexachlorobutadiene for 90 days. *Toxicol. appl. Pharmacol.*, **30**, 255–265

Stott, W.T., Quast, J.F. & Watanabe, P.G. (1981) Differentiation of the mechanisms of oncogenicity of 1,4-dioxane and 1,3-hexachlorobutadiene in the rat. *Toxicol. appl. Pharmacol.*, **60**, 287–300

Trevisan, A., Cristofori, P., Fanelli, G., Bicciato, F. & Stocco, E. (1998) Glutamine transaminase K intranephron localization in rats determined by urinary excretion after treatment with segment specific nephrotoxicants. *Arch. Toxicol.*, **72**, 531–535

Vamvakas, S., Kordowich, F.J., Dekant, W., Neudecker, T. & Henschler, D. (1988a) Mutagenicity of hexachloro-1,3-butadiene and its S-conjugates in the Ames test—role of activation by the mercapturic acid pathway and its nephrocarcinogenicity. *Carcinogenesis*, **9**, 907–910

Vamvakas, S., Müller, D.A., Dekant, W. & Henschler, D. (1988b) DNA-binding of sulfur-containing metabolites from ^{35}S-(pentachlorobutadienyl)-L-cysteine in bacteria and isolated renal tubular cells. *Drug Metab. Drug Interactions*, **6**, 349–358

Van Duuren, B.L., Goldschmidt, B.M., Loewengart, G., Smith, A. C., Melchionne, S., Seidman, I. & Roth, D. (1979) Carcinogenicity of halogenated olefinic and aliphatic hydrocarbons in mice. *J. natl Cancer Inst.*, **63,** 1433–1439

Verschueren, K. (1996) *Handbook of Environmental Data on Organic Chemicals*, 3rd Ed., New York, Van Nostrand Reinhold Co., pp. 1070–1072

Werner, M., Guo, Z., Birner, G., Dekant, W. & Guengerich, F.P. (1995) The sulfoxidation of the hexachlorobutadiene metabolite *N*-acetyl-*S*-(1,2,3,4,4-pentachlorobutadienyl)-L-cysteine is catalyzed by human cytochrome P450 3A enzymes. *Chem. Res. Toxicol.*, **8**, 917–923

WHO (1993) *Guidelines for Drinking Water Quality*, 2nd Ed., Vol. 1, *Recommendations*, Geneva, pp. 73–74

WHO (1994) *Hexachlorobutadiene* (Environmental Health Criteria 156), Geneva, International Programme on Chemical Safety

Wild, D., Schütz, S. & Reichert, D. (1986) Mutagenicity of the mercapturic acid and other S-containing derivates of hexachloro-1,3-butadiene. *Carcinogenesis,* **7**, 431–434

Wolf, C.R., Berry, P.N., Nash, J.A., Green, T. & Lock, E.A. (1984) Role of microsomal and cytosolic glutathione *S*-transferases in the conjugation of hexachloro-1:3-butadiene and its possible relevance to toxicity. *J. Pharmacol. exp. Ther.*, **228**, 202–208

Woodruff, R.C., Mason, J.M., Valencia, R. & Zimmering, S. (1985) Chemical mutagenesis testing in *Drosophila*. V. Results of 53 coded compounds tested for the National Toxicology Program. *Environ. Mutag.*, **7**, 677–702

HEXACHLOROETHANE

This substance was considered by previous working groups, in 1978 (IARC, 1979) and 1987 (IARC, 1987). Since that time, new data have become available and these have been incorporated into the monograph and taken into consideration in the present evaluation.

1. Exposure Data

1.1 Chemical and physical data

1.1.1 *Nomenclature*

Chem. Abstr. Serv. Reg. No.: 67-72-1
Chem. Abstr. Name: Hexachloroethane
IUPAC Systematic Name: Hexachloroethane
Synonyms: Ethane hexachloride; 1,1,1,2,2,2-hexachloroethane; hexachloroethylene

1.1.2 *Structural and molecular formulae and relative molecular mass*

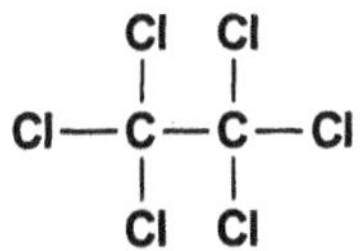

C_2Cl_6 Relative molecular mass: 236.74

1.1.3 *Chemical and physical properties of the pure substance*

(*a*) *Description*: Crystals; camphorous odour (Budavari, 1996)
(*b*) *Boiling-point*: Triple-point sublimation temperature, 187°C (Lide, 1997)
(*c*) *Density*: 2.091 g/cm^3 at 20°C (Lide, 1997)
(*d*) *Solubility*: Insoluble in water; very soluble in ethanol and diethyl ether; soluble in benzene (Lide, 1997)
(*e*) *Volatility*: Vapour pressure, 53.2 Pa at 20°C; relative vapour density (air = 1), 8.16 (Verschueren, 1996)
(*f*) *Octanol/water partition coefficient (P)*: log P, 3.4 (Verschueren, 1996)
(*g*) *Conversion factor*: mg/m^3 = 9.68 × ppm

1.2 Production and use

Information available in 1995 indicated that hexachloroethane was produced in Brazil, China, India, Japan, the Russian Federation and the United States (Chemical Information Services, 1995).

Hexachloroethane is used in metallurgy for refining aluminium alloys, removing impurities from molten metals and recovering metal from ores or smelting products. It is used as a degassing agent for magnesium and to inhibit the explosiveness of methane and combustion of ammonium perchlorate. It is also used as a smoke generator in grenades, in pyrotechnics, as an ignition suppressant, as a component of fire extinguishing fluids, as a polymer additive, as a flame-proofing agent, as a vulcanizing agent and in the production of synthetic diamonds (Budavari, 1996).

1.3 Occurrence

1.3.1 *Natural occurrence*

Hexachloroethane is not known to occur naturally.

1.3.2 *Occupational exposure*

According to the 1981–83 National Occupational Exposure Survey (National Institute for Occupational Safety and Health, 1998), approximately 8500 workers in the United States were potentially exposed to hexachloroethane. Occupational exposure to hexachloroethane may occur during its production and during its use as a refining agent, degassing agent, explosive inhibitor, smoke generator, ignition suppressant, component of fire extinguishing fluids, polymer additive, flame-proofing agent or vulcanizing agent (Budavari, 1996).

1.3.3 *Environmental occurrence*

Hexachloroethane has been detected occasionally in drinking-water systems and at low concentrations (nanograms per cubic meter) in the atmosphere. Limited data indicate that the typical background air concentrations in the northern hemisphere range from 48 to 68 ng/m^3. Hexachloroethane is rarely detected in surface waters or biota and has not been reported in ambient soil, sediments or commercial food products (Agency for Toxic Substances and Disease Registry, 1997).

According to the Environmental Protection Agency Toxic Chemical Release Inventory for 1987, 2600 kg hexachloroethane were released into the air, 89 kg were disposed of by underground injection and 230 kg were released onto the land from manufacturing and processing facilities in the United States. By 1996, 1300 kg were released into the air, 15 kg were released into water and 920 kg were disposed of by underground injection. These figures do not include releases from the manufacture and use of military smoke and pyrotechnic devices, since Federal facilities in the United States are not required to report releases (National Library of Medicine, 1998).

1.4 Regulations and guidelines

The American Conference of Governmental Industrial Hygienists (1997) has recommended 9.7 mg/m^3 as the 8-h time-weighted average threshold limit value, with a skin notation for potential dermal absorption, for exposure to hexachloroethane in workplace air. Values of 9.7–100 mg/m^3 have been used as standards or guidelines in other countries (International Labour Office, 1991).

No international guidelines have been established for hexachloroethane in drinking-water (WHO, 1993).

2. Studies of Cancer in Humans

One cohort study has been conducted of exposure to hexachloroethane (Seldén *et al.*, 1997), which was a retrospective follow-up study of cancer incidence during 1958–92 among 6454 workers at aluminium foundries and secondary aluminium smelters in Sweden, hexachloroethane being one of the agents to which some of the workers were exposed. No significant excess and no significant trend over duration of employment in the incidences of anorectal, liver or lung cancers or malignant lymphomas was found among the 1880 male workers who were considered to have been most heavily exposed to hexachloroethane and its by-products. The standardized incidence ratio for liver cancer among these workers was 1.1 (95% CI, 0.13–3.8), based on two cases with less than one year's employment. Malignant lymphomas were found in excess in this group (standardized incidence ratio, 2.3), but the excess was not significant (95% CI, 0.93–4.7; seven exposed cases). Confounding by agents such as polycyclic aromatic hydrocarbons, silica dust or hexachlorobenzene cannot be ruled out, and the power of the study was low, in particular for liver cancer.

3. Studies of Cancer in Experimental Animals

Previous evaluation

Hexachloroethane was tested in one experiment in mice and one in rats by oral administration. It produced hepatocellular carcinomas in male and female mice. In rats, no statistically significant excess of tumours was observed; however, a marginal increase in the incidence of renal tubular tumours, rarely seen in control animals, was found in male rats (IARC, 1979).

New studies

3.1 Oral administration

Rat: Groups of 50 male and 50 female Fischer 344/N rats, seven weeks of age, were given hexachloroethane (purity, > 99%) by oral gavage in corn oil at doses of 0, 10 or 20 mg/kg bw for males and 0, 80 or 160 mg/kg bw for females, on five days per week for 104 weeks. The survival rates at the end of the study were 31/50, 29/50 and 26/50 in males and 32/50, 27/50 and 32/50 in females at the three doses, respectively. Hexachloroethane increased the incidence of renal tubular adenomas and carcinomas combined in male rats at the high dose, the incidences being 1/50 (control), 2/50 (low dose) and 7/50 (high dose).

When adjusted for intercurrent mortality, the renal tumour incidences in male rats (expressed as percentages) were 2.6, 5.9 and 24% in the control, low-dose and high-dose groups, respectively. Male rats at the high dose also had a significant increase in the incidence of renal tubular hyperplasia. None of the females had renal tumours even though they were exposed to eightfold higher doses than the males. The incidence of phaeochromocytomas of the adrenal gland was marginally increased in males at the low dose (control, 15/50; low dose, 28/45; and high dose, 21/49). The incidence rates of phaeochromocytoma adjusted for survival were 41, 82 and 62% for the control, low-dose and high-dose male groups, respectively; none was observed in the females (National Toxicology Program, 1989).

3.2 Administration with known carcinogens or modifying factors

Rat: Hexachloroethane was tested in an initiation–promotion protocol in rats in which the end-point was development of foci of hepatocellular alteration, regarded as putative preneoplastic lesions predictive of liver tumour development. In an initiation study, groups of 10 male Osborne-Mendel rats weighing 180–230 g underwent a two-thirds hepatectomy and 24 h later received 500 mg/kg bw hexachloroethane (purity, 98%) by oral gavage in corn oil. Six days after the partial hepatectomy, phenobarbital was administered in the diet as a promoting agent at a concentration of 0.05% for seven weeks, followed by control diet for a further seven days before sacrifice. Positive controls were given an initiating dose of 30 mg/kg bw *N*-nitrosodiethylamine intraperitoneally, followed by the phenobarbital-containing diet as described above. Negative controls were given 2 mL/kg bw corn oil by gavage, followed by control diet. In the promotion phase of this study, groups of 10 male Osborne-Mendel rats were initiated with 30 mg/kg bw *N*-nitrosodiethylamine intraperitoneally or given 5 mL/kg bw water 24 h after a two-thirds hepatectomy. Six days later, the rats were given 500 mg/kg bw hexachloroethane in corn oil by gavage on five days per week for seven weeks or, for control rats, corn oil alone. The rats were killed one week after the end of the promotion phase. Foci of hepatocellular alteration were identified by morphological examination or immunohistochemical staining for γ-glutamyltranspeptidase. Hexachloroethane showed no evidence of initiating activity but significantly increased ($p < 0.05$) the number of liver foci in the promotion phase of the study (Story *et al.*, 1986; Milman *et al.*, 1988).

4. Other Data Relevant to and Evaluation of Carcinogenicity and its Mechanisms

4.1 Absorption, distribution, metabolism and excretion

4.1.1 *Humans*

No data were available to the Working Group.

4.1.2 *Experimental systems*

After hexachloroethane was administered in the feed of male and female Fischer 344 rats at 62 mg/kg bw per day for eight weeks, the ratio of its concentration in blood: liver:kidney:fat was 1:1:20–40:100. The concentrations decreased in all organs examined in an apparent first-order manner, with half-lives of approximately 2.5 days (Gorzinski *et al.*, 1985).

4.2 Toxic effects

4.2.1 *Humans*

The possible short-term adverse effects of hexachloroethane were investigated in a group of 11 munition workers who were exposed to hexachloroethane at concentrations of 10–20 mg/m^3 or more for five weeks. They were compared with a sex- and age-matched unexposed control group. Mild skin and mucous membrane irritation were reported in the exposed group, but clinical and laboratory examinations revealed no adverse effects on blood, liver, kidney or lung function (Seldén *et al.*, 1994).

4.2.2 *Experimental systems*

Rats exposed by inhalation to 2500 mg/m^3 hexachloroethane for 8 h showed no adverse effects during exposure or for 14 days thereafter. In contrast, two of six rats exposed to 57 000 mg/m^3 died at the end of the 8-h exposure, and the body weights of the surviving animals were reduced. Subacute diffuse interstitial pneumonitis was diagnosed after 14 days, but no other gross lesions were observed. Male and female Sprague-Dawley rats, male beagle dogs, male Hartley guinea-pigs and male and female quail (*Coturnix japonica*) were treated with 15, 48 or 260 ppm (140, 460 and 2500 mg/m^3) hexachloroethane vapour for 6 h a day on five days a week for six weeks. No effects were seen with the two lower doses, while the dose of 260 ppm affected mainly the nervous system of dogs and to a lesser extent that of rats. The dogs developed tremor, facial muscular fasciculations and hypersalivation. The oxygen consumption of rats at the high dose was reduced, but pulmonary function tests showed no difference from reported normal values. The rats showed tremor, ruffled pelt and red exudate around the eyes but no changes in either avoidance performance or spontaneous motor activity. The only other adverse effects were increased organ:body-weight ratios for the kidney, spleen and testis in male rats and the liver in female rats. Guinea-pigs receiving the high dose showed body-weight reduction. No signs of toxicity were seen in quail. In the same study, hexachloroethane was given to groups of five male rabbits daily by gavage for 12 days; the experiment was terminated four days after the last dose. A dose of 100 mg/kg bw was not toxic, while doses of 320 and 1000 mg/kg bw reduced body weights, caused liver degeneration and necrosis and renal tubular nephrocalcinosis and decreased the serum potassium and glucose concentrations (Weeks *et al.*, 1979).

Hexachloroethane was administered in the diet at approximate doses of 0, 1, 15 and 62 mg/kg bw per day for 16 weeks to male and female Fischer 344 rats. The high dose was toxic to the kidney, as manifested by slightly increased kidney weights in males, but not in females, and tubular atrophy, degeneration, hypertrophy and/or dilatation in males and to a lesser extent in females. The livers of both males and females at the high dose were heavier, while histopathological swelling of hepatocytes was observed only in males at the two higher doses (Gorzinski *et al.*, 1985).

In a 16-day study in Fischer 344 rats, oral administration of 187 or 375 mg/kg bw hexachloroethane produced hyaline droplet formation in the cytoplasm of the renal tubular epithelium in male rats, with tubular-cell regeneration. No renal effects were observed in female rats (National Toxicology Program, 1989).

In male and female rats dosed orally with 0, 47, 94, 188, 375 or 750 mg/kg bw hexachloroethane on five days a week for 13 weeks, the compound-related effects included increased relative weights of the liver, heart, kidney and brain in males and females at the highest dose. Renal changes were seen in all treated males (9/10 at the lowest dose), including increased hyaline droplet formation, tubular regeneration and tubular casts, and their severity was dose-related. No renal changes were observed in female rats. Hepatocellular necrosis was observed in females at 188 mg/kg bw and in both males and females at the two highest doses (National Toxicology Program, 1989).

A study of the effects of hexachloroethane on replicative DNA synthesis in hepatocytes from eight-week-old male B6C3F$_1$ mice that had been given a dose of 1000 mg/kg bw by gavage gave inconclusive results (Miyagawa *et al.*, 1995).

4.3 Reproductive and developmental effects

4.3.1 *Humans*

Hexachloroethane was detected at a mean concentration of 427 ppt [ng/mL] in 20% of samples of ovarian follicular fluid obtained from 150 Canadian women. It was not detected in serum (Foster *et al.*, 1996).

4.3.2 *Experimental systems*

In a study of developmental toxicity, groups of 22 female Sprague Dawley received 0, 50, 100 or 500 mg/kg bw hexachloroethane (purity, 99.8%) by gavage in corn oil or 0, 15, 48 or 260 ppm (0, 140, 460 or 2500 mg/m^3) via inhalation on days 6–16 of gestation. Tremors and decreased body-weight gain were observed after exposure to the high dose by either route. After oral exposure to 500 mg/kg bw, increased resorptions and decreased live litter size were noted (Weeks *et al.*, 1979). [The Working Group noted that few actual experimental results were contained in this summary article of research by the United States Army.]

Hexachloroethane was one of a number of organic chemicals present in three samples of materials used or originating in the manufacture of semiconductors that were tested for developmental toxicity. The concentrations of hexachloroethane in the three mixtures ranged from 0.30 to 10.95 mg/kg, which were low in comparison with those of the other organic chemicals present. The mixtures were administered to mice of three strains by oral gavage on days 6–15 of gestation. Two of the mixtures resulted in dose-related embryonic deaths, fetal growth retardation and malformations, primarily cleft palate, in all strains.

The authors suggested that the effects were the result of the presence of titanocene dichloride-like contaminants (Schmidt *et al.*, 1995).

4.4 Genetic and related effects

4.4.1 *Humans*

No data were available to the Working Group.

4.4.2 *Experimental systems* (see Table 1 for references)

Hexachloroethane did not cause differential toxicity in the *Bacillus subtilis* rec system or SOS DNA repair in *Salmonella typhimurium*. It was not mutagenic to *S. typhimurium* TA100, TA98, TA1535 or TA1537 or *Saccharomyces cerevisiae*. Gene conversion was induced in *S. cerevisiae* in the absence of exogenous metabolic activation whereas crossing-over and aneuploidy were not induced in *Aspergillus nidulans*. Hexachlorethane induced somatic mutations in *Drosophila melanogaster*.

Hexachloroethane induced sister chromatid exchange, but not chromosomal aberrations in Chinese hamster ovary cells in culture. It did not induce micronuclei in human cells *in vitro* and did not transform BALB/c 3T3 mouse cells.

Hexachloroethane was reported to bind to DNA *in vitro* in the presence of an exogenous metabolic system. After a single intraperitoneal injection to mice and rats *in vivo*, it was bound to DNA, RNA and protein. The binding to DNA was weak but was greatest in mouse liver; it was very weak in mouse kidney, lung and stomach and in all organs of rats.

4.5 Mechanistic considerations

Hexachloroethane produces a spectrum of histopathological effects in the kidneys of male rats, but not of female rats or of mice, which are consistent with those typically induced by chemicals that cause α_{2u}-globulin nephropathy. It is structurally similar to pentachloroethane, which also causes renal tumours in male rats (National Toxicology Program, 1983). Pentachloroethane has been shown to increase the renal cortical concentrations of α_{2u}-globulin and stimulate renal cell proliferation (Goldsworthy *et al.*, 1988). Although these comparisons suggest that hexachloroethane acts through an α_{2u}-globulin-associated mechanism, the available data are insufficient to fulfil the criteria for establishing this mechanism (Capen *et al.*, 1999).

5. Summary of Data Reported and Evaluation

5.1 Exposure data

Exposure to hexachloroethane may occur during its production and use in metal refining, in fire suppression and in other minor uses.

Table 1. Genetic and related effects of hexachloroethane

Test system	Results[a]		Dose[b] (LED or HID)	Reference
	Without exogenous metabolic system	With exogenous metabolic system		
Prophage, induction of SOS repair, strand breaks, cross-links	–	–	42	Nakamura *et al.* (1987)
Bacillus subtilis rec, differential toxicity	–	NT	10 μg/plate	Kinae *et al.* (1981)
Salmonella typhimurium, forward mutation, arabinose resistance (Ara[r])	–	–	7100 μg/plate	Roldán-Arjona *et al.* (1991)
Salmonella typhimurium TA100, TA98, TA1535, TA1537, reverse mutation	–	–	10000 μg/plate	Haworth *et al.* (1983)
Salmonella typhimurium TA100, TA98, TA1537, reverse mutation	–	–	10 μg/plate	Kinae *et al.* (1981)
Saccharomyces cerevisiae, gene conversion	+	–	1200	Bronzetti *et al.* (1989)
Saccharomyces cerevisiae, reverse mutation	–	–	3000	Bronzetti *et al.* (1989)
Aspergillus nidulans, crossing-over	–	NT	800	Crebelli *et al.* (1988)
Aspergillus nidulans, aneuploidy	–	NT	800	Crebelli *et al.* (1988)
Drosophila melanogaster, somatic mutation	+		2400 feed	Vogel & Nivard (1993)
Sister chromatid exchange, Chinese hamster ovary cells *in vitro*	–	+	350	Galloway *et al.* (1987)
Chromosomal aberrations, Chinese hamster ovary cells *in vitro*	–	–	NR	Galloway *et al.* (1987)
Cell transformation, BALB/c 3T3 mouse cells	–	NT	20	Tu *et al.* (1985)
Micronucleus formation, human lymphoblastoid AHH-1, MCL-5 and h2E1 cells *in vitro*	–	NT	24	Doherty *et al.* (1996)
Binding (covalent) to calf thymus DNA *in vitro*	NT	+	13	Lattanzi *et al.* (1988)
Binding (covalent) to DNA, male rat and mouse liver, kidney, lung and stomach cells *in vivo*	+		2 ip × 1	Lattanzi *et al.* (1988)
Binding (covalent) to RNA or protein, male rat and mouse liver, kidney, lung and stomach cells *in vivo*	+		2 ip × 1	Lattanzi *et al.* (1988)

[a] +, positive; –, negative; NT, not tested

[b] LED, lowest effective dose; HID, highest ineffective dose; unless otherwise stated, in-vitro test, : μg/mL; in-vivo study, mg/kg bw per day; NR, not reported; ip, intraperitoneal

5.2 Human carcinogenicity data

One cohort study of workers at aluminium foundries and aluminium smelters in Sweden showed no significant association between exposure to hexachloroethane and cancer incidence.

5.3 Animal carcinogenicity data

Hexachloroethane was tested in one experiment in mice and two experiments in rats by oral administration. It produced liver tumours in mice of each sex. In rats, it produced a statistically significantly increased incidence of renal tubular tumours in males in one study and a marginal increase in the incidence of renal tubular tumours in another study, also only in males. In a two-stage liver initiation–promotion assay in rats, hexachloroethane showed promoting but no initiating activity.

5.4 Other relevant data

No data were available to the Working Group on the absorption, distribution, metabolism or excretion of hexachloroethane in humans. It is absorbed in rats after oral administration, is concentrated in kidney and fat and is excreted by apparent first-order kinetics.

In humans, exposure by inhalation to hexachloroethane (10–20 mg/m^3) produced mild irritation of the skin and mucous membrane. Inhalation produced respiratory irritation in rodents.

After short-term exposure, hexachloroethane caused renal toxicity in male rats and hepatocellular necrosis in both male and female rats.

The data on reproductive toxicity were inadequate for evaluation.

No data were available on the genetic and related effects of hexachloroethane in humans. Hexachloroethane was found to bind to DNA in mouse liver after intraperitoneal injection; no other data were available on its genetic effects in experimental systems *in vivo*. It induced sister chromatid exchange in one study but did not induce chromosomal damage in mammalian cells *in vitro*. It induced gene mutation in *Drosophila* and yeast but was not mutagenic to bacteria.

5.5 Evaluation

There is *inadequate evidence* in humans for the carcinogenicity of hexachloroethane.

There is *sufficient evidence* in experimental animals for the carcinogenicity of hexachloroethane.

Overall evaluation

Hexachloroethane is *possibly carcinogenic to humans (Group 2B)*.

6. References

Agency for Toxic Substances and Disease Registry (1997) *Toxicological Profile for Hexachloroethane*, Atlanta, GA, Department of Health and Human Services

American Conference of Governmental Industrial Hygienists (1997) *1997 TLVs® and BEIs®*, Cincinnati, OH, p. 26

Bronzetti, G., Morichetti, E., del Carratore, R., Rosellini, D., Paolilni, M., Cantelli-Forti, G., Grilli, S. & Vellosi, R. (1989) Tetrachloroethane, pentachloroethane, and hexachloroethane. Genetic and biochemical studies. *Teratog. Carcinog. Mutag.*, **9**, 349–357

Budavari, S., ed. (1996) *The Merck Index*, 12th Ed., Whitehouse Station, NJ, Merck & Co., Inc., p. 800

Capen, C.C., Dybing, E., Rice, J.M. & Wilbourn, J.D., eds (1999) *Species Differences in Thyroid, Kidney and Urinary Bladder Carcinogenesis* (IARC Scientific Publications No. 147), Lyon, IARC

Chemical Information Services (1995) *Directory of World Chemical Producers 1995/96 Standard Edition*, Dallas, TX, p. 386

Crebelli, R., Benigni, R., Franekic, J., Conti, G., Conti, L. & Carere, A. (1988) Induction of chromosome malsegregation by halogenated organic solvents in Aspergillus nidulans: Unspecific or specific mechanism? *Mutat Res.*, **201**, 401–411

Doherty, A.T., Ellard, S., Parry, E.M. & Parry, J.M. (1996) An investigation into the activation and deactivation of chlorinated hydrocarbons to genotoxins in metabolically competent human cells. *Mutagenesis*, **11**, 247–274

Foster, W.G., Jarrell, J.F., Younglai, E.V., Wade, M.G., Arnold, D.L. & Jordan, S. (1996) An overview of some reproductive toxicology studies conducted at Health Canada. *Toxicol. ind. Health*, **12**, 447–459

Galloway, S.M., Armstrong, M.J., Reuben, C., Colman, S., Brown, B., Cannon, C., Bloom, A.D., Nakamura, F., Ahmed, M., Duk, S., Rimpo, J., Margolin, B.H., Resnick, M.A., Anderson, B. & Zeiger, E. (1987) Chromosome aberrations and sister chromatid exchanges in Chinese hamster ovary cells: Evaluations of 108 chemicals. *Environ. mol. Mutag.*, **10** (Suppl. 1), 1–175

Goldsworthy, T.L., Lyght, O., Burnett, V.L. & Popp, J.A. (1988) Potential role of α-2u-globulin, protein droplet accumulation, and cell replication in the renal carcinogenicity of rats exposed to trichloroethylene, perchloroethylene and pentachloroethane. *Toxicol. appl. Pharmacol.*, **96**, 367–379

Gorzinski, S.J., Nolan, R.J., McCollister, S.B., Kociba, R.J. & Mattsson, J.L. (1985) Subchronic oral toxicity, tissue distribution and clearance of hexachloroethane in the rat. *Drug Chem. Toxicol.*, **8**, 155–169

Haworth, S., Lawlor, T., Mortelmans, K., Speck, W. & Zeiger, E. (1983) Salmonella mutagenicity test results for 250 chemicals. *Environ. Mutag.*, **5** (Suppl. 5), 3–142

IARC (1979) *IARC Monographs on the Evaluation of the Carcinogenic Risk of Chemicals to Humans*, Vol. 20, *Some Halogenated Hydrocarbons*, Lyon, pp. 467–476

IARC (1987) *IARC Monographs on the Evaluation of Carcinogenic Risks to Humans*, Suppl. 7, *Overall Evaluations of Carcinogenicity: An Updating of* IARC Monographs *Volumes 1 to 42*, Lyon, p. 64

International Labour Office (1991) *Occupational Exposure Limits for Airborne Toxic Substances*, 3rd Ed. (Occupational Safety and Health Series No. 37), Geneva, pp. 216–217

Kinae, N., Hashizume, T., Makita, T., Tomita, I., Kumura, I. & Kanamori, H. (1981) Studies on the toxicity of pulp and paper mill effluents—II. Mutagenicity of the extracts of the liver from spotted sea trout (*Nibea mitsukurii*). *Water Res.*, **15**, 25–30

Lattanzi, G., Colacci, A., Grilli, S., Mazzullo, M., Prodi, G., Taningher, M. & Turina, M.P. (1988) Binding of hexachloroethane to biological macromolecules from rat and mouse organs. *J. Toxicol. environ. Health*, **24**, 403–411

Lide, D.R., ed. (1997) *CRC Handbook of Chemistry and Physics*, 78th Ed., Boca Raton, FL, CRC Press, p. 3-155

Milman, H.A., Story, D.L., Riccio E.S., Sivak, A., Tu, A.S., Williams, G.M., Tong, C. & Tyson, C.A. (1988) Rat liver foci and *in vitro* assays to detect initiating and promoting effects of chlorinated ethanes and ethylenes. *Ann. N.Y. Acad. Sci.*, **534**, 521–530

Miyagawa, M., Takasawa, H., Sugiyama, A., Inoue, Y., Murata, T., Uno, Y. & Yoshikawa, K. (1995) The in vivo-in vitro replicative DNA synthesis (RDS) test with hepatocytes prepared from male B6C3F1 mice as an early prediction assay for putative nongenotoxic (Ames-negative) mouse hepatocarcinogens. *Mutat Res.*, **343**, 157–183

Nakamura, S., Oda, Y., Shimada, T., Oki, I. & Sugimoto, K. (1987) SOS-inducing activity of chemical carcinogens and mutagens in Salmonella typhimurium TA135/pSK1002: Examination with 151 chemicals. *Mutat Res.*, **192**, 239–246

National Institute for Occupational Safety and Health (1998) *National Occupational Exposure Survey (1981–1983)*, Cincinnati, OH

National Library of Medicine (1998) *Toxic Chemical Release Inventory 1987 and 1996* (TRI87 and TRI96), Bethesda, MD

National Toxicology Program (1983) *NTP Technical Report on the Carcinogenesis Bioassay of Pentachloroethane (CAS No. 76-01-7) in F344/N Rats and B6C3F$_1$ Mice (Gavage Study)* (NTP 81-34; NIH Publ. No. 83-1788; NTP TR 232), Research Triangle Park, NC

National Toxicology Program (1989) *Toxicology and Carcinogenesis Studies of Hexachloroethane (CAS No. 67-72-1) in F344/N Rats (Gavage Studies)* (Tech. Rep. Ser. No. 361; NIH Publication No. 89-2816), Research Triangle Park, NC

Roldán-Arjona, T., Carcía-Pedrajas, M.D., Luque-Romero, F.L., Hera, C. & Pueyo, C. (1991) An association between mutagenicity of the Ara test of Salmonella typhimurium and carcinogenicity in rodents for 16 halogenated aliphatic hydrocarbons. *Mutagenesis*, **6**, 199–205

Schmidt, R., Scheufler, H., Bauer, S., Wolff, L., Pelzing, M. & Herzschuh, R. (1995) Toxicological investigations in the semiconductor industry. III. Studies on prenatal toxicity caused by waste products from aluminum plasma etching process. *Toxicol. ind. Health*, **11**, 49–61

Seldén, A., Kvarnlöf, A., Bodin, L. & Spangberg, O. (1994) Health effects of low level occupational exposure to hexachloroethane. *J. occup. Med. Toxicol.*, **3**, 61–67

Seldén, A.I., Westberg, H.B. & Axelson, O. (1997) Cancer morbidity in workers at aluminum foundries and secondary aluminum smelters. *Am. J. ind. Med.*, **32**, 467–477

Story, D.L., Meierhenry, E.F., Tyson, C.A. & Milman, H.A. (1986) Differences in rat liver enzyme-altered foci produced by chlorinated aliphatics and phenobarbital. *Toxicol. ind. Health*, **2**, 351–362

Tu, A., Murray, T.A., Hatch, K.M., Sivak, A. & Milman, H.A. (1985) In vitro transformation of BALB/c-3T3 cells by chlorinated ethanes and ethylenes. *Cancer Lett.*, **28**, 85–92

Verschueren, K. (1996) *Handbook of Environmental Data on Organic Chemicals*, 3rd Ed., New York, Van Nostrand Reinhold Co., pp. 1092–1093

Vogel, E.W. & Nivard, M.J.M. (1993) Performance of 181 chemicals in a Drosophila assay predominantly monitoring interchromosomal mitotic recombination. *Mutagenesis*, **8**, 57–81

Weeks, M.H., Angerhofer, R.A., Bishop, R., Thomasino, J. & Pope, C.R. (1979) The toxicity of hexachloroethane in laboratory animals. *Am. ind. Hyg. Assoc. J.*, **40**, 187–199

WHO (1993) *Guidelines for Drinking Water Quality*, 2nd Ed., Vol. 1, *Recommendations*, Geneva

d-LIMONENE

This substance was considered by a previous working group, in 1992 (IARC, 1993). Since that time, new data have become available, and these have been incorporated into the monograph and taken into consideration in the present evaluation.

1. Exposure Data

1.1 Chemical and physical data

1.1.1 *Nomenclature*

Chem. Abstr. Serv. Reg. No.: 5989-27-5
Chem. Abstr. Name: (R)-1-Methyl-4-(1-methylethenyl)cyclohexene
IUPAC Systematic Name: (R)-(+)-*para*-Mentha-1,8-diene
Synonyms: (+)-Dipentene; (R)-4-isopropenyl-1-methyl-1-cyclohexene; D-limonene; d-(+)-limonene; D-(+)-limonene; (+)-limonene; (+)-α-limonene; (+)-(R)-limonene; (+)-(4R)-limonene; (R)-limonene; (R)-(+)-limonene; (4R)-(+)-limonene; (+)-*para*-mentha-1,8-diene; (R)-*p*-mentha-1,8-diene; (R)-(+)-*para*-mentha-1,8-diene

1.1.2 *Structural and molecular formulae and relative molecular mass*

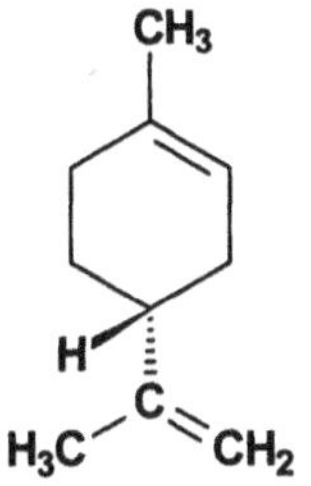

$C_{10}H_{16}$ Relative molecular mass: 136.24

1.1.3 *Chemical and physical properties of the pure substance*

(*a*) *Description*: Colourless liquid with characteristic citrus odour (National Toxicology Program, 1991)
(*b*) *Boiling-point*: 175.5–176°C (Budavari, 1996)
(*c*) *Melting-point*: –96.9°C (National Toxicology Program, 1991); –74.3°C has also been reported (Lide, 1991)
(*d*) *Density*: 0.8411 g/cm^3 at 20°C (National Toxicology Program, 1991)

(*e*) *Solubility*: Slightly soluble in water (13.8 mg/mL at 25°C); soluble in acetone, dimethyl sulfoxide and ethanol (National Toxicology Program, 1991; National Library of Medicine, 1998)

(*f*) *Volatility*: Vapour pressure, 133 Pa at 14°C and 665 Pa at 40.4°C; relative vapour density (air = 1), 4.69 (National Toxicology Program, 1991)

(*g*) *Conversion factor*: mg/m^3 = 5.57 × ppm

1.2 Production and use

Information available in 1995 indicated that *d*-limonene was produced in Australia, Brazil, Germany, Japan and the United States (Chemical Information Services, 1995).

d-Limonene has been used for many years as a flavour and fragrance additive in foods, beverages and consumer products. It is increasingly used as a solvent. It is also used in the manufacture of resins, as a wetting and dispersing agent and in insect control (National Toxicology Program, 1991; IARC, 1993; Budavari, 1996).

d-Limonene and its metabolite perillyl alcohol are currently undergoing clinical trials for use in treatment of breast cancer and other tumours, and chemoprevention trials are under consideration (Gould, 1995; O'Shaugnessy, 1996; Vigushin *et al.*, 1998).

1.3 Occurrence

1.3.1 *Natural occurrence*

d-Limonene is one of the most common terpenes in nature, occurring in citrus and a wide variety of other plant species. It is a major constituent of oil of citrus rind, dill oil, oil of cumin, neroli, bergamot and caraway (National Toxicology Program, 1991) [see IARC (1993) for a detailed discussion of its occurrence].

1.3.2 *Occupational exposure*

According to the 1981–83 National Occupational Exposure Survey (National Institute for Occupational Safety and Health, 1998), approximately 138 300 workers in the United States were potentially exposed to *d*-limonene. Occupational exposure to *d*-limonene may occur during its production and use, notably as an industrial solvent.

1.3.3 *Environmental occurrence*

The average daily dietary intake of *d*-limonene has been estimated to be about 0.3 mg/kg bw (Flavor and Extract Manufacturers' Association, 1991).

d-Limonene has been detected in indoor and outdoor air in various locations (IARC, 1993; National Library of Medicine, 1998).

1.4 Regulations and guidelines

The 8-h time-weighted exposure limit for *d*-limonene in Sweden is 150 mg/m^3 and the short-term (15 min) exposure limit is 300 mg/m^3 (National Board of Occupational Safety and Health, 1996).

No international guidelines for *d*-limonene in drinking-water have been established (WHO, 1993).

2. Studies of Cancer in Humans

No data were available to the Working Group.

3. Studies of Cancer in Experimental Animals

Previous evaluation

d-Limonene was tested for carcinogenicity by oral gavage in one study in mice and one study in rats. In mice and female rats, there were no treatment-related tumours, but male rats had renal tubular hyperplasia and a significantly increased combined incidence of renal tubular adenomas and carcinomas. In a two-stage experiment, oral treatment with *d*-limonene after administration of *N*-nitrosoethylhydroxyethylamine enhanced the development of renal tubular hyperplasia and renal tubular adenomas in male Fischer rats, which synthesize α_{2u}-globulin in the liver in large quantities, but not in male NBR rats, which do not (IARC, 1993). [The present Working Group reconfirmed the adequacy of the bioassays of *d*-limonene in male and female mice and rats conducted by the National Toxicology Program as cited in IARC (1993), noting the convincing renal tumour response in male rats and the absence of renal tumours in female rats.]

New studies

3.1 Administration with known carcinogens

Mouse: In a model of lung carcinogenesis, groups of 25 female A/J mice, six to seven weeks of age, were fed *d*-limonene in the diet at a concentration of 0.63% for 17 weeks. One week after commencement of treatment, the mice received an intraperitoneal injection of 10 μmol 4-(methylnitrosamino)-1-(3 pyridyl)-1-butanone (NNK) in 0.1 mL saline. *d*-Limonene treatment significantly reduced the number of lung tumours per mouse, from 8.1 in mice given NNK alone to 2.4 ($p < 0.05$), although the percentage of mice with lung tumours was not significantly different between those given NNK (100%) and those given *d*-limonene (96%) (El-Bayoumy *et al.*, 1996).

Rat: In a model of putative colonic preneoplasia, groups of 12 male Fischer 344 rats, five weeks of age, were given 0.5% *d*-limonene in the drinking-water (equivalent to 0.67% in the diet) for five weeks. One week after the start of treatment, the rats received subcutaneous injections of 15 mg/kg bw azoxymethane once a week for three weeks and were killed at 10 weeks of age. In rats given azoxymethane and *d*-limonene, the frequencies of aberrant crypt foci and the numbers of aberrant crypts per focus and of aberrant crypts per colon were significantly decreased ($p < 0.01$ to $p < 0.001$) when compared with the group given azoxymethane alone (Kawamori *et al.*, 1996).

In a multi-organ model of carcinogenesis, groups of 20 Fischer 344 male rats aged five weeks were treated sequentially with *N*-nitrosodiethylamine (100 mg/kg bw by intraperitoneal injection as a single dose at the beginning of the study), *N*-methyl-*N*-nitrosourea (20 mg/kg bw by intraperitoneal injection four times during weeks 1 and 2), *N*-nitrosobutyl-*N*-(4-hydroxybutyl)amine (0.05% in drinking-water during weeks 1 and 2), 1,2-dimethylhydrazine (40 mg/kg bw by subcutaneous injection four times during weeks 3 and 4) and *N*-nitrosodihydroxydipropylamine (0.1% in drinking-water during weeks 3 and 4). From the end of week 4, *d*-limonene at doses of 0.5, 1 or 2% was administered in the diet for 24 weeks, when surviving rats were sacrificed (i.e. 28 weeks after the start of the study). A group receiving 2% *d*-limonene but no initiating carcinogen schedule was also included. The number of rats with renal tubular adenomas was statistically significantly increased ($p < 0.01$) at the high dose of *d*-limonene: 13/19 with the carcinogen schedule plus 2% *d*-limonene and 4/19 with the carcinogen schedule alone. This increase in renal tumour incidence was accompanied by an increased number of atypical tubules (a preneoplastic lesion) per rat. None of the rats fed 2% *d*-limonene alone had a renal tumour. No modification of carcinogenesis was observed in any other organ (Kimura *et al.*, 1996).

Hamster: In a model of pancreatic carcinogenesis, groups of 25 Syrian golden hamsters, five weeks of age, were given subcutaneous injections of 15 mg/kg bw *N*-nitrosobis(2-oxopropyl)amine in 0.9% saline once a week for five weeks and simultaneously fed chow pellets containing 0, 1 or 2% *d*-limonene for up to 26 weeks, when the animals were killed. The high dose of *d*-limonene significantly decreased the number of pancreatic carcinomas, from 0.74 ± 0.15 in the animals given the carcinogen alone to 0.25 ± 0.12 in the animals given carcinogen plus 2% *d*-limonene ($p < 0.05$) (Nakaizumi *et al.*, 1997).

4. Other Data Relevant to an Evaluation of Carcinogenicity and its Mechanisms

4.1 Absorption, distribution, metabolism and excretion

4.1.1 *Humans*

d-Limonene is absorbed from the gastrointestinal tract. Two male volunteers given 1.6 g [^{14}C]*d*-limonene orally excreted 52–83% of the dose in their urine within 48 h. The major urinary metabolite isolated was 8-hydroxy-*para*-menth-1-en-9-yl-β-D-glucopyranosiduronic acid (Kodama *et al.*, 1976).

The toxicokinetics of *d*-limonene were studied in volunteers exposed by inhalation for 2 h to 10, 225 or 450 mg/m^3 *d*-limonene and to a workload of 50 W to simulate light physical activity; 10 mg/m^3 was considered to be the control concentration. The relative pulmonary uptake was approximately 70% of the amount supplied. Three linear phases of elimination could be distinguished in the time studied: a terminal phase of slope γ for slow elimination (320–1300 min after exposure), an intermediate phase of slope β for rapid elimination (16–319 min after exposure) and an initial phase of slope α (0–15 min after exposure). The plasma half-life of *d*-limonene was approximately 2.6 min for the α phase, 32 min for the β phase and 75 min for the γ phase. The lung clearance rate in 4 h was 1.1 L/kg per h for 225 mg/m³ and 1.4 L/kg per h for 450 mg/m³, and the lung clearance rate in 21 h was 1.1 L/kg per h for 450 mg/m³ (Falk-Filipsson *et al.*, 1993).

A pilot study was conducted in healthy volunteers (five women, two men) to investigate the metabolism and the toxicity of pharmacologically (supradietary) administered *d*-limonene. After the subjects had ingested 100 mg/kg *d*-limonene in a custard, their blood was drawn at 0 and 24 h for blood chemistry and at 0, 4 and 24 h for analysis of metabolites. Gas chromatography–mass spectrometry indicated the presence of five *d*-limonene metabolites in plasma: two major peaks were identified as dihydroperillic acid and perillic acid and a third major peak was limonene-1,2-diol; limonene itself was only a minor component. Two minor peaks were found to be the respective methyl esters of the acids. In all subjects, the metabolite concentrations were higher at 4 h than at 24 h, but a half-life value was not determined (Crowell *et al.*, 1994).

The toxicokinetics of *d*-limonene were studied in two women with breast cancer and one man with colorectal cancer. The patients received 0.5–12 g/m² body surface area per day orally for 21 days, and plasma and urine samples were collected on days 1 and 21. The metabolites were characterized and their structures elucidated by liquid chromatography–mass spectrometry and nuclear magnetic resonance spectrometry. Five major metabolites were detected in plasma: limonene-1,2-diol, limonene-8,9-diol, perillic acid, an isomer of perillic acid and dihydroperillic acid. The urinary metabolites comprised the glucuronides of the two isomers of perrilic acid, limonene-8,9-diol and a monohydroxylated limonene. The results are consistent with those of previously published studies in humans and in animals, but this study was the first in which limonene-8,9-diol and an additional isomer of perillic acid were identified (Poon *et al.*, 1996).

In a phase I clinical trial of orally administered *d*-limonene, 17 women and 15 men aged 35–78 (median, 57), with advanced metastatic solid tumours received an average of three treatment cycles of 21 days (one dose on day 1, then three daily doses on days 4–21) at doses ranging from 0.5 to 12 g/m² body surface area. *d*-Limonene was slowly absorbed, the maximal plasma concentration being attained at 1–6 h. The mean peak plasma concentrations of *d*-limonene were 11–20 μmol/L, and the predominant metabolites were perillic acid (21–71 μmol/L), dihydroperillic acid (17–28 μmol/L), limonene-1,2-diol (10–21 μmol/L), uroterpinol (14–45 μmol/L) and an isomer of perillic acid. After reaching these peaks, the plasma concentrations decreased according to first-order kinetics. The values for the integrated area under the curve for time–concentration showed little variation with administered dose. There was no accumulation of the parent or metabolites after a treatment cycle (Vigushin *et al.*, 1998).

4.1.2 *Experimental systems*

[^{14}C]*d*-Limonene was absorbed rapidly after administration by gavage of 800 mg/kg bw (4.15 μCi/animal) to male Wistar rats. The radiolabel concentration in blood was maximal after 2 h, and large amounts of radiolabel were also observed in the liver (maximal after 1 h) and kidneys (maximal after 2 h). Negligible concentrations were found in blood and organs after 48 h (Igimi *et al.*, 1974).

Urinary recovery of [^{14}C]*d*-limonene was 77–96% within three days in rats, guinea-pigs, hamsters and dogs. Faecal recovery was 2–9% within three days (Kodama *et al.*, 1976). Bile-duct-cannulated rats given *d*-limonene orally excreted 25% of the dose in the bile within 24 h (Igimi *et al.*, 1974).

After oral administration of *d*-limonene to rabbits, the urinary metabolites isolated were *para*-mentha-1,8-dien-10-ol (M-I on Figure 1), *para*-menth-1-ene-8,9-diol (M-II), perillic acid (M-III), perillic acid-8,9-diol (M-IV), *para*-mentha-1,8-dien-10-yl-β-D-glucopyranosiduronic acid (M-V) and 8-hydroxy-*para*-menth-1-en-9-yl-β-D-glucopyranosiduronic acid (M-VI) (Kodama *et al.*, 1974). After oral administration of *d*-limonene to dogs and rats, five other urinary metabolites were isolated: 2-hydroxy-*para*-menth-8-en-7-oic acid (M-VII), perillylglycine (M-VIII), perillyl-β-D-glucopyranosiduronic acid (MIX), *para*-mentha-1,8-dien-6-ol (M-X) and probably *para*-menth-1-ene-6,8,9-triol (M-XI). The major urinary metabolite was M-IV in rats and rabbits, M-IX in Syrian hamsters, M-II in dogs and M-VI in guinea-pigs (Kodama *et al.*, 1976). The possible metabolic pathways of *d*-limonene are shown in Figure 1.

Under alkaline extraction conditions, *d*-limonene was metabolized by rat liver microsomes *in vitro* to the glycols *d*-limonene 8,9-diol and *d*-limonene 1,2-diol *via* the 8,9- and 1,2-epoxides (Watabe *et al.*, 1980, 1981). Under neutral extraction conditions, no hydrolysis of *d*-limonene-1,2-epoxide to its corresponding diol was observed (Lehman-McKeeman *et al.*, 1989). In rat liver microsomes, epoxidation of *d*-limonene at the 1,2 double bond occurs only in the *cis* orientation, whereas in mouse liver microsomes both *cis* and *trans* isomers of this epoxide are formed (Lehman-McKeeman & Caudill, 1992a).

When [^{14}C]*d*-limonene was administered orally to male and female Sprague-Dawley rats at a dose of 409 mg/kg bw, the renal concentration of *d*-limonene equivalents was about 2.5 times higher in males than females, and approximately 40% of the radiolabel in male rat kidneys was bound reversibly to renal proteins. The major metabolite bound to the renal protein fraction was identified as *d*-limonene-1,2-epoxide (> 80%), parent *d*-limonene and the 1,2-diol representing minor components of the protein-bound moieties. The renal protein to which these metabolites bound was identified as α_{2u}-globulin by high-performance liquid chromatography (Lehman-McKeeman *et al.*, 1989).

4.2 Toxic effects

4.2.1 *Humans*

Five healthy adult male volunteers who received a single oral dose of 20 g *d*-limonene all developed transient proteinuria, non-bloody diarrhoea and tenesmus. The results of functional tests of the liver, kidney and pancreas were normal (Igimi *et al.*, 1976).

In the study of volunteers treated by inhalation, described in section 4.1.1, no irritating or central nervous system-related symptoms were found. A 2% decrease in lung vital capacity was found after exposure to 450 mg/m^3 when compared with 10 mg/m^3; this difference was statistically but not clinically significant (Falk-Filipsson *et al.*, 1993).

Figure 1. Possible metabolic pathways of *d*-limonene

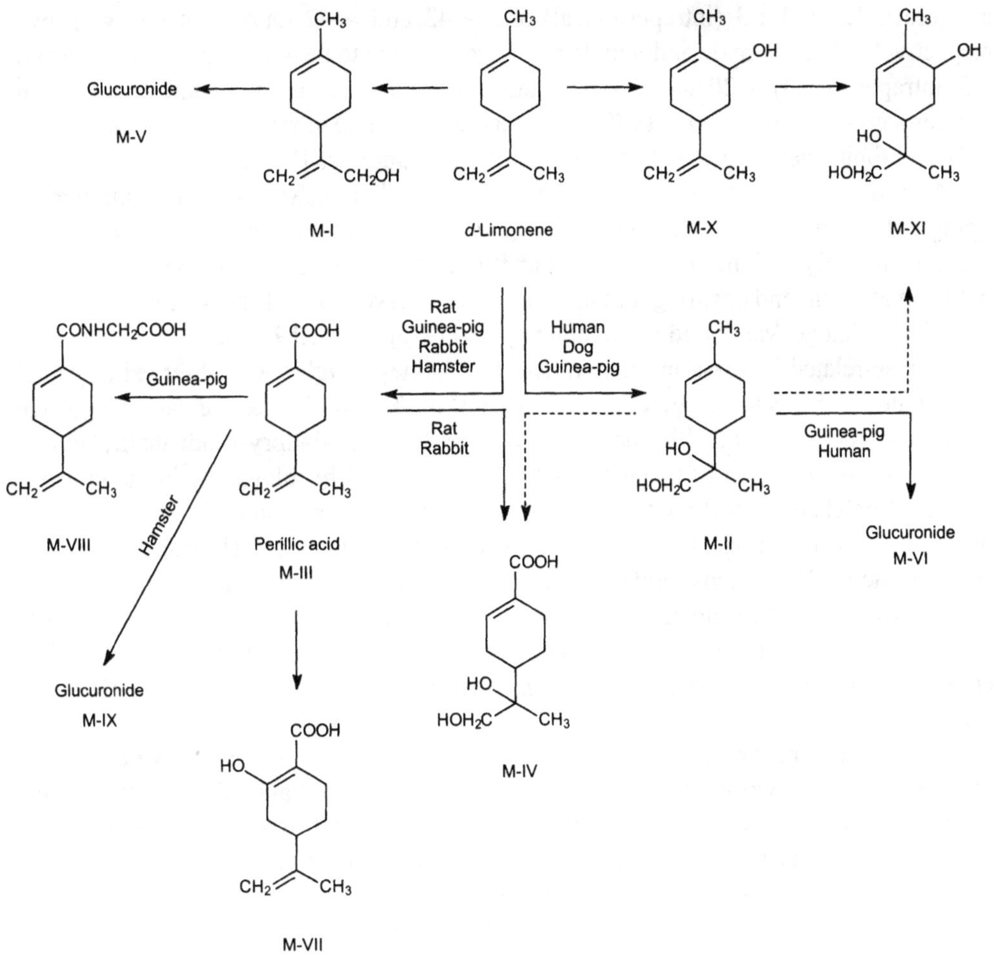

From Kodama *et al.* (1976)
M-I, *p*-Mentha-1,8-dien-10-ol; M-II, *p*-menth-1-ene-8,9-diol; M-IV, perillic acid-8,9-diol; M-V, *p*-mentha-1,8-dien-10-yl-β-D-glucopyranosiduronic acid; M-VI, 8-hydroxy-*p*-menth-1-en-9-yl-β-D-glucopyranosiduronic acid; M-VII, 2-hydroxy-*p*-menth-8-en-7-oic acid; M-VIII, perillylglycine; M-IX, perillyl-β-D-glucopyranosiduronic acid; M-X, *p*-mentha-1,8-dien-6-ol; M-XI, *p*-menth-1-ene-6,8,9-triol

In the phase-I clinical trial of orally administered *d*-limonene described in section 4.1.1, toxicity was limited to gastrointestinal symptoms (irritation, nausea, diarrhoea) and was dose-related over the range 6.5–12 g/m^2 body surface area per day (Vigushin *et al.*, 1998).

4.2.2 *Experimental systems*

The LD_{50} values for *d*-limonene in male and female mice were reported to be 5.6 and 6.6 (oral), 1.3 and 1.3 (intraperitoneal) and > 42 and > 42 (subcutaneous) g/kg bw, respectively; those in male and female rats were reported to be 4.4 and 5.1 (oral), 3.6 and 4.5 (intraperitoneal), > 20 and > 20 (subcutaneous) and 0.12 and 0.11 (intravenous) g/kg bw, respectively (Tsuji *et al.*, 1975a). The acute oral LD_{50} in rats and the acute dermal LD_{50} in rabbits were reported to exceed 5 g/kg bw (Opdyke, 1975).

After daily administration of *d*-limonene at 277–2770 mg/kg bw to male and female Sprague-Dawley rats for one month, the highest dose was found to have caused a slight decrease in body weight and food consumption. On histological examination (staining with hematoxylin and eosin), granular casts were observed in the kidney of males, but no significant change was found in the other organs (Tsuji *et al.*, 1975a).

A dose-related increase in relative liver and kidney weights was observed in young adult male Fischer 344 rats given 75, 150 or 300 mg/kg bw *d*-limonene daily by gavage on five days per week and killed on study days 6 or 27. With Mallory-Heidenhain staining, a dose-related formation of hyaline droplets was observed histologically in the kidneys. Hyaline droplet nephropathy was associated with increased concentrations of α_{2u}-globulin in renal cortical homogenates separated by two-dimensional gel electrophoresis. The concentrations of other renal proteins were not increased by *d*-limonene treatment. Alterations considered to be sequelae of the hyaline droplet response, including granular casts in the outer zone of the medulla and multiple cortical changes collectively classified as chronic nephrosis, were observed in the kidneys of all rats killed on day 27 (Kanerva *et al.*, 1987).

Oral administration of 75 or 150 mg *d*-limonene to male Fischer 344/N rats on five days per week for two years was associated with dose-related alterations to the kidney, such as increased incidences of mineralization and epithelial hyperplasia and increased severity of chronic progressive nephropathy. In the same study, no signs of toxicity, including renal hyaline droplet formation, were observed in female Fischer 344/N rats dosed at 300 or 600 mg/kg bw (National Toxicology Program, 1990).

Male and female $B6C3F_1$ mice were treated orally on five days a week for two years with doses of 250 or 500 and 500 or 1000 mg/kg bw, respectively. The mean body weights of females at the high dose were 5–15% lower than those of controls after week 28, but no compound-related toxicity was observed in animals of either sex (National Toxicology Progam, 1990).

In beagle dogs, oral doses of more than 340 mg/kg bw (bitches) and 1000 mg/kg bw (dogs) per day for six months resulted in protein casts in the renal tubules. Daily doses of more than 1000 mg/kg bw (bitches) and 3024 mg/kg bw (dogs) resulted in slight weight loss due to frequent vomiting in some animals (Tsuji *et al.*, 1975b).

In another study in adult beagle dogs, *d*-limonene at 100 or 1000 mg/kg bw (maximal tolerated dose for emesis) per day by gavage twice daily for six months increased kidney weights but induced no histopathological changes, hyaline droplet accumulation or nephropathy (Webb *et al.*, 1990).

d-Limonene given orally for four days at 1650 mg/kg bw per day caused no renal toxicity in male NCI Black Reiter rats, which do not synthesize the α_{2u}-globulin that is normally present in hyaline droplets found in male Fischer 344 rats with *d*-limonene-induced nephrotoxicity (Dietrich & Swenberg, 1991a).

The ability of *d*-limonene to cause hyaline droplet nephropathy was evaluated in C57BL/6-derived transgenic mice engineered to express α_{2u}-globulin. These mice excreted approximately 30% less α_{2u}-globulin than male rats. α_{2u}-Globulin was detected in the kidney by immunoblotting; after *d*-limonene treatment at 150 mg/kg bw for three days, the concentration of α_{2u}-globulin was increased threefold relative to untreated controls. Spontaneous hyaline droplet formation was not seen in control transgenic mice, but small droplets were observed after *d*-limonene treatment (Lehman-McKeeman & Caudill, 1994).

d-Limonene at 150 mg/kg bw increased renal-cell proliferation in male Fischer 344 rats, particularly in the P_2 segment of the renal proximal tubular epithelium, after 4 or 31 weeks of exposure. Cell proliferation, determined by bromodeoxyuridine labelling, was increased approximately fivefold over that in control rats. No increase in renal-cell proliferation was observed in male NBR rats treated similarly in the same experiment (Dietrich & Swenberg, 1991b).

d-Limonene increased renal-cell proliferation in response to hyaline droplet exacerbation in Fischer 344 rats dosed orally for 91 days at 0, 5, 30, 75 or 150 mg/kg bw. No exacerbation of hyaline droplets was noted at the lowest dose, and there was no increase in proliferating cell nuclear antigen-labelled renal proximal tubular cells. At doses of 30 mg/kg bw *d*-limonene and higher, both hyaline droplet formation and the percentage of labelled cells were increased. At the highest dose, the percentage of antigen-labelled cells was increased by about six times over that in controls, and the cells were localized to the P_2 segment of the proximal tubule (Lehman-McKeeman, 1995).

mRNA for α_{2u}-globulin was markedly reduced or was undetectable in the livers of male rats [strain not specified] fed diets containing the peroxisome proliferator and lipid-lowering agent ciprofibrate (0.025% wt/wt) for seven weeks. This finding was confirmed by immunoblot analysis with antibodies against α_{2u}-globulin, although immunohistochemical staining and in-situ hybridization showed the presence of a few cells that contained α_{2u}-globulin protein and its m-RNA. The α_{2u}-globulin m-RNA reappeared in the liver two weeks after cessation of ciprofibrate treatment. Feeding of ciprofibrate for two weeks, followed by simultaneous feeding of ciprofibrate and *d*-limonene (150 mg/kg bw per day, six days a week), showed that ciprofibrate prevented α_{2u}-globulin accumulation and the nephrotoxicity associated with binding of *d*-limonene to this protein (Alvares *et al.*, 1996).

4.3 Reproductive and developmental effects

4.3.1 *Humans*

No data were available to the Working Group.

4.3.2 *Experimental systems*

Studies in mice, rats and rabbits exposed by oral administration during organogenesis showed impaired weight gains in the dams and a transient reduction in the growth of the offspring. Anomalies of the ribs were observed in offspring of mice and rats (IARC, 1993).

It was reported in an abstract that *d*-limonene was not teratogenic to frog embryos (*Xenopus laevis*) although a teratogenic effect was reported at the lowest concentration (0.00114 mg/L) (Holck *et al.*, 1991).

4.4 Genetic and related effects

4.4.1 *Humans*

No data were available to the Working Group.

4.4.2 *Experimental systems* (see Table 1 for references)

d-Limonene was not mutagenic to *Salmonella typhimurium*. In single studies, it did not induce sister chromatid exchange, chromosomal aberrations, trifluorothymidine resistance or transformation of rodent cells *in vitro*. *d*-Limonene gave negative results in the mammalian spot test even at toxic doses.

d-Limonene has been found to inhibit gap-junctional intercellular communication in mouse primary keratinocytes and derived cell lines.

The metabolite *d*-limonene-1,2-oxide gave negative results in the SOS chromotest. It was not mutagenic to *S. typhimurium* and did not induce unscheduled DNA synthesis in rat hepatocytes *in vitro*. Essential oils containing *d*-limonene did not induce differential toxicity in *Bacillus subtilis*, nor did they induce reverse mutation in *S. typhimurium*.

d-Limonene did not inhibit the transformation of rat tracheal epithelial cells by benzo[*a*]pyrene (Steele *et al.*, 1990).

4.5 Mechanistic considerations

4.5.1 *Renal tumours in male rats*

The criteria for establishing that an agent causes renal tumours in male rats through a response associated with α_{2u}-globulin (Capen *et al.*, 1999) are as follows:

- lack of genotoxic activity (the agent and/or a metabolite) on the basis of an overall evaluation of results obtained *in vitro* and *in vivo*;
- nephropathy and renal tumorigenicity seen only in male rats;
- induction in shorter studies of the characteristic sequence of histopathological changes, of which protein droplet accumulation is obligatory;
- identification of the protein that accumulates in tubular cells as α_{2u}-globulin;
- reversible binding of the chemical or metabolite to α_{2u}-globulin;
- induction of sustained increased cell proliferation in the renal cortex; and
- similarities in dose–response relationship of the tumour outcome with those for histopathological end-points (protein droplets, α_{2u}-globulin accumulation, cell proliferation).

Table 1. Genetic and related effects of *d*-limonene and its metabolites

Test system	Results[a]		Dose[b] (LED or HID)	Reference
	Without exogenous metabolic system	With exogenous metabolic system		
***d*-Limonene**				
Salmonella typhimurium TA100, TA98, TA1535, TA1537, TA1538, reverse mutation	–	–	2720 μg/plate	Watabe *et al.* (1981)
Salmonella typhimurium TA100, TA98, TA1535, TA1537, reverse mutation	–	–	3333 μg/plate	Haworth *et al.* (1983)
Gene mutation, mouse lymphoma L5178Y cells, *tk* locus *in vitro*	–	–	60	National Toxicology Program (1990)
Sister chromatid exchange, Chinese hamster ovary cells *in vitro*	–	–	162	National Toxicology Program (1990)
Chromosomal aberrations, Chinese hamster ovary cells *in vitro*	–	–	500	National Toxicology Program (1990)
Inhibition of intercellular communication mouse 3PC cells *in vitro*	+	NT	136	Jansen & Jongen (1996)
Cell transformation, Syrian hamster embryo cells	–	NT	50	Oshiro *et al.* (1998)
Mammalian spot test, mouse *in vivo*	–		215 ip × 3	Fahrig (1982)
***d*-Limonene-1,2-oxide**				
Escherichia coli PQ37, induction of SOS repair	–	–	500	von der Hude *et al.* (1990a)
Salmonella typhimurium TA100, TA1535, reverse mutation	–	–	500 μg/plate	von der Hude *et al.* (1990a)
Unscheduled DNA synthesis, primary rat hepatocytes *in vitro*	–	NT	15	von der Hude *et al.* (1990b)

Table 1 (contd)

Test system	Results[a]		Dose[b] (LED or HID)	Reference
	Without exogenous metabolic system	With exogenous metabolic system		
Essential oils containing *d*-limonene				
Bacillus subtilis rec strains, differential toxicity	–	NT	30 μL/plate	Zani *et al.* (1991)
Salmonella typhimurium TA100, TA98, TA1535, TA1537 reverse mutation	–	–	2.5 μL/plate	Zani *et al.* (1991)

[a] +, positive; –, negative; NT, not tested

[b] LED, lowest effective dose; HID, highest ineffective dose; unless otherwise stated, in-vitro test, μg/mL; in-vivo test, mg/kg bw per day; ip, intraperitoneal

These criteria are met by *d*-limonene, which produces hyaline droplet nephropathy and causes renal tubular tumours in male rats through an α_{2u}-globulin-associated response.

d-Limonene causes a renal syndrome that occurs exclusively in male rats. Male rats are unique in that they exhibit a background of spontaneous protein droplets in the proximal tubule, particularly within the cells of the P_2 segment. *d*-Limonene exacerbates the formation of these droplets, and it was shown by two-dimensional gel electrophoresis that the only protein accumulating was α_{2u}-globulin (Alden *et al.*, 1984; Kanerva *et al.*, 1987).

α_{2u}-Globulin is synthesized in the liver, secreted into the general circulation and reabsorbed by renal proximal tubule cells. Hepatic synthesis of α_{2u}-globulin occurs only in adult male rats (Roy *et al.*, 1966). The critical role of α_{2u}-globulin in the renal effects of *d*-limonene is demonstrated by the absence of histopathological changes in female rats and in species that do not synthesize α_{2u}-globulin. Thus, *d*-limonene shows no renal toxicity in female rats, in male NBR rats or in other species studied, including male and female mice and dogs (Chatterjee *et al.*, 1989; Dietrich & Swenberg, 1991a). *d*-Limonene also has no renal toxicity in ciprofibrate-treated male rats in which synthesis of α_{2u}-globulin is repressed (Alvares *et al.*, 1996). Whereas mice do not develop hyaline droplet nephropathy, transgenic mice that synthesize α_{2u}-globulin develop these lesions (Lehman-McKeeman & Caudill, 1994).

The mechanism by which *d*-limonene causes α_{2u}-globulin accumulation in the male rat kidney has been elucidated. The prerequisite step in the development of the nephropathy is the binding to α_{2u}-globulin of an agent, which in the case of *d*-limonene is the 1,2-epoxide (Lehman-McKeeman *et al.*, 1989). This binding is specific for α_{2u}-globulin and reversible, with a binding affinity (K_d) of approximately 5.6×10^{-7} mol/L (Borghoff *et al.*, 1991; Lehman-McKeeman & Caudill, 1992a). Binding of this ligand to α_{2u}-globulin reduces the rate of its lysosomal degradation relative to that of native protein, thereby causing it to accumulate. Lysosomal cathepsin activity towards other protein substrates is not altered (Lehman-McKeeman *et al.*, 1990).

Whereas accumulation of α_{2u}-globulin can be observed after a single oral dose of *d*-limonene, continued treatment results in additional histological changes in the kidney. Phagolysosomes become enlarged, engorged with protein and show polyangular crystalloid inclusions. After three to four weeks of dosing, progressive renal injury, characterized by single-cell degeneration and necrosis in the P_2 segment of the renal proximal tubule, is noted. Dead cells are sloughed into the lumen of the nephron, contributing to the development of granular casts at the cortico-medullary junction (Swenberg & Lehman-McKeeman, 1999). Renal functional perturbations, including reduced uptake of organic anions, cations and amino acids and mild proteinuria resulting from a large increase in the amount of α_{2u}-globulin excreted in urine, are observed. These functional changes occur only in male rats and only at doses that exacerbate the protein droplet formation (Swenberg & Lehman-McKeeman, 1999). In response to the cell death and functional changes, there is a compensatory increase in cell proliferation in the kidney, most notably in the P_2 segment of the proximal tubules, the site of protein accumulation

(Dietrich & Swenberg, 1991b; Swenberg & Lehman-McKeeman, 1999). With continued treatment, the cell proliferation persists, but it does not restore renal function. The increase in cell proliferation is linked to the development of renal tubular tumours (Dietrich & Swenberg, 1991b). α_{2u}-Globulin nephropathy and renal-cell proliferation occur at doses consistent with those that produce renal tubular tumours.

The link between α_{2u}-globulin nephropathy and renal-cell proliferation was established for *d*-limonene in comparative studies of male NBR and Fischer 344 rats. Cell proliferation in renal tubules was increased by *d*-limonene in Fischer 344 rats after 4 or 31 weeks of exposure to *d*-limonene but not in NBR rats which do not develop α_{2u}-globulin nephropathy. Thus, the increase in cell proliferation was shown to be totally dependent on the presence of α_{2u}-globulin. Furthermore, when evaluated in an initiation–promotion study with *N*-nitrosoethyl-*N*-hydroxyethylamine, *d*-limonene treatment increased the incidence of renal adenomas in Fischer 344 rats, whereas no renal tumours occurred in NBR rats (Dietrich & Swenberg, 1991b).

The available data indicate that renal tubular tumours in male rats develop by a secondary, non-DNA reactive mechanism. Histopathological, biochemical and cell proliferation investigations provide compelling evidence that *d*-limonene produces a syndrome that begins acutely as accumulation of α_{2u}-globulin but represents a continuum of changes that progress ultimately to renal tubular tumours (Swenberg *et al.*, 1989; Flamm & Lehman-McKeeman, 1991; Hard *et al.*, 1993; Hard & Whysner, 1994; Swenberg & Lehman-McKeeman, 1999).

Relevance to humans

The requisite step in the development of α_{2u}-globulin nephropathy is binding of *d*-limonene, and particularly the 1,2-epoxide, to α_{2u}-globulin. α_{2u}-Globulin is a member of a superfamily of proteins that bind and transport a variety of ligands. Many of these proteins are synthesized in mammalian species, including humans. Therefore, the question of whether a similar mechanism occurs in humans can be addressed by determining whether these structurally homologous proteins function in humans in a manner analogous to α_{2u}-globulin. This question has been answered both qualitatively and quantitatively.

The protein content of human urine is very different from that of rat urine, as humans excrete very little protein (about 1% of the concentration found in urine of male rats). Human urinary protein is also predominantly a species of high molecular mass, and there is no protein in human plasma or urine identical to α_{2u}-globulin (Olson *et al.*, 1990). No α_{2u}-globulin-like protein has been detected in human kidney tissue (Borghoff & Lagarde, 1993). Saturable binding of *d*-limonene-1,2-epoxide to α_{2u}-globulin can be shown *in vitro*, but other superfamily proteins, particularly those synthesized by humans, do not bind this agent (Lehman-McKeeman & Caudill, 1992b).

The unique specificity of the syndrome of renal toxicity in male rats due to α_{2u}-globulin is demonstrated by the lack of toxicity and of renal tumours in mice. Mice synthesize mouse urinary protein, which shares nearly 90% sequence identity to α_{2u}-globulin; however, *d*-limonene-1,2-epoxide does not bind to the mouse protein and it does not produce a similar syndrome in mice. Additionally, the lack of a response in female rats, which synthesize many other proteins of the superfamily, demonstrates that these proteins are unlikely to contribute to renal toxicity.

The X-ray crystal structure of α_{2u}-globulin has been derived and indicates that although α_{2u}-globulin may share amino acid sequence with many other proteins it has a unique ligand-binding pocket. Other superfamily proteins are characterized by flattened, elongated binding pockets, whereas the ligand-binding site in α_{2u}-globulin is distinguished by a spherical, non-restrictive shape. The elongated, flattened binding pockets in mouse urinary protein and in superfamily proteins synthesized by humans preclude the binding of *d*-limonene-1,2-epoxide to these proteins (Lehman-McKeeman, 1997).

From a quantitative perspective, adult male rat kidneys reabsorb about 35 mg α_{2u}-globulin per day. Female rats synthesize less than 1% of the amount of α_{2u}-globulin reabsorbed by male rats, but no α_{2u}-globulin is detected in female rat kidney and female rats do not develop nephropathy. The most abundant α_{2u}-globulin superfamily protein in human kidney and plasma is α_1-acid glycoprotein, and this protein does not bind to agents that induce α_{2u}-globulin nephropathy in rats.

Taken together, there is no evidence that any human protein can contribute to a renal syndrome similar to α_{2u}-globulin nephropathy, and thus no evidence that *d*-limonene is carcinogenic in humans by a mechanism similar to α_{2u}-globulin nephropathy.

The induction of renal-cell tumours in male rats by agents that act through an α_{2u}-globulin-associated response is not predictive of carcinogenic hazard to humans (Capen *et al.*, 1999). This conclusion is based on extensive evidence that the presence of α_{2u}-globulin is an absolute requirement for the carcinogenic activity and that neither α_{2u}-globulin nor any protein that can function like α_{2u}-globulin is synthesized by humans (Swenberg & Lehman-McKeeman, 1999).

d-Limonene has no carcinogenic activity at any other site in male rats. Consequently, all of the mechanistic data support the conclusion that the renal tumours in male rats produced by *d*-limonene are not relevant to humans.

5. Summary of Data Reported and Evaluation

5.1 Exposure data

d-Limonene is a terpene which occurs naturally in citrus and a variety of other plants. Exposure occurs from its presence in foods and its use as a solvent. It is being evaluated in clinical trials for use as a cancer chemotherapeutic agent.

5.2 Human carcinogenicity data

No data were available to the Working Group.

5.3 Animal carcinogenicity data

d-Limonene was tested for carcinogenicity by oral gavage in mice and rats and in several two-stage experiments with multi-organ carcinogens. It significantly increased the incidence of renal tubular tumours (adenomas and carcinomas) and induced atypical renal tubular hyperplasia in male rats, which normally synthesize α_{2u}-globulin in the liver, but not in female rats or in mice of either sex. It consistently enhanced the incidences of renal tubular tumours and atypical renal tubular hyperplasia initiated by carcinogens in two-stage carcinogenesis assays in male rats of a strain conventionally used in bioassays, but not in a strain that lacks hepatic synthesis of α_{2u}-globulin.

d-Limonene was tested as a cancer-preventive agent in other experimental models with known carcinogens. It inhibited lung carcinogenesis in mice, preneoplastic stages of colon carcinogenesis in rats and pancreatic carcinogenesis in hamsters.

5.4 Other relevant data

d-Limonene is metabolized in humans and experimental animals to a variety of metabolites, including perillic acid and *d*-limonene-1,2-diol. *d*-Limonene causes a male rat-specific nephrotoxicity resulting from accumulation of the male rat-specific protein α_{2u}-globulin. *d*-Limonene-1,2-epoxide binds reversibly to α_{2u}-globulin. *d*-Limonene causes sustained cell proliferation in renal proximal tubular cells, and the dose–response relationships for tumour outcome, enhanced cell proliferation and other histopathological end-points typical of α_{2u}-globulin nephropathy are similar. Female rats, male rats of strains that do not express this protein and other species are not susceptible to the nephrotoxic action of *d*-limonene.

Developmental toxicity in the form of delayed prenatal growth has been observed in mice, rats and rabbits exposed to *d*-limonene during gestation. Skeletal anomalies have also been observed in the fetuses of exposed mice and rabbits.

The few available data indicate that *d*-limonene and its 1,2-epoxide metabolite are not genotoxic.

5.5 Evaluation

There is *inadequate evidence* in humans for the carcinogenicity of *d*-limonene.

There is *sufficient evidence* in experimental animals for the carcinogenicity of *d*-limonene.

Overall evaluation

In making its overall evaluation of the carcinogenicity to humans of *d*-limonene, the Working Group concluded that *d*-limonene produces renal tubular tumours in male rats by a non-DNA-reactive mechanism, through an α_{2u}-globulin-associated response. Therefore, the mechanism by which *d*-limonene increases the incidence of renal tubular tumours in male rats is not relevant to humans.

d-Limonene is *not classifiable as to its carcinogenicity to humans (Group 3).*

6. References

Alden, C.L., Kanerva, R.L., Ridder, G. & Stone, L.C. (1984) The pathogenesis of the nephrotoxicity of volatile hydrocarbons in the male. In: Mehlman, M.A., Hemstreet, C.P., Thorpe, J.J. & Weaver, N.K., eds, *Advances in Modern Environmental Toxicology*, Vol. 7, *Renal Effects of Petroleum Hydrocarbons*, Princeton, NJ, Princeton Scientific Publishers, pp. 107–120

Alvares, K., Subbarao, V., Rao, M.S. & Reddy, J.K. (1996) Ciprofibrate represses alpha(2u)-globulin expression in liver and inhibits d-limonene nephrotoxicity. *Carcinogenesis*, **17**, 311–316

American Industrial Hygiene Association (1993) *Workplace Environmental Exposure Level Guides: d-Limonene*, Fairfax, VA

Borghoff, S.J. & Lagarde, W.H. (1993) Assessment of binding of 2,4,4-trimethyl-2-pentanol to low molecular weight proteins isolated from kidneys of male rats and humans. *Toxicol. appl. Pharmacol.*, **119**, 228–235

Borghoff, S.J., Miller, A.B., Bowen, J.P. & Swenberg, J.A. (1991) Characteristics of chemical binding to α_{2u}-globulin *in vitro*—Evaluating structure activity relationships. *Toxicol. appl. Pharmacol.*, **107**, 228–238

Budavari, S., ed. (1996) *The Merck Index*, 12th Ed., Whitehouse Station, NJ, Merck & Co., p. 938

Capen, C.C., Dybing, E., Rice, J.M. & Wilbourn, J.D., eds (1999) *Species Differences in Thyroid, Kidney and Urinary Bladder Carcinogenesis* (IARC Scientific Publications No. 147), Lyon, IARC

Chatterjee, B., Demyan, W.F., Spong, C.S., Garg, B.D. & Roy, A.K. (1989) Loss of androgenic induction of α_{2u}-globulin gene family in the liver of NIH Black rats. *Endocrinology*, **125**, 1385–1388

Chemical Information Services (1995) *Directory of World Chemical Producers 1995/96 Standard Edition*, Dallas, TX, p. 452

Crowell, P.L., Elson, C.E., Bailey, H.H., Elegbede, A., Haag, J.D. & Gould, M.N. (1994) Human metabolism of the experimental cancer therapeutic agent d-limonene. *Cancer Chemother. Pharmacol.*, **35**, 31–37

Dietrich, D.R. & Swenberg, J.A. (1991a) NCI-Black-Reiter (NBR) male rats fail to develop renal disease following exposure to agents that induce α-2u-globulin nephropathy. *Fundam. appl. Toxicol.*, **16**, 719–762

Dietrich, D.R. & Swenberg, J.A. (1991b) The presence of α_{2u}-globulin is necessary for *d*-limonene promotion of male rat kidney tumors. *Cancer Res.*, **51**, 3512–3521

El-Bayoumy, K., Upadhyaya, P., Desai, D.H., Amin, S., Hoffmann, D. & Wynder, E.L. (1996) Effects of 1,4-phenylenebis(methylene)selenocyanate, phenethyl isothiocyanate, indole-3-carbinol, and *d*-limonene individually and in combination on the tumorigenicity of the tobacco-specific nitrosamine 4-(methylnitrosamino)-1-(3-pyridyl)-1-butanone in A/J mouse lung. *Anticancer Res.*, **16**, 2709–2712

Fahrig, R. (1982) Effects of food additives in the mammalian spot test. *Prog. clin. biol. Res.*, **109**, 334–348

Falk-Filipsson, A., Löf, A., Hagberg, M., Hjelm, E.W. & Wang, Z. (1993) d-Limonene exposure to humans by inhalation: Uptake, distribution, elimination, and effects on the pulmonary function. *J. Toxicol. environ. Health*, **38**, 77–88

Flamm, W.G. & Lehman-McKeeman, L.D. (1991) The human relevance of the renal tumor-inducing potential of d-limonene in male rats: Implications for risk assessment. *Regul. Toxicol. Pharmacol.*, **13**, 70–86

Flavor and Extract Manufacturers' Association (1991) *d-Limonene Monograph*, Washington DC, pp. 1–4

Gould, M.N. (1995) Prevention and therapy of mammary cancer by monoterpenes. *J. cell. Biochem.*, **22** (Suppl.), 139–144

Hard, G.C. & Whysner, J. (1994) Risk assessment of d-limonene: An example of male rat-specific renal tumorigens. *Crit. Rev. Toxicol.*, **24**, 231–254

Hard, G.C., Rodgers, L.S., Baetcke, K.P., Richards, W.L., McGaughy, R.E. & Valcovic, L.R. (1993) Hazard evaluation of chemicals that cause α_{2u}-globulin, hyaline droplet nephropathy, and tubule neoplasia in the kidneys of male rats. *Environ. Health Perspectives*, **99**, 313–349

Haworth, S., Lawlor, T., Mortelmans, K., Speck, W. & Zeiger, E. (1983) *Salmonella* mutagenicity test results for 250 chemials. *Environ. Mutag.*, **Suppl. 1**, 3–142

Holck, A.R., Estep, J.E. & Hemeyer, R.D. (1991) Teratogenicity of d-limonene to Xenopus embryos (Abstract no. P20). *J. Am. Coll. Toxicol.*, **10**, 624

von der Hude, W., Seelbach, A. & Basler, A. (1990a) Epoxides: Comparison of the induction of SOS repair in *Escherichia coli* PQ37 and the bacterial mutagenicity in the Ames test. *Mutat. Res.*, **231**, 205–218

von der Hude, W., Mateblowski, R. & Basler, A. (1990b) Induction of DNA-repair synthesis in primary rat hepatocytes by epoxides. *Mutat. Res.*, **245**, 145–150

IARC (1993) *IARC Monographs on the Evaluation of Carcinogenic Risks to Humans*, Vol. 56, *Some Naturally Occurring Substances: Food Items and Constituents, Heterocyclic Aromatic Amines and Mycotoxins*, Lyon, pp. 135–162

Igimi, H., Nishimura, M., Kodama, R. & Ide, H. (1974) Studies on the metabolism of *d*-limonene (*p*-mentha-1,8-diene). I. The absorption, distribution and excretion of *d*-limonene in rats. *Xenobiotica*, **4**, 77–84

Igimi, H., Hisatsugu, T. & Nishimura, M. (1976) The use of *d*-limonene preparation as a dissolving agent of gallstones. *Dig. Dis.*, **21**, 926–939

Jansen, L.A.M. & Jongen, W.M.F. (1996) The use of initiated cells as a test system for the detection of inhibitors of gap junctional intercellular communication. *Carcinogenesis*, **17**, 333–339

Kanerva, R.L., Ridder, G.M., Lefever, F.R. & Alden, C.L. (1987) Comparison of short-term renal effects due to oral administration of decalin or *d*-limonene in young adult male Fischer-344 rats. *Food chem. Toxicol.*, **25**, 345–353

Kawamori, T., Tanaka, T., Hirose, Y., Ohnishi, M. & Mori, H. ((1996) Inhibitory effects of *d*-limonene on the development of colonic aberrant crypt foci induced by azoxymethane in F344 rats. *Carcinogenesis*, **17**, 369–372

Kimura, J., Takahashi, S., Ogiso, T., Yoshida, Y., Akagi, K., Hasegawa, R., Kurata, M., Hirose, M. & Shirai, T. (1996) Lack of chemoprevention effects of the monoterpene *d*-limonene in a rat multi-organ carcinogenesis model. *Jpn. J. Cancer Res.*, **87**, 589–594

Kodama, R., Noda, K. & Ide, H. (1974) Studies on the metabolism of *d*-limonene (*p*-mentha-1,8-diene). II. The metabolic fate of *d*-limonene in rabbits. *Xenobiotica*, **4**, 85–95

Kodama, R., Yano, T., Furukawa, K., Noda, K. & Ide, H. (1976) Studies on the metabolism of *d*-limonene (*p*-mentha-1,8-diene). IV. Isolation and characterization of new metabolites and species differences in metabolism. *Xenobiotica*, **6**, 377–389

Lehman-McKeeman, L.D. (1997) α_{2u}-Globulin nephropathy. In: Sipes, I.G., McQueen, C.A. & Gandolfi, A.J., eds, *Comprehensive Toxicology*, Vol. 7, *Renal Toxicology*, New York, Pergamon Press, pp. 677–692

Lehman-McKeeman, L.D. & Caudill, D. (1992a) Biochemical basis for mouse resistance to hyaline droplet nephropathy: Lack of relevance of the α2u-globulin protein superfamily in this male rat-specific syndrome. *Toxicol. appl. Pharmacol.*, **112**, 214–221

Lehman-McKeeman, L.D. & Caudill, D. (1992b) α_{2u}-Globulin is the only member of the lipocalin protein superfamily that binds to hyaline droplet inducing agents. *Toxicol. appl. Pharmacol.*, **116**, 170–176

Lehman-McKeeman, L.D. & Caudill, D. (1994) d-Limonene induced hyaline droplet nephropathy in alpha 2u-globulin transgenic mice. *Fundam. appl. Toxicol.*, **23**, 562–568

Lehman-McKeeman, L.D., Rodriguez, P.A., Takigiku, R., Caudill, D. & Fey, M.L. (1989) *d*-Limonene-induced male rat-specific nephrotoxicity: Evaluation of the association between *d*-limonene and α_{2u}-globulin. *Toxicol. appl. Pharmacol.*, **99**, 250–259

Lehman-McKeeman, L.D., Rivera-Torres, M.I. & Caudill, D. (1990) Lysosomal degradation of α2u-globulin and α2u-globulin–xenobiotic conjugates. *Toxicol. appl. Pharmacol.*, **103**, 539–548

Lide, D.R., ed. (1991) *CRC Handbook of Chemistry and Physics*, 72nd Ed., Boca Raton, FL, CRC Press, p. 3-308

Nakaizumi, A., Baba, M., Uehara, H., Iishi, H. & Tatsuta, M. (1997) *d*-Limonene inhibits *N*-nitrosobis(2-oxopropyl)amine induced hamster pancreatic carcinogenesis. *Cancer Lett.*, **117**, 99–103

National Board of Occupational Safety and Health (1996) *Occupational Exposure Limit Values*, Solna

National Institute for Occupational Safety and Health (1998) *National Occupational Exposure Survey (1981–1983)*, Cincinnati, OH

National Library of Medicine (1998) *Hazardous Substances Data Bank (HSDB)*, Bethesda, MD [Record No. 4186]

National Toxicology Program (1990) *NTP Technical Report on the Toxicology and Carcinogenesis Studies of d-Limonene (CAS No. 5989-27-5) in F344/N Rats and B6C3F1 Mice (Gavage Studies)* (NTP TR 347), Research Triangle Park, NC, National Institutes of Health, pp. 145–151

National Toxicology Program (1991) *NTP Chemical Repository Data Sheet: d-Limonene*. Research Triangle Park, NC

O'Shaughnessy, J.A. (1996) Chemoprevention of breast cancer. *J. Am. med. Assoc.*, **275**, 1349–1353

Olson, M.J., Johnson, J.T. & Reidy, C.A. (1990) A comparison of male rat and human urinary proteins: Implications for human resistance to hyaline droplet nephropathy. *Toxicol. appl. Pharmacol.*, **102**, 524–536

Opdyke, D.L.J. (1975) *d*-Limonene. *Food Cosmet. Toxicol.*, **13** (Suppl.), 825–826

Oshiro, Y., Balwierz, P.S., Eurell, T.E., Morris, D.L. & Alden, C.L. (1998) Exploration of the transformation potential of a unique male rat protein alpha$_{2u}$-globulin using hamster embryonic cells. *Toxicol. Pathol.*, **26**, 381–387

Poon, G.K., Vigushin, D., Griggs, L.J., Rowlands, M.G., Coombes, R.C. & Jarman, M. (1996) Identification and characterization of limonene metabolites in patients with advanced cancer by liquid chromatography/mass spectrometry. *Drug Metab. Disposition*, **24**, 565–571

Roy, A.K., Neuhaus, O.W. & Harmison, C.R. (1966) Preparation and characterization of a sex-dependent rat urinary protein. *Biochim. biophys. Acta*, **127**, 72–81

Saito, K., Uwagawa, S., Kaneko, H., Shiba, K., Tomigahara, Y. & Nakatsuka, I. (1996) alpha(2u)-Globulins in the urine of male rats: A reliable indicator for alpha(2u)-globulin accumulation in the kidney. *Toxicology*, **106**, 149–157

Steele, V.E., Kelloff, G.J., Wilkinson, B.P. & Arnold, J.T (1990) Inhibition of transformation in cultured rat tracheal epithelial cells by potential chemopreventive agents. *Cancer Res.*, **50**, 2068–2074

Swenberg, J.A. & Lehman-McKeeman, L.D. (1999) α_{2u}-Urinary globulin-associated nephropathy as a mechanism of renal tubular cell carcinogenesis in male rats. In: Capen, C.C., Dybing, E., Rice, J.M. & Wilbourn, J.D., eds, *Species Differences in Thyroid, Kidney and Urinary Bladder Carcinogenesis* (IARC Scientific Publications No. 147), Lyon, IARC, pp. 95–118

Swenberg, J.A., Short, B.G., Borghoff, S.J., Strasser, J. & Charbonneau, M. (1989) The comparative pathobiology of α_{2u}-globulin nephropathy. *Toxicol. appl. Pharmacol.*, **97**, 35–46

Tsuji, M., Fujisaki, Y., Arikawa, Y., Masuda, S., Kinoshita, S., Okubo, A., Noda, K., Ide, H. & Iwanage, Y. (1975a) [Studies on *d*-limonene, as gallstone solubilizer. II. Acute and subacute toxicities.] *Oyo Yakuri*, **9**, 387–401 (in Japanese)

Tsuji, M., Fujisaki, Y., Arikawa, Y., Masuda, S., Tanaka, T., Sato, K., Noda, K., Ide, H. & Kikuchi, M. (1975b) [Studies on *d*-limonene, as gallstone solubilizer. IV. Chronic toxicity in dogs.] *Oyo Yakuri*, **9**, 775–808 (in Japanese)

Vigushin, D.M., Poon, G.K., Boddy, A., English, J., Halbert, G.W., Pagonis, C., Jarman, M. & Coombes, R.C. (1998) Phase I and pharmacokinetic study of D-limonene in patients with advanced cancer. *Cancer Chemother. Pharmacol.*, **42**, 111–117

Watabe, T., Hiratsuka, A., Isobe, M. & Ozawa, N. (1980) Metabolism of *d*-limonene by hepatic microsomes to non-mutagenic epoxides toward *Salmonella typhimurium*. *Biochem. Pharmacol.*, **29**, 1068–1071

Watabe, T., Hiratsuka, A., Ozawa, N. & Isobe, M. (1981) A comparative study of the metabolism of *d*-limonene and 4-vinylcyclohex-1-ene by hepatic microsomes. *Xenobiotica*, **11**, 333–344

Webb, D.R., Kanerva, R.L., Hysell, D.K., Alden, C.L. & Lehman-McKeeman, L.D. (1990) Assessment of the chronic oral toxicity of *d*-limonene in dogs. *Food chem. Toxicol.*, **28**, 669–675

WHO (1993) *Guidelines for Drinking Water Quality*, 2nd Ed., Vol. 1, *Recommendations*, Geneva

Zani, F., Massimo, G., Benvenuti, S., Bianchi, A., Albasini, A., Meleari, M., Vampa, G., Beilotti, A. & Mazza, P. (1991) Studies on the genotoxic properties of essential oils with *Bacillus subtilis rec*-assay and *Salmonella*/microsome reversion assay. *Planta med.*, **57**, 237–241

MELAMINE

This substance was considered by previous working groups, in 1985 (IARC, 1986) and 1987 (IARC, 1987). Since that time, new data have become available, and these have been incorporated into the monograph and taken into consideration in the present evaluation.

1. Exposure Data

1.1 Chemical and physical data

1.1.1 *Nomenclature*

Chem. Abstr. Serv. Reg. No.: 108-78-1

Deleted CAS Reg. Nos.: 504-18-7; 65544-34-5; 67757-43-1; 68379-55-5; 70371-19-6; 94977-27-2

Chem. Abstr. Name: 1,3,5-Triazine-2,4,6-triamine

IUPAC Systematic Name: Melamine

Synonyms: Cyanuramide; cyanurotriamide; cyanurotriamine; isomelamine; triaminotriazine; 2,4,6-triaminotriazine; triamino-*s*-triazine; 2,4,6-triamino-1,3,5-triazine; 2,4,6-*s*-triazinetriamine; 1,3,5-triazine-2,4,6(1H,3H,5H)-triimine

1.1.2 *Structural and molecular formulae and relative molecular mass*

H2N NH2 N N N NH2

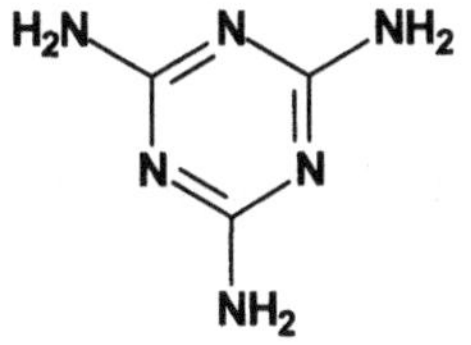

$C_3H_6N_6$ Relative molecular mass: 126.12

1.1.3 *Chemical and physical properties of the pure substance*

(*a*) *Description*: Monoclinic prisms (Budavari, 1996)

(*b*) *Melting-point*: 345°C; decomposes (Lide, 1997)

(*c*) *Density*: 1.573 g/cm^3 at 16°C (Lide, 1997)

(*d*) *Solubility*: Slightly soluble in water and ethanol; insoluble in diethyl ether (Lide, 1997)

(*e*) *Octanol/water partition coefficient (P)*: log P, –1.14 (Verschueren, 1996)

(*f*) *Conversion factor*: mg/m^3 = 5.16 × ppm

1.2 Production and use

Information available in 1995 indicated that melamine was produced in 14 countries (Chemical Information Services, 1995).

Melamine forms synthetic resins with formaldehyde (Budavari, 1996). It is used in the manufacture of melamine resins, laminates, surface coating resins, plastic moulding compounds, textile resins, bonding resins, gypsum–melamine resin mixtures, orthopaedic casts, rubber additives and paper products (National Toxicology Program, 1991).

1.3 Occurrence

1.3.1 *Natural occurrence*

Melamine is not known to occur naturally.

1.3.2 *Occupational exposure*

According to the 1981–83 National Occupational Exposure Survey (National Institute for Occupational Safety and Health, 1998), approximately 43 000 workers in the United States were potentially exposed to melamine. Occupational exposure to melamine may occur during its production and during its use in the manufacture of synthetic resins with formaldehyde.

1.3.3 *Environmental occurrence*

According to the Environmental Protection Agency Toxic Chemical Release Inventory for 1987, 82 000 kg melamine were released into the air, 240 000 kg were discharged into water, 11 000 kg were disposed of by underground injection and 2500 kg were released onto the land from manufacturing and processing facilities in the United States (National Library of Medicine, 1998). Exposure to melamine in the environment has been judged to be low (Environmental Protection Agency, 1988), but few quantitative data are available.

1.4 Regulations and guidelines

No international guidelines for melamine in drinking-water have been established (WHO, 1993).

2. Studies of Cancer in Humans

No data were available to the Working Group.

3. Studies of Cancer in Experimental Animals

Previous evaluation

Melamine was tested for carcinogenicity by oral administration in the diet in one study in mice and in one study in rats, and for initiating activity by skin application in one study in mice. No neoplasm related to treatment was observed after oral administration to mice. Male rats fed diets containing melamine developed transitional-cell tumours of the urinary bladder; with one exception, all tumour-bearing animals had bladder stones probably consisting of melamine. This finding precluded a clear interpretation of the results. In a two-stage mouse-skin assay in which melamine was tested at one dose, it did not show initiating activity (IARC, 1986). [The present Working Group noted the occurrence of urinary bladder hyperplasia associated with toxicity in male mice treated with melamine in the diet.]

New studies

Oral administration

Rat: Groups of 20 male Fischer 344 rats, six weeks of age, were fed diets containing 0.3, 1 or 3% melamine (purity, > 99%) for a total of 36 weeks and were killed four weeks later. Carcinomas of the urinary bladder were observed in 0/20, 1/20 and 15/19 rats at the low, intermediate and high doses and papillomas in 0/20, 1/20 and 12/19 rats, respectively. One carcinoma and three papillomas of the ureter were also induced in 19 rats at the high dose. The findings of tumours correlated with the formation of calculi (see section 4; Okumura *et al.*, 1992).

Groups of 20 male Fischer 344 rats, six weeks of age, were fed diets containing 1.0 or 3.0% melamine (purity, 99.94%), with or without 5 or 10% sodium chloride (NaCl) for a total of 36 weeks and were killed at week 40. Urinary bladder carcinomas were observed in 4/19, 18/20 and 18/20 rats given 1% melanine alone, 3% melamine alone or 3% melamine plus 5% NaCl, respectively. No carcinomas were observed in the groups receiving 3% melamine plus 10% NaCl or 1% melamine plus 5 or 10% NaCl. The incidences of papillomas were similarly decreased by NaCl. In contrast to the incidence of 10/20 in the group given 3% melamine alone, 5/20 and 3/20 rats receiving 3% melamine plus 5% NaCl or 10% NaCl, respectively, developed papillomas. Papillomas developed in 8/19 rats receiving 1% melamine alone. The occurrence of tumours correlated with calculus (melamine–uric acid salt) formation and papillomatosis (Ogasawara *et al.*, 1995).

4. Other Data Relevant to an Evaluation of Carcinogenicity and its Mechanisms

4.1 Absorption, distribution, metabolism and excretion

4.1.1 *Humans*

The urinary metabolites recovered after administration of hexamethylmelamine to two patients indicated that the *s*-triazine ring is very stable and does not undergo cleavage *in vivo* (Worzalla *et al.*, 1974).

4.1.2 *Experimental systems*

Fifty per cent of a single oral dose of 250 mg/kg bw melamine was recovered from the urine of rats within 6 h (Lipschitz & Stokey, 1945).

The urinary metabolites, including melamine, recovered after administration of hexamethylmelamine to rats indicated that the *s*-triazine ring is very stable and does not undergo cleavage *in vivo* (Worzalla *et al.*, 1974).

After administration of a single oral dose of 0.38 mg [^{14}C]-melamine to adult male Fischer 344/N rats, 90% of the administered dose was excreted in the urine within the first 24 h. An elimination half-life of 3 h and a renal clearance of 2.5 mL/min were calculated. Most of the radiolabel was concentrated in the kidney and bladder, and negligible amounts were detected in exhaled air and faeces. Virtually no residual radiolabel was observed in tissues after 24 h. Chromatography of the radiolabelled material found in plasma and urine indicated that melamine was not metabolized in rats (Mast *et al.*, 1983).

4.2 Toxic effects

4.2.1 *Humans*

No data were available to the Working Group.

4.2.2 *Experimental systems*

The LD_{50} values for melamine given in corn oil by gavage were reported to be 3.3 and 7.0 g/kg bw in male and female B6C3F$_1$ mice, respectively, and 3.2 and 3.8 g/kg bw in male and female Fischer 344/N rats (National Toxicology Program, 1983).

Male and female Fischer 344 rats and B6C3F$_1$ mice were fed diets containing 5000–30 000 ppm [250–1500 mg/kg bw per day for rats and 750–4500 mg/kg bw per day for mice] melamine (purity, 97%) for 14 days. A hard crystalline solid was found in the urinary bladder in most male rats receiving 10 000 ppm or more and in all treated male mice; in females, this solid was found at doses of ≥ 20 000 ppm in all rats and in 2/5 mice given 30 000 ppm. In a subsequent study, diets containing 0, 6000, 9000, 12 000, 15 000 or 18 000 ppm melamine were fed to groups of 12 male and 12 female rats and to groups of 10 male and 10 female mice for 13 weeks. Stones were found in the urinary bladders of most male rats in a dose-related manner and in the bladders of some female rats receiving ≥ 15 000 ppm. Bladder stones were observed in both male and female mice receiving ≥ 12 000 ppm. Ulceration of the urinary bladder was also seen in treated mice of each sex fed ≥ 12 000 ppm; 60% of the mice that had bladder ulcers also had stones. The distribution of bladder ulcers and stones was not considered to provide evidence for an association between ulceration and bladder stones in animals of either sex. In another study of the same duration, diets containing 750, 1500, 3000, 6000 or 12 000 ppm [37.5, 75, 150, 300 and 600 mg/kg bw per day] melamine were fed to rats. Hyperplasia of the bladder epithelium was noted in male rats receiving ≥ 3000 ppm, but in none of the female rats. Urinary bladder stones were not observed in treated or control female rats, but the incidence among male rats increased in a dose-related manner from the lowest dose (2/10) to the highest (9/9) (National Toxicology Program, 1983; Melnick *et al.*, 1984).

Male Fischer 344 rats and B6C3F$_1$ mice were fed diets containing 0, 2250 or 4500 ppm melamine and female rats received 0, 4500 or 9000 ppm melamine in the diet for 103 weeks. Twenty per cent of the males at the high dose, only 2% at the low dose and none of the controls had bladder stones. Seven of the eight urinary bladders with transitional-cell carcinomas and three of the remaining 41 bladders without neoplasms had stones. There was therefore a statistically significant ($p < 0.001$) correlation between the presence of bladder stones and bladder tumours. Although 4% of the controls and 85 and 93% of the treated male mice had bladder stones, none developed bladder tumours (National Toxicology Program, 1983; Melnick *et al.*, 1984).

Groups of 20 male Fischer 344 rats were fed diets containing 0, 0.3, 1 or 3% melamine in the diet for 36 weeks followed by a four-week recovery period. Ten animals per group underwent exploratory laparotomy at the end of week 36, and all animals were killed at week 40. The weight of the bladder was threefold greater in rats receiving 3% in the diet than in controls. The incidences of papillary or nodular hyperplasia were 0 in controls, 5% with 0.3% melamine, 30% with 1% melamine and 63% with 3% melamine; those of papillomatosis were 0, 0, 25 and 89% and those of calculi were 0, 0, 70 and 100% at 36 weeks and 0, 20, 45 and 42% at 40 weeks. The correlation between calculus formation at week 36 and tumour incidence at week 40 was highly significant ($p = 0.0065$) (Okumura *et al.*, 1992).

The incidence and composition of urinary bladder calculi after exposure for 36 weeks to melamine with and without additional NaCl in the diet was studied in five-week-old male male Fischer 344/DuCrj rats. Water intake, as a surrogate for urinary output, was increased in groups exposed to 3% melamine with or without 5 or 10% NaCl, in groups exposed to 1% melamine with 5 or 10% NaCl and in a group exposed to 10% NaCl only; water intake was not increased in animals exposed to 1% melamine only. The incidences of calculi and papillomatosis were 30 and 75% with 3% melamine, 75 and 85% with 3% melamine plus 5% NaCl, 30 and 10% with 3% melamine plus 10% NaCl, 37 and 47% with 1% melamine, 11 and 11% with 1% melamine plus 5% NaCl, 5 and 0% with 1% melamine plus 10% NaCl. No calculi or papillomatosis were reported in controls or with 10% NaCl alone. Therefore, the addition of NaCl to 1% melamine decrease the incidences of calculi and papillomatosis, in parallel with a decrease in the incidence of neoplasia. With 3% melamine, NaCl did not affect the induction of calculi or papillomatosis but decreased the incidence of neoplasia. Thus, with the lower concentration of melamine NaCl appeared to increase urinary output and decrease the incidences of hyperplasia, calculus formation and neoplasia. Chemical analysis of the calculi showed that they contained approximately equal amounts of melamine and uric acid on a molar basis, which together accounted for 61–81% of the weight (Ogasawara *et al.*, 1995).

4.3 Reproductive and developmental effects

No data were available to the Working Group.

4.4 Genetic and related effects

4.4.1 *Humans*

No data were available to the Working Group.

4.4.2 *Experimental systems* (see Table 1 for references)

Melamine induced λ prophage in *Escherichia coli* WP2s(λ) but did not induce reverse mutation in *Salmonella typhimurium* in the presence or absence of an exogenous metabolic activation system. Sex-linked recessive lethal mutations were not induced in *Drosophila melanogaster*. Melamine did not induce gene mutation in mouse lymphoma L5178Y $tk^{+/-}$ cells.

It was reported in abstracts that melamine did not induce gene mutation in *S. typhimurium*, sister chromatid exchange in Chinese hamster ovary cells *in vitro* or micronuclei in mouse bone marrow *in vivo* (Mast *et al.*, 1982a,b).

4.5 Mechanistic considerations

No biotransformation of melamine has been reported. A highly statistically significant, consistent relationship between bladder neoplasia in male rats and calculus formation has been found: in one bioassay, all but one rat with urinary bladder tumours also had bladder stones. The ability of rodents to eliminate bladder stones may account for the absence of stones in the one rat. The bladder stones contained melamine and uric acid in equal molar amounts, as well as other components. Melamine also produced a dose-related increase in the incidence of urinary bladder hyperplasia and papillomatosis but only at doses that also produced calculi. The addition of NaCl to the diets, which increased water consumption, inhibited the formation of bladder calculi, bladder hyperplasia and neoplasia in male rats exposed to 1% [500 mg/kg bw per day] melamine, which is similar to the dose that produces bladder tumours (Teelmann & Niemann, 1979). Although bladder tumours related to calculus formation are not considered to be species-specific, they are related to administration of high doses (Capen *et al.*, 1999).

5. Summary of Data Reported and Evaluation

5.1 Exposure data

Exposure to melamine may occur during its production and use in the manufacture of synthetic resins with formaldehyde.

5.2 Human carcinogenicity data

No data were available to the Working Group.

5.3 Animal carcinogenicity data

Melamine has been studied for carcinogenicity in mice and rats of each sex by oral administration. It produced urinary bladder and ureteral carcinomas in male rats but only

Table 1. Genetic and related effects of melamine

Test system	Results[a]		Dose[b] (LED or HID)	Reference
	Without exogenous metabolic system	With exogenous metabolic system		
Prophage induction, *Escherichia coli* WP2s (λ)	+	+	78 µg/well	Rossman *et al.* (1991)
Salmonella typhimurium TA100, TA98, TA1535, TA1537, reverse mutation	–	–	1110 µg/plate	Haworth *et al.* (1983)
Drosophila melanogaster, sex-linked recessive lethal mutations	–		1% feed	Röhrborn (1962)
Gene mutation, mouse lymphoma L5178Y cells, *tk* locus *in vitro*	–	–	160 µg/mL	McGregor *et al.* (1988)

[a] +, positive; –, negative
[b] LED, lowest effective dose; HID, highest ineffective dose

urinary bladder hyperplasia in male mice. The occurrence of urinary bladder tumours in male rats correlated strictly with calculus formation and exposure to high doses. The dose dependence was confirmed by subsequent studies in male rats in which concomitant administration of sodium chloride to increase urinary output resulted in a decreased tumour yield.

5.4 Other relevant data

There is no evidence that melamine undergoes biotransformation. The urinary bladder tumours seen in male rats exposed to high doses of melamine appear to be produced by a non-DNA-reactive mechanism involving epithelial hyperplasia secondary to the presence of melamine-containing bladder stones. Consequently, bladder tumours would not be expected in either rodents or humans except at doses that produce bladder calculi.

No data were available on the reproductive or developmental toxicity of melamine.

No data were available on the genetic and related effects of melamine in humans. It was not genotoxic in experimental systems.

5.5 Evaluation

There is *inadequate evidence* in humans for the carcinogenicity of melamine.

There is *sufficient evidence* in experimental animals for the carcinogenicity of melamine under conditions in which it produces bladder calculi.

Overall evaluation

In making its overall evaluation, the Working Group noted that the non-DNA-reactive mechanism by which melamine produced urinary bladder tumours in male rats occurred only under conditions in which calculi were produced.

Melamine is *not classifiable as to its carcinogenicity to humans (Group 3).*

6. References

Budavari, S., ed. (1996) *The Merck Index*, 12th Ed., Whitehouse Station, NJ, Merck & Co., p. 990

Capen, C.C., Dybing, E., Rice, J.M. & Wilbourn, J.D., eds (1999) *Species Differences in Thyroid, Kidney and Urinary Bladder Carcinogenesis*, Lyon, IARC

Chemical Information Services (1995) *Directory of World Chemical Producers 1995/96 Standard Edition*, Dallas, TX, p. 462

Environmental Protection Agency (1988) Melamine; toxic chemical release reporting; community right-to-know. *Fed. Reg.*, **53**, 23128–23133

Haworth, S., Lawlor, T., Mortelmans, K., Speck, W. & Zeiger, E. (1983) *Salmonella* mutagenicity test results for 250 chemials. *Environ. Mutag.*, **Suppl. 1**, 3–142

IARC (1986) *IARC Monographs on the Evaluation of the Carcinogenic Risk of Chemicals to Humans*, Vol. 39, *Some Chemicals Used in Plastics and Elastomers*, Lyon, pp. 333–346

IARC (1987) *IARC Monographs on the Evaluation of Carcinogenic Risks to Humans*, Suppl. 7, *Overall Evaluations of Carcinogenicity: An Updating of* IARC Monographs *Volumes 1 to 42*, Lyon, p. 65

Lide, D.R., ed. (1997) *CRC Handbook of Chemistry and Physics*, 78th Ed., Boca Raton, FL, CRC Press, p. 3-323

Lipschitz, W.L. & Stokey, E. (1945) The mode of action of three new diuretics: Melamine, adenine and formoguanamine. *J. Pharmacol. exp. Ther.*, **83**, 235–249

Mast, R.W., Friedman, M.A. & Finch, R.A. (1982a) Mutagencity testing of melamine (Abstract No. 602). *Toxicologist*, **2**, 172

Mast, R.W., Naismith, R.W. & Friedman, M.A. (1982b) Mouse micronucleus assay of melamine (Abstract No. Bi-8). *Environ. mol. Mutag.*, **4**, 340–341

Mast, R.W., Jeffcoat, A.R., Sadler, B.M., Kraska, R.C. & Friedman, M.A. (1983) Metabolism, disposition and excretion of [^{14}C]melamine in male Fischer 344 rats. *Food chem. Toxicol.*, **21**, 807–810

McGregor, D.B., Brown, A., Cattanach, P., Edwards, I., McBride, D., Riach, C. & Caspary, W.J. (1988) Responses of the L5178Y tk^{+}/tk^{-} mouse lymphoma cell forward mutation assay: III. 72 coded chemicals. *Environ. mol. Mutag.*, **12**, 85–154

Melnick, R.L., Boorman, G.A., Haseman, J.K., Montali, R.J. & Huff, J. (1984) Urolithiasis and bladder carcinogenicity of melamine in rodents. *Toxicol. appl. Pharmacol.*, **72**, 292–303

National Institute for Occupational Safety and Health (1998) *National Occupational Exposure Survey (1981–83)*, Cincinnati, OH

National Library of Medicine (1998) *Toxic Chemical Release Inventory 1987* (TRI87), Bethesda, MD

National Toxicology Program (1983) *Carcinogenesis Bioassay of Melamine (CAS No. 108-78-1) in F344/N Rats and B6C3F1 Mice (Feed Study)* (Technical Report No. 245), Research Triangle Park, NC

National Toxicology Program (1991) *NTP Chemical Repository Data Sheet: Melamine*, Research Triangle Park, NC

Ogasawara, H., Imaida, K., Ishiwata, H., Toyoda, K., Kawanishi, T., Uneyama, C., Hayashi, S., Takahashi, M. & Hayashi, Y. (1995) Urinary bladder carcinogenesis induced by melamine in F344 male rats: Correlation between carcinogenicity and urolith formation. *Carcinogenesis*, **16**, 2773–2777

Okumura, M., Hasegawa, R., Shirai, T., Ito, M., Yamada, S. & Fukushima, S. (1992) Relationship between calculus formation and carcinogenesis in the urinary bladder of rats administered the non-genotoxic agents, thymine or melamine. *Carcinogenesis*, **13**, 1043–1045

Röhrborn, G. (1962) [Chemical constitution and mutagenic activity. II. Triazine derivatives.] *Z. Verfbungslehre*, **93**, 1–6 (in German)

Rossman, T.G., Molina, M., Meyer, L., Boone, P., Klein, C.B., Wang, Z., Li, F., Lin, W.C. & Kinney, P.L. (1991) Performance of 133 compounds in the lambda prophage induction end-point of the Microscreen assay and a comparison with S. typhimurium mutagenicity and rodent carcinogenicity assay. *Mutat. Res.*, **260**, 349–367

Teelmann, K. & Niemann, W. (1979) The short term fate of dischargeable glass beads implanted surgically in the mouse urinary bladder. *Arch. Toxicol.*, **42**, 51–61

Verschueren, K. (1996) *Handbook of Environmental Data on Organic Chemicals*, 3rd Ed., New York, Van Nostrand Reinhold Co., pp. 1213–1214

WHO (1993) *Guidelines for Drinking Water Quality*, 2nd Ed., Vol. 1, *Recommendations*, Geneva

Worzalla, J., Kaiman, B.D., Johnson, B.M., Ramirez, G. & Bryan, G.T. (1974) Metabolism of hexamethylmelamine-ring-^{14}C in rats and man. *Cancer Res.*, **34**, 2669–2674

METHYL *tert*-BUTYL ETHER

1. Exposure Data

1.1 Chemical and physical data

1.1.1 *Nomenclature*

Chem. Abstr. Serv. Reg. No.: 1634-04-4
Chem. Abstr. Name: 2-Methoxy-2-methyl-propane
IUPAC Systematic Name: *tert*-Butyl methyl ether
Synonyms: *t*-Butyl methyl ether; *tert*-butoxymethane; 1,1-dimethylethyl methyl ether; methyl 1,1-dimethylethyl ether; 2-methyl-2-methoxypropane; methyl tertiary butyl ether; MTBE

1.1.2 *Structural and molecular formulae and relative molecular mass*

$$H_3C-O-\underset{CH_3}{\overset{CH_3}{\overset{|}{\underset{|}{C}}}}-CH_3$$

$C_5H_{12}O$ Relative molecular mass: 88.15

1.1.3 *Chemical and physical properties of the pure substance*

(*a*) *Description*: Colourless liquid with a terpene-like odour (Lewis, 1993; Agency for Toxic Substances and Disease Registry, 1996)
(*b*) *Boiling-point*: 55.2°C (Lide, 1997)
(*c*) *Melting-point*: –108.6°C (Lide, 1997)
(*d*) *Density*: 0.7405 g/cm^3 at 20°C (Lide, 1997)
(*e*) *Spectroscopy data*: Infrared (prism [46183], grating [31183]) and nuclear magnetic resonance (proton [19010], C-13 [4377]) spectral data have been reported (Sadtler Research Laboratories, 1980).
(*f*) *Solubility*: Soluble in water (48 g/L); very soluble in ethanol and diethyl ether (Budavari, 1996; Lide, 1997)
(*g*) *Volatility*: Vapour pressure: 3.26×10^4 Pa at 25°C (Budavari, 1996); relative vapour density (air = 1), 3.1 (Environmental Protection Agency, 1994)
(*h*) *Explosive limits*: Upper, 8.4 %; lower, 1.65%, by volume in air (Scholz *et al.*, 1990)
(*i*) *Octanol/water partition coefficient (P)*: log P, 0.94 (Hansch *et al.*, 1995)
(*j*) *Conversion factor*: mg/m^3 = $3.60 \times$ ppm

1.1.4 *Technical products and impurities*

The typical purity of commercial methyl *tert*-butyl ether is 98–99 wt %. The contaminants may include *tert*-butanol and diisobutenes, residual methanol and, depending on the quality of the C-4 feedstock mixture, also C-5 and C-6 hydrocarbons. The typical composition of methyl *tert*-butyl ether adopted for use in fuels is: purity, 98–99 wt %; alcohols (methanol, *tert*-butanol), 0.5–1.5 wt %; hydrocarbons (C-5 and C-6, diisobutenes), 0.1–1.0 wt %; water, 50–1500 mg/kg; total sulfur (max.), 10 mg/kg; and residue on evaporation (max.), 10 mg/kg. For special applications, 99.95% pure methyl *tert*-butyl ether is marketed under the trade name Driveron S (Scholz *et al.*, 1990).

1.1.5 *Analysis*

Pure methyl *tert*-butyl ether is analysed by gas chromatography, preferably in capillary columns with a highly polar stationary phase, e.g. 1,2,3-tris(2-cyanoethoxy)propane, Carbowax 20 M or DX-1. For gas chromatographic analysis of methyl *tert*-butyl ether-containing fuels, an oxygen-specific flame ionization detector or a column combination technique can be used (Scholz *et al.*, 1990). The National Institute for Occupational Safety and Health recommends Method 1615 for sampling and analysis of methyl *tert*-butyl ether, which involves sampling with standard-sized coconut charcoal tubes, desorbing the sample with carbon disulfide, and analysis by gas chromatography–flame ionization detector; the estimated limit of detection is 0.02 mg/sample (Palassis, 1994).

Method 524.2 of the Environmental Protection Agency (1992) is a general-purpose purge-and-trap gas chromatography–mass spectrometry method for the identification and simultaneous measurement of purgeable volatile organic compounds, including methyl *tert*-butyl ether, in surface water, groundwater and drinking-water in any stage of treatment. The limit of detection for methyl *tert*-butyl ether is 0.09 μg/L. The United States Geological Survey (1995) recommended a similar method for determining methyl *tert*-butyl ether in whole water, with a detection limit of 0.06 μg/L.

Methyl *tert*-butyl ether is readily analysed in a variety of direct reading instruments, which can be used for real-time analysis and for the determination of instantaneous air concentrations. Direct reading instruments that have been successfully used to measure methyl *tert*-butyl ether are combustible gas indicators, infrared spectrophotometers, flame ionization detectors and photoionization detectors (Arco Chemical Co., 1993).

1.2 Production and use

1.2.1 *Production*

Extensive studies during the Second World War demonstrated the qualities of methyl *tert*-butyl ether as a high-octane fuel component; however, it was not until 1973 that the first commercial plant was in operation in Italy. Reduction in the lead content of gasoline in the mid-1970s led to a drastic increase in the demand for octane enhancers, and methyl *tert*-butyl ether is used increasingly in this way (Scholz *et al.*, 1990).

In 1987, the production volume of methyl *tert*-butyl ether in the United States was 1.6 million tonnes (Scholz *et al.*, 1990), and by 1995 it was 8.0 million tonnes (Kirschner,

1996). The production and consumption of methyl *tert*-butyl ether in 1995 and 1996 in Asia are presented in Table 1.

Table 1. Production and consumption of methyl *tert*-butyl ether in Asia in 1995 and 1996 (barrels/day)

Country or region	Production/consumption	
	1995	1996
China	5200/4500	6295/5100
Taiwan	2500/8750	3480/10 700
India	200/250	500/500
Indonesia	0/200	0/800
Japan	6100/6000	7500/6900
Republic of Korea	5900/7000	10 800/8500
Malaysia	4900/200	6199/238
Philippines	0/100	0/300
Singapore	1600/3000	2200/3500
Thailand	0/2000	0/3500
Asia Pacific Region	26 400/32 000	36 974/40 038

From Anon. (1997)

Methyl *tert*-butyl ether is currently produced by the acid-catalysed addition of methanol to isobutene. Suitable catalysts are solid acids such as bentonites and, especially, macroporous acidic ion-exchange resins. In 1990, 54 methyl *tert*-butyl ether plants with a total installed capacity of 7.3 million tonnes were in operation worldwide (Scholz *et al.*, 1990).

Information available in 1994 indicated that methyl *tert*-butyl ether was produced in 21 countries (Chemical Information Services, 1995).

1.2.2 *Use*

Methyl *tert*-butyl ether was first used commercially in Europe in 1973 for gasoline blending. It has been used in the United States since 1979, mainly as an octane enhancer in gasoline. It is the main oxygenate, which was present in 1997 in more than 30% of gasoline sold in the United States. It typically represents about 15% of the content of oxygenated fuels sold during winter months to reduce carbon monoxide in areas where there is heavy pollution by carbon monoxide (Piel, 1995; Stern & Kneiss, 1997). After 1992, it represented approximately 12% of the content of reformulated gasolines sold year-round in 37 areas with ozone pollution associated with emissions of volatile organic compounds.

More than 95% of the methyl *tert*-butyl ether produced is used as a component of gasoline. The market for fuels, amounting to approximately 100 million tonnes/year in western Europe and 320 million tonnes/year in the United States, has a capacity for methyl *tert*-butyl ether that will exceed production for some time to come (Scholz *et al.*, 1990). Methyl *tert*-butyl ether is used extensively in the Republic of Korea, Taiwan and Thailand, where the oxygenate content and environmental concerns are both intense. It is also used in significant quantities in China and Japan (Miller, 1998).

In Canada, where methylcyclopentadienyl manganese bicarbonyl is used as an octane enhancer, methyl *tert*-butyl ether-blended gasoline (6.5–9.6% content) accounts for only 2% of the total unleaded gasoline used (Government of Canada, 1992).

The importance of methyl *tert*-butyl ether is based primarily on its exceptionally good octane-enhancing properties when used as a gasoline blendstock. Depending on the composition of the base gasoline, blend octane numbers of 115–135 (research octane number) and 98–120 (motor octane number) can be achieved. The highest blend values are obtained with saturated, paraffin-rich gasolines and the lowest with olefin-rich gasolines. The lead and aromatics content also influence the blend octane numbers of methyl *tert*-butyl ether (Scholz *et al.*, 1990).

Besides increasing the octane number, methyl *tert*-butyl ether also reduced the fuel vapour pressure (Reid vapour pressure), so that the vapour emissions during automobile fuelling and operation are reduced. Addition of methyl *tert*-butyl ether reduces exhaust emissions, particularly carbon monoxide, unburnt hydrocarbons, polycyclic aromatics and particulate carbon. Although methyl *tert*-butyl ether has a somewhat lower heat of combustion than gasoline, addition of up to 20 vol% neither impairs motor power nor increases fuel consumption (Scholz *et al.*, 1990).

Methyl *tert*-butyl ether is also used in the petrochemical industry. Production of isobutene from the splitting of methyl *tert*-butyl ether is the only application that has been exploited on an industrial scale. By reversing its formation reaction, methyl *tert*-butyl ether can be cracked to isobutene and methanol on acidic catalysts at temperatures above 100°C. The methanol obtained as a co-product is recycled to synthesize methyl *tert*-butyl ether. Methyl *tert*-butyl ether can also be used in a number of chemical reactions, for example the production of methacrolein, methacrylic acid and isoprene. The lack of acidic hydrogen atoms makes methyl *tert*-butyl ether a suitable solvent for chemical reactions such as Grignard reactions. Because of its negligible tendency to form peroxides, its high ignition temperature and its narrow explosion limits, methyl *tert*-butyl ether is a good solvent for analytical use. It is also used as an extractant, for example in solvent dewaxing of hydrocarbon oils (Scholz *et al.*, 1990).

Methyl *tert*-butyl ether is being evaluated for clinical use to dissolve gallstones (Agency for Toxic Substances and Disease Registry, 1996).

1.3 Occurrence

1.3.1 *Natural occurrence*

Methyl *tert*-butyl ether is not known to occur naturally.

1.3.2 *Occupational exposure*

Occupational exposure to methyl *tert*-butyl ether may occur by inhalation and dermal absorption during its production, formulation, distribution, use and disposal, either as pure methyl *tert*-butyl ether or blended into gasoline (Agency for Toxic Substances and Disease Registry, 1996). The estimated numbers of exposed workers in the United States are 900 000 professional drivers, 300 000 mechanics, 150 000 gasoline station workers, 7700 distribution workers, 1500 transport workers, 1800 blending workers and 880 manufacturing workers (Brown, 1997).

Tables 2 and 3 present the concentrations of methyl *tert*-butyl ether in worksite air collated by petroleum industry associations in Europe and the United States. In the European companies, the average full-shift concentrations to which workers in gasoline-related activities were exposed were 1.1–2.8 mg/m³; the average shorter-term concentration was ≤ 86 mg/m³ for top loading, which was four times higher than that for bottom loading. Even higher concentrations were measured during maintenance. In activities in which workers were exposed to undiluted methyl *tert*-butyl ether, ship-loading operations were associated

Table 2. Occupational exposure to methyl *tert*-butyl ether in the European petroleum industry; personal monitoring, 1981–95

Job or activity	Sampling (min)	No. of samples	Arithmetic mean (mg/m³)	Range (mg/m³)
From gasoline				
Driver bottom loading	480	49	2.8	0.01–10
Supervisor		45	2.2	≤ 14
Maintenance worker		13	2.3	≤ 20
Laboratory technician		10	1.1	≤ 3.2
Tetraethyllead operator	126–420	10	< 3.6	≤ 3.6
Area operator		6	< 3.6	< 3.6
Ship loading		7	< 3.6	< 3.6
Bottom loading	2–99	14	21	7.2–36
Top loading		6	86	29–160
Sampling		6	< 3.6	< 3.6–36
Filter change laboratory		2	23	14–32
From undiluted methyl *tert*-butyl ether				
Plant operator	100–390	10	2.4	0.08–19
Plant operator		5	< 3.6	< 3.6
Ship loading		2	46	45–46
Plant operator	15–40	3	< 3.6	< 3.6
Check tank levels		2	2.7	1.2–4.2
Hose disconnection		2	23	8.3–38

From McKee & Molyneux (1997)

Table 3. Occupational exposure to methyl *tert*-butyl ether in the United States petroleum industry, 1983–93

Operation	Exposure type	No. of samples	Geometric mean (mg/m³)	Range (mg/m³)
Manufacture, routine operations	Short-term[a]	27	2.4	0.58–28
	8-h TWA[b]	76	0.22	0.04–900
Manufacture, routine maintenance/turnaround	Short-term	8	4.0	1.8–26
	8-h TWA	4	0.47	0.14–2.5
Blending: undiluted methyl *tert*-butyl ether	Short-term	35	17	0.00–350
	Task[c]	13	7.4	0.76–260
	8-h TWA	12	6.2	0.14–320
Blending: fuel mixtures	Short-term	98	1.5	0.07–360
	Task	19	0.43	0.11–7.1
	8-h TWA	112	0.36	0.07–50
Transport: undiluted methyl *tert*-butyl ether	Short-term	66	43	1.1–3800
	Task	27	8.4	0.14–2500
	8-h TWA	10	1.1	0.11–2600
Transport: fuel mixtures	Short-term	64	14	0.00–1800
	Task	92	1.8	0.07–210
	8-h TWA	42	0.58	0.04–94
Distribution: fuel mixtures	Short-term	129	1.7	0.00–50
	Task	10	3.6	0.93–15
	8-h TWA	87	0.43	0.04–7.9

From McCoy & Johnson (1995); TWA, time-weighted average
[a] Duration, < 30 min
[b] Duration, 6–9 h
[c] Duration, 30 min–6 h

with an average exposure of 45 mg/m³ (McKee & Molyneux, 1997). In a study of gasoline road-tanker drivers in Finland, top loading (without vapour recovery) was associated with the highest short-term (15–40 min) levels, with a mean of 91 mg/m³, whereas that for bottom loading was 13 mg/m³. During unloading at service stations, the corresponding mean levels were 16 mg/m³ in northern and 71 mg/m³ in southern Finland (Hakkola & Saarinen, 1996). Essentially similar results were obtained during a later study by the same group (Saarinen *et al.*, 1998).

In the United States, the highest shift-long exposure was in blending undiluted methyl *tert*-butyl ether (mean, 6.2 mg/m³), while the highest short-term exposure was in transporting undiluted methyl *tert*-butyl ether (mean, 43 mg/m³). In general, the short-term concentrations were 3–10 times higher than the shift-long concentrations. Operations involving exposure to undiluted methyl *tert*-butyl ether resulted in concentrations 3–20 times higher than those involving exposure to fuel mixtures. Of the short-term exposures, transport involved higher concentrations than blending activities. Methyl *tert*-butyl ether manufacture was associated with the lowest exposures during routine operations, while the concentration increased during routine maintenance and turnaround operations and were highest during spills, leaks and upsets (McCoy & Johnson, 1995). A series of 38 personal air samples (15 min) taken in a petroleum refinery to evaluate the geometric mean of the concentrations of methyl *tert*-butyl ether in operations where there were potentially high exposures during short periods was 8.8 mg/m^3 (< 3.2–130 mg/m^3); concentrations > 36 mg/m^3 were found during sampling of railroad cars and connecting and disconnecting valves to them. The average full-shift concentration was 2.1 mg/m^3 (< 0.15–6.3 mg/m^3; $n = 9$). Individual exposures to > 3.6 mg/m^3 were found during laboratory testing and unloading of methyl *tert*-butyl ether from railroad cars (Lillquist & Zeigle, 1998).

Table 4 presents the concentrations to which workers in the United States are exposed in occupations related to automobile refuelling and servicing. As expected, exposure was higher when oxygenated fuels were used. The mean exposure of service station attendants, the most heavily exposed, during a full shift was < 3.6 mg/m^3, and individual values were rarely > 0.5–1 mg/m^3. In areas where methyl *tert*-butyl ether is used at a small percentage in gasoline, the concentrations to which service station attendants were exposed were usually below the limit of detection (about 0.11 mg/m^3). Workers who spent most of their work day in a vehicle had no detectable exposure, even in areas of oxygenated fuel use. This finding is consistent with the evaluation of Brown (1997) of a geometric mean exposure of 40 μg/m^3 for professional drivers in areas of the United States where methyl *tert*-butyl ether is used. Few data are available on peak exposures. Short-term (< 30 min) exposure was found to be an order of magnitude greater than the 8-h values for refuelling activities (McCoy & Johnson, 1995). Real-time video monitoring of total exposure to hydrocarbons indicated that peak concentrations of methyl *tert*-butyl ether (> 100 times the average for 1–2 s) occur during refuelling, even in the presence of vapour recovery systems (Cook & Kovein, 1997). The effect of spills has not been quantified (Hartle, 1993), while the effect of vehicle exhaust emissions seems to be minimal as engines are shut off during refuelling (Cook & Kovein, 1997).

The concentration of methyl *tert*-butyl ether in blood at the end of a shift and the difference between post- and pre-shift concentrations have been found to correlate with the concentrations in air (Moolenaar *et al.*, 1994; Mannino *et al.*, 1995; White *et al.*, 1995). In an area where oxygenated fuels were used, the median concentration in the blood of gasoline pump attendants was approximately 15 μg/L, which was 10 times higher than that of car repair workers and 100 times higher than that of commuters (White *et al.*, 1995). A decrease from 1.8 to 0.24 μg/L in the median blood concentration of methyl *tert*-butyl ether was observed in Alaskan workers exposed to gasoline vapours and engine exhausts after discontinuation of the use of oxygenated fuels (Moolenaar *et al.*, 1994). Saarinen *et al.* (1998) reported that the time-weighted average exposure was strongly related to the urinary concentration of methyl *tert*-butyl ether in samples collected 1–3 h after a workshift, whereas urinary *tert*-butyl alcohol was not a reliable indicator of exposure.

Table 4. Occupational exposure to methyl *tert*-butyl ether in United States service stations and automobile repair centres

Occupation/type of fuel	Year, location	Air concentration (mg/m³)		Sample type and duration	No. of samples	Reference
		Mean	Range			
Service station attendants and operators	1990			Personal 4 h		Hartle (1993)
Low methyl *tert*-butyl ether (0.03–0.13%)	Cincinnati, OH		ND–0.58[a]		32	
Oxygenated fuel (12–13% methyl *tert*-butyl ether)	Phoenix, AZ	1.1	0.14–14		41	
Equipped with stage II vapour recovery (0.03–2.1% methyl *tert*-butyl ether)	Los Angeles, CA	0.50	0.07–2.6[b]		48	
Various jobs, oxygenated fuel (13–17% methyl *tert*-butyl ether)	1993, Stamford, CT			Personal 8 h		Buchta (1993a)
Mechanics		0.40 (GM)	< 0.11–43		28	
Commuters[c]		ND	ND		7	
Supervisors		0.18 (GM)	< 0.11–0.54		4	
Various jobs, methyl *tert*-butyl ether up to 10%	1993, Albany,			Personal 8 h		Almaguer (1993)
Mechanics	NY	0.11 (median)	< 0.11–0.50		8	
Parking-lot attendants			< 0.11		8	
Service station attendants, oxygenated fuel (15–18% methyl *tert*-butyl ether)	1994, Newark, NJ	1.4 (GM)	0.29–4.6	Personal 3–10 h	21	Cook & Kovein (1995)
Various workers exposed routinely to motor vehicle exhaust or gasoline fumes	1992, 1993, Fairbanks, AK			Area 8 h		Moolenaar *et al.* (1994)
During oxygenated fuel programme (15% methyl *tert*-butyl ether)		0.37 (median)	0.02–2.9		18	
After oxygenated fuel programme (0.4–5% methyl *tert*-butyl ether)		0.13 (median)	ND–0.51		28	

Table 4 (contd)

Occupation/type of fuel	Year, location	Air concentration (mg/m^3)		Sample type and duration	No. of samples	Reference
		Mean	Range			
Various workers, low methyl *tert*-butyl ether (< 1%)	1993, Fairbanks, AK			Personal, full-shift		Buchta (1993b)
Mechanics		0.22 (GM)	< 0.11–1.6		26	
Commuters[c]			< 0.11		6	
Service and parts advisors			< 0.14		5	
Refuelling activities, various fuels	1983–93, USA			Personal and area		McCoy & Johnson (1995)
		2.8 (GM)	0.32–120	8 h	13	
		17 (GM)	0.58–490	< 30 min	11	

ND, not detected; GM, geometric mean
[a] Only one of 32 samples above the limit of detection
[b] Only 15 of 48 samples above the limit of detection
[c] Workers spending most of the work day inside a vehicle

Gasoline is a complex mixture, and workers exposed to methyl *tert*-butyl ether in occupations with exposure to gasoline or engine exhaust are exposed concurrently to several substances. Correlations were found in various studies between the air or blood concentrations of methyl *tert*-butyl ether and those of benzene, toluene, ethylbenzene, xylene and carbon monoxide (Moolenaar *et al.*, 1994; Mannino *et al.*, 1995; White *et al.*, 1995). Exposure of service station attendants to benzene does not seem to be affected by the addition of up to 13% methyl *tert*-butyl ether to gasoline (Hartle, 1993). 1,3-Butadiene was not detected in a bulk sample of methyl *tert*-butyl ether collected from a petroleum refinery storage tank (Lillquist & Zeigle, 1998).

1.3.3 *Environmental occurrence*

Methyl *tert*-butyl ether enters the environment (principally air and water) during all phases of the petroleum fuel cycle, which includes production refinery stack releases, storage tank releases, pipeline leaks and significant releases from underground storage tanks, evaporative losses from gasoline stations and vehicles and, to a much smaller degree, from small gasoline engines in lawn mowers and recreational watercraft. Methyl-*tert*-butyl ether has been reported (generally at low concentrations) in air, rainwater, surface water, groundwater, drinking-water and human tissues (Environmental Protection Agency, 1994; Environment Canada, 1995; Agency for Toxic Substances and Disease Registry, 1996; Environmental Protection Agency, 1996; Health Effects Institute, 1996; National Research Council, 1996; National Science and Technology Council, 1996; Zogorski *et al.*, 1996; Brown, 1997; National Science and Technology Council, 1997; National Library of Medicine, 1998; Squillace *et al.*, 1998; WHO, 1998). Human exposure to methyl *tert*-butyl ether has been estimated by modelling multiple exposure pathways (Long *et al.*, 1994; Agency for Toxic Substances and Disease Registry, 1996; Health Effects Institute, 1996; Brown, 1997; Stern & Tardiff, 1997; WHO, 1998).

(*a*) *Air*

Total industrial releases of methyl *tert*-butyl ether from refineries and manufacturers in Canada in 1994 were approximately 28 000 kg, the bulk of which (98.1%) was released into the air (Environment Canada, 1995).

In 1994, 190 industrial facilities in the United States reported air emissions of methyl *tert*-butyl ether to the Environmental Protection Agency Toxic Chemical Release Inventory, totalling 1.4 million kg, which represents 96.2% of the total methyl *tert*-butyl ether releases from these sources (National Library of Medicine, 1998). Industrial releases of methyl *tert*-butyl ether reported in 1993 totalled about 1.7 million kg, about 84% of which were from refineries (Zogorski *et al.*, 1996).

Methyl *tert*-butyl ether discharged into the air remains principally in air, with smaller amounts entering water (Agency for Toxic Substances and Disease Registry, 1996; Zogorski *et al.*, 1996; WHO, 1998). Because of dispersion, mixing and the relatively short half-life of methyl *tert*-butyl ether in the atmosphere (1–11 days), the concentrations in the atmosphere and in precipitation would be expected to decrease with distance from the source. Methyl *tert*-butyl ether in air tends to partition into atmospheric water, including precipitation, and thus contributes to its concentrations in surface and groundwater (Zogorski *et al.*, 1996; Squillace *et al.*, 1998).

The presence of methyl *tert*-butyl ether in ambient air and microenvironments has been reported since its introduction into reformulated gasolines, especially from Canada and the United States and to a much lesser degree from Europe (in particular Finland), reflecting the principal use patterns (Agency for Toxic Substances and Disease Registry, 1996; Health Effects Institute, 1996; Zogorski *et al.*, 1996; WHO, 1998; Zogorski *et al.*, 1998).

(i) *Ambient air*

In Porto Alegre, Brazil, the concentrations of methyl *tert*-butyl ether in ambient air between March 1996 and April 1997 ranged from 0.72 to 62 μg/m^3 (average, 24 ± 16 μg/m^3). The rate of emission of methyl *tert*-butyl ether from vehicle exhausts was estimated to be 1700 ± 190 tonnes per year since 15% of the vehicles in the area run on fuels containing methyl *tert*-butyl ether (Grosjean *et al.*, 1998).

The concentrations of methyl *tert*-butyl ether in ambient air at various locations in nine Canadian cities (Edmonton, Halifax, Montreal, St John, Stouffville, Toronto, Vancouver, Windsor and Winnipeg) between 1995 and 1996 were reported. The locations included petroleum refineries, gasoline processing and storage plants, pipeline transfer points and urban areas. The concentrations of methyl *tert*-butyl ether in the urban areas were generally very low, ranging from the detection limit (0.1 μg/m^3) to < 0.4 μg/m^3. In the vicinity of petroleum refineries, methyl *tert*-butyl ether concentrations ranged from 0.81 to 11 μg/m^3 in Edmonton and from 0.23 to 1.5 μg/m^3 in Montreal. In the vicinity of Vancouver gasoline processing and storage plants, the concentrations were generally in the range 0.39–3.4 μg/m^3. The methyl *tert*-butyl ether concentrations at the boundary of a petroleum refinery in St John during a period of complaints about odours in 1995 ranged from 15 to 280 μg/m^3 in four sampling periods (WHO, 1998).

The results of monitoring of methyl *tert*-butyl ether in air in the United States are considered inadequate to characterize the concentrations to be expected in ambient air (Zogorski *et al.*, 1996). The annual mean methyl *tert*-butyl ether concentration in ambient air in the United States during the late 1980s was estimated to be < 0.7 μg/m^3 (Environmental Protection Agency, 1994; Agency for Toxic Substances and Disease Registry, 1996). Twenty-four-hour ambient air sampling in 1990–91 at various sites in Boston, MA, and Houston, TX, where methyl *tert*-butyl ether was used at < 5% volume in gasoline showed concentrations of < 0.7–1.8 μg/m^3 and < 0.7–10 μg/m^3, respectively. In both Boston and Houston, the median concentration was < 0.7 μg/m^3 (Kelly *et al.*, 1993).

An analysis of indoor and ambient air samples was undertaken in Fairbanks, Alaska, during the winter of 1992–93 after a series of complaints of ill health after the introduction of methyl *tert*-butyl ether as an oxygenate in gasoline. Both ambient outdoor air and air in workplaces, schools, post offices and one residence were sampled in December 1992 when methyl *tert*-butyl ether was introduced and in February 1993 when it was no longer used in gasolines. At a major intersection in Fairbanks, the mean concentrations in ambient air were 16 mg/m³ in December 1992 and 4.0 mg/m³ in February 1993. The mean concentrations at those times were 17 and 1.9 μg/m³ at an elementary school, 27 and 3.6 μg/m³ in a private residence, 1100 and 220 μg/m³ in some garage and 300 and 41 μg/m³ inside vehicles (Gordian & Guay, 1995).

The median concentration of methyl *tert*-butyl ether in the ambient air of Fairbanks, AK, Milwaukee, WI, Albany, NY, Stamford, CT, Boston, MA, and Houston, TX ranged from 0.47 to 17 μg/m³, with the highest median value measured in Fairbanks. When the value for Fairbanks was excluded, the maximum concentration measured in ambient air was 15 μg/m³ in Milwaukee, and the median ambient air concentrations in the five cities other than Fairbanks were < 3.6 μg/m³ (1 ppb). The concentrations of methyl *tert*-butyl ether in air near gasoline stations, roadways, parking lots, garages and blending and distribution facilities were higher than those in ambient urban air (Health Effects Institute, 1996; Zogorski *et al.*, 1996).

The results of two monitoring surveys carried out in 1995–96 indicated that the average ambient air concentrations of methyl *tert*-butyl ether after 3-h sampling at four southern California locations were 2.2–26 μg/m³ and those at seven California locations after 24-h sampling were 4.7–17 μg/m³ (Poore *et al.*, 1997; WHO, 1998).

A regional study of air from the Houston Regional Monitoring Corporation, which included the Houston Ship Channel industrial complex in Texas and some of the largest methyl *tert*-butyl ether manufacturing facilities, during the period September 1987 to September 1988 showed a mean ambient air concentration below the detection limit of 0.7 μg/m³ (0.2 ppb) in 24-h time-averaged samples. The total yearly emissions of methyl *tert*-butyl ether in the Harris and Chambers counties were suggested to be 280 tonnes (LaGrone, 1991).

In a study of ambient air in Milwaukee, WI, where reformulated gasoline containing approximately 11% by volume of methyl *tert*-butyl ether was used, 11 weekly 24-h samples collected at an air sampling station from January to March 1995 showed concentrations of methyl *tert*-butyl ether ranging from < 0.36 to 15 μg/m³; the concentration in 45% of the samples was below the detection limit of 0.36 μg/m³ (0.1 ppb). The median concentration was 0.47 μg/m³ (0.13 ppb). The concentrations in control samples from the nearby cities of Madison and Green Bay where reformulated gasoline was not mandated were below the detection limit (WHO, 1998). In the same study, the mean concentrations of methyl *tert*-butyl ether in air samples were 1.9 μg/m³ in three samples collected near a freeway interchange, 3.8 μg/m³ in two samples from a busy intersection and 1.8 μg/m³ in two samples from a roadway in Milwaukee (Allen *et al.*, 1996; WHO, 1998).

Measurements at an enclosed parking ramp in Milwaukee were conducted in February 1995 to determine the effect on ambient concentrations of methyl *tert*-butyl ether of starting cold engines. Concentrations of < 72 μg/m³ with a mean of 7.4 μg/m³ were found in eight samples. The highest concentrations were found when a large number of vehicles were started while cold within a short period (WHO, 1998).

At one refinery in the United States, the 24-h concentration of methyl *tert*-butyl ether was 20 μg/m³ in one of nine samples taken downwind from the perimeter of a rural refinery, which was reported to release approximately 33 tonnes of methyl *tert*-butyl ether into the air yearly. During the same period, methyl *tert*-butyl ether was not detected in 26 other downwind and upwind samples. Methyl *tert*-butyl ether was not detected (detection limit, 6 μg/m³) in 54 24-h samples taken at two other refineries [the annual emissions from these refineries to the air were not provided] (American Petroleum Institute, 1989).

(ii) *Refuelling operations*

Non-occupational and consumer exposures to methyl *tert*-butyl ether have been measured in a number of studies. The general public has the greatest exposure to methyl *tert*-butyl ether during vehicle refuelling. The concentrations are generally higher at service stations where there is no vapour recovery system, and the concentrations usually decrease from the personal breathing zone of the customer or attendant to the pump island to the station perimeter. The heaviest exposure tended to be short. The median concentrations in the customer breathing zone during refuelling were typically 1.1–22 μg/m³ and occasionally higher. Concentrations of 0.04–0.36 μg/m³ were measured inside vehicles during this time, reflecting potential exposure of passengers (Allen *et al.*, 1996; Health Effects Institute, 1996; Zogorski *et al.*, 1996; WHO, 1998).

In April 1993, air samples were taken inside vehicles during refuelling and suburban commuting in New Jersey, New York and Connecticut (United States), where gasoline containing 10–15% by volume methyl *tert*-butyl ether was sold. The concentrations of methyl *tert*-butyl ether inside vehicles immediately before, during and after refuelling were 24–110 μg/m³, 130–310 μg/m³ and 31–150 μg/m³, respectively, in three cars, with average concentrations of 54, 200 and 72 μg/m³, respectively. Short-term peak concentrations of methyl *tert*-butyl ether occurred during refuelling. The 60-min air concentrations of methyl *tert*-butyl ether inside 20 suburban commuter vehicles in stop–start traffic ranged from 4 to 580 μg/m³ with a mean of 21 μg/m³, most values being < 20 μg/m³ and higher values being associated with the use of high-emission vehicles (Lioy *et al.*, 1994).

Finland is the only European country where methyl *tert*-butyl ether is used in reformulated gasoline as an octane enhancer and oxygenate source at 11% of gasoline blend throughout the year since 1994. The concentrations of methyl *tert*-butyl ether at the perimeter and pump island of two self-service stations (one at an urban roadside and one at a simple roadside equipped with 'stage I' vapour recovery systems) were ascertained during the period May–June and October, 1995. The service stations studied represented typical Nordic stations in size, location and design. The measurements in the customer breathing zone showed a wide distribution, the lowest exposures being the most frequent. Measurements in the breathing zone showed concentrations of < 0.2–240 mg/m³ in 313 individual samples. On average, customers were exposed to a concentration of 6 mg/m³ during a 1-min refuelling time. The average range in perimeter air samples at both service stations was 0.5–120 μg/m³ methyl *tert*-butyl ether. The mean concentrations measured at the centre of the pump island ranged from 250 to 1350 μg/m³ (n = 15) (Vainiotalo *et al.*, 1996a,b). An additional study to assess the exposure of customers at service stations to methyl *tert*-butyl ether from gasolines with lower concentrations (average, 2.7%) showed an overall average concentration in the breathing zone of 3.3 mg/m³ (0.02–51 mg/m³; $n = 167$), which was higher than that expected from studies of gasoline containing 11% methyl *tert*-butyl ether (Vainiotalo *et al.*, 1997).

Exposure to methyl *tert*-butyl ether in 1991–92 at 16 service stations in Italy belonging to a single company was compared with that at 42 service stations belonging to all companies operating in Italy in 1995. The overall arithmetic mean concentrations, taken as a conservative estimate of personal exposure, were: 710 μg/m³ in summer ($n = 76$) and 370 μg/m³ in winter ($n = 128$) in 1991–92 and 260 μg/m³ in summer ($n = 347$) in 1995 (Giacomello, 1996).

(*b*) *Water*

Methyl *tert*-butyl ether has been found in storm-water, groundwater, reservoir water and drinking-water, especially in areas where it is used extensively in gasoline and where methyl *tert*-butyl ether could be released more readily to air and water (Agency for Toxic Substances and Disease Registry, 1996; Davidson, 1996; Delzer *et al.*, 1996; Environmental Protection Agency, 1996; Health Effects Institute, 1996; National Science and Technology Council, 1996; Squillace *et al.*, 1996; Zogorski *et al.*, 1996; National Science and Technology Council, 1997; Squillace *et al.*, 1997; WHO, 1998; Zogorski *et al.*, 1998). Although methyl *tert*-butyl ether released from non-point sources (e.g., precipitation and small surface spills) can enter water, the primary concern with regard to contamination of water by this chemical is substantial surface spills and leakage from underground storage tanks. Because it is highly soluble in water, methyl *tert*-butyl ether can partition readily from gasoline into water, resulting in high aqueous concentrations. In shallow groundwater below underground storage tanks, concentrations up to 200 000 μg/L have been found (Davidson, 1996; National Research Council, 1996; National Science and Technology Council, 1997).

Methyl *tert*-butyl ether was detected in storm-water runoff in about 7% of 592 samples from 16 United States cities with populations greater than 100 000 during 1991–95. The concentrations ranged from 0.2 to 8.7 μg/L with a median of 1.5 μg/L (limit of detection, 0.2 μg/L). Eighty-three per cent of the detectable methyl *tert*-butyl ether was found during winter. It was detected both in cities where oxygenated gasoline was used to reduce carbon monoxide concentrations and in cities presumed to have used methyl *tert*-butyl ether in gasoline for octane enhancement (Zogorski *et al.*, 1996).

Storm-water runoff may be an important non-point source of methyl *tert*-butyl ether to groundwater. In a United States Geological Survey, storm-water runoff samples were collected in Phoenix, AZ, Denver/Lakewood, CO, and Colorado Springs, CO. Methyl *tert*-butyl ether was detected in 17% of the 94 storm-water samples collected between October 1991 and September 1994 during the summer, with a median concentration of 1.5 μg/L (Squillace *et al.*, 1996).

Methyl *tert*-butyl ether is a potentially important groundwater contaminant because of its mobility and persistence. It persists in groundwater under both aerobic and anaerobic conditions because it resists physical, chemical and microbial degradation (Squillace *et al.*, 1996; Zogorski *et al.*, 1996; National Science and Technology Council, 1997; Squillace *et al.*, 1998; WHO, 1998; Zogorski *et al.*, 1998).

Methyl *tert*-butyl ether was the second most frequently detected of 60 volatile organic chemicals in samples of shallow ambient water collected from urban areas in the United States during 1993–94 as part of the Geological Survey's National Water-Quality Assessment Program. Only concentrations of ≥ 0.2 μg/L were reported. It was detected more frequently in shallow groundwater in urban areas (27% of 210 wells and springs sampled in eight urban areas) than in shallow groundwater in agricultural areas (1.3% of 549 shallow agricultural wells sampled in 21 areas) or deeper groundwater in major aquifiers (1% of 412 wells sampled in nine areas). Methyl *tert*-butyl ether was most frequently detected in shallow groundwater in Denver, CO, and in urban areas in New England (Squillace *et al.*, 1996; Zogorski *et al.*, 1996, 1998).

In shallow urban groundwater, methyl *tert*-butyl ether is generally not found with benzene, toluene, ethylbenzene or xylene which are commonly associated with gasoline spills, as methyl *tert*-butyl ether is much more soluble in water (Squillace *et al.*, 1996: Zogorski *et al.*, 1996). Measurements of methyl *tert*-butyl ether and benzene between 1993 and 1998 in a shallow, sandy aquifer located near Beaufort, SC, suggested that the concentrations of methyl *tert*-butyl ether are lower than those of benzene because of the natural attenuation processes of dilution and dispersion in less contaminated groundwater rather than biodegradation at this point-source of gasoline release (Landmeyer *et al.*, 1998).

In an analysis of data on methyl *tert*-butyl ether in surface and groundwater systems of Long Island, NY, and New Jersey, methyl *tert*-butyl ether was one of the most frequently detected volatile organic compounds. Point and non-point sources of contamination are distinguished by seasonal patterns of detection, frequent detection of low concentrations and associations with land use and population size. When only concentrations ≥ 0.5 μg/L were reported, methyl *tert*-butyl ether was the third most frequently detected volatile organic compound (9%) in 208 wells monitored in Suffolk County, NY, with concentrations ranging from 0.6 to 47 μg/L, and was the second most frequently detected volatile organic compound in streams, occurring in 29% of 93 streams in Suffolk County at concentrations ranging from 0.6 to 20 μg/L. It was detected more frequently in samples collected during winter (33%) than summer (26%), corresponding to the expected increase in both the use of oxygenated fuels and the concentrations of methyl *tert*-butyl ether in precipitation during winter (Stackelberg *et al.*, 1997). Methyl *tert*-butyl ether was detected in all of 42 surface water samples collected from streams on Long Island, NY, and in New Jersey during 27–30 January 1997. The median and maximum concentrations detected were 0.36 μg/L and 8.7 μg/L, respectively. The highest concentrations of methyl *tert*-butyl ether were measured in the most intensely developed parts of the area, in streams draining basins with the highest percentages of urban land use (O'Brien *et al.*, 1997).

In an analysis of methyl *tert*-butyl ether in public groundwater systems in five states where the compound was being used, 2.5% of the 2500 systems sampled had concentrations above the detection limit but below 10 μg/L, but one system had concentrations of 10–20 μg/L; the median limit of detection was 0.5 μg/L (Davidson, 1996).

According to the Environmental Protection Agency's Toxic Release Inventory, about 93.5% of the methyl *tert*-butyl ether released from industries in the United States in 1992 was released into the atmosphere, 3.5% was discharged into surface water and 2.5% was injected into wells (Environmental Protection Agency, 1994). In 1994, 190 facilities in the United States reported the discharge of 41 tonnes of methyl *tert*-butyl ether into surface water (National Library of Medicine, 1998).

Although methyl *tert*-butyl ether has been detected in public and private drinking-water supplies derived from groundwater in the United States, the available data are inadequate to characterize its occurrence in drinking-water nationwide, since the Federal Government does not require routine monitoring of methyl *tert*-butyl ether in drinking-water. However, it was detected in 51 public drinking-water systems in all states that provided information (Colorado, Iowa, Illinois, New Jersey and Texas). The concentration of methyl *tert*-butyl ether in nearly all these systems (47 of 51; 92%) was < 20 μg/L (Zogorski *et al.*, 1996).

In an analysis of groundwater used as a drinking-water supply in six sampling areas in the lower Susquehannna River Basin (in the states of Pennsylvania and Maryland) in 1993–95, methyl *tert*-butyl ether was the most commonly detected of 60 volatile organic compounds. It was found in 16/118 wells at concentrations ranging from 0.11 to 51 μg/L (Daly & Lindsey, 1996).

No data on methyl *tert*-butyl ether in drinking-water were available from other countries (WHO, 1998).

(*c*) *Soil and sediments*

As methyl *tert*-butyl ether sorbs only weakly to subsurface solids, sorption does not substantially retard its transport by groundwater (Squillace *et al.*, 1997). No quantitative estimates of the release of methyl *tert*-butyl ether to soil or sediment were available (Agency for Toxic Substances and Disease Registry, 1996; WHO, 1998).

In 1994, about 1000 kg of methyl *tert*-butyl ether were released onto the land from 190 industrial facilities in the United States, representing < 1% of the total environmental releases from these facilities (National Library of Medicine, 1998).

(*d*) *Human tissues and secreta*

The concentration of methyl *tert*-butyl ether in the blood of commuters in Fairbanks, AK (United States) decreased from 0.18 μg/L (range, 0.05–0.3 μg/L) to 0.09 μg/L (range, < 0.05–0.41 μg/L) after discontinuation of the use of oxygenated fuels (Moolenaar *et al.*, 1994).

The exposure of 14 commuters to methyl *tert*-butyl ether from oxygenated gasolines in Stamford, CT (United States), was measured in 1993. The median blood concentration was 0.11 μg/L and the range was < 0.05–2.6 μg/L. The blood concentrations correlated strongly with those in personal breathing zone samples, with estimated correlation coefficients of 0.80 between air and blood for methyl *tert*-butyl ether and 0.70 between methyl *tert*-butyl ether in air and *tert*-butyl alcohol in blood (White *et al.*, 1995).

1.4 Regulations and guidelines

The American Conference of Governmental Industrial Hygienists (1997) recommended 144 mg/m^3 as the 8-h time-weighted average (TWA) threshold limit value for exposure to methyl *tert*-butyl ether in workplace air. The TWA in the Czech Republic is 100 mg/m^3, with a short-term exposure limit (STEL) of 200 mg/m^3. The STEL in the Russian Federation is 100 mg/m^3. The 8-h TWA in Sweden is 180 mg/m^3, and the STEL is 250 mg/m^3 (United Nations Environment Programme, 1998). The 8-h TWA in Finland is 180 mg/m^3 (Finnish Institute of Occupational Health, 1998).

No international guidelines for methyl *tert*-butyl ether in drinking-water have been established (WHO, 1993).

2. Studies of Cancer in Humans

No data on exposure to methyl *tert*-butyl ether itself were available to the Working Group. Exposure to gasoline and in petroleum refining has been evaluated in previous monographs (IARC, 1989).

3. Studies of Cancer in Experimental Animals

3.1 Oral administration

Rat: Groups of 60 male and 60 female Sprague-Dawley rats, eight weeks of age, were given gastric instillations of 0, 250 or 1000 mg/kg bw methyl *tert*-butyl ether (purity, > 99%) in 1 mL olive oil once a day on two days with one day's rest and for another two days with two days' rest, each week for 104 weeks and were kept under observation until they died. The survival rate of males at the high dose was increased beyond 80 weeks after the start of treatment and was dose-dependently decreased in females beyond 16 weeks after the start of treatment [statistical significance not indicated; mean survival times not given]. No relevant differences in male and female body weights were observed. At necropsy, multiple organs were examined histopathologically, and a statistically significant increase ($p = 0.05$) in the incidence of Leydig-cell testicular adenomas was found in males at the high dose: control, 2/26; low dose, 2/25; high dose, 11/32 [group sizes indicate the number of rats alive at 96 weeks of age, when the first Leydig-cell tumour was observed]. A dose-related increase in the incidence of lymphomas and leukaemias was seen in female rats: control, 2/58; low dose, 6/51; high dose, 12/47 ($p < 0.01$ at both doses) [groups sizes refer to the number of rats alive at 56 weeks of age, when the first leukaemia was observed]. There was no increase in the incidence of lymphomas or leukaemias in males: control, 10/59; low dose, 9/59; high dose, 7/58

(Belpoggi *et al.*, 1995, 1998). [The Working Group noted that the dosing schedule was unusual, that animals were allowed to live out their natural lifespan and that mortality-adjusted analysis was not performed; therefore, estimates of effective group numbers and tumour incidences were difficult to analyse.]

3.2 Inhalation exposure

Mouse: Groups of 50 male and 50 female CD-1 mice, seven to eight weeks of age, were exposed to 0, 400, 3000 or 8000 ppm [0, 1400, 11 000 and 29 000 mg/m³] methyl *tert*-butyl ether vapour (purity, > 99%) in air for 6 h a day on five days per week for 18 months, when the experiment was terminated. The daily doses were estimated to be 340, 2600 and 6800 mg/kg bw at the three exposure levels, respectively. Males and females at the high dose had reduced body-weight gain and earlier mortality due to toxicity. The survival time decreased from 510 days in control males to 438 days in animals at the high dose and in females from 519 to 489 days. The incidence of hepatocellular adenomas was increased in females at the high dose: control, 2/50; low dose, 1/50; intermediate dose, 2/50; high dose, 10/50 ($p < 0.01$). The incidence of hepatocellular carcinoma was not increased. In males, no significant changes in hepatocellular tumours (adenomas and carcinomas) were noted, but the incidence of carcinomas showed a tendency to increase: control, 2/49; low dose, 4/50; intermediate dose 3/50; high dose, 8/49 (Bird *et al.*, 1997; Mennear, 1997). [The Working Group noted that mortality-adjusted analysis was not performed and that therefore the tumour incidence in the high-dose group may have been underestimated. They also noted that groups at the intermediate and low doses were not subjected to complete histopathological examination unless the animals died spontaneously or were killed when moribund.]

Rat: Groups of 50 male and 50 female Fischer 344 rats, seven to eight weeks of age, were exposed for 6 h a day on five days per week to 0, 400, 3000 or 8000 ppm [0, 1400, 11 000 and 29 000 mg/m³] methyl *tert*-butyl ether vapour (purity, > 99%) in air for 24 months. The doses were estimated to be 220, 1700 and 4400 mg/kg bw at the three exposure levels, respectively. Males at the high and intermediate doses were killed at week 82 and week 97, respectively, due to excess mortality from severe progressive nephrosis. The other groups were killed at 24 months. The mean survival times for the males at the low dose and controls were 617 and 632 days; the survival times of control females and those at the low, intermediate and high doses were 697, 683, 697 and 676 days, respectively. The incidence of renal tubular-cell tumours was increased in males at the two higher doses: adenomas—control, 1/50; low dose, 0/50; intermediate dose, 5/50; high dose, 3/50; carcinomas—control, 0/50; low dose, 0/50; intermediate dose, 3/50; high-dose, 0/50. The combined incidence in males at the intermediate dose (8/50) was statistically significantly different from that of controls and was outside the range of the historical controls. Female rats showed no significant increase in the incidence of renal tumours. The incidence and size of interstitial-cell adenomas of the testis were significantly increased in rats at the two higher doses ($p < 0.05$), with incidences of 32/50 controls, 35/50 at the low dose, 41/50 at the intermediate dose and 47/50 at the high dose

(Bird *et al.*, 1997; Mennear, 1997). [The Working Group noted the unusually low incidence of interstitial adenomas of the testis in control rats when compared with the historical control incidence in that laboratory and that mortality-adjusted analysis was not performed.]

3.3 Administration with known carcinogens or modifying factors

Mouse: In a model of liver carcinogenesis, groups of 12 female B6C3F$_1$ mice, 12 days of age, received a single intraperitoneal injection of 5 mg/kg bw *N*-nitrosodiethylamine or saline. Beginning at eight weeks of age, mice were exposed by inhalation to 0 or 8000 ppm [29 000 mg/m^3] methyl *tert*-butyl ether (purity, > 99.95%) in air for 6 h per day on five days per week and were killed after 16 or 32 weeks. Exposure to methyl *tert*-butyl ether for 16 or 32 weeks after treatment with *N*-nitrosodiethylamine did not enhance the development of altered hepatic foci or increase the numbers of hepatocellular adenomas or carcinomas. No hepatic foci occurred in the group receiving methyl *tert*-butyl ether alone (Moser *et al.*, 1996a).

3.4 Carcinogenicity of metabolites

Mouse: Groups of 60 male and 60 female B6C3F$_1$ mice, approximately seven weeks of age, were given 0, 5, 10 or 20 mg/mL *tert*-butyl alcohol in their drinking-water for two years, providing average daily doses of approximately 540, 1000 and 2100 mg/kg bw *tert*-butyl alcohol to males and approximately 510, 1000 and 2100 mg/kg bw to females. The survival rate of males at the high dose was significantly lower than that of controls, but the final mean body weights of exposed males were similar to those of controls. The mean body weights of females at the high dose were 10–15 % lower than those of controls from 13 weeks to the end of the study. The incidence of thyroid gland follicular-cell hyperplasia was significantly increased in all exposed male groups and in females at the two higher doses. The incidence of follicular-cell adenoma or carcinoma (combined) was higher in males at the intermediate dose but was not significantly increased (control, 1/60; low dose, 0/59; intermediate dose, 4/59; high dose, 2/57). The incidence of follicular-cell adenoma was significantly increased in females at the high dose: control, 2/58; low dose, 3/60; intermediate dose, 2/59; high dose, 9/59 ($p = 0.039$) (Cirvello *et al.*, 1995; National Toxicology Program, 1995).

Rat: Groups of 60 male and 60 female Fischer 344/N rats, approximately seven weeks of age, were given 0, 1.25, 2.5 or 5 mg/mL (males) or 0, 2.5, 5 or 10 mg/mL (females) *tert*-butyl alcohol in their drinking-water for two years, providing average daily doses of approximately 90, 200 and 420 mg/kg bw for males and 180, 330 and 650 mg/kg bw for females. Ten rats per group were evaluated after 15 months of treatment. The survival rates of males and females at the high dose were significantly lower than those of controls, due to toxicity. The final mean body weights of exposed males were 15–24 % lower than those of controls, and the final mean body weight of females at the high dose was 21% lower than that of controls. Water consumption was increased dose-dependently in males and decreased in females. The incidence of renal adenomas and carcinomas combined, based on a single section of each kidney was not increased, being 1/50 (control), 3/50 (low dose), 4/50 (intermediate dose) and 3/50 (high dose). When step-sections including the single section were used, the kidney tumour incidences were increased significantly in males at the intermediate dose: 8/50 (control), 13/50 (low dose), 19/50 (intermediate dose; $p < 0.01$) and 13/50 (high dose). The incidence of focal renal tubule hyperplasia was also increased in males at the high dose (Cirvello *et al.*, 1995; National Toxicology Program, 1995).

4. Other Data Relevant to an Evaluation of Carcinogenicity and its Mechanisms

4.1 Absorption, distribution, metabolism and excretion

The metabolism of methyl *tert*-butyl ether has been reviewed (WHO, 1998). A scheme for the metabolism of methyl *tert*-butyl ether is presented in Figure 1.

4.1.1 *Humans*

One 25-year-old man weighing 102.5 kg with a ventilation volume of 10.82 L/min and one 21-year-old woman weighing 66.5 kg with a ventilation volume of 8.65 L/min were exposed to 5.01 mg/m^3 methyl *tert*-butyl ether vapour for 1 h. Breath, blood and urine samples were collected before and up to 580 min after exposure. The blood concentrations of methyl *tert*-butyl ether at the end of exposure were 8.2 μg/L in the man and 14 μg/L in the woman. The concentrations in breath and blood decayed rapidly after exposure but were still elevated 7 h after exposure when compared with those before exposure. The blood concentration of *tert*-butyl alcohol, a metabolite of methyl *tert*-butyl ether, increased gradually during exposure and remained elevated up to 7 h after exposure; the highest concentrations measured were 9.5 μg/L in the man and 10 μg/L in the woman. Urinary elimination accounted for < 1% of the total methyl *tert*-butyl ether eliminated (Buckley *et al.*, 1997).

Cain *et al.* (1996) exposed two men and two women, aged 18–26 years, to 1.7 ppm [6.1 mg/m^3] methyl *tert*-butyl ether for at least 1 h. Blood samples were taken before, during and after exposure and analysed for methyl *tert*-butyl ether. The mean concentration in blood at the end of exposure was 17 μg/L.

Ten men aged 23–51 years and weighing 70–90 kg were exposed to 5, 25 or 50 ppm [18, 90 and 180 mg/m^3] methyl *tert*-butyl ether during 2 h of light exercise (50 W) on three occasions separated by at least two weeks. Methyl *tert*-butyl ether and *tert*-butyl alcohol were monitored in exhaled breath, blood and urine. The average concentrations of methyl *tert*-butyl ether in blood were proportional to the exposure and were 1.4, 6.5 and 15 μmol/L [120, 570 and 1100 μg/L] at the end of exposure to the three concentrations, respectively. Elimination of methyl *tert*-butyl ether in blood occurred in four phases with half-lives of 1 min, 10 min, 1.5 h and 19 h. The integrated area under the curve of the blood concentration of methyl *tert*-butyl ether over time was linearly related to the exposure, suggesting

Figure 1. Metabolism of methyl *tert*-butyl ether

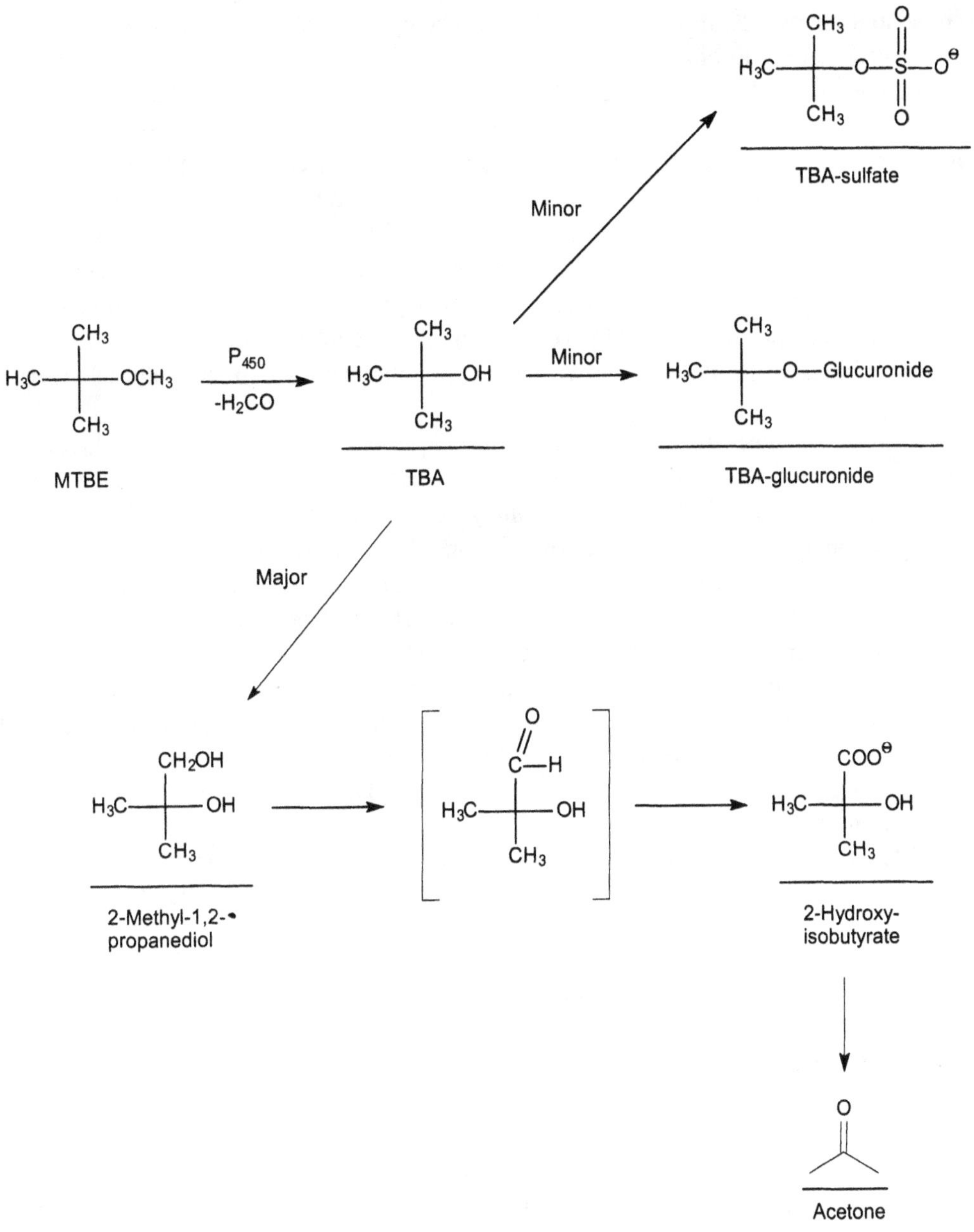

From Bernauer *et al.* (1998); metabolites excreted in urine are underlined.
TBA, *tert*-butyl alcohol; MTBE, methyl-*tert*-butyl ether

linear kinetics up to 50 ppm. Elimination of methyl *tert*-butyl ether in urine occurred in two linear phases with half-lives of 20 min and 3 h. The amount of methyl *tert*-butyl ether excreted in urine over 22 h represented ~0.1% of the uptake. Linear kinetics was observed for *tert*-butyl alcohol in blood at doses up to 50 ppm. The elimination half-lives of *tert*-butyl alcohol in blood and urine were 10 and 8.2 h, respectively. The blood concentration of *tert*-butyl alcohol, unlike that of methyl *tert*-butyl ether, increased slowly during exposure and remained high for several hours after exposure. Renal clearance of *tert*-butyl alcohol was calculated to be low, suggesting extensive blood protein binding or extensive tubular reabsorption. The 22-h cumulative excretion of *tert*-butyl alcohol in urine represented approximately 1% of the uptake of methyl *tert*-butyl ether (Nihlén *et al.*, 1998a).

A single subject was exposed by inhalation to 1 ppm [3.6 mg/m^3] methyl *tert*-butyl ether for 10 min. Approximately 0.9% of the amount of the inhaled dose was excreted unchanged in urine, with 2.4% excreted as *tert*-butyl alcohol within 10 h after exposure (Lee & Weisel, 1998).

One male volunteer aged 44 and weighing 80 kg was given [^{13}C]*tert*-butyl alcohol orally in a gel capsule at a dose of 5 mg/kg bw (Bernauer *et al.*, 1998). His urine was collected at 12-h intervals for 48 h and analysed by ^{13}C nuclear magnetic resonance. 2-Hydroxyisobutyrate (α-hydroxybutyric acid) and 2-methyl-1,2-propanediol were identified in the urine samples as major metabolites; minor urinary metabolites were *tert*-butyl alcohol and *tert*-butyl alcohol glucuronide. The sulfate conjugate of *tert*-butyl alcohol was present only in trace amounts.

White *et al.* (1995) obtained blood samples from 44 people in Stamford, CT, United States, who were either occupationally exposed to methyl *tert*-butyl ether or exposed to it while commuting. The blood levels of methyl *tert*-butyl ether ranged from a median of 15 μg/L (7.6–29 μg/L) for gasoline service station attendants to 1.7 μg/L (0.17–37 μg/L) for car repair workers and 0.11 μg/L (0.05–2.6 μg/L) for commuters. The *tert*-butyl alcohol levels reflected the same trend. The concentrations of methyl *tert*-butyl ether in blood correlated strongly with those in the breathing zone (correlation coefficient, 0.8; $p = 0.004$).

4.1.2 *Experimental systems*

(*a*) *Whole animals*

A number of studies of the pharmacokinetics and disposition of methyl *tert*-butyl ether conducted in male and female Fischer 344 rats after intravenous, oral or dermal administration of methyl *tert*-butyl ether or by inhalation were described by Miller *et al.* (1997). With few exceptions, the pharmacokinetics and disposition of methyl *tert*-butyl ether were the same in male and female rats after all types of administration, but only data for male rats were reported. In one study, rats received methyl *tert*-butyl ether either by intravenous injection into the caudal vein (40 mg/kg bw), by oral gavage (40 or 400 mg/kg bw), by dermal application (40 or 400 mg/kg bw in occluded chambers), by a single nose-only 6-h exposure to 400 or 8000 ppm [1400 and 29 000 mg/m^3] or by repeated exposure to 400 ppm for 15 days. Plasma samples were analysed for methyl *tert*-butyl ether and *tert*-butyl alcohol by gas chromatography at various times after exposure to methyl *tert*-butyl ether, and the data collected were used to assess pharmacokinetics. Comparisons of the integrated area under the blood concentration–time curve for methyl *tert*-butyl ether after intravenous or oral administration indicate that methyl *tert*-butyl ether is rapidly and completely absorbed from the gastrointestinal tract. Dermal absorption represented approximately 16 and 34% of the low and high dose, respectively. Metabolism did not appear to be saturated after oral or dermal doses of 40 and 400 mg/kg bw; however, the data suggested that the metabolism of methyl *tert*-butyl ether was saturated after exposure by inhalation to 8000 ppm for 6 h. The pharmacokinetics of methyl *tert*-butyl ether and *tert*-butyl alcohol were similar after intravenous, oral and inhalation exposure and were best described by an open one-compartment model. The half-lives for the clearance of methyl *tert*-butyl ether from plasma after intravenous and oral (40 mg/kg bw) administration and inhalation ranged from 0.45 to 0.57 h. After oral administration of 400 mg/kg bw methyl *tert*-butyl ether, its half-life was 0.79 h. Plasma elimination of methyl *tert*-butyl ether after dermal application was best described by a two-compartment model, and the elimination half-life was 1.8–2.3 h. The half-lives for elimination of *tert*-butyl alcohol ranged from 0.92 after intravenous injection to 3.4 h after inhalation. Repeated exposure to methyl *tert*-butyl ether for 15 days had no effect on its clearance from plasma.

Miller *et al.* (1997) also described the disposition of [^{14}C]methyl *tert*-butyl ether in male Fischer 344 rats up to seven days after intravenous injection of 40 mg/kg bw or dermal application of 40 or 400 mg/kg bw, and in male and female rats after a single nose-only exposure by inhalation to 400 or 8000 ppm [1400 or 29 000 mg/m^3] or after repeated exposure by inhalation to 400 ppm [^{14}C]methyl *tert*-butyl ether for 6 h per day for 15 days. Total radiolabel was determined in tissues, urine, faeces and exhaled air, and the composition of the radiolabelled material was analysed in exhaled air and urine samples. Relatively little difference was observed between male and female rats in the disposition of [^{14}C]methyl *tert*-butyl ether after inhalation. The total recovery of ^{14}C measured in excreta, expired air and tissues of rats 48 h after exposure represented 91–105% of the dose. Most of the absorbed radiolabel (86–98%) was recovered in expired air and urine within 48 h, and only a small amount (< 2%) was excreted in faeces. Within the first 3 h after exposure, the proportion of radiolabel that was eliminated in exhaled air was 60% after intravenous dosing, 9–19% after dermal application, 21–54% after a single inhalation dose and 17% after repeated inhalation. Most of the exhaled radiolabel was associated with methyl *tert*-butyl ether itself: > 95% after intravenous and dermal administration and 66–80% after inhalation. Methyl *tert*-butyl ether was metabolized first to *tert*-butyl alcohol, which was either exhaled or further metabolized and eliminated in the urine. A dose-dependent shift in metabolism and route of elimination was observed after inhalation, with a greater proportion of the dose recovered in expired air as parent compound after the high dose and a larger proportion of the dose recovered in urine after the low dose. Repeated exposure to methyl *tert*-butyl ether did not affect its disposition. Of the four metabolites identified in urine, α-hydroxybutyric acid accounted for approximately 70% of the total urinary radiolabel found after inhalation, and 2-methyl-1,2-

propanediol accounted for approximately 14%. Two unidentified metabolites accounted for about 10 and 5% of the excreted radioactivity. Neither methyl *tert*-butyl ether nor *tert*-butyl alcohol was detected in urine samples from male and female Fischer 344 rats exposed to methyl *tert*-butyl ether.

Bernauer *et al.* (1998) identified urinary metabolites of methyl *tert*-butyl ether and *tert*-butyl alcohol in rats exposed to 2000 ppm [2-^{13}C]methyl *tert*-butyl ether for 6 h. Urine was collected up to 48 h after exposure and analysed by ^{13}C nuclear magnetic resonance and gas chromatography–mass spectrometry. The metabolism of *tert*-butyl alcohol was evaluated in rats given the unlabelled compound or [^{13}C]*tert*-butyl alcohol by gavage at a dose of 250 mg/kg bw in corn oil. Urine was collected up to 72 h after dosing. 2-Methyl-1,2-propanediol, 2-hydroxyisobutyrate (α-hydroxybutyric acid) and an unidentified conjugate of *tert*-butyl alcohol presumed to be a sulfate were the major urinary metabolites of methyl *tert*-butyl ether; small amounts of *tert*-butyl alcohol and its glucuronide were also identified. Rats dosed with [^{13}C]*tert*-butyl alcohol eliminated [^{13}C]acetone, *tert*-butyl alcohol and its glucuronide as minor metabolites.

Male ddY mice were given a single intraperitoneal dose of 50, 100 or 500 mg/kg bw methyl *tert*-butyl ether in corn oil. The amount of methyl *tert*-butyl ether exhaled depended on the dose administered and ranged from 23 to 69% of the dose. More than 90% of the methyl *tert*-butyl ether excreted through the lungs was eliminated within 3 h (Yoshikawa *et al.*, 1994).

Male Wistar rats were exposed to 50, 100 or 300 ppm [180, 360 or 1100 mg/m^3] methyl *tert*-butyl ether vapour for 6 h per day on five days per week for 2, 6, 10 or 15 weeks. The rats were killed immediately after exposure, and their blood, cerebral hemispheres and perirenal fat were analysed for methyl *tert*-butyl ether and *tert*-butyl alcohol. The liver and kidneys were also excised and microsomes were prepared. The blood concentrations of methyl *tert*-butyl ether were dose-dependent and did not change with the number of weeks of exposure. The *tert*-butyl alcohol concentrations in blood were dose-dependent and were highest after six weeks of exposure. Methyl *tert*-butyl ether, but not *tert*-butyl alcohol, was detected in perirenal fat. The exposure caused a transient increase in microsomal UDP-glucuronosyltransferase activity in liver and kidneys, but no effect on liver or kidney microsomal 7-ethoxycoumarin *O*-deethylase activity and minor, transient induction of kidney microsomal NADPH-cytochrome c reductase activity (Savolainen *et al.*, 1985).

(*b*) *In vitro*

Human liver microsomes (eight samples) were found to metabolize methyl *tert*-butyl ether to *tert*-butyl alcohol with activities ranging from 86 to 175 pmol formed per minute per milligram of total protein (Hong *et al.*, 1997a). The metabolizing activity of methyl *tert*-butyl ether was approximately twofold greater in rat and mouse liver microsomes (284–288 pmol *tert*-butyl alcohol formed/min per mg of protein) than in human microsomes. Human cytochrome P450 (CYP) 2A6 and CYP 2E1 cDNAs were individually co-expressed with human cytochrome P450 reductase by a baculovirus expression system, and the expressed enzymes (microsomal preparations of infected Sf9 cells) were used to assess the metabolism of methyl *tert*-butyl ether. The expressed CYP 2A6 was found to be more active than CYP 2E1 in metabolizing methyl *tert*-butyl ether to *tert*-butyl alcohol.

The metabolism of methyl *tert*-butyl ether to formaldehyde and *tert*-butyl alcohol was evaluated in liver microsomes prepared from male Sprague-Dawley rats treated with acetone or phenobarbital and in controls. Acetone and phenobarbital induce CYP 2E1 and CYP 2B1, respectively. Equimolar amounts of *tert*-butyl alcohol and formaldehyde were formed. Both acetone and phenobarbital induced the metabolism of methyl *tert*-butyl ether. A monoclonal antibody to CYP 2E1 inhibited the metabolism of methyl *tert*-butyl ether by liver microsomes prepared from acetone-induced rats by 35%. Methyl *tert*-butyl ether treatment resulted in a 50-fold increase in liver microsomal pentoxyresorufin dealkylase activity with no change in *N*-nitrosodimethylamine demethylase activity, suggesting an increase in CYP 2B1 but not in CYP 2E1 activity. The activities of these enzymes concord with the results of immunoblot analysis, which showed higher activity of CYP 2B1 and no change in that of CYP 2E1 when compared with controls (Brady *et al.*, 1990). In liver microsomes prepared from male Sprague-Dawley rats and exposed to purified rat CYPs (2B1, 2E1, 2C11, 1A1), CYP 2B1 was the main enzyme involved in the oxidation of methyl *tert*-butyl ether, CYP 2E1 having a lesser role (Turini *et al.*, 1998).

Microsomes prepared from nasal mucosae, including olfactory and respiratory epithelium, and liver, lung, kidney and olfactory bulbs of male Sprague-Dawley rats were used to compare the metabolic activity of these tissues towards methyl *tert*-butyl ether (Hong *et al.*, 1997b). The activity was measured *in vitro* by analysing *tert*-butyl alcohol headspace concentration by gas chromatography. The olfactory mucosa showed the highest activity in metabolizing methyl *tert*-butyl ether, and the activity was 46-fold higher than in liver. No detectable activity was found in microsomes prepared from lungs, kidneys or olfactory bulbs of the brain. [The Working Group noted that measuring *tert*-butyl alcohol levels in the headspace by gas chromatography is not a sensitive method for assessing the metabolism of methyl *tert*-butyl ether in tissues with low enzyme activity.]

tert-Butyl alcohol, a metabolite of methyl *tert*-butyl ether, was found to be oxidatively demethylated, producing formaldehyde in liver microsomes prepared from Sprague-Dawley rats (Cederbaum & Cohen, 1980). Casanova and Heck (1997) demonstrated that the metabolism of methyl *tert*-butyl ether to formaldehyde in hepatocytes prepared from female CD-1 mice, male B6C3F$_1$ mice and male Fischer 344 rats approached saturation at concentrations below 0.33 mmol/L. Formaldehyde production in the metabolism of methyl *tert*-butyl ether was evaluated by measuring the formation of DNA–protein cross-links and RNA–formaldehyde adducts. No increases were detected at concentrations of methyl *tert*-butyl ether up to 6.75 mmol/L. Induction of methyl *tert*-butyl ether metabolism did not change the yields of either of these adducts, and no species or strain differences were seen.

4.2 Toxic effects

The toxicity of methyl *tert*-butyl ether has been reviewed (WHO, 1998).

4.2.1 *Humans*

(*a*) *Controlled studies*

Nineteen men and 18 women were exposed to 1.39 ppm [5.0 mg/m^3] methyl *tert*-butyl ether for 1 h on several occasions, each separated by at least one week, and each subject completed a questionnaire on symptoms before and during exposure. Cognitive testing and objective measures of ocular and nasal irritation were also evaluated. There was no significant effect upon headache, nasal irritation or odour intensity, and no evidence of ocular inflammation was apparent as measured by polymorphonuclear neutrophils on the eye surface, tear film break-up time and mRNA coding for interleukin-6 or interleukin-8 in cells removed from the eye. The numbers of inflammation mediators and neutrophils were not significantly different in the nasal lavage fluid of control and treated volunteers. The subjects did not report any adverse symptoms due to this exposure (Prah *et al.*, 1994).

Of 43 people who were evaluated for the acute effects of exposure to 1.7 ppm [6 mg/m^3] methyl *tert*-butyl ether for 1 h, 22 men aged 18–32 and 21 women aged 18–34 remained throughout the study. Symptoms such as irritation, headache and mental fatigue were evaluated, and eye irritation (by tear-film breakup, eye redness) and nasal inflammation (by measurement of polymorphonuclear neutrophilic leukocytes) were measured before and after exposure. No increase in such symptoms was observed (Cain *et al.*, 1996).

Ten white men aged 23–51 years were exposed by inhalation to 5, 25 or 50 ppm [18, 90 and 180 mg/m^3] methyl *tert*-butyl ether vapour for 2 h on three occasions, with an interval of at least two weeks between exposures, during 2 h of light (50 W) physical exercise. The subjects rated the degree of irritative symptoms, discomfort and central nervous system effects before, during and after exposure on a questionnaire. The only rating noted was that of solvent smell, which increased greatly as the subject entered the chamber and with exposure concentration. Ocular changes (redness and tear film break-up time, conjunctival epithelial damage and blinking frequency) and nasal measurements such as peak expiratory flow, acoustic rhinometry to assess nasal swelling (5 and 25 ppm) and levels of inflammatory markers in nasal lavages (50 ppm) were evaluated. No effect on any of the eye measurements was associated with exposure to methyl *tert*-butyl ether. Although some nasal changes where reported, they were not related to the concentration. Nasal airway resistance, calculated from peak expiratory flows, increased significantly after exposure, but the increase did not exhibit any relationship to concentration. Overall, this study showed no or minimal acute effects of methyl *tert*-butyl ether at these concentrations (Nihlén *et al.*, 1998b).

(*b*) *Occupational exposure*

The relationships between exposure to methyl *tert*-butyl ether and acute human health effects have been reviewed (Borak *et al.*, 1998).

A study was conducted to assess neuropsychological symptoms among 101 road tanker drivers in Finland exposed to gasoline containing 10% methyl *tert*-butyl ether. The control group in this study consisted of 100 milk delivery drivers from the same locations. Interviews based on standardized symptom questionnaires were carried out before and at the end of the same work week. Tanker drivers were found to have a higher fatigue score then the control groups, and 20% of the tanker drivers reported headaches or nausea (Hakkola *et al.*, 1997). [The Working Group noted that specific exposure to methyl *tert*-butyl ether was not evaluated in this study.]

In New Jersey (United States), 237 garage workers were evaluated to determine whether a higher prevalence of acute adverse health effects was associated with exposure to methyl *tert*-butyl ether. The workers were divided into those with low and high exposure to methyl *tert*-butyl ether on the basis of the region of New Jersey from which they came; thus, 122 workers exposed after oxygenated fuels had been phased out were considered to have low exposure, and 115 workers who were exposed during implementation of the oxygenated fuels programme were considered to have high exposure. The workers completed questionnaires including questions on symptoms experienced during the previous 30 days. No adverse health effects were attributed to methyl *tert*-butyl ether (Mohr *et al.*, 1994).

A study was conducted to determine whether symptoms associated with exposure to methyl *tert*-butyl ether were reported at an increased rate among 14 people with 'multiple chemical sensitivities', five with 'chronic fatigue syndrome' and six controls in situations where exposure was likely to be highest (i.e. in service stations and while driving a car). The participants were interviewed by telephone. Enclosed shopping centres elicited the most symptoms among the patients; while a significant rate of methyl *tert*-butyl ether-associated symptoms was reported by the patients when they were in service stations, similar rates were seen in other situations, such as in grocery shops. Thus, the study did not provide clear evidence that an usually high rate of symptoms occurred only where methyl *tert*-butyl ether was most prevalent (Fiedler *et al.*, 1994).

The percentage of apoptotic cells in peripheral blood lymphocytes of 60 men and women exposed to methyl *tert*-butyl ether and benzene from water that had been contaminated for five to eight years was reported to be greater than that in a group of people who had no exposure to these chemicals. The concentrations of methyl *tert*-butyl ether and benzene in the water samples were reported to be 1–76 and 0.2–14 μg/L, respectively. The proportions of apoptotic lymphocytes were 26 ± 1.8 (SE)% in the exposed and 12 ± 1.3% in the unexposed groups, respectively (Vojdani *et al.*, 1997a). [The Working Group noted that the concentrations were not measured over the period in which the water was reported to have been contaminated. Furthermore, exposure to methyl *tert*-butyl ether and benzene was not characterized, so that the response observed cannot be attributed to either chemical.]

The generation of immunoglobulin (Ig)G, IgM, IgA and IgE antibodies against methyl *tert*-butyl ether was investigated in 18 men and six women who had been employed as gasoline service station attendants for at least two years and in eight men and four women otherwise employed. Significant increases in IgG and IgM antibodies against methyl *tert*-butyl ether were noted in seven exposed and one control person. The antibody titres did not correlate with the severity or number of reported adverse symptoms, i.e. headaches, shortness of breath, burning eyes, nose and throat, muscle fatigue, memory loss and difficulty in concentrating (Vojdani *et al.*, 1997b).

Effects on the immune system were measured by monitoring plasma interleukin-6 at the beginning and end of a single workday in 22 mechanics exposed to automobile emissions derived from fuels containing methyl *tert*-butyl ether. Interleukin-6 is involved in the differentiation of B cells to IgG-secreting plasma cells and is also an inducer of acute-phase proteins and cytotoxic T cells. No change in interleukin-6 was detected (Duffy, 1994). [The Working Group noted that exposure to methyl *tert*-butyl ether was not characterized in this study.]

Blood samples were obtained from volunteers in Fairbanks, Alaska (United States), and methyl *tert*-butyl ether was analysed by gas chromatography–mass spectrometry. The first phase of the study, involving 18 people, was conducted in early December 1992 during implementation of the oxygenated fuels programme, in which methyl *tert*-butyl ether constituted about 15% w/v of gasoline, and the second, involving 28 people, was conducted in February 1993, two months after the programme had been discontinued. The concentrations of methyl *tert*-butyl ether in the blood of workers (including service station attendants, garage workers, drivers and mechanics after a work shift were approximately seven times higher during phase I (median, 1.8 μg/L; range, 0.2–37 μg/L) than during phase II (median, 0.24 μg/L; range, 0.05–1.4 μg/L; $p = 0.0001$). As expected, the blood concentrations were higher in workers at the end than at the beginning of a workshift. The highest concentration measured was 37 μg/L in a worker at the end of a shift in phase I. Higher blood concentrations correlated with heavier exposure. Standardized questionnaires were administered to the workers at the end of the workshift on the same day that blood samples were obtained, eliciting information on key symptoms that have been associated with exposure to methyl *tert*-butyl ether, such as headache, eye irritation, burning of the nose or throat and cough, and other specific health complaints. A much higher prevalence of these symptoms was noted during phase I than phase II; however, the relationship between blood concentrations of methyl *tert*-butyl ether and symptoms was not statistically significant. The authors recognized several limitations to this pilot study (Moolenaar *et al.*, 1994).

(*c*) *Instillation into the gall-bladder*

A number of studies of the potential use of methyl-*tert*-butyl ether to dissolve gall-bladder stones have been reported and reviewed (Borak *et al.*, 1998). Dissolution of gall-bladder stones in humans involves injection through a catheter into the gall-bladder. In one study in which the concentrations of methyl *tert*-butyl ether in blood were measured, the peak concentrations in patients with gall-bladder stones were about 1000-fold higher than those in workers exposed by inhalation (Leuschner *et al.*, 1991). Although methyl *tert*-butyl ether and its metabolite *tert*-butyl alcohol were measured in the blood and urine of these patients and elimination took several days, no clinical reactions were reported.

4.2.2 *Experimental systems*

The lethality of methyl *tert*-butyl ether has been studied in rats and rabbits. The oral LD_{50} in rats was 4 mL/kg bw, the inhalation LC_{50} in rats was 86 mg/L (4 h), and the dermal LD_{50} in rabbits was > 10 mL/kg bw (Clayton & Clayton, 1981).

The neurotoxicity of methyl *tert*-butyl ether was evaluated in nine-week-old male and female Fischer 344 rats exposed to 0, 800, 4000 or 8000 ppm [0, 2900, 14 000 or 29 000 mg/m³] methyl *tert*-butyl ether for 6 h, with evaluation of their behaviour 1, 6 and 24 h later. At 1 h after exposure, animals exposed to the highest dose showed a variety of sensorimotor changes indicative of central nervous system depression. The most frequent findings were ataxia, duck-walk, increased lachrymation, laboured respiration, decreased muscle tone, lowered body temperature and decreased hind-leg grip strength. No changes were observed 6 or 24 h after exposure. In a longer study, animals were exposed to 0, 800, 4000 or 8000 ppm methyl *tert*-butyl ether for 6 h per day on five days a week for 13 weeks. Any neurobehavioural changes were neither persistent nor cumulative. The body and brain weights of rats at the highest dose were decreased, but no histological changes were seen in the brain or peripheral nervous tissue. The authors concluded that any neurotoxic effects caused by methyl *tert*-butyl ether exposure at concentrations up to 8000 ppm were minimal (Daughtrey *et al.*, 1997).

Five-week-old Fischer 344 rats were exposed to 0, 800, 4000 or 8000 ppm [0, 2900, 14 000 or 29 000 mg/m³] methyl *tert*-butyl ether for 6 h a day on five days a week for 13 weeks. Animals at the high dose had decreased body weights throughout the study. The activities of aspartate aminotransferase and alanine aminotransferase were decreased in all exposed males and in females at the high dose. Increased corticosterone levels, indicative of stress, were found in male rats at the high dose, but there was no exposure-related effect on the levels of aldosterone and adrenocorticotropic hormone. The absolute and relative weights of the liver, kidney and adrenal gland were significantly increased and brain weights were significantly decreased in male and female rats at the high concentration. No histological changes were observed, with the exception of a mild increase in hyaline droplet formation in the kidneys, increased haemosiderosis in the spleen and an increased incidence of hyperplasia in the lymph nodes in exposed male rats (Lington *et al.*, 1997).

Groups of 10 male and 10 female Fischer 344 rats and CD-1 mice were exposed to 0, 400, 3000 or 8000 ppm [0, 1400, 11 000 and 29 000 mg/m³] methyl *tert*-butyl ether for 6 h a day on five days a week for four weeks, with additional groups of five rodents of each species and each sex assigned to the control and high-dose groups and retained for a 16-day recovery period. Osmotic mini-pumps containing 5-bromo-2′-deoxyuridine were implanted 24 and 48 h before necropsy in rats and mice, respectively, to assess DNA synthesis on study day 5 and at the end of the exposure. Absolute body weight and body-weight gain were decreased in female mice after 1 week and in male and female rats throughout study in groups receiving the high dose. Increased renal DNA synthesis was found in male rats exposed to 3000 ppm on study day 5 and in those at 3000 and 8000 ppm methyl *tert*-butyl ether at the end of the study. No changes in DNA synthesis were observed in the kidneys of exposed female rats or in male or female rats at the end of the 16-day recovery period. In mice, the labelling indices in the liver were increased significantly following five days of exposure to 8000 ppm methyl *tert*-butyl ether, but there was no significant increase in male mice. No effects were observed at the end of the treatment period or after the 16-day recovery period (Bird *et al.*, 1997).

In a study of the ability of methyl *tert*-butyl ether to induce protein droplet accumulation, α_{2u}-globulin accumulation and renal-cell proliferation, male and female Fischer 344 rats were exposed to 0, 413, 1516 or 3013 ppm [0, 250, 5500 and 11 000 mg/m³] methyl *tert*-butyl ether for 6 h a day for 10 consecutive days. Microscopic lesions in the kidneys of exposed male rats were characterized by epithelial-cell necrosis, protein droplet accumulation and karyomegaly within the proximal tubules; in addition, occasional epithelial cell exfoliation into the tubular lumen was observed. In male rat kidney sections stained with Mallory Heidenhain stain, protein droplet accumulation increased in a concentration-related manner. Immunohistochemical staining of kidney sections from male rats for α_{2u}-globulin showed greater amounts in exposed male rats than in controls, but the exposure–response relationship was not linear. A statistically significant positive trend was found by enzyme-linked immunosorbent assay in the exposure-related increase in renal α_{2u}-globulin concentration, and this change was significant in male rats exposed to 3013 ppm methyl *tert*-butyl ether when compared with unexposed males. The labelling indices, measured by 5-bromo-2′-deoxyuridine incorporation, indicated an exposure-dependent increase in cell proliferation in the renal cortexes of male but not female rats. A strong positive correlation ($r = 0.994$) was demonstrated between the mean labelling index and the mean α_{2u}-globulin concentration. The results of this study indicate that methyl *tert*-butyl ether is a mild inducer of α_{2u}-globulin nephropathy and enhanced renal-cell proliferation in male but not female rats (Prescott-Mathews *et al.*, 1997).

Groups of 12-week-old male and female Sprague-Dawley rats were given 0, 357, 714, 1071 or 1428 mg/kg bw methyl *tert*-butyl ether orally in corn oil. Mild anaesthesia and diarrhoea were observed in treated animals. All treated females had decreased lung weights, with increased blood urea nitrogen and decreased creatinine concentrations at the highest dose. Males had an increased creatinine concentration at the highest dose and increased serum aspartate aminotransferase and lactate dehydrogenase activities at doses ≥ 1071 mg/kg bw. Nephropathy, characterized by increased hyaline droplets within the cytoplasm of proximal tubular epithelial cells, was recorded in 88% of the males given the highest dose and in 40% of the male controls. [The Working Group noted that the slides were stained with haematoxylin and eosin. Although droplets can be visualized with this stain, it is not specific for protein. Also, the criteria for scoring these lesions were not presented.] In a longer study, rats were treated with 0, 100, 300, 900 or 1200 mg/kg bw methyl *tert*-butyl ether in corn oil. The blood urea nitrogen concentration was decreased and that of cholesterol increased in all treated females, whereas the blood urea nitrogen concentration was decreased in treated male rats. The relative kidney weights of female rats were significantly increased at doses ≥ 300 mg/kg bw. There was a trend to increased liver and kidney weights in treated male rats, and chronic nephropathy was common in both controls and males at the high dose. The tubular degeneration that characterizes nephropathy was graded as more severe in the treated rats. [The Working Group noted that the authors did not distinguish between chronic nephropathy and hyaline droplet nephropathy.] Fifty per cent of the male rats at the highest dose had a small number of tubules plugged with granular casts, and all had slightly increased numbers of cytoplasmic hyaline droplets in proximal tubular epithelial cells. After either 14 or 90 days of treatment, significant microscopic findings were restricted to the kidneys of male rats (Robinson *et al.*, 1990).

Eight-week-old female B6C3F$_1$ mice were exposed to 7814 ppm [28 000 mg/m^3] methyl *tert*-butyl ether for 6 h a day on five days a week for 3 or 21 days. The relative weight of the uterus was decreased in both treated groups, and the relative liver weight was higher after three days but not after 21 days. The activity of pentoxyresorufin-*O*-dealkylase, a marker enzyme for the CYP 2B family which is commonly induced by many tumour promoters, was increased by 5- and 14-fold after 3 and 21 days of exposure to methyl *tert*-butyl ether, respectively. 7-Ethoxyresorufin activity was increased two- to threefold at both 3 and 21 days. The hepatic labelling index, as measured by 5-bromo-2′-deoxyuridine incorporation, was significantly increased in exposed mice at 3 but not at 21 days. This transient increased occurred in the absence of hepatotoxicity, indicating that methyl *tert*-butyl ether is a hepatic mitogen. Mild centrilobular to midzonal swelling of hepatocytes was also observed. In the same report, it was shown that the rate of 17β-oestradiol metabolism to water-soluble metabolites was significantly increased in hepatocytes isolated from female B6C3F$_1$ mice treated by gavage with methyl *tert*-butyl ether at 1800 mg/kg bw per day for three consecutive days (Moser *et al.*, 1996b).

Exposure of female B6C3F$_1$ mice to 8000 ppm [28 000 mg/m^3] methyl *tert*-butyl ether by inhalation for 6 h per day on five days per week for 3, 16 or 32 weeks caused a significant decrease in body weight at 16 and 32 weeks when compared with controls. Treatment also significantly increased the liver weight and hepatic microsomal P450 activity, with no indication of cytotoxic or hepatic necrosis. Other changes observed were decreased ovary, pituitary and uterine weights after 16 and 32 weeks of exposure; increased length of the oestrous cycle (numbers of days in both oestrus and non-oestrus stages) after 32 weeks; a decreased number of uterine glands and decreased uterine glandular and luminal epithelial DNA synthesis after 3 or 21 days or 16 or 32 weeks; and a decreased number of epithelial layers in the cervix and vagina at all times. Neither methyl *tert*-butyl ether nor its metabolite *tert*-butyl alcohol inhibited the binding of [^{3}H]17β-oestradiol to a recombinant human receptor. Treatment of HepG2 cells with methyl *tert*-butyl ether did not induce oestrogen receptor activity or antagonize a maximally inducing dose of 17β-oestradiol. In mice exposed to methyl *tert*-butyl ether, oestrogen levels in serum were not affected. The authors suggested that these results indicate that methyl *tert*-butyl ether-induced endocrine effects are not mediated through the oestrogen receptor (Moser *et al.*, 1998).

Male Wistar rats, 12 weeks of age, were exposed to 50, 100 or 300 ppm [180, 360 or 1100 mg/m^3] methyl *tert*-butyl ether for 6 h a day on five days a week for 2, 10 or

15 weeks, and microsomes were prepared from liver and kidney. A transient increase in UDP-glucuronosyl transferase activity was found in liver and kidney microsomes, but there was almost no effect on the hepatic cytochrome P450 concentration and only minor induction of renal cytochrome P450. Muscle creatine kinase activity, which is associated with contractile capacity, was decreased after two weeks of exposure, had returned to control levels at 10 weeks and then increased after exposure to 100 or 200 ppm for 15 weeks (Savolainen *et al.*, 1985).

Male and female Fischer 344 rats and CD-1 mice were exposed to 0, 400, 3000 or 8000 ppm [0, 1400, 10 000 or 28 000 mg/m^3] methyl *tert*-butyl ether for 6 h a day on five days a week for either 24 months (rats) or 18 months (mice). At the highest concentration, clinical signs of prostration, eye twitching, hypoactivity, lack of startle reflex and ataxia were observed in both mice and rats. Body-weight gain was significantly reduced by the end of the study in animals at the high dose, with decreases of 16% in male mice, 24% in female mice, 29% in male rats and 22% in female rats. At necropsy, a statistically significant decrease in the incidence of cystic endometrial-cell hyperplasia was seen in female mice and an increase in hepatocellular hypertrophy in mice of each sex at 3000 and 8000 ppm. An exposure-related increase in the incidence and severity of renal changes associated with chronic progressive nephropathy was seen in all treated male rats and to a lesser extent in female rats at 3000 and 8000 ppm. In male rats at 3000 and 8000 ppm, chronic progressive nephropathy was the major cause of death (Bird *et al.*, 1997).

Eight-week-old male and female Sprague-Dawley rats were given 0, 250 or 1000 mg/kg bw methyl *tert*-butyl ether in olive oil by gavage on four days a week for 104 weeks and were maintained until they died. Body weights were unaffected. After 88 weeks of age, the survival rate of male rats treated with 1000 mg/kg bw was increased, and the survival rate of females showed a dose–dependent decrease. There was no evidence of behavioural changes, and no relevant non-neoplastic changes were detected either grossly or histologically (Belpoggi *et al.*, 1995).

Toxicity of metabolites

Male and female Fischer 344 rats and B6C3F$_1$ mice were exposed to *tert*-butyl alcohol in their drinking-water for 94–95 days at doses of 0, 0.25, 0.5, 1, 2 or 4% (w/v) [providing doses of approximately 240–3600 mg/kg bw per day for rats and approximately 320–7500 mg/kg bw per day for mice] (Lindamood *et al.*, 1992). Of the 10 animals per sex at the highest dose, all of the males and six of the females died before the end of the study. Body-weight gain was depressed in male rats at all doses and in female rats and male and female mice at the highest dose. Ataxia and hypoactivity were observed in treated animals. Treated mice showed hyperplasia of the transitional epithelium and inflammation of the urinary bladder. In rats, gross lesions were also observed in the urinary tract, accompanied by urinary tract calculi, dilatation of the urethra and renal pelvis and thickening of the urinary bladder mucus; they also had increased severity of mineralization of the kidney. A treatment-associated increase in hyaline (protein) droplets was seen in male rats at 0.25–2% *tert*-butyl alcohol and a decrease in rats at 4%. Male rats at 1 or 2% *tert*-butyl alcohol showed a significant increase in proliferating cell nuclear antigen-stained S-phase nuclei, but those at 4% showed a significant decrease. The results for proliferating cell nuclear antigen-positive nuclei in female kidneys were inconclusive.

4.3 Reproductive and developmental effects

4.3.1 *Humans*

No data were available to the Working Group.

4.3.2 *Experimental systems*

Groups of 30 pregnant CD-1 mice and 25 pregnant Sprague-Dawley rats were exposed to methyl *tert*-butyl ether (purity, 95.03–98.93%) by inhalation at target concentrations of 0, 250, 1000 or 2500 ppm [0, 9000, 3600 and 90 000 mg/m^3] on gestation days 6–15; the fetuses were examined by routine teratological techniques on day 18 (mice) or 20 (rats) of gestation. In rats, the only significant effect seen in either dams or offspring was a transient reduction in food consumption at the start of exposure; fetal body weight was stated to be unaffected. Pregnant mice showed a slight increase in the frequency of lachrymation but no significant dose-related reduction in food consumption or body weight. No significant effects were observed in the fetuses in terms of viability, growth or morphology (Conaway *et al.*, 1985). [The Working Group noted that no quantitative data were presented.]

Groups of 30 pregnant CD-1 mice and 15 pregnant New Zealand white rabbits were exposed to methyl *tert*-butyl ether (purity, 99%) vapour by inhalation at 0, 1000, 4000 or 8000 ppm [0, 3600, 14 000 and 28 000 mg/m^3] for 6 h per day on gestation days 6–15 and 6–18, respectively. The high dose represented 50% of the lower explosive limit. The pregnant females and their fetuses were examined by routine teratological techniques. In mice, maternal toxicity was seen at 4000 ppm (hypoactivity and ataxia) and 8000 ppm (hypoactivity, ataxia and reduced food consumption and body-weight gain). Late resorptions and dead fetuses and the incidence of cleft palate were increased at 8000 ppm, while fetal body weight was lower, and the incidence of skeletal variations (poorly ossified phalanges, vertebral arches and centra, reduced number of caudal segments) was increased at 4000 and 8000 ppm. Post-implantation deaths were seen mainly among male offspring. The authors noted that maternal stress may have contributed to the developmental effects, as exposure to similar concentrations is known to increase corticosterone activity, which, in turn, could produce similar outcomes. In rabbits, no effects on development were observed, although maternal weight gain and food consumption were reduced at the two higher doses and relative liver weights were reduced at 8000 ppm (Bevan *et al.*, 1997a).

Groups of 15 male and 30 female CD rats, approximately eight weeks old, were exposed to measured concentrations of methyl *tert*-butyl ether (purity, 95–99%) of about 0, 300, 1200 or 2900 ppm [0, 1100, 4400 and 10 000 mg/m^3] for 6 h per day for 12 and

3 weeks, respectively, prior to breeding. Exposure of males was continued during the mating period, while females were exposed on seven days a week for 6 h per day on days 0–20 of gestation and on days 5–20 of lactation. The offspring were not directly exposed. A second mating was conducted after the first litter had been weaned to yield an F_{1b} generation. Four of 30 dams at 300 ppm and 5/30 at 2900 ppm had dilated renal pelvises, while the incidences were 1/30 in controls and 0/30 at 1200 ppm. No effects were reported on growth, the weights of the reproductive organs, the histological appearance of the gonads of animals of either sex or reproductive performance and fertility in the parental generation. There were no significant effects on the growth of offspring in the F_{1a} or F_{1b} litters, although there was a slight but significant decrease in pup viability in F_{1a} litters at the low and intermediate doses between days 0 and 4 of lactation. The incidence of dilated renal pelvis was slightly elevated in the F_{1a} offspring at the low and intermediate doses that were examined at weaning (Biles *et al.*, 1987).

In a two-generation study, groups of 25 male and 25 female Sprague Dawley rats were exposed to 0, 400, 3000 or 8000 ppm [0, 1400, 11 000 and 29 000 mg/m³] methyl *tert*-butyl ether for 6 h per day for 10 weeks before mating. Parental females were exposed during mating, gestation and from day 5 of lactation. F_1 animals were exposed from day 28; after eight weeks, adults were mated within treatment groups to yield an F_2 group. F_1 and F_2 animals at the high dose showed ataxia, hypoactivity and reduced body weights; the effects were less severe and/or transient at the intermediate dose. In the F_1 generation, increased liver weights were reported in animals of each sex at the high dose and in the males at the intermediate dose. The histological appearance of the liver was reported to be unchanged by exposure. The number of dead F_2 pups was increased on postnatal day 4, and the growth of F_1 and F_2 pups at the two higher doses was decreased during the preweaning period (Bevan *et al.*, 1997b).

4.4 Genetic and related effects

4.4.1 *Humans*

No data were available to the Working Group.

4.4.2 *Experimental systems* (see Table 5 for references)

Methyl *tert*-butyl ether was not mutagenic to *Salmonella typhimurium* TA98, TA100, TA104 or TA1535 in the presence and absence of an exogenous activation system. Methyl *tert*-butyl ether induced gene mutation in mouse lymphoma L5178Y $tk^{+/-}$ cells in the presence of exogenous activation. The mutagenicity was eliminated when formaldehyde dehydrogenase was added to the assay system.

Methyl *tert*-butyl ether did not induce sex-linked recessive lethal mutation in *Drosophila melanogaster*. It did not induce unscheduled DNA synthesis in the liver of mice exposed by inhalation and did not induce micronuclei in mouse bone marrow or chromosomal aberrations in rat bone marrow. Negative results were also obtained for micronucleus formation in mice treated by intraperitoneal injection with doses near the lethal concentration.

Table 5. Genetic and related effects of methyl *tert*-butyl ether

Test system	Results[a]		Dose[b] (LED or HID)	Reference
	Without exogenous metabolic system	With exogenous metabolic system		
Salmonella typhimurium TA100, TA98, TA104, TA1535, reverse mutation	–	–	7400 μg/plate	Kado *et al.* (1998)
Drosophila melanogaster, sex-linked recessive lethal mutations	–		0.3% feed	McKee *et al.* (1997)
Gene mutation, mouse lymphoma L5178Y cells, *tk* locus *in vitro*	NT	+	740 μg/mL	Mackerer *et al.* (1996)
Unscheduled DNA synthesis, male and female CD-1 mouse hepatocytes *in vivo*	–		8000 ppm inh, 6 h/d × 2 d	McKee *et al.* (1997)
Micronucleus formation, male and female CD-1 mouse bone-marrow cells *in vivo*	–		8000 ppm inh, 6 h/d × 2 d	McKee *et al.* (1997)
Micronucleus formation, male and female Swiss-Webster mouse bone-marrow cells *in vivo*	–		1750 ip × 1	Kado *et al.* (1998)
Chromosomal aberrations, male and female Fischer 344 rat bone-marrow cells *in vivo*	–		8000 ppm inh, 6 h/d × 5 d	McKee *et al.* (1997)

[a] +, positive; –, negative; NT, not tested

[b] LED, lowest effective dose; HID, highest ineffective dose; unless otherwise stated, in-vivo test, mg/kg bw per day; inh, inhalation; d, day; ip, intraperitoneal

5. Summary of Data Reported and Evaluation

5.1 Exposure data

Methyl *tert*-butyl ether is a volatile synthetic chemical that has been used widely since the 1980s in proportions up to 15% as a component of gasolines for its octane-enhancing and air pollution-reducing properties. Exposure to methyl *tert*-butyl ether may occur through inhalation and skin contact during its production, formulation, distribution and use, either as methyl *tert*-butyl ether or in gasoline. In the petroleum industry, the average exposure is generally below 5 ppm (20 mg/m^3), although higher exposure occurs during some operations. In service stations where fuels containing > 10% methyl *tert*-butyl ether are delivered, the average concentration to which attendants are exposed is about 0.5 ppm (2 mg/m^3). The ambient air concentrations in regions where methyl *tert*-butyl ether-rich gasoline is used are usually 1–5 ppb (4–20 μg/m^3), while in other regions they are below 1 ppb (4 μg/m^3). During self-service refuelling, individuals may be exposed to levels up to 10 ppm (40 mg/m^3) or more for a few minutes. Methyl *tert*-butyl ether has been detected in a small percentage of drinking-water samples in the United States.

5.2 Human carcinogenicity data

Although methyl *tert*-butyl ether has been in commercial use for gasoline blending since the 1970s, no analytical epidemiological studies have addressed a possible association of methyl *tert*-butyl ether with human cancer.

5.3 Animal carcinogenicity data

Methyl *tert*-butyl ether was tested for carcinogenicity in a non-standard protocol in rats by gavage. The incidences of Leydig-cell tumours of the testis in males and of lymphomas and leukaemias combined in females were increased. Methyl *tert*-butyl ether was tested by inhalation in one experiment in mice and in one experiment in rats. It increased the incidence of hepatocellular adenomas in female mice and that of renal tubular tumours in male rats in a non-dose-related manner.

tert-Butyl alcohol, a metabolite of methyl *tert*-butyl ether, marginally increased the incidence of follicular-cell adenomas of the thyroid in female mice.

5.4 Other relevant data

Methyl *tert*-butyl ether is metabolized in humans and rodents to *tert*-butyl alcohol. In both species, methyl *tert*-butyl ether is cleared from blood rapidly whereas *tert*-butyl alcohol accumulates and is cleared at a slower rate than the parent compound. In rats exposed to methyl *tert*-butyl ether, the metabolites identified in urine include *tert*-butyl alcohol, its sulfate and glucuronide conjugates, 2-methyl-1,2-propanediol and 2-hydroxyisobutyrate.

No significant acute effects on human health were seen after exposure of volunteers by inhalation to methyl *tert*-butyl ether itself or of service-station attendants to gasoline.

In male rats, methyl *tert*-butyl ether-induced kidney lesions were associated with α_{2u}-globulin nephropathy, a male rat-specific response. Exposure of female mice to 8000 ppm [29 g/m^3] methyl *tert*-butyl ether in air was mitogenic to the liver and caused changes in oestrogen-regulated tissues.

Methyl *tert*-butyl ether did not induce developmental toxicity in rats or rabbits exposed via inhalation to concentrations that affected maternal food consumption. In one study in mice, increased incidences of postimplantation loss and cleft palate were seen at doses that also induced hypoactivity, ataxia and reduced food consumption in the dams. Another study in mice, conducted at lower doses that were less toxic to dams, did not provide evidence of developmental toxicity.

No data were available on the genetic and related effects of methyl *tert*-butyl ether in humans. The few available data indicate that methyl *tert*-butyl ether is not genotoxic in experimental systems.

5.5 Evaluation

There is *inadequate evidence* in humans for the carcinogenicity of methyl *tert*-butyl ether.

There is *limited evidence* in experimental animals for the carcinogenicity of methyl *tert*-butyl ether.

Overall evaluation

Methyl *tert*-butyl ether is *not classifiable as to its carcinogenicity to humans (Group 3).*

6. References

Agency for Toxic Substances and Disease Registry (1996) *Toxicological Profile for Methyl* tert-*Butyl Ether*, Atlanta, GA

Allen, K.M., Grande, D. & Foley, T. (1996) Monitoring reformulated gasoline in Milwaukee, Wisconsin. In: *A&WMA Conference on the Measurement of Toxic and Related Air Pollutants, Research Triangle Park, NC, May 7–9 1996*, Madison, WI, Wisconsin Department of Natural Resources

Almaguer, D. (1993) *NIOSH Health Hazard Evaluation Report* (Report No. HETA 93-0884-2344), Cincinnati, OH, National Institute for Occupational Safety and Health

American Conference of Governmental Industrial Hygienists (1997) *1997 TLVs® and BEIs®* Cincinnati, OH, p. 29

American Petroleum Institute (1989) *Monitoring Near Refineries for Airborne Chemicals*, Vol. 1, *Validated Ambient Air Concentrations around Three Refineries* (Publ. No. 4484), Washington DC

Anon. (1997) MTBE—The quest for cleaner air. *Asian chem. News*, **May 12**

Arco Chemical Co. (1993) *Product Safety Bulletin: Methyl Tertiary Butyl Ether*, Newtown Square, PA, Environmental Health and Safety Department

Belpoggi, F., Soffritti, M. & Maltoni, C. (1995) Methyl-tertiary-butyl ether (MTBE)—a gasoline additive—causes testicular and lymphohaematopoietic cancers in rats. *Toxicol. ind. Health*, **11**, 119–149

Belpoggi, F., Soffritti, M. & Maltoni, C. (1998) Pathological characterization of testicular tumours and lymphomas–leukaemias, and of their precursors observed in Sprague-Dawley rats exposed to methyl-tertiary-butyl-ether (MTBE). *Eur. J. Oncol.*, **3**, 201–206

Bernauer, U., Amberg, A., Scheutzow, D. & Dekant, W. (1998) Biotransformation of ^{12}C- and 2-^{13}C-labeled methyl *tert*-butyl ether, ethyl *tert*-butyl ether, and *tert*-butyl alcohol in rats: Identification of metabolites in urine by ^{13}C nuclear magnetic resonance and gas chromatography/mass spectrometry. *Chem. Res. Toxicol.*, **11**, 651–658

Bevan, C., Tyl, R.W., Neeper-Bradley, L., Fisher, L.C., Panson, R.D., Douglas, J.F. & Andews, L.S. (1997a) Developmental toxicity evaluation of methyl tertiary-butyl ether (MTBE) by inhalation in mice and rabbits. *J. appl. Toxicol.*, **17** (Suppl. 1), S21–S29

Bevan, C., Neeper-Bradley, T.L., Tyl, R.W., Fisher, L.C., Panson, R.D., Kneiss, J.J. & Andrews, L.S. (1997b) Two-generation reproductive toxicity study of methyl tertiary-butyl ether (MTBE) in rats. *J. appl. Toxicol.*, **17** (Suppl. 1), S13–S19

Biles, R.W., Schroeder, R.E. & Holdsworth, C.E. (1987) Methyl tertiary butyl ether inhalation in rats: a single generation reproduction study. *Toxicol. ind. Health*, **3**, 519–533

Bird, M.G., Burleigh-Flayer, H.D., Chun, J.S., Douglas, J.F., Kneiss, J.J. & Andrews, L.S. (1997) Oncogenicity studies of inhaled methyl tertiary-butyl ether (MTBE) in CD-1 mice and F-344 rats. *J. appl. Toxicol.*, **17**, S45–S55

Borak, J., Pastides, H., Van Ert, M., Russi, M. & Herzstein, J. (1998) Exposure to MTBE and acute human health effects: A critical literature review. *Hum. ecol. Risk Assess.*, **4**, 177–200

Brady, J.F., Xiao, F., Ning, S.M. & Yang, C.S. (1990) Metabolism of methyl *tertiary*-butyl ether by rat hepatic microsomes. *Arch. Toxicol.*, **64**, 157–160

Brown, S.L. (1997) Atmospheric and potable water exposures to methyl *tert*-butyl ether (MTBE). *Regul. Toxicol. Pharmacol.*, **25**, 256–276

Buchta, T.M. (1993a) *NIOSH Health Hazard Evaluation Report* (Report No. HETA 93-802-2338), Cincinnati, OH, National Institute for Occupational Safety and Health

Buchta, T.M. (1993b) *NIOSH Health Hazard Evaluation Report* (Report No. HETA 93-606-2336), Cincinnati, OH, National Institute for Occupational Safety and Health

Buckley, T.J., Prah, J.D., Ashley, D., Zweidinger, R.A. & Wallace, L.A. (1997) Body burden measurements and models to assess inhalation exposure to methyl tertiary butyl ether (MTBE). *J. Air Waste Manage. Assoc.*, **47**, 739–752

Budavari, S., ed. (1996) *The Merck Index*, 12th Ed., Whitehouse Station, NJ, Merck & Co., p. 1032

Cain, W.S., Leaderer, B.P., Ginsberg, G.L., Andrews, L.S., Cometto-Muñiz, J.E., Gent, J.F., Buck, M., Berglund, L.G., Mohsenin, V., Monahain, E. & Kjaergaard, S. (1996) Acute exposure to low-level methyl tertiary-butyl ether (MTBE): Human reactions and pharmacokinetic response. *Inhal. Toxicol.*, **8**, 21–48

Casanova, M. & d'A. Heck, H. (1997) Lack of evidence for the involvement of formaldehyde in the hepatocarcinogenicity of methyl *tertiary* butyl ether in CD-1 mice. *Chem.-biol. Interactions*, **105**, 131–143

Cederbaum, A.I. & Cohen, G. (1980) Oxidative demethylation of *t*-butyl alcohol by rat liver microsomes. *Biochem. biophys. Res. Comm.*, **97**, 730–736

Chemical Information Services (1995) *Directory of World Chemical Producers 1995/96 Standard Edition*, Dallas, TX, p. 138

Cirvello, J.D., Radovsky, A., Heath, J.E., Farnell, D.R. & Lindamood, C. (1995) Toxicity and carcinogenicity of *t*-butyl alcohol in rats and mice following chronic exposure in drinking water. *Toxicol. ind. Health*, **11**, 151–165

Clayton, G. & Clayton, F., eds (1981) *Patty's Industrial Hygiene and Toxicology*, 3rd Ed., Vol. 2A, New York, Wiley-Interscience, p. 2503

Clegg, E.D., Cook, J.C., Chapin, R.E., Foster, P.M. & Daston, G.P. (1997) Leydig cell hyperplasia and adenoma formation: Mechanisms and relevance to humans. *Reprod. Toxicol.*, **11**, 107–121

Conaway, C.C., Schroeder, R.E. & Snyder, N.K. (1985) Teratology evaluation of methyl tertiary butyl ether in rats and mice. *J. Toxicol. environ. Health*, **16**, 797–809

Cook, C.K. & Kovein, R.J. (1995) *NIOSH Health Hazard Evaluation Report* (Report No. HETA 94-0220-2526), Cincinnati, OH, National Institute for Occupational Safety and Health

Cook, C.K. & Kovein, R.J. (1997) Exposure of service station attendants to oxygenated gasoline containing methyl *tert*-butyl ether. *Appl. occup. environ. Hyg.*, **12**, 571–576

Daly, M.H. & Lindsey, B.D. (1996) *Occurrence and Concentrations of Volatile Organic Compounds in Shallow Ground Water in the Lower Susquehanna River Basin, Pennsylvania and Maryland* (United States Geological Survey Water-Resources Investigations Report No. 96-4141), Denver, CO, United States Geological Survey

Daughtrey, W.C., Gill, M.W., Pritts, I.M., Douglas, J.F., Kneiss, J.J. & Andrews, L.S. (1997) Neurotoxicological evaluation of methyl tertiary-butyl ether in rats. *J. appl. Toxicol.*, **17**, S57–S64

Davidson, J.M. (1996) Fate and transport of MTBE: The latest data. In: *Proceedings of the Petroleum Hydrocarbons & Organic Chemicals in Ground Water Conference, Houston, TX, November 30, 1995*, Dublin, OH, National Ground Water Association, pp. 285–301

Delzer, G.C., Zogorski, J.S., Lopes, T.J. & Bosshart, R.L. (1996) *Occurrence of the Gasoline Oxygenate MTBE and BTEX Compounds in Urban Stormwater in the United States, 1991–1995* (United States Geological Survey Water-Resources Investigation Report No. 96-4145), Rapid City, SD, United States Geological Survey

Duffy, L.K. (1994) Oxyfuel in Alaska: Use of interleukins to monitor effects on the immune system. *Sci. total Environ.*, **151**, 253–256

Environment Canada (1995) *National Pollutant Release Inventory Summary Report 1994—Canadian Environmental Protection Act*, Hull, Québec, Minister of Supply and Services Canada

Environmental Protection Agency (1992) Method 524.2—Measurement of purgeable organic compounds in water by capillary column gas chromatography/mass spectrometry (Revision 4.0), Cincinnati, OH, Environmental Monitoring Systems Laboratory

Environmental Protection Agency (1994) *Chemical Summary for Methyl-tert-Butyl Ether* (EPA-749/F-94-017a), Washington DC, Office of Pollution Prevention and Toxics

Environmental Protection Agency (1996) *Drinking Water Regulations and Health Advisories* (EPA 822-B-96-002), Washington DC, Office of Water

Fiedler, N., Mohr, S.N., Kelly-McNeil, K. & Kipen, H.M. (1994) Response of sensitive groups to MTBE. *Inhal. Toxicol.*, **6**, 539–552

Finnish Institute of Occupational Health (1998) *Finnish Occupational Exposure Limits 1998*, Helsinki, Ministry of Social Affairs and Health [http://www.occuphealth.fi/ttl/projekti/htp/english/oel_eng.htm]

Giacomello, P. (1996) MTBE exposures in service stations. In: *7th European Fuel Oxygenates Association Conference, Sodehotel, 24–25 October, 1996*, Brussels, European Fuel Oxygenates Association

Gordian, M.E. & Guay, G. (1995) Benzene in Alaska. *Alaska Med.*, **37**, 25–36

Government of Canada (1992) *Methyl* tertiary-*Butyl Ether* (Priority Substances List Assessment Report No. 5), Ottawa, Canada Communication Group

Grosjean, E., Grosjean, D., Gunawardena, R. & Rasmussen, R.A. (1998) Ambient concentrations of ethanol and methyl *tert*-butyl ether in Porto Alegre, Brazil, March 1996–April 1997. *Environ. Sci. Technol.*, **32**, 736–742

Hakkola, M. & Saarinen, L. (1996) Exposure of tanker drivers to gasoline and some of its components. *Ann. occup. Hyg.*, **40**, 1–10

Hakkola, M., Honkasalo, M.-L. & Pulkkinen, P. (1997) Changes in neuropsychological symptoms and moods among tanker drivers exposed to gasoline during a work week. *Occup. Med.*, **47**, 344–348

Hansch, C., Leo, A. & Hoekman, D. (1995) *Exploring QSAR: Hydrophobic, Electronic, and Steric Constants*, Washington DC, American Chemical Society, p. 15

Hartle, R. (1993) Exposure to methyl *tert*-butyl ether and benzene among service station attendants and operators. *Environ. Health Perspectives*, **101** (Suppl. 6), 23–26

Health Effects Institute (1996) *The Potential Health Effects of Oxygenates Added to Gasoline. A Review of the Current Literature. A Special Report of the Institute's Oxygenates Evaluation Committees*, Cambridge, MA

Hong, J.-Y., Yang, C.S., Lee, M., Wang, Y.-Y., Huang, W., Tan, Y., Pattern, C.J. & Bondoc, Y. (1997a) Role of cytochrome-P450 in the metabolism of methyl *tert*-butyl ether in human livers. *Arch. Toxicol.*, **71**, 266–269

Hong, J.-Y., Wang, Y.Y., Bondoc, F.Y., Yang, C.S., Lee, M. & Huang, W.Q. (1997b) Rat olfactory mucosa displays a high activity in metabolizing methyl *tert*-butyl ether and other gasoline ethers. *Fundam. appl. Toxicol.*, **40**, 205–210

IARC (1989) *IARC Monographs on the Evaluation of Carcinogenic Risks to Humans*, Vol. 45, *Occupational Exposures in Petroleum Refining; Crude Oil and Major Petroleum Fuels*, Lyon

Kado, N.Y., Kuzmicky, P.A., Loarca-Pina, G.L. & Mumtaz, M.M. (1998) Genotoxicity testing of methyl tertiary-butyl ether (MTBE) in the Salmonella microsuspension assay and mouse bone marrow micronucleus test. *Mutat. Res.*, **412**, 131–138

Kelly, T.J., Callahan, P.J., Piell, J. & Evans, G.F. (1993) Method development and field measurements for polar volatile organic compounds in ambient air. *Environ. Sci. Technol.*, **27**, 1146–1153

Kirschner, E.M. (1996) Growth of top 50 chemicals slowed in 1995 from very high 1994 rate. *Chem. Eng. News*, **74**, 16–20

LaGrone, F.S. (1991) Potential community exposure to toxic chemicals. *Environ. Sci. Technol.*, **25**, 366–368

Landmeyer, J.E., Chapelle, F.H., Bradley, P.M., Pankow, J.F., Church, C.D. & Tratnyek, P.G. (1998) Fate of MTBE relative to benzene in a gasoline-contaminated aquifer (1993–1998). *Ground Water Monit. Remed.*, **18**, 93–102

Lee, C.-W. & Weisel, C.P. (1998) Determination of methyl *tert*-butyl ether and *tert*-butyl alcohol in human urine by high-temperature purge-and-trap gas chromatography–mass spectrometry. *J. anal. Toxicol.*, **22**, 1–5

Leuschner, U., Hellstern, A., Schmidt, K., Fischer, H., Guldutuna, S., Hübner, K. & Leuschner, M. (1991) Gallstone dissolution with methyl *tert*-butyl ether in 120 patients—Efficacy and safety. *Dig. Dis. Sci.*, **36**, 193–199

Lewis, R.J., Jr (1993) *Hawley's Condensed Chemical Dictionary*, 12th Ed., New York, Van Nostrand Reinhold Co., p. 760

Lide, D.R., ed. (1997) *CRC Handbook of Chemistry and Physics*, 78th Ed., Boca Raton, FL, CRC Press, p. 3-275

Lillquist, D. R. & Zeigle, K.L. (1998) Assessment of occupational methyl tertiary butyl ether vapor exposures to petroleum refinery and transport loading rack facility employees. *Appl. occup. environ. Hyg.*, **13**, 53–57

Lindamood, C., III, Farnell, D.R., Giles, H.D., Prejean, J.D., Collins, J.J., Takahashi, K. & Maronpot, R.R. (1992) Subchronic toxicity studies of *t*-butyl alcohol in rats and mice. *Fundam. appl. Toxicol.*, **19**, 91–100

Lington, A.W., Dodd, D.E., Ridlon, S.A., Douglas, J.F., Kneiss, J.J. & Andrews, L.S. (1997) Evaluation of 13-week inhalation toxicity study on methyl *t*-butyl ether (MTBE) in Fischer 344 rats. *J. appl. Toxicol.*, **17** (Suppl. 1), S37–S44

Lioy, P.J., Weisel, C.P., Jo, W.-K., Pellizzari, E. & Raymer, J.H. (1994) Microenvironmental and personal measurements of methyl-tertiary butyl ether (MTBE) associated with automobile use activities. *J. Expos. Anal. environ. Epidemiol.*, **4**, 427–441

Long, G., Meek, M.E. & Savard, S. (1994) Methyl *tertiary*-butyl ether: Evaluation of risks to health from environmental exposure in Canada. *Environ. Carcinog. ecotoxicol. Rev.*, **C12**, 389–395

Mackerer, C.R., Angelosanto, F.A., Blackburn, G.R. & Schreiner, C.A. (1996) Identification of formaldehyde as the metabolite responsible for the mutagenicity of methyl tertiary-butyl ether in the activated mouse lymphoma assay. *Proc. soc. exp. biol. Med.*, **212**, 338–341

Mannino, D.M., Schreiber, J., Aldous, K., Ashley, D., Moolenar, R. & Almaguer, D. (1995) Human exposure to volatile organic compounds: A comparison of organic vapor monitoring badge levels with blood levels. *Int. Arch. occup. environ. Health*, **67**, 59–64

McCoy, M. & Johnson, T. (1995) *Petroleum Industry Data Characterizing Occupational Exposures to Methyl Tertiary Butyl Ether (MTBE) 1983–1993* (API Publication No. 4622), Washington DC, American Petroleum Institute

McKee, R. & Molyneux, M. (1997) *The Health Hazards and Exposures Associated with Gasoline Containing MTBE*, Brussels, CONCAWE

McKee, R.H., Vergnes, J.S., Galvin, J.B., Douglas, J.R., Kneiss, J.J. & Andrews, L.S. (1997) Assessment of the *in vivo* mutagenic potential of methyl tertiary-butyl ether. *J. appl. Toxicol.*, **17**, S31–S36

Mennear, J.H. (1997) Carcinogenicity studies on MTBE: Critical review and interpretation. *Risk Anal.*, **17**, 673–681

Miller, K.D. (1998) Gasoline demand growth in Asia—Opportunities for MTBE. *World Oxygen. Mthly*, **April/May**

Miller, M.J., Ferdinandi, E.S., Klan, M., Andrews, L.S., Douglas, J.F. & Kneiss, J.J. (1997) Pharmacokinetics and disposition of methyl *t*-butyl ether in Fischer-344 rats. *J. appl. Toxicol.*, **17** (Suppl. 1), S3–S12

Mohr, S.N., Fiedler, N., Weisel, C. & Kelly-McNeil, K. (1994) Health effects of MTBE among New Jersey garage workers. *Inhal. Toxicol.*, **6**, 553–562

Moolenaar, R.L, Hefflin, B.J., Ashely, D.L., Middaugh, J.P. & Etzel, R.A. (1994) Methyl tertiary butyl ether in human blood after exposure to oxygenated fuel in Fairbanks, Alaska. *Arch. environ. Health*, **49**, 402–409

Moser, G.J., Wong, B.A., Wolf, D.C., Fransson-Steen, R.L. & Goldsworthy, T.L. (1996a) Methyl tertiary butyl ether lacks tumor-promoting activity in *N*-nitrosodiethylamine-initiated B6C3F1 female mouse liver. *Carcinogenesis*, **17**, 2753–2761

Moser, G.J., Wong, B.A., Wolf, D.C., Moss, O.R. & Goldsworthy, T.L. (1996b) Comparative short-term effects of methyl tertiary butyl ether and unleaded gasoline vapor in female B6C3F1 mice. *Fundam. appl. Toxicol.*, **31**, 173–183

Moser, G.J., Wolf, D.C., Sar, M., Gaido, K.W., Janszen, D. & Goldsworthy, T.L. (1998) Methyl tertiary butyl ether-induced endocrine alterations in mice are not mediated through the estrogen receptor. *Toxicol. Sci.*, **41**, 77–87

National Library of Medicine (1998) *Toxic Chemical Release Inventory 1994* (TRI94), Bethesda, MD

National Research Council (1996) *Toxicological and Performance Aspects of Oxygenated Motor Vehicle Fuels*, Washington DC, National Academy Press

National Science and Technology Council (1996) *Interagency Assessment of Potential Health Risks Associated with Oxygenated Gasoline*, Washington DC, Executive Office of the President of the United States

National Science and Technology Council (1997) *Interagency Assessment of Oxygenated Fuels*, Washington DC, Executive Office of the President of the United States

National Toxicology Program (1995) *Toxicology and Carcinogenesis Studies of t-Butyl Alcohol in F344/N Rats and B6C3F1 Mice* (Tech. Rep. Ser. No. 436; NIH Publ. No. 95-3167), Research Triangle Park, NC

Nihlén, A., Löf, A. & Johanson, G. (1998a) Experimental exposure to methyl *tertiary*-butyl ether. I. Toxicokinetics in humans. *Toxicol. appl. Pharmacol.*, **148**, 274–280

Nihlén, A., Wålinder, R., Löf, A. & Johanson, G. (1998b) Experimental exposure to methyl tertiary-butyl ether: II. Acute effects in humans. *Toxicol. appl. Pharmacol.*, **148**, 281–287

O'Brien, A.K, Reiser, R.G. & Gylling, H. (1997) *Spatial Variability of Volatile Organic Compounds in Streams on Long Island, New York and in New Jersey* (Fact Sheet FS-194-97), West Trenton, NJ, United States Geological Survey

Palassis, J. (1994) Method 1615: Methyl *tert*-butyl ether. In: Eller, P.M., ed., *NIOSH Manual of Analytical Methods (NMAM)* (DHHS (NIOSH) Publication No. 94-113), 4th Ed., Cincinnati, OH, National Institute for Occupational Safety and Health

Piel, W.J. (1995) Historical perspective on the use of ethers in fuels. In: *EPA Proceedings of the Conference on MTBE and Other Oxygenates*, Washington DC, Environmental Protection Agency, pp. 16–20

Poore, M., Chang, B., Niyati, F. & Madden, S. (1997) Sampling and analysis of methyl *t*-butyl ether in ambient air at selected locations in California. In: *Abstracts of Papers (Part 1)—213rd ACS National Meeting, San Francisco, CA, April 13–17, 1997*, Washington DC, American Chemical Society, Paper ENVR 215

Prah, J.D., Goldstein, G.M., Devlin, R., Otto, D., Ashley, D., House, D., Cohen, K.L. & Gerrity, T. (1994) Sensory, symptomatic, inflammatory, and ocular responses to and the metabolism of methyl tertiary butyl ether in a controlled human exposure experiment. *Inhal. Toxicol.*, **6**, 521–538

Prescott-Mathews, J.S., Wolf, D.C., Wong, B.A. & Borghoff, S.J. (1997) Methyl *tert*-butyl ether causes α2u-globulin nephropathy and enhanced renal cell proliferation in male Fischer-344 rats. *Toxicol. appl. Pharmacol.*, **143**, 301–314

Robinson, M., Bruner, R.H. & Olson, G.R. (1990) Fourteen- and ninety-day oral toxicity studies of methyl tertiary-butyl ether in Sprague-Dawley rats. *J. Am. Coll. Toxicol.*, **9**, 525–540

Saarinen, L., Hakkola, M., Pekari, K., Lappalainen, K. & Aitio, A. (1998) Exposure of gasoline road-tanker drivers to methyl *tert*-butyl ether and methyl *tert*-amyl ether. *Int. Arch. occup. environ. Health*, **71**, 143–147

Sadtler Research Laboratories (1980) *Standard Spectra Collection, 1980 Cumulative Index*, Philadelphia, PA

Savolainen, H., Pfäffli, P. & Elovaara, E. (1985) Biochemical effects of methyl *tertiary*-butyl ether in extended vapour exposure of rats. *Arch. Toxicol.*, **57**, 285–288

Scholz, B., Butzert, H., Neumeister, J. & Nierlich, F. (1990) Methyl *tert*-butyl ether. In: Elvers, B., Hawkins, S. & Schulz, G., eds, *Ullmann's Encyclopedia of Industrial Chemistry*, 5th rev. Ed., Vol. A16, New York, VCH Publishers, pp. 543–550

Squillace, P.J., Zogorski, J.S., Wilber, W.G. & Price, C.V. (1996) Preliminary assessment of the occurrence and possible sources of MTBE in ground water in the United States, 1993–1994. *Environ. Sci. Technol.*, **30**, 1721–1730

Squillace, P.J., Pankow, J.F., Korte, N.C. & Zogorski, J.S. (1997) Review of the environmental behavior and fate of methyl *tert*-butyl ether. *Environ. Toxicol. Chem.*, **16**, 1836–1844

Squillace, P.J., Pankow, J.F., Korte, N.E. & Zogorski, J.S. (1998) *Environmental Behavior and Fate of Methyl* tert-*Butyl Ether (MTBE)* (United States Geological Fact Sheet FS-203-96 (Revised 2/98)), Rapid City, SD, United States Geological Survey

Stackelberg, P.E., O'Brien, A.K. & Terracciano, S.A. (1997) Occurrence of MTBE in surface and ground water, Long Island, New York and New Jersey. In: *Proceedings of the 213rd ACS National Meeting, San Francisco, CA, April 13–17, 1997*, Washington DC, American Chemical Society, pp. 394–397

Stern, B.R. & Kneiss, J.J. (1997) Methyl tertiary-butyl ether (MTBE): Use as an oxygenate in fuels. *J. appl. Toxicol.*, **17**, S1–S2

Stern, B.R. & Tardiff, R.G. (1997) Risk characterization of methyl *tertiary* butyl ether (MTBE) in tap water. *Risk Anal.*, **17**, 727–743

Turini, A., Amato, G., Longo, V. & Gervasi, P.G. (1998) Oxidation of methyl- and ethyl-tertiary-butyl ethers in rat liver microsomes: Role of the cytochrome P450 isoforms. *Arch. Toxicol.*, **72**, 207–214

United Nations Environment Programme (1998) *UNEP Chemicals (IRPTC) Data Bank Legal File, Recommendations and Legal Mechanisms*, Geneva, World Health Organization

United States Geological Survey (1995) *Method for Methyl* tert-*Butyl Ether and Other Fuel Oxygenates* (Fact Sheet FS-219-95), Denver, CO, National Water Quality Laboratory

Vainiotalo, S., Peltonen, Y. & Pfäffli, P. (1996a) MTBE exposure in service stations. In: *7th European Fuel Oxygenates Association Conference, Sodehotel, 24–25 October, 1996*, Brussels, European Fuel Oxygenates Association

Vainiotalo, S., Peltonen, Y. & Pfäffli, P. (1996b) *Driver Exposure to MTBE During Gasoline Refueling, and Levels of MTBE in Ambient Air in the Vicinity of Service Stations* (Final Report to BIT/EFOA), Helsinki, Finnish Institute of Occupational Health

Vainiotalo, S., Peltonen, Y., Ruonakangas, A. & Pfäffli, P. (1997) *Customer Exposure to MTBE, TAME and C_6 Alkyl Methyl Ethers During Gasoline Refueling* (Final report to Neste Oy), Helsinki, Finnish Institute of Occupational Health

Vojdani, A., Mordechai, E. & Brautbar, N. (1997a) Abnormal apoptosis and cell cycle progression in humans exposed to methyl tertiary-butyl ether and benzene contaminating water. *Hum. exp. Toxicol.*, **16**, 485–494

Vojdani, A., Namatalla, G. & Brautbar, N. (1997b) Methyl tertiary-butyl ether antibodies among gasoline service station attendants. *Ann. N.Y. Acad. Sci.*, **837**, 96–104

White, M.C., Johnson, C.A., Ashley, D.L., Buchta, T.M. & Pelletier, D.J. (1995) Exposure to methyl *tertiary*-butyl ether from oxygenated gasoline in Stamford, Connecticut. *Arch. environ. Health*, **50**, 183–189

WHO (1993) *Guidelines for Drinking Water Quality*, 2nd Ed., Vol. 1, *Recommendations*, Geneva

WHO (1998) *Methyl* tertiary-*Butyl Ether* (Environmental Health Criteria 206), Geneva, International Programme on Chemical Safety

Yoshikawa, M., Arashidani, K., Katoh, T., Kawamoto, T. & Kodama, Y. (1994) Pulmonary elimination of methyl *tertiary*-butyl ether after intraperitoneal administration in mice. *Arch. Toxicol.*, **68**, 517–519

Zogorski, J.S., Morduchowitz, A., Baehr, A.L., Bauman, B.J., Dwayne, L., Drew, R.T., Korte, N.E., Lapham, W.W., Pankow, J.F. & Washington, E.R. (1996) *Fuel Oxygenates and Water Quality: Current Understanding of Sources, Occurrence in Natural Waters, Environmental Behavior, Fate and Significance* (Final Report), Washington DC, Office of Science and Technology Policy, Executive Office of the President

Zogorski, J.S., Delzer, G.C., Bender, D.A., Squillace, P.J., Lopes, T.J., Baehr, A.L., Stackelberg, P.E., Landmeyer, J.E., Boughton, C.J., Lico, M.S., Pankow, J.F., Johnson, R.L. & Thomson, N.R. (1998) MTBE: Summary findings and research by the US Geological Survey. In: *Proceedings of the Annual Conference of the American Water Works Association, Dallas, 1998*, Denver, American Water Works Association, pp. 287–309

NITRILOTRIACETIC ACID AND ITS SALTS

This substance was considered by a previous working group, in 1989 (IARC, 1990). Since that time, new data have become available, and these have been incorporated into the monograph and taken into consideration in the present evaluation.

1. Exposure Data

1.1 Chemical and physical data

1.1.1 *Nomenclature*

Nitrilotriacetic acid

Chem. Abstr. Serv. Reg. No.: 139-13-9
Deleted CAS Reg. No.: 26627-44-1; 26627-45-2; 80751-51-5
Chem. Abstr. Name: *N,N*-Bis(carboxymethyl)glycine
IUPAC Systematic Name: Nitrilotriacetic acid
Synonyms: Nitrilo-2,2′,2″-triacetic acid; nitrilotris(methylenecarboxylic acid); NTA; triglycine; triglycollamic acid; α,α′,α″-trimethylaminetricarboxylic acid

Nitrilotriacetic acid, sodium salt

Chem. Abstr. Serv. Reg. No.: 10042-84-9
Chem. Abstr. Name: *N,N*-Bis(carboxymethyl)glycine, sodium salt
IUPAC Systematic Name: Nitrilotriacetic acid, sodium salt
Synonyms: Nitrilotriacetic acid sodium salt; NTA sodium salt; NTA, sodium salt; sodium aminotriacetate; sodium nitriloacetate; sodium nitrilotriacetate; sodium NTA

Nitrilotriacetic acid, monosodium salt

Chem. Abstr. Serv. Reg. No.: 18994-66-6
Chem. Abstr. Name: *N,N*-Bis(carboxymethyl)glycine, monosodium salt
IUPAC Systematic Name: Nitrilotriacetic acid, monosodium salt
Synonyms: Monosodium nitrilotriacetate; NTA, monosodium salt

Nitrilotriacetic acid, disodium salt

Chem. Abstr. Serv. Reg. No.: 15467-20-6
Chem. Abstr. Name: *N,N*-Bis(carboxymethyl)glycine, disodium salt
IUPAC Systematic Name: Nitrilotriacetic acid, disodium salt
Synonyms: Disodium hydrogen nitrilotriacetate; disodium nitrilotriacetate; nitrilotriacetic acid disodium salt; NTA, disodium salt

Nitrilotriacetic acid, disodium salt, monohydrate

Chem. Abstr. Serv. Reg. No.: 23255-03-0
Chem. Abstr. Name: *N,N*-Bis(carboxymethyl)glycine, disodium salt, monohydrate
IUPAC Systematic Name: Nitrilotriacetic acid, disodium salt, monohydrate
Synonyms: Disodium nitrilotriacetic acid monohydrate; NTA, disodium salt, monohydrate

Nitrilotriacetic acid, trisodium salt

Chem. Abstr. Serv. Reg. No.: 5064-31-3
Deleted CAS Reg. No.: 37291-81-9
Chem. Abstr. Name: *N,N*-Bis(carboxymethyl)glycine, trisodium salt
IUPAC Systematic Name: Nitrilotriacetic acid, trisodium salt
Synonyms: Nitrilotriacetic acid trisodium salt; NTA trisodium salt; NTA, trisodium salt; trisodium nitrilotriacetate; trisodium 2,2′,2″-nitrilotriacetate; trisodium NTA

Nitrilotriacetic acid, trisodium salt, monohydrate

Chem. Abstr. Serv. Reg. No.: 18662-53-8
Chem. Abstr. Name: *N,N*-Bis(carboxymethyl)glycine, trisodium salt, monohydrate
IUPAC Systematic Name: Nitrilotriacetic acid, trisodium salt, monohydrate
Synonyms: NTA, trisodium salt, monohydrate; trisodium nitrilotriacetate monohydrate

1.1.2 *Structural and molecular formulae and relative molecular mass*

$$HO-C(=O)-CH_2-N(CH_2-C(=O)-OH)(CH_2-C(=O)-OH)$$

$C_6H_9NO_6$ Relative molecular mass: 191.14

Monosodium salt

$C_6H_8NO_6.Na$ Relative molecular mass: 213.14

Disodium salt

$C_6H_7NO_6.2Na$ Relative molecular mass: 235.13

Disodium salt, monohydrate

$C_6H_7NO_6.2Na.H_2O$ Relative molecular mass: 253.11

Trisodium salt

$C_6H_6NO_6.3Na$ Relative molecular mass: 257.13

Trisodium salt, monohydrate

$C_6H_6NO_6.3Na.H_2O$ Relative molecular mass: 275.11

1.1.3 *Chemical and physical properties of the pure substance*

(*a*) *Description*: White crystalline powder (Lewis, 1993)

(*b*) *Melting-point*: 242°C (decomposes) (Lide, 1997)

(*c*) *Solubility*: Slightly soluble in water; soluble in ethanol (Lide, 1997)

(*d*) *Conversion factor*: mg/m³ = 7.82 × ppm

1.2 Production and use

Information available in 1995 indicated that nitrilotriacetic acid was produced in 10 countries (Chemical Information Services, 1995).

Nitrilotriacetic acid is used as a chelating and sequestering agent, and as a builder in synthetic detergents (Budavari, 1996). It is also used as an eluting agent in the purification of rare earth elements (Lewis, 1993), as a boiler feedwater additive, in water and textile treatment, in metal plating and cleaning and in pulp and paper processing (National Toxicology Program, 1991).

1.3 Occurrence

1.3.1 *Natural occurrence*

Nitrilotriacetic acid and its salts and complexes are not known to occur naturally.

1.3.2 *Occupational exposure*

According to the 1981–83 National Occupational Exposure Survey (National Institute for Occupational Safety and Health, 1998), approximately 270 000 workers in the United States were potentially exposed to nitrilotriacetic acid and its trisodium salts. Occupational exposure to these compounds may occur in their production and use. Workers involved in detergent formulation were estimated to be exposed to concentrations up to 4.6 μg/kg bw per day (Universities Associated for Research and Education in Pathology, 1985), and lifetime average daily doses were estimated to be less than 1 μg/kg bw for all workers formulating or using nitrilotriacetic acid-containing products (CanTox, 1996).

1.3.3 *Environmental occurrence*

Four major assessments have been conducted of exposure to nitrilotriacetic acid: by the Midwest Research Institute (1979), the Environmental Protection Agency (1980), the Universities Associated for Research and Education in Pathology (1985) and CanTox (1996). Although different methods were used and slightly different results were obtained, all four studies indicate that daily exposure of consumers to all possible sources of nitrilotriacetic acid is generally < 1 µg/kg bw. Among the sources specifically considered were drinking-water, showering and bathing, wearing clothes washed with nitrilotriacetic acid-containing detergents, inhalation of detergents, skin contact with washwater from laundry or dishes and ingestion of residues on hand-washed dishes.

According to the Environmental Protection Agency Toxic Chemical Release Inventory for 1987, 800 kg of nitrilotriacetic acid were released into the air, 2300 kg were discharged into water, 860 000 kg were disposed of by underground injection and 2300 kg were released onto the land from manufacturing and processing facilities in the United States. By 1996, the levels were 5 kg released into the air, 35 kg released into water and 680 kg disposed of by underground injection (National Library of Medicine, 1998).

1.4 Regulations and guidelines

WHO (1993) has established an international drinking-water guideline for nitrilotriacetic acid of 200 µg/L.

2. Studies of Cancer in Humans

No data were available to the Working Group.

3. Studies of Cancer in Experimental Animals

Previous evaluation

Nitrilotriacetic acid was tested for carcinogenicity by oral administration in the diet in mice and rats. It induced renal-cell adenocarcinomas in mice of each sex, renal-cell tumours in male rats and transitional-cell and squamous-cell carcinomas of the urinary bladder, hepatocellular adenomas and adrenal phaeochromocytomas in female rats.

Nitrilotriacetic acid, trisodium salt was tested for carcinogenicity in mice and rats by oral administration. When administered in the diet as the monohydrate, it induced haematopoietic tumours in male mice and benign and malignant tumours of the urinary system (kidney, ureter and bladder) in rats of each sex. When administered in drinking-water to male rats, it induced renal adenomas and adenocarcinomas.

In two-stage carcinogenicity studies in male rats by oral administration, nitrilotriacetic acid and its trisodium salt increased the incidence of urinary-tract tumours after pretreatment with various *N*-nitrosamines (IARC, 1990).

New studies

No new data on nitriloacetic acid and its salts were available to the Working Group.

4. Other Data Relevant to an Evaluation of Carcinogenicity and its Mechanisms

4.1 Absorption, distribution, metabolism and excretion

4.1.1 *Humans*

No new data were available to the Working Group.

4.1.2 *Experimental systems*

Nitrilotriacetic acid and its sodium salt are absorbed in mammals; the parent compound is not metabolized and is excreted rapidly by filtration in the kidney. The information on the absorption, distribution and excretion of nitrilotriacetic acid and its salts has been reviewed previously (IARC, 1990).

4.2 Toxic effects

The toxic effects of nitrilotriacetic acid and its salts have been reviewed previously (IARC, 1990).

4.2.1 *Humans*

No data were available to the Working Group.

4.2.2 *Experimental systems*

Renal tubular cells show evidence of toxicity in rats and mice given high doses of nitrilotriacetic acid or its sodium salt corresponding to the doses that produce renal-cell tumours in these species. Regenerative proliferation ensues. The toxicity correlates with plasma and urinary accumulation of Zn^{++}, considered to occur secondary to the chelating properties of nitrilotriacetic acid. Administration of zinc nitrilotriacetic acid or co-administration of zinc salts with nitrilotriacetic acid accentuates this effect (Anderson *et al.*, 1985).

The urothelial effects of nitrilotriacetic acid and its sodium salt occur in rats but not in mice, and sex differences are seen, depending on the experimental treatment. Urothelial tumours (renal pelvis, ureters, bladder) occur in animals of each sex. In contrast to the effect in renal tubules, the urothelial effects are not due to accumulation of zinc but rather appear to be related to depletion of calcium. This occurs at doses higher than those required for the nephrotoxicity produced by nitrilotriacetic acid, and the doses correspond to those that produce urothelial toxicity and regenerative hyperplasia. Although nitrilotriacetic acid-containing microcrystalluria occurs, this was not considered to be a sufficient explanation for the urothelial toxic and regenerative effects (Anderson *et al.*, 1985).

Nitrilotriacetic acid did not mediate efficient oxidative production of single- and double-strand breaks in DNA *in vitro* in supercoiled plasmid pZ189 (Toyokuni & Sagripanti, 1993).

It increased the incidence of liver-cell nodules but not carcinomas in female rats (IARC, 1990).

4.3 Reproductive and developmental effects

4.3.1 *Humans*

No data were available to the Working Group.

4.3.2 *Experimental systems*

The developmental and reproductive effects of nitrilotriacetic acid have been reviewed (Anderson *et al.*, 1985). No significant maternal, embryonic or fetal effects were reported in rats exposed to up to 0.5% in the diet, rabbits exposed by oral gavage to up to 250 mg/kg bw per day or in mice exposed via the drinking-water at 0.2%. Addition of heavy metals such as mercury and cadmium did not change the response. Similarly, studies of reproductive toxicity did not indicate an effect on neonatal development.

Nitrilotriacetic acid was used to assess the predictive value of two assays for mammalian teratogenesis *in vitro*: an assay for inhibition of the growth of embryonic palatal mesenchymal cells, which evaluates effects on proliferative potential, and an assay for inhibition of the attachment of mouse ascites tumour cells to concanavalin A-coated surfaces. The concentrations of nitrilotriacetic acid that inhibited growth or attachment by 50% were > 1 mmol/L in both assays, and the authors considered the results to be negative (Steele *et al.*, 1988).

Exposure of developing *Drosophila* larvae to nitrilotriacetic acid caused a dose-related increase in gross wing defects and extra bristles in adults, but the authors did not consider these effects predictive of developmental toxicity in mammals (Lynch *et al.*, 1991).

Nitrilotriacetic acid was evaluated for effects on amphibian embryogenesis in the frog embryo teratogenesis assay *Xenopus laevis* (FETAX) assay. The concentration that caused the deaths of 50% of the embryos was reported to be 540 mg/L, the concentration that induced terata in 50% of the surviving embryos was 530 mg/mL, and the teratogenic index was 1.0 mg/mL. The authors considered the effects to be due to disruption and osmoregulation and not to teratogenic potential (Dawson *et al.*, 1989).

4.4 Genetic and related effects

4.4.1 *Humans*

No data were available to the Working Group.

4.4.2 *Experimental systems* (see Table 1 for references)

Nitrilotriacetic acid did not induce reverse mutation in *Escherichia coli* and did not induce gene mutation in either *Saccharomyces cerevisiae* or *Schizosaccharomyces pombe*. It did not induce sex-linked recessive lethal mutation or dominant lethal mutation but induced aneuploidy in *Drosophila melanogaster*. It did not induce sister chromatid exchange or chromosomal aberrations in Chinese hamster cells *in vitro*. It did not induce dominant lethal mutation but induced aneuploidy in mice *in vivo*.

Table 1. Genetic and related effects of nitrilotriacetic acid and its salts

Test system	Results[a]		Dose[b] (LED or HID)	Reference
	Without exogenous metabolic system	With exogenous metabolic system		
Nitrilotriacetic acid				
Escherichia coli WP2, reverse mutation	–	NT	4000	Zetterberg (1970)
Saccharomyces cerevisiae, forward mutation	–	NT	4000	Zetterberg (1970)
Saccharomyces cerevisiae, reverse mutation	–	NT	4000	Zetterberg (1970)
Schizosaccharomyces pombe, reverse mutation	–	NT	4000	Zetterberg (1970)
Drosophila melanogaster, sex-linked recessive lethal mutations	–		1900 inj	Kramers (1976)
Drosophila melanogaster, sex-linked recessive lethal mutations	–		4000	Woodruff *et al.* (1985)
Drosophila melanogaster, dominant lethal mutations	–		1900 inj	Kramers (1976)
Drosophila melanogaster, aneuploidy, germ cells	+		9600	Costa *et al.* (1988)
Drosophila melanogaster, aneuploidy, germ cells	+		4000	Ramel & Magnusson (1979)
Sister chromatid exchange, Chinese hamster ovary cells *in vitro*	–	–	5	Loveday *et al.* (1989)
Chromosomal aberrations, Chinese hamster ovary cells *in vitro*	–	–	5	Loveday *et al.* (1989)
Dominant lethal mutation, mice *in vivo*	–		125	Epstein *et al.* (1972)
Aneuploidy, mouse germ cells *in vivo*	+		275	Costa *et al.* (1988)
Nitrilotriacetic acid, disodium salt				
Gene mutation, mouse lymphoma L5178Y cells, *tk* locus *in vitro*	–	NT	941	Toyokuni *et al.* (1995)
Sister chromatid exchange, Chinese hamster lung V79 cells *in vitro*	–	NT	358	Hartwig *et al.* (1993)
DNA damage (8-hydroxydeoxyguanosine formation), rat kidney *in vivo*	–		100 ip × 1	Umemura *et al.* (1990)
Nitrilotriacetic acid, trisodium salt				
Echerichia coli PQ37, SOS chromotest	–	–	NR	Venier *et al.* (1987)
Escherichia coli WP2, differential toxicity	+	+	250	Venier *et al.* (1987)
Salmonella typhimurium TA100, TA98, TA1535, TA1537, TA1538, reverse mutation	–	–	10 000 μg/plate	Dunkel *et al.* (1985)

Table 1 (contd)

Test system	Results[a]		Dose[b] (LED or HID)	Reference
	Without exogenous metabolic system	With exogenous metabolic system		
Nitrilotriacetic acid, trisodium salt (contd)				
Salmonella typhimurium TA100, TA98, TA1535, TA1537, TA1538, reverse mutation	–	–	870 μg/plate	Loprieno *et al.* (1985)
Salmonella typhimurium TA100, reverse mutation	–	–	870 μg/plate	Venier *et al.* (1987)
Escherichia coli WP2 *uvr*A, reverse mutation	–	–	10 000 μg/plate	Dunkel *et al* (1985)
Escherichia coli WP2 *uvr*A, reverse mutation (fluctuation test)	–	–	100 000	Venier *et al.* (1987)
Saccharomyces cerevisiae, gene conversion	–	–	40	Loprieno *et al.* (1985)
Aspergillus nidulans, genetic crossing-over	–	NT	10 930	Crebelli *et al.* (1986)
Schizosaccharomyces pombe, forward mutation	–	–	40	Loprieno *et al.* (1985)
Aspergillus nidulans, forward mutation	–	NT	18 510	Crebelli *et al.* (1986)
Aspergillus nidulans, aneuploidy	–	NT	10 930	Crebelli *et al.* (1986)
Allium cepa, micronuclei	+	NT	550	De Marco *et al.* (1986)
Vicia faba, chromosomal aberrations	+	NT	1375	Kihlman & Sturelid (1970)
Drosophila melanogaster, somatic mutation (and recombination)	(+)		1336	Zordan *et al.* (1991)
Micronucleus formation, Chinese hamster lung Cl-1 cells *in vitro*	+	NT	514	Modesti *et al.* (1995)
Unscheduled DNA synthesis, rat primary hepatocytes *in vitro*	–	NT	1000	Williams *et al.* (1982)
Gene mutation, Chinese hamster lung V79 cells, *hprt* locus *in vitro*	–	NT	1.5	Celotti *et al.* (1987)
Gene mutation, mouse lymphoma L5178Y cells, *tk* locus *in vitro*	–	–	2350	Mitchell *et al.* (1988)
Sister chromatid exchange, Chinese hamster ovary cells *in vitro*	–	NT	1.9	Loprieno *et al.* (1985)
Sister chromatid exchange, Chinese hamster ovary cells *in vitro*	–	NT	1.0	Venier *et al.* (1985)
Sister chromatid exchange, Chinese hamster ovary cells *in vitro*	–	NT	275	Ved Brat & Williams (1984)
Sister chromatid exchange, Chinese hamster ovary cells *in vitro*	–	NT	514	Montaldi *et al.* (1985)
Sister chromatid exchange, mouse lymphocytes *in vitro*	–	NT	257	Montaldi *et al.* (1985)
Chromosomal aberrations, rat kangaroo kidney PT K1 cells *in vitro*	+	NT	688	Kihlman & Sturelid (1970)
Gene mutation, human EUE cells DT^R, *in vitro*	+	NT	3	Grilli & Capucci (1985)

Table 1 (contd)

Test system	Results[a]		Dose[b] (LED or HID)	Reference
	Without exogenous metabolic system	With exogenous metabolic system		
Nitrilotriacetic acid, trisodium salt (contd)				
Sister chromatid exchange, human lymphocytes *in vitro*	–	NT	275	Ved Brat & Williams (1984)
Chromosomal aberrations, human lymphocytes *in vitro*	–	NT	2063	Montaldi *et al.* (1988)
Sister chromatid exchange, mouse bone-marrow cells *in vivo*	–		275 ip × 1	Russo *et al.* (1989)
Aneuploidy, mouse bone-marrow cells *in vivo*	–		275 ip × 1	Russo *et al.* (1989)
Micronucleus formation, mouse bone-marrow cells *in vivo*	–		400 ip × 1	Montaldi *et al.* (1988)

[a] +, positive; (+), weakly positive; –, negative; NT, not tested

[b] LED, lowest effective dose; HID, highest ineffective dose; unless otherwise stated, in-vitro test, μg/mL; in-vivo test, mg/kg bw per day; inj, injection; ip, intraperitoneal; NR, not reported

Nitrilotriacetic acid, disodium salt did not induce gene mutation in mouse lymphoma L5178Y *tk*$^{+/-}$ cells or sister chromatid exchange in Chinese hamster lung V79 cells *in vitro*. It did not induce oxidative DNA damage in rat kidney cells *in vivo*.

Nitrilotriacetic acid, trisodium salt gave negative results in the bacterial SOS DNA repair assay but induced differential toxicity in various repair-deficient *Escherichia coli* WP2 strains. It did not induce gene mutation in *Salmonella typhimurium* TA100, TA1535, TA1537, TA1538 or TA98 or in *E. coli* WP2 *uvrA* with or without exogenous metabolic activation. It did not induce gene conversion, crossing-over, forward mutation or aneuploidy in yeast and fungi without exogenous metabolic activation or gene conversion or forward mutation with exogenous metabolic activation. Nitrilotriacetic acid, trisodium salt induced micronuclei and chromosomal aberrations in plant cells, but it did not give rise to micronuclei in Chinese hamster lung cells *in vitro*. It weakly induced somatic mutation in *D. melanogaster*. It did not induce unscheduled DNA synthesis in rat primary hepatocytes in the absence of metabolic activation. Nitrilotriacetic acid, trisodium salt did not induce gene mutation at the *hprt* locus of Chinese hamster lung V79 cells without exogenous metabolic activation or at the *tk* locus of mouse lymphoma L5178Y cells with or without exogenous metabolic activation. It did not induce sister chromatid exchange in Chinese hamster ovary cells or mouse lymphocytes *in vitro*. Nitrilotriacetic acid, trisodium salt induced chromosomal aberrations in rat-kangaroo kidney cells *in vitro* without exogenous metabolic activation and gene mutation in human cells *in vitro*. It did not induce sister chromatid exchange or chromosomal aberration in human lymphocytes *in vitro*. It did not induce micronuclei or aneuploidy *in vivo* in mice treated with a single intraperitoneal injection.

4.5 Mechanistic considerations

The nephrocarcinogenic effects of nitrilotriacetic acid in rats and mice appear to be related to dose-dependent changes in Zn^{++} homeostasis. Orally administered nitrilotriacetic acid and its trisodium salt were nephrotoxic to rats and mice of each sex. The toxicity occurs at high doses and appears to be due to Zn^{++} accumulation secondary to the chelating properties of nitrilotriacetic acid. Administration of zinc nitrilotriacetic acid or Zn^{++} accentuated the nephrotoxicity of nitrilotriacetic acid.

Nitrilotriacetic acid has urothelial effects only in rats and at doses higher than those required for nephrotoxicity and proliferative effects. Although the mechanism of induction of the urothelial effects is not known, they are not related to Zn^{++} homeostasis but rather correlate with depletion of cellular calcium and possibly the formation of nitrilotriacetic acid-containing microcrystals.

The renal and urothelial effects of nitrilotriacetic acid are associated with cellular toxicity and regenerative hyperplasia. Its toxic, regenerative proliferative and tumorigenic effects occur only at high doses. No direct genotoxic effect appears to be involved.

None of 12 renal-cell carcinomas in rats treated with ferric nitrilotriacetate acid had mutations in codons 12, 13 or 61 of the H-, K- and N-*ras* genes. Only one high-grade tumour contained a CGC→CTC transversion in codon 246 of the *p53* gene (Nishiyama *et al.*, 1995).

5. Summary of Data Reported and Evaluation

5.1 Exposure data

Exposure to nitrilotriacetic acid and its salts occurs during their production, formulation and use in synthetic laundry and dishwashing detergents and related products as metal chelating and sequestering agents.

5.2 Human carcinogenicity data

No data were available to the Working Group.

5.3 Animal carcinogenicity data

Nitrilotriacetic acid was tested for carcinogenicity by oral administration in the diet to mice and rats. It induced renal tubular tumours (adenomas and adenocarcinomas) in mice of each sex and in male rats and transitional-cell and squamous-cell carcinomas of the urinary bladder, hepatocellular adenomas and adrenal phaeochromocytomas in female rats.

The trisodium salt was tested for carcinogenicity in mice and rats by oral administration. When administered in the diet as the monohydrate, it induced haematopoietic tumours in male mice and benign and malignant tumours of the urinary system (kidney, ureter and bladder) in rats of each sex. When administered in drinking-water to male rats, it induced renal tubular adenomas and adenocarcinomas.

In two-stage studies of carcinogenicity in male rats treated by oral administration, nitrilotriacetic acid and its trisodium salt increased the incidence of urinary-tract tumours after pretreatment with various *N*-nitrosamines.

5.4 Other relevant data

Nitrilotriacetic acid is absorbed in mammals, but it is not metabolized and is excreted rapidly by filtration in the kidney.

Orally administered nitrilotriacetic acid and its trisodium salt were nephrotoxic to rats and mice of each sex. Toxicity occurs at high doses and appears to be due to Zn^{++} accumulation secondary to the chelating properties of nitrilotriacetic acid; administration of Zn^{++} accentuated the nephrotoxicity of the acid. Urothelial cytotoxicity and regenerative hyperplasia were seen in male and female rats but not in mice, and only at doses higher than those that produced nephrotoxicity. The mechanism is unclear but appears to involve cellular Ca^{++} depletion secondary to the chelating effect of nitrilotriacetic acid. Urinary microcrystals were also produced.

Nitrilotriacetic acid does not induce developmental toxicity in rats, rabbits or mice exposed during gestation and gave negative results in short-term assays to screen for teratogenesis in two cellular assays in *Drosophila* larvae and frog embryos.

No data were available on the genetic and related effects of nitrilotriacetic acid or its salts in humans. Nitrilotriacetic acid and its disodium and trisodium salts were not genotoxic in experimental systems *in vivo*, except that the acid induced aneuploidy in mouse germ cells. Neither the acid nor its salts were genotoxic in mammalian cells *in vitro* and they were not mutagenic to bacteria.

5.5 Evaluation

There is *inadequate evidence* in humans for the carcinogenicity of nitrilotriacetic acid and its salts.

There is *sufficient evidence* in experimental animals for the carcinogenicity of nitrilotriacetic acid and its salts.

Overall evaluation

Nitrilotriacetic acid and its salts *are possibly carcinogenic to humans (Group 2B)*.

6. References

Anderson, R.L., Bishop, W.E. & Campbell, R.L. (1985) A review of the environmental and mammalian toxicology of nitrilotriacetic acid. *CRC crit. Rev. Toxicol.*, **15**, 1–102

Budavari, S., ed. (1996) *The Merck Index*, 12th Ed., Whitehouse Station, NJ, Merck & Co., p. 1131

CanTox (1996) *Assessment of Human Exposure to Sodium Nitrilotriacetate Monohydrate from the Use of Various Industrial/Institutional and Consumer Products*, Mississauga, Ontario

Celotti, L., Furlan, D., Seccati, L. & Levis, A.G. (1987) Interactions of nitrilotriacetic acid (NTA) with Cr(IV) Compounds in the induction of gene mutations in cultured mammalian cells. *Mutat. Res.*, **190**, 35–39

Chemical Information Services (1995) *Directory of World Chemical Producers 1995/96 Edition*, Dallas, TX, p. 524

Costa, R., Russo, A., Zordan, M., Pacchierotti, A., Tavella, A. & Levis, A.G. (1988) Nitrilotriacetic acid (NTA) induces aneuploidy in *Drosophila* and mouse germ-line cells. *Environ. mol. Mutag.*, **12**, 397–407

Crebelli, R., Bellincampi, D., Conti, G., Conti, L., Morpurgo, G. & Carere, A. (1986) A comparative study on selected chemical carcinogens for chromosome malsegregation, mitotic crossing-over and forward mutation induction in *Aspergillus nidulans*. *Mutat. Res.*, **172**, 139–149

Dawson, D.A., Fort, D.J., Newell, D.L. & Bantle, J.A. (1989) Developmental toxicity testing with FETAX: Evaluation of five compounds. *Drug chem. Toxicol.*, **12**, 67–75

De Marco, A., Romanelli, M., Stzi, M.A. & Vitagliano, E. (1986) Induction of micronucleated cells in *Vicia faba* and *Allium cepa* root tips treated with nitrilotriacetic acid (NTA). *Mutat. Res.*, **171**, 145–148

Dunkel, V.C., Zeiger, E., Brusick, D., McCoy, E., McGregor, D., Mortelmans, K., Rosenkranz, H.S. & Simmon, F.G. (1985) Reproducibility of microbial mutagenicity assays: II. Testing of carcinogens and noncarcinogens in *Salmonella typhimurium* and *Escherichia coli*. *Environ. Mutag.*, **7** (Suppl. 5), 1–248

Environmental Protection Agency (1980) *Final Report: NTA*, Washington DC

Epstein, S.S., Arnold, E., Andrea, S., Bass, W. & Bishop, Y. (1972) Detection of chemical mutagens by the dominant lethal assay in the mouse. *Toxicol. appl. Pharmacol.*, **23**, 288–325

Grilli, M.P. & Capucci, A. (1985) Mutagenic effect of nitrilotriacetic acid on cultured human cells. *Toxicol. Lett.*, **25**, 137–141

Hartwig, A., Klyszcz-Nasko, H., Schlepegrell, R. & Beyersmann, D. (1993) Cellular damage by ferric nitrilotriacetate and ferric citrate in V79 cells: Interrelationship between lipid peroxidation, DNA strand breaks and sister chromatid exchanges. *Carcinogenesis*, **14**, 107–112

IARC (1990) *IARC Monographs on the Evaluation of Carcinogenic Risks to Humans*, Vol. 48, *Some Flame Retardants and Textile Chemicals, and Exposure in the Textile Manufacturing Industry*, Lyon, pp. 181–212

Kihlman, B.A. & Sturelid, S. (1970) Nitrilotriacetic acid (NTA) and chromosome breakage. *Environ. Mutag. Soc. Newsl.*, **3**, 32–33

Kramers, P.G.N. (1976) Mutagenicity studies with nitrilotriacetic acid and Citrex S-5 in *Drosophila*. *Mutat. Res.*, **40**, 277–280

Lewis, R.J., Sr (1993) *Hawley's Condensed Chemical Dictionary*, 12th Ed., New York, Van Nostrand Reinhold Co., p. 824

Lide, D.R., ed. (1997) *CRC Handbook of Chemistry and Physics*, 78th Ed., Boca Raton, FL, CRC Press, p. 3-173

Loprieno, N., Bonacristiani, G., Venier, P., Montaldi, A., Majone, F., Bianchi, V., Paglialunga, S. & Levis, A.G. (1985) Increased mutagenicity of chromium compounds by nitrilotriacetic acid. *Environ. Mutag.*, **7**, 185–200

Loveday, K.S., Lugo, M.H., Resnick, M.A., Anderson, B.E. & Zeige, E. (1989) Chromosome aberration and sister chromatid exchange tests in Chinese hamster ovary cells *in vitro*. II. Results with 20 chemicals. *Environ. mol. Mutag.*, **13**, 60–94

Lynch, D.W., Schuler, R.L., Hood, R.D. & Davis, D.G. (1991) Evaluation of *Drosophila* for screening developmental toxicants: Test results with eighteen chemicals and presentation of a new *Drosophila* bioassay. *Teratog. Carcinog. Mutag.*, **11**, 147–173

Midwest Research Institute (1979) *Chemical Technology and Economics in Environmental Perspective. Task IV. Potential Worker and Consumer Exposure to Nitrilotriacetic Acid (NTA) in Detergents* (US EPA Report No. EPA-560/11-79-008/US NTIS PB297753), Kansas City, MO

Mitchell, A.D., Rudd, C.J. & Caspary, W.J. (1988) Evaluation of the L5178Y mouse lymphoma cell mutagenesis assay: Intralaboratory results for sixty-three coded chemicals tested at SRI International. *Environ. mol. Mutag.*, **12** (Suppl. 13), 37–101

Modesti, D., Tanzarella, C. & Degrassi, F. (1995) Genotoxic activity of nitrilotriacetic acid in Chinese hamster cells. *Mutat. Res.*, **343**, 1–6

Montaldi, A., Zentilin, L., Venier, P., Gola, I., Bianchi, V., Paglialunga, S. & Levis, A.G. (1985) Interaction of nitrilotriacetic acid with heavy metals in the induction of sister chromatid exchanges in cultured mammalian cells. *Environ. Mutag.*, **7**, 381–390

Montaldi, A., Mariot, T., Zordan, M., Paleologo, M. & Levis, A.G. (1988) Nitrilotriacetic acid (NTA) does not induce chromosomal damage in mammalian cells either *in vitro* or *in vivo. Mutat. Res.*, **208**, 95–100

National Institute for Occupational Safety and Health (1998) *National Occupational Exposure Survey (1981–1983)*, Cincinnati, OH

National Library of Medicine (1998) *Toxic Chemical Release Inventory 1987 & 1996* (TRI87 & TRI96), Bethesda, MD

National Toxicology Program (1991) *NTP Chemical Repository Data Sheet: Nitrilotriacetic Acid (NTA)*, Research Triangle Park, NC

Nishiyama, Y., Suwa, H., Okamoto, K., Fukumoto, M., Hiai, H. & Toyokuni, S. (1995) Low incidence of point mutation in H-, K- and N-ras oncogenes and p53 tumor suppressor gene in renal cell carcinoma and peritoneal mesothelioma of Wistar rats induced by ferric nitrilotriacetate. *Jpn. J. Cancer Res.*, **86**, 1150–1158

Ramel, C. & Magnusson, J. (1979) Chemical induction of non-disjunction in Drosophila. *Environ. Health Perspectives*, **31**, 59–66

Russo, A., Pacchierotti, F., Bassani, B. & Levis, A.G. (1989) Lack of induction of somatic aneuploidy in the mouse by nitrilotriacetic acid (NTA). *Mutat. Res.*, **226**, 111–114

Steele, V.E., Morrissey, R.E., Elmore, E.L., Gurganus-Rocha, D., Wilkinson, B.P., Curren, R.D., Schmetter, B.S., Louie, A.T., Lamb, J.C., IV & Yang, L.L. (1988) Evaluation of two *in vitro* assays to screen for potential developmental toxicants. *Fundam. appl. Toxicol.*, **11**, 673–684

Toyokuni, S. & Sagripanti, J.-L. (1993) DNA single- and double-strand breaks produced by ferric nitrilotriacetate in relation to renal tubular carcinogenesis. *Carcinogenesis*, **14**, 223–227

Toyokuni, S., Sagripanti, J.-L. & Hitchins, V.M. (1995) Cytotoxic and mutagenic effects of ferric nitrilotriacetate on L5178Y mouse lymphoma cells. *Cancer Lett.*, **88**, 157–162

Umemura, T., Sai, K., Takagi, A., Hasegawa, R. & Kurokawa, Y. (1990) Formation of 8-hydroxydeoxyguanosine (8-OH-dG) in rat kidney DNA after intraperitoneal administration of ferric nitrilotriacetate (Fe-NTA). *Carcinogenesis*, **11**, 345–347

Universities Associated for Research and Education in Pathology (1985) *Assessment of the Practical Risk to Human Health from the Use of Nitrilotriacetic Acid (NTA) in Household Laundry Products*, Rockville, MD

Ved Brat, S. & Williams, G.M. (1984) Nitrilotriacetic acid does not induce sister-chromatid exchanges in hamster or human cells. *Food chem. Toxicol.*, **22**, 211–215

Venier, P., Montaldi, A., Gava, C., Zentilin, L., Tecchio, G., Bianchi, V., Paglialunga, S. & Levis, A.G. (1985) Effects of nitrilotriacetic acid on the induction of gene mutations and sister-chromatid exchanges by insoluble chromium compounds. *Mutat. Res.*, **156**, 219–228

Venier, P., Gava, C., Zordan, M., Bianchi, V., Levis, A.G., De Flora, S., Benicelli, C. & Camoirano, A. (1987) Interactions of chromium with nitrilotriacetic acid (NTA) in the induction of genetic effects in bacteria. *Toxicol. environ. Chem.*, **14**, 201–218

WHO (1993) *Guidelines for Drinking Water Quality*, 2nd Ed., Vol. 1, *Recommendations*, Geneva, pp. 74–75

Williams, G.M., Laspia, M.F. & Dunkel, B.C. (1982) Reliability of the hepatocyte primary culture/DNA repair test in testing of coded carcinogens and noncarcinogens. *Mutat. Res.*, **97**, 359–370

Woodruff, R.C., Mason, J.M., Valencia, R. & Zimmering, S. (1985) Chemical mutagenesis testing in *Drosophila*. V. Results of 53 coded compounds tested for the National Toxicology Program. *Environ. Mutag.*, **7**, 677–702

Zetterberg, G. (1970) Negative results with nitrilotriacetic acid (NTA) as an inducer of gene mutation in some microorganisms. *Environ. Mutat. Soc. Newsl.*, **3**, 31–32

Zordan, M., Graf, U., Singer, D., Bfeltrame, C., Valle, L.D., Osti, M., Costa, R. & Levis, A.G. (1991) The genotoxicity of nitrilotriacetic acid (NTA) in a somatic mutation and recombination test in Drosophila melanogaster. *Mutat. Res.*, **262**, 253–261

PARACETAMOL

This substance was considered by a previous working group, in 1989 (IARC, 1990). Since that time, new data have become available, and these have been incorporated into the monograph and taken into consideration in the present evaluation.

1. Exposure Data

1.1 Chemical and physical data

1.1.1 *Nomenclature*

Chem. Abstr. Serv. Reg. No.: 103-90-2
Deleted CAS Reg. No.: 8055-08-1
Chem. Abstr. Name: *N*-(4-Hydroxyphenyl)acetamide
IUPAC Systematic Name: 4′-Hydroxyacetanilide
Synonyms: 4-Acetamidophenol; acetaminophen; 4-acetaminophenol; 4-(acetylamino)-phenol; 4-(*N*-acetylamino)phenol; 4-hydroxyacetanilide; 4′-hydroxyacetanilide; *N*-(4-hydroxyphenyl)acetamide

1.1.2 *Structural and molecular formulae and relative molecular mass*

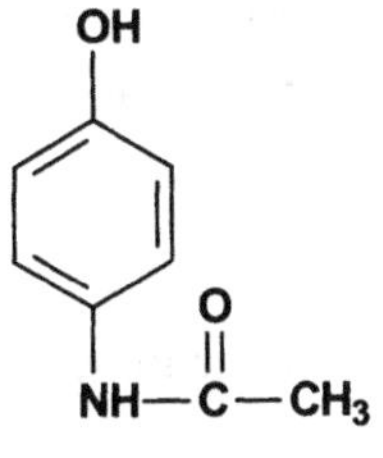

$C_8H_9NO_2$ Relative molecular mass: 151.17

1.1.3 *Chemical and physical properties of the pure substance*

(*a*) *Description*: White crystalline powder (Verschueren, 1996)
(*b*) *Melting-point*: 170°C (Lide, 1997)
(*c*) *Density*: 1.293 g/cm^3 at 21°C (Lide, 1997)
(*d*) *Solubility*: Insoluble in water; very soluble in ethanol (Lide, 1997)
(*e*) *Octanol/water partition coefficient (P)*: log P, 0.31 (Hansch *et al.*, 1995)
(*f*) *Conversion factor*: mg/m^3 = 6.18 × ppm

1.2 Production and use

Information available in 1995 indicated that paracetamol was produced in 19 countries (Chemical Information Services, 1995).

Paracetamol is used as an analgesic and antipyretic, in the treatment of a wide variety of arthritic and rheumatic conditions involving musculoskeletal pain and in other painful disorders such as headache, dysmenorrhoea, myalgia and neuralgia. It is also indicated as an analgesic and antipyretic in diseases accompanied by generalized discomfort or fever, such as the common cold and other viral infections. Other uses include the manufacture of azo dyes and photographic chemicals, as an intermediate for pharmaceuticals and as a stabilizer for hydrogen peroxide (National Toxicology Program, 1991).

Demand for bulk paracetamol in the United States in 1997 was estimated to be 30 000–35 000 tonnes, more than half of worldwide consumption (Mirasol, 1998).

The conventional oral dose of paracetamol for adults is 325–1000 mg (650 mg rectally); the total daily dose should not exceed 4000 mg. For children, the single dose is 40–480 mg, depending on age and weight; no more than five doses should be administered within 24 h. For infants under three months of age, a dose of 10 mg/kg bw is recommended (Insel, 1996; Reynolds, 1996).

1.3 Occurrence

1.3.1 *Natural occurrence*

Paracetamol is not known to occur naturally.

1.3.2 *Occupational exposure*

According to the 1981–83 National Occupational Exposure Survey (National Institute for Occupational Safety and Health, 1998), approximately 65 000 workers in the United States were potentially exposed to paracetamol. Occupational exposure may occur during its production and during its use as an analgesic and antipyretic, chemical intermediate or stabilizer.

1.3.3 *Environmental occurrence*

No information on the environmental occurence of paracetamol was available to the Working Group.

1.4 Regulations and guidelines

No international guidelines for paracetamol in drinking-water have been established (WHO, 1993).

2. Studies of Cancer in Humans

Previous evaluation

An association between use of paracetamol and cancer of the ureter (but not of other sites in the urinary tract) was observed in one Australian case–control study. None of three other case–control studies evaluated previously (IARC, 1990) showed an association between use of paracetamol and cancer in the urinary tract. Table 1 summarizes the results of these studies and those of case–control studies that have been published subsequently.

New studies

2.1 Cohort studies

A number of studies have been reported of patients with rheumatoid arthritis, osteoarthrosis, back pain or rheumatic disease, who were assumed to have greater than average use of analgesic and anti-rheumatoid drugs. As use specifically of paracetamol could not be separated from use of other drugs in these studies, they were considered not to be useful in evaluating the carcinogenicity of paracetamol.

2.2 Case–control studies

2.2.1 *Cancers of the urinary tract*

A population-based case–control study was conducted in Ontario, Canada, involving all histologically confirmed cases of renal-cell carcinoma newly diagnosed in 1986 or 1987 among residents aged 25–69 years (Kreiger *et al.*, 1992). Cases were ascertained through the files of the Ontario Cancer Registry, and control subjects were randomly selected from the same geographic area and frequency-matched to cases by age and sex. A self-administered questionnaire was completed for 513 of the patients with renal-cell carcinoma (81%) and 1369 of the controls (72%) either directly by the subjects themselves or by their next-of-kin (10% of cases and 0.4% of controls). Only 21 cases (4.1%) and 75 controls (5.4%) reported use of paracetamol, defined as use of any type of a paracetamol-containing analgesic at least every other day for one month or more prior to 1980, yielding odds ratios (adjusted for age, smoking habits and body mass index) of 0.9 (95% confidence interval [CI], 0.4–1.8) for men and 0.6 (95% CI, 0.4–1.6) for women. [The Working Group noted that no estimates of cumulative lifetime use among exposed subjects were available.]

In a population-based case–control study in New South Wales, Australia (McCredie *et al.*, 1993), all residents aged 20–79 years in whom cancer of the renal parenchyma or renal pelvis had been diagnosed during 1989–90 were identified from records of the New South Wales Central Cancer Registry, supplemented by surveillance of records from urological units of the State. Control subjects were selected from the electoral rolls and frequency matched on age. A personal or telephone interview was completed for 489 patients (310 men and 179 women) with renal-cell cancer (66% of all eligible patients), 147 (58 men and 89 women) with renal pelvis cancer (74% of eligible cases) and 523 (231 men and 292 women) of the control subjects (72% of eligible controls). The questionnaire sought information about lifetime consumption of prescription and non-prescription analgesics before 1987 in addition to other known or suspected risk factors for urinary tract cancer. Consumers of analgesics were defined as those who had taken this type of drug at least 20 times in their lifetime. Study subjects had often taken more

Table 1. Case–control studies of paracetamol by cancer site

Reference and location	Subjects	Estimated exposure (lifetime intake, kg)	Odds ratio (95% CI)	Comments
Renal-cell cancer				
McLaughlin *et al.* (1985)[a]	313 male patients	Ever		Adjusted for age and cigarette smoking
Minnesota, United States	182 female patients	Men	0.7 (0.5–1.0)	
	697 controls	Women	1.2 (0.8–1.9)	
		Regular, > 36 months		
		Men	0.7 (0.1–3.4)	
		Women	1.2 (0.3–4.6)	
McCredie *et al.* (1988)[a]	229 male patients	Regular use (≥ 0.1 kg)	1.2 (0.8–1.8)	Adjusted for age, sex, smoking and intake of other analgesics
New South Wales, Australia	131 female patients			
	985 controls			
Kreiger *et al.* (1992)	312 male patients	Any[b]		Adjusted for age, cigarette smoking and body mass index
Ontario, Canada	201 female patients	Men	0.9 (0.4–1.8)	
	1369 controls	Women	0.6 (0.4–1.6)	
McCredie *et al.* (1993)	310 male patients	Any[c], men and women	1.5 (1.0–2.3)	Adjusted for age, sex, cigarette smoking, obesity and intake of phenacetin
New South Wales, Australia	179 female patients	≤ 0.48 kg	1.9 (1.0–3.6)	
	523 controls	0.49–1.36 kg	0.9 (0.4–1.9)	
		≥ 1.37 kg	1.7 (0.9–3.3)	
Mellemgaard *et al.* (1994)	226 male patients	Any[d]		Adjusted for age, smoking, history of hypertension and socioeconomic status
Denmark	142 female patients	Men	1.1 (0.5–3.0)	
	396 controls	Women	1.0 (0.4–2.5)	
		> 1 kg		
		Men	0.9 (0.2–4.0)	
		Women	0.5 (0.1–1.8)	

Table 1 (contd)

Reference and location	Subjects	Estimated exposure (lifetime intake, kg)	Odds ratio (95% CI)	Comments
***Renal-cell cancer* (contd)**				
Chow *et al.* (1994)	277 male patients	Regular use[d], men	[0.8] [0.5–1.4]	Unadjusted
Minnesota, United States	163 female patients	0.1–1 kg	0.7 (0.3–1.9)	Adjusted for age, smoking and body
	691 controls	1.1–5 kg	0.7 (0.2–1.8)	mass index
		> 5 kg	0.4 (0.0–4.2)	
		Regular use[d], women	[1.0] [0.6–1.9]	Unadjusted
		0.1–1 kg	1.0 (0.3–2.8)	Adjusted for age, smoking and body
		1.1–5 kg	0.9 (0.4–2.1)	mass index
		> 5 kg	0.9 (0.2–4.6)	
McCredie *et al.* (1995)[e]	1732 patients	Regular use[f]	1.1 (0.9–1.5)	Adjusted for centre, age, sex, cigarette
New South Wales (Australia),	[distribution by sex not	0.1–1 kg	1.1 (0.8–1.6)	smoking and body mass index
Sweden, Germany, Minnesota	given]	1.1–5 kg	0.9 (0.6–1.5)	
(USA), Denmark	2309 controls	> 5 kg	1.9 (0.9–3.9)	
		Men	1.0 (0.7–1.4)	
		Women	1.3 (0.9–2.0)	
Rosenberg *et al.* (1998)	258 male patients	Non-cancer controls		Adjusted for age, sex, interview year
United States	125 female patients	Regular use[d]	1.2 (0.7–2.1)	and geographic area
	8149 non-cancer	< 5 years	1.3 (0.6–2.7)	
	controls	≥ 5 years	1.1 (0.5–2.6)	
	6499 cancer controls	Cancer controls		
		Regular use[d]	1.1 (0.6–2.0)	
		< 5 years	1.2 (0.6–2.6)	
		≥ 5 years	1.1 (0.4–2.5)	

Table 1 (contd)

Reference and location	Subjects	Estimated exposure (lifetime intake, kg)	Odds ratio (95% CI)	Comments
Renal cancer, not otherwise specified				
Derby & Jick (1996)	222 patients	No. of prescriptions		Crude odds ratio
United States	[distribution by sex not	< 10 (< 0.2 kg)	[1.2] [0.8–1.6]	
	given]	10–19 (0.2–0.4 kg)	1.3 (0.6–2.8)	
	885 controls	20–39 (0.5–0.9 kg)	1.9 (0.7–5.6)	
		≥ 40 (≥ 1 kg)	2.6 (1.1–6.0)	
Renal pelvis				
McLaughlin *et al.* (1985)[a]	50 male patients	Ever		Adjusted for age and cigarette smoking
United States	24 female patients	Men	1.2 (0.6–2.5)	
	697 controls	Women	2.2 (0.8–5.8)	
		Regular use, > 36		
		months	2.5 (0.3–18)	
		Men	5.8 (0.8–40)	
		Women		
McCredie & Stewart (1988)[a]	31 male patients	Regular use		Adjusted for sex, tobacco smoking and
New South Wales, Australia	42 female patients	≥ 0.1 kg	1.2 (0.6–2.3)	phenacetin use
	689 controls	≥ 1 kg	0.8 (0.4–1.7)	
McCredie *et al.* (1993)	58 male patients	Any[c], men and women	1.3 (0.7–2.4)	Adjusted for age, sex, cigarette
New South Wales, Australia	89 female patients	≤ 0.48 kg	0.9 (0.2–3.0)	smoking, educational level and intake
	523 controls	0.49–1.36 kg	0.9 (0.3–2.5)	of phenacetin
		≥ 1.37 kg	2.0 (0.9–4.4)	

Table 1 (contd)

Reference and location	Subjects	Estimated exposure (lifetime intake, kg)	Odds ratio (95% CI)	Comments
Renal pelvis and ureter				
Ross *et al.* (1989)[a] Los Angeles, United States	127 male patients 60 female patients 187 controls	Regular use (> 30 days/year)	1.3 [0.76–2.2]	Variables used in adjustment not indicated
Linet *et al.* (1995) United States	331 male patients 171 female patients 496 controls	Regular use ≤ 1 kg > 1 kg	1.0 (0.6–1.8) 1.1 (0.5–2.1) 1.0 (0.4–2.3)	Adjusted for age, sex, cigarette smoking and geographic area
Ureter				
McCredie *et al.* (1988)[a] New South Wales, Australia	39 male patients 16 female patients 689 controls	Regular use ≥ 0.1 kg ≥ 1 kg	 2.5 (1.1–5.9) 2.0 (0.8–4.5)	Adjusted for sex, tobacco smoking and phenacetin use
Urinary bladder				
Piper *et al.* (1985)[a] New York, United States	173 female patients 173 controls	Regular use, only (> 30 days/year)	1.5 (0.4–7.2)	Matched-pair analysis
McCredie & Stewart (1988)[a] New South Wales, Australia	307 male patients 381 female patients	Regular use ≥ 0.1 kg ≥ 1 kg	 0.7 (0.4–1.3) 0.7 (0.4–1.3)	Adjusted for sex, tobacco smoking and phenacetin use
Derby & Jick (1996) United States	504 patients [distribution by sex not given] 2009 controls	No. of prescriptions < 10 (< 0.2 kg) 10–19 (0.2–0.4 kg) 20–39 (0.5–0.9 kg) ≥ 40 (≥ 1 kg)	 [1.0] [0.8–1.2] 1.1 (0.6–2.0) 1.1 (0.6–2.3) 1.3 (0.6–2.8)	Crude odds ratio

Table 1 (contd)

Reference and location	Subjects	Estimated exposure (lifetime intake, kg)	Odds ratio (95% CI)	Comments
Lower urinary tract (mainly bladder)				
Steineck *et al.* (1995) Stockholm, Sweden	325 patients [distribution by sex not given] 393 controls	Any use	1.6 (1.1–2.3)	Summary estimate, adjusted for sex, year of birth, smoking and use of other types of analgesics. According to the authors, 'no details in the exposure substantiated the finding'
Rosenberg *et al.* (1998) United States	384 male patients 114 female patients 8149 non-cancer controls 6499 cancer controls	Non-cancer controls		Adjusted for age, sex, interview year, and geographic area
		Regular use[d]	1.1 (0.6–1.9)	
		< 5 years	1.1 (0.5–2.3)	
		≥ 5 years	1.1 (0.5–2.6)	
		Cancer controls		
		Regular use[d]	0.9 (0.5–1.6)	
		< 5 years	0.8 (0.4–1.8)	
		≥ 5 years	1.0 (0.4–2.4)	
Ovary				
Cramer *et al.* (1998) United States	563 patients 523 controls	Continuous use[g]	0.5 (0.3–0.9)	Adjusted for age, study centre, education, religion, parity, use of oral contraceptives and certain types of pain

[a] Evaluated previously (IARC, 1990)
[b] At least every other day for one month or more
[c] At least 20 times during lifetime
[d] At least twice weekly for a month
[e] Includes patient material from the studies of McCredie *et al.* (1993), Mellemgaard *et al.* (1994) and Chow *et al.* (1994)
[f] Lifetime intake of at least 0.1 kg
[g] At least once a week for at least six months

than one type of analgesic, a substantial proportion having used phenacetin-containing compounds (21% of patients and 9% of controls). Use of paracetamol in any form was reported by 73 patients with renal-cell carcinoma (15%), 40 patients with cancer of the renal pelvis (27%) and by 55 controls (11%). When adjusted for age, sex, cigarette smoking, obesity, educational level and use of other types of analgesics, use of paracetamol as a single drug was associated with a nonsignificant odds ratio for renal-cell carcinoma of 1.5 (95% CI, 0.9–2.4), and use of paracetamol in any form gave a nonsignificant odds ratio of 1.5 (95% CI, 1.0–2.3); the odds ratios for cancer of the renal pelvis were 1.3 (95% CI, 0.6–2.7) for paracetamol as a single drug and 1.3 (95% CI, 0.7–2.4) in any form. No dose–response relationship was found between lifetime consumption of paracetamol (highest category, ≥ 1.37 kg) taken in any form and the occurrence of either cancer. When the analysis was confined to the subset of subjects who had never taken phenacetin or aspirin analgesics, regular consumption of paracetamol as a single drug was associated with a relative risk for renal-cell cancer of 1.6 (95% CI, 1.0–2.8) based on 38 exposed cases and 30 exposed controls. The authors noted that before 1968 in Australia most users of analgesics took phenacetin-containing preparations, indicating that residual confounding from this drug may have influenced the results of this study.

In a population-based study, Mellemgaard *et al.* (1994) included all histologically confirmed cases of renal-cell carcinoma diagnosed between 1989 and 1991 in Danish inhabitants aged 20–79 years at the time of diagnosis. Control subjects were randomly selected from computerized files of the national Central Population Register with frequency matching by sex, age and place of residence at 1 April 1968. Personal interviews including detailed information on lifetime use of analgesics prior to diagnosis were completed with 368 of the eligible patients (76%) and 396 of the eligible controls (79%). A drug–exposure matrix for prescribed and non-prescribed analgesics was applied in which information on past and current brand names obtained from study subjects was converted to information on active ingredients. Minimal consumption was defined as use twice weekly for a month. Any such consumption of paracetamol was reported for 22 cases (6%) and 24 controls (6%). The odds ratios for renal-cell carcinoma, adjusted for age, smoking, history of hypertension and socioeconomic status, were 1.1 (95% CI, 0.5–3.0) in men and 1.0 (95% CI, 0.4–2.5) in women. Among the study subjects with the highest life-long intake of paracetamol (> 1 kg), the odds ratios were 0.9 (95% CI, 0.2–4.0) for men and 0.5 (95% CI, 0.1–1.8) for women, based on a total of 10 exposed cases and 22 exposed controls.

Chow *et al.* (1994) studied 591 patients in the population of Minnesota, United States, aged 20–79 years, in whom renal-cell carcinoma had been newly diagnosed during 1988–90 and were identified through an existing State cancer surveillance system, and 691 control subjects, who were identified by random-digit dialling (aged 64 years or younger) or from the files of the Health Care Financing Administration of the State (aged 65 years or older) and matched to the cases by age and sex. Information on use of prescription and non-prescription analgesics, height, weight, medical conditions, smoking habits, alcohol use and occupational histories was collected at personal interviews with the study subjects or their next-of-kin. The response rates were 87% for cases and approximately 85% for controls. Interviews were conducted with next-of-kin for 151 (26%) of the cases and none of the controls; however, the risk estimates were based only on information from the 440 (74%) directly interviewed cases and the 691 (100%) directly interviewed controls. Exposure to paracetamol, phenacetin and other analgesic ingredients was assessed by means of a drug-exposure linkage system, in which information on brand names obtained from study subjects was converted on an annual basis into information on the type and amount of active ingredients. Total life-long use was estimated by summing annual exposure of subjects before 1987. Any regular use of paracetamol, defined as two or more times per week for one month or longer, was reported by 43 patients (10%) and 70 controls (10%). When users were compared with study participants who reported no or irregular use of any analgesics, use of paracetamol was associated with crude odds ratios of [0.8] [95% CI, 0.5–1.4] for men and [1.0] [95% CI, 0.6–1.9] for women. After adjustment for age, smoking status and body mass index, there was no trend to increasing risk with increasing lifetime consumption of paracetamol, salicylates or phenacetin for either men or women. Lifetime intake of paracetamol amounting to 0.1–1, 1.1–5 or > 5 kg was associated with odds ratios of 0.7 (95% CI, 0.3–1.9), 0.7 (95% CI, 0.2–1.8) and 0.4 (95% CI, 0.0–4.2), respectively, among men and 1.0 (95% CI, 0.3–2.8), 0.9 (95% CI, 0.4–2.1) and 0.9 (95% CI, 0.2–4.6), respectively, among women. A statistically nonsignificant excess risk was found for women (odds ratio, 2.1; 95% CI, 0.6–6.9) who had used only paracetamol-containing analgesics, on the basis of seven exposed cases, but there was no corresponding increase among men (odds ratio, 1.2; 95% CI, 0.5–3.2; eight exposed cases). [The Working Group noted that different proportions of patients and controls were interviewed directly and thus included in the analysis, which might have resulted in biased selection of cases.]

McCredie *et al.* (1995) reported on the results of a large international case–control study of renal-cell carcinoma which, in addition to the previously described study materials from New South Wales, Australia (McCredie *et al.*, 1993), Denmark (Mellemgaard *et al.*, 1994) and Minnesota, United States (Chow *et al.*, 1994), also included study materials from Uppsala, Sweden, and from Berlin and Heidelberg, Germany. In the Swedish study, patients aged 20–79 years with histologically confirmed renal-cell carcinoma diagnosed in the Uppsala Health Care Region during 1989–91 were identified in a population-based cancer registry, preceded by a rapid ascertainment system; patients in the German study were identified by monitoring all hospitals and pathology departments of the Berlin and Heidelberg study areas but keeping an upper age limit of 75 years. Controls, frequency-matched to cases by age and sex, were taken from registries covering the entire background population. The three sets of previously unpublished material from Sweden and Germany comprised approximately 30% of the material in this pooled, international analysis, which covered a total of 1732 patients with renal-cell carcinoma and 2309 controls. These figures resulted from overall response rates of 72% and 75%

among cases and controls, respectively. Personal interviews were conducted with essentially the same questionnaire in all of the study centres, and estimates of lifetime intake of prescription and non-prescription paracetamol, phenacetin and other analgesics were derived from a jointly developed drug-exposure matrix specifying the amount and composition of active ingredients in each analgesic on sale in the five countries during the study period. Significant exposure to analgesics was defined as life-long intake of at least 0.1 kg which is equivalent to two 500-mg paracetamol tablets twice a week for one year. When compared with study participants who reported cumulative intake of less than 0.1 kg of any analgesic and with adjustment for centre, age, sex, cigarette smoking and body mass index, intake of 0.1 kg or more of paracetamol was associated with odds ratios of 1.0 (95% CI, 0.7–1.4; 55 exposed cases) for men and 1.3 (95% CI, 0.9–2.0; 64 exposed cases) for women and 1.1 (95% CI, 0.9–1.5) for the two sexes combined, on the basis of a total of 119 exposed patients and 142 exposed controls. Life-time intake of paracetamol of 0.1–1, 1.1–5 and > 5 kg (the two sexes combined) was associated with odds ratios of 1.1 (95% CI, 0.8–1.6), 0.9 (95% CI, 0.6-1.5) and 1.9 (95% CI, 0.9–3.9). The risk of the subset of women with a total consumption of > 5 kg paracetamol was statistically significantly increased, at 2.5 (95% CI, 1.0–6.2), based on 14 exposed cases and eight exposed controls, but there was no corresponding increase among men (odds ratio, 1.1; 95% CI, 0.3–4.0; six exposed cases). Adjustment for consumption of phenacetin did not alter the risk. The odds ratios for regular use exclusively of paracetamol were 0.6 (95% CI, 0.3–1.3) for men and 1.3 (95% CI, 0.6–2.6) for women; the risk did not increase with dose. [The Working Group noted that inclusion in the reference exposure category of cumulative doses up to 0.1 kg might have reduced the risk estimates.]

In a population-based study, Steineck *et al.* (1995) included incident cases of squamous- or transitional-cell carcinoma of the urinary tract diagnosed in the Stockholm area, Sweden, during the period 1985–87. Cases were identified from the files of the city hospitals, and controls, frequency-matched by sex and year of birth, were chosen at random from a computerized register covering the population of Stockholm. A postal questionnaire supplemented by a telephone interview was completed for 325 patients (78%), comprising 305 with cancer of the urinary bladder, six with cancer of the ureter, 11 with cancer of the renal pelvis and three with cancer at multiple sites in the lower urinary tract, and with 393 controls (77%). The questionnaire contained questions about use of paracetamol, aspirin and phenacetin, each categorized according to total intake (1–99 or ≥ 100 tablets) in each of three specified decades (1950–79), and about the subjects' medical history and smoking habits. Any use of paracetamol was reported by 119 cases (37%) and 119 controls (30%), yielding an odds ratio adjusted for sex, year of birth, tobacco smoking and other use of analgesics of 1.6 (1.1–2.3). The authors reported that analyses by duration and amount did not substantiate the finding [data were not given].

In a hospital-based study, Rosenberg *et al.* (1998) studied 498 patients with a histologically confirmed transitional-cell cancer of the urinary tract (440 patients with bladder cancer, 41 with renal pelvis cancer and 17 with cancer of the ureter or urethra) and 383 patients with a histologically confirmed renal-cell cancer from among the population of adult patients under the age of 70 years who had been admitted to hospitals located in various cities of the United States over the years 1977–96 for any of a variety of malignant and non-malignant conditions. Two control groups were selected from the same population of adult patients under surveillance, i.e. one admitted for a non-malignant condition judged to be unrelated to use of paracetamol (8149 control patients) and the other for a cancer at one of a number of selected sites (6499 control patients). Information on use of prescription and non-prescription medications was obtained from patients and controls at personal interviews conducted by nurses during hospitalization on the basis of answers to questions about a number of indications for use of paracetamol and other analgesics, which included pain and muscle ache. Information on personal characteristics, medical and reproductive history and smoking habits was also collected. The overall response rate in the surveillance study was 95%. Any regular use of paracetamol, defined as use on two or more days a week for at least a month, that had begun at least one year before admission for the index disease was reported by 15 patients with transitional-cell cancer (3.0%), 14 patients with renal-cell carcinoma (3.7%), 294 non-cancer controls (3.6%) and 191 cancer controls (2.9%). The odds ratios for transitional-cell cancer, adjusted for age, sex, interview year and geographic area, were 1.1 (95% CI, 0.6–1.9) in the study with non-cancer controls and 0.9 (95% CI, 0.5–1.6) in the study with cancer controls when compared with study participants who reported no use of paracetamol. The corresponding relative risk estimates were 1.1 (95% CI, 0.5–2.6) and 1.0 (95% CI, 0.4–2.4) for five or more years of regular use and 1.1 (95% CI, 0.9–1.4) and 1.2 (95% CI, 0.9–1.5) for irregular use of paracetamol. The odds ratios for renal-cell cancer were 1.2 (95% CI, 0.7–2.1) in the study with non-cancer controls and 1.1 (95% CI, 0.6–2.0) in the study with cancer controls for regular use of paracetamol when compared with no use and 1.1 (95% CI, 0.5–2.6) and 1.1 (95% CI, 0.4–2.5) for long-term use (five years or more). Essentially identical relative risk estimates were seen for the group of irregular users of paracetamol. [The Working Group noted that hospital controls are more likely than population controls to have a condition that leads to use of paracetamol.]

In a population of about 380 000 members of a cooperative health insurance organization in Washington, United States, Derby and Jick (1996) studied 222 patients, aged 20 years or older, with cancer of the kidney and 504 with cancer of the urinary bladder, which had been diagnosed during the period 1980–91 at hospitals maintained by the insurance organization. Groups of 885 and 2009 control subjects were selected from among all members of the organization and matched to the cases of kidney and bladder cancer, respectively, on sex, age and duration of membership of the organization; they had to be free of cancer at the date of diagnosis of the corresponding case. Information on over-the-counter drugs and prescribed medications obtained by study subjects at one of the pharmacies maintained by the insurance organization was available from 1974 onwards. Information on smoking habits, coffee drinking, height, weight, occupation and history of urinary tract infections was taken from outpatient medical records, if available. Study subjects were categorized according to number of prescriptions for paracetamol ever filled at the pharmacy, and the cumulative amount taken by the subject was estimated as follows: 1 prescription, 2–9 (< 0.2 kg), 10–19 (0.2–0.4 kg), 20–39 (0.5–0.9 kg) and > 40 (≥ 1 kg). The crude odds ratios were 0.9 (0.6–1.5), 1.3 (0.9–1.9), 1.3 (0.6–2.8), 1.9 (0.7–5.6) and 2.6 (1.1–6.0; nine exposed patients), respectively, compared with those with no prescription filled (*p* for trend, 0.01). Multivariate analysis with adjustment, whenever possible, for smoking, body mass index and history of urinary tract infection further increased the odds ratio for kidney cancer associated with 40 or more paracetamol prescriptions to 4.5 (95% CI, 0.7–30). The crude odds ratios for bladder cancer were 1.0 (0.8–1.4), 1.0 (0.8–1.3), 1.1 (0.6–2.0), 1.1 (0.6–2.3) and 1.3 (0.6–2.8) for subjects who filled 1, 2–9, 10–19, 20–39 and 40 or more paracetamol prescriptions, respectively, compared with those with no prescription filled. Analysis after adjustment for smoking, coffee drinking and occupation, whenever the information was available, gave essentially the same results. [The Working Group noted that potential confounders were not adjusted for in estimating several of the odds ratios reported above, including those for which the 95% confidence intervals excluded unity.]

In a multi-centre case–control study in New Jersey, Iowa and California, United States, Linet *et al.* (1995) included all histologically confirmed cases of cancer of the renal pelvis or ureter diagnosed between 1983 and 1986 among white residents aged 20–79 years. Controls for cases under the age of 65 at the time of diagnosis were chosen by random-digit dialling, while controls for cases aged 65 and older were selected from Medicare files maintained by the Health Care Financing Administration. Controls were frequency-matched to cases by age, sex and study centre. Personal interviews, conducted in the homes of subjects, were completed for 502 cases (62% of all eligible patients) and 496 controls (approximately 60% of eligible individuals), in which detailed information was sought on regular use of a large number of over-the-counter and prescription analgesics, excluding the five-year period before the interview. Lifetime cumulative use of paracetamol, salicylates and phenacetin was assessed by means of a drug-exposure matrix for analgesics in which information on past and current brand names obtained from study subjects was converted to information on amounts and types of active ingredients. Any regular use of paracetamol, defined as a minimum of two or more doses per week for at least one month, was reported for 35 patients (7%) and 31 controls (6.2%), which yielded an odds ratio for cancers of the renal pelvis and ureter, adjusted for age, sex, study centre and cigarette smoking, of 1.0 (95% CI, 0.6–1.8). Exclusive consumption of paracetamol was associated with an odds ratio of 0.8 (95% CI, 0.3–2.3), and lifetime intake of ≤ 1 kg or > 1 kg paracetamol was associated with odds ratios of 1.1 (95% CI, 0.5–2.1) and 1.0 (95% CI, 0.4–2.3), respectively. [The Working Group noted that, although 12 controls (2.4%) had had lifetime exposure to more than 1 kg phenacetin, no association was seen in this study between cancers of the renal pelvis and ureter and use of phenacetin. Analgesic mixtures containing phenacetin are a recognized human carcinogen with the renal pelvis as the target tissue (IARC, 1987).]

2.2.2 *Ovarian cancer*

Cramer *et al.* (1998) reported on a population-based case–control study of women with a diagnosis of epithelial ovarian cancer or a lesion of borderline malignancy who were residents of eastern Massachusetts or all of New Hampshire (United States) at the date of diagnosis in 1992–97; the cases were identified from state cancer registries. Control subjects, matched to cases by age and geographical area, were identified through random-digit dialling, or—for cases in Massachusetts aged 60 years or older—from lists of all residents in towns. Of 1080 notified cases of ovarian cancer, only 563 (52%) were included in the analysis together with 523 control subjects [57%], after exclusion for various reasons. Interviews, usually completed at the subject's home, included questions about demographics, menstrual and reproductive history, medical and family history and personal habits. Continuous use of over-the-counter and prescribed analgesics, defined as at least once a week for at least six months, was assessed for paracetamol, aspirin and ibuprofen until one year before diagnosis. Any continuous use of over-the-counter paracetamol was reported by 26 patients with ovarian cancer (4.6%) and 46 control subjects (8.8%), yielding an odds ratio, adjusted for age, study centre, education, religion, parity, use of oral contraceptives and menstrual, arthritic or headache pain, of 0.5 (95% CI, 0.3–0.9). The lowest risks for ovarian cancer were seen for women who had used paracetamol daily (odds ratio, 0.4; 95% CI, 0.2–0.7; 16 cases, 35 controls), for more than 10 years (odds ratio, 0.4; 95% CI, 0.2–0.9; 10 cases, 24 controls) and for more than 20 tablet–years, defined as the number of tablets per day multiplied by the number of years of use (odds ratio, 0.5; 95% CI, 0.2–1.0; 10 cases, 20 controls). Inverse associations between use of paracetamol and risk were seen for all the histological subtypes of ovarian cancer included in the study. [The Working Group noted that the overall response rate among cases and controls was very low and that there were a number of substantial differences in demographic variables between cases and controls, suggesting that the results may have been influenced by biased selection of study subjects.]

3. Studies of Cancer in Experimental Animals

Previous evaluation

Paracetamol was tested for carcinogenicity by oral administration in mice and rats. In one strain of mice, a significant increase in the incidence of multiple liver carcinomas and adenomas was observed in animals of each sex at a markedly toxic dose; in two studies on another strain, no increase in the incidence of any tumour was observed at a well-tolerated dose that was approximately half that in the preceding study. Administration of paracetamol to two different strains of rats did not increase tumour incidence. In a further strain of rats, the incidence of neoplastic liver nodules was increased in animals of each sex given the higher dose; the combined incidence of bladder papillomas and carcinomas (mostly papillomas) was significantly greater in high-dose male and in low-dose female rats. Although treatment increased the incidence of bladder calculi in treated rats, there was no relationship between the presence of calculi and of either hyperplasia or tumours in the bladder. Oral administration of paracetamol to rats also enhanced the incidence of renal adenomas induced by *N*-nitroso-*N*-ethyl-*N*-hydroxyethylamine (IARC, 1990). [The present Working Group noted that in the study in rats in which tumours were induced (Flaks *et al.*, 1985) no tumours were found in either male or female controls, which is a highly unusual finding and raises questions about the interpretation of the findings.]

New studies

3.1 Oral administration

3.1.1 *Mouse*

Groups of 50 male and 50 female B6C3F$_1$ mice, eight to nine weeks old, were given paracetamol (purity, > 99%) in the diet at concentrations of 0, 600, 3000 or 6000 mg/kg diet (ppm) for up to 104 weeks. There was no difference in survival between control and exposed mice, but a dose-related depression in body-weight gain was recorded in animals of each sex. Under the conditions of this study, there was no evidence of carcinogenic activity. The incidence of thyroid gland follicular-cell hyperplasia was increased in a dose-related manner in both males and females (National Toxicology Program, 1993).

3.1.2 *Rat*

Groups of 50 male and 50 female Fischer 344/N rats, seven to eight weeks old, were given paracetamol (purity, > 99%) in the diet at concentrations of 0, 600, 3000 or 6000 mg/kg diet (ppm) for up to 104 weeks. There was no difference in survival between control and exposed groups and no effect of treatment on body-weight gain. No treatment-related increase in tumour incidence was found in male rats, but an increase in the incidence of mononuclear cell leukaemia was observed in females at the high dose (9/50, 17/50, 15/50, 24/50 for the four groups respectively) (National Toxicology Program, 1993). [The Working Group noted the high and variable incidence of mononuclear-cell leukaemia between and within studies with Fischer rats and considered that this was not a treatment-related effect.]

3.2 Administration with known carcinogens or modifying factors

Rat: In a model of urinary bladder carcinogenesis, groups of 10 or 20 male Fischer 344 rats, six weeks of age, were treated with 0.1% *N*-nitrosodi(2-hydroxypropyl)amine in the drinking-water and 3.0% uracil in the diet for the first four weeks as an initiating schedule and, one week later, were given either a diet containing 0.8% paracetamol or a basal (control) diet for 35 weeks, at which point the animals were killed. Paracetamol did not significantly increase the incidences of tumours of the renal tubules, renal pelvis, ureter or urinary bladder when compared with the initiated control group (Shibata *et al.*, 1995).

In a model of intestinal carcinogenesis, six groups of 27 (controls) or 48 male Fischer 344 rats, approximately eight weeks of age, were given paracetamol (purity, 99%) in the diet at concentrations of 0, 250 or 5000 mg/kg (ppm) for 44 weeks, when the animals were killed. Commencing two weeks after the start of paracetamol feeding, 50 mg/kg bw

3,2-dimethyl-4-aminobiphenyl (DMAB) were injected subcutaneously once weekly for 20 weeks. Vehicle controls were given 1 mL/kg bw corn oil by the same route and for the same period as DMAB but no DMAB or paracetamol. There was also an untreated control group (no corn oil, paracetamol or DMAB), a group receiving paracetamol alone and a group receiving DMAB alone. Less than 50% of the animals receiving DMAB survived, the deaths being due mainly to intestinal obstruction from tumour growth. No intestinal tumours occurred in the controls or those receiving paracetamol alone. The incidence of intestinal tumours in those given DMAB alone was 73%, which was significantly reduced to 50% ($p < 0.05$) by paracetamol at each dose (Williams & Iatropoulos, 1997).

In a short-term model of fatty liver and liver cirrhosis, groups of 8–22 male Fischer 344 rats, six weeks of age, were fed either a choline-deficient or a choline-supplemented diet for four weeks, followed by a single oral gavage of paracetamol at doses of 0, 0.5, 1 or 1.5 mg/kg bw in 0.2% tragacanth gum solution. Four hours after paracetamol treatment, the rats were subjected to a two-thirds hepatectomy, followed by a two-week recovery period, and then two weeks of feeding of 0.02% of 2-acetylaminofluorene coupled with a single gavage of carbon tetrachloride at the mid-point. The rats were killed nine weeks after the beginning of the study after an 18-h fast. A positive control group received a single intraperitoneal injection of *N*-nitrosodiethylamine in the place of paracetamol. Foci of hepatocellular alteration were assayed by immunohistochemical staining for γ-glutamyltranspeptidase or the placental form of glutathione-S-transferase. Paracetamol did not significantly alter the number or size of liver foci when compared with the relevant control values (Maruyama *et al.*, 1990).

In a long-term model of fatty liver and liver cirrhosis, groups of 8–13 male Fischer 344 rats, six weeks of age, were fed either a choline-deficient diet for 27 weeks to produce liver cirrhosis or a choline-supplemented diet as a control group. From 27 weeks, the rats were fed a diet containing 0, 0.05, 0.45 or 0.9% paracetamol, basal diet or choline-supplemented diet, until week 52, at which time the surviving animals were killed. Foci of hepatocellular alteration were assayed by immunohistochemical staining for γ-glutamyltranspeptidase or the placental form of glutathione-S-transferase. Paracetamol did not alter the number or size of liver foci when compared with the relevant control groups (Maruyama *et al.*, 1990).

4. Other Data Relevant to an Evaluation of Carcinogenicity and its Mechanisms

4.1 Absorption, distribution, metabolism and excretion

4.1.1 *Humans*

After oral administration, paracetamol is absorbed rapidly from the small intestine, while absorption from the stomach is negligible. The rate of absorption depends on the rate of gastric emptying (Clements *et al.*, 1978). First-pass metabolism of paracetamol is dose-dependent: the systemic availability after oral administration ranges from 90% of

1–2 g to 63% of 0.5 g. The plasma concentrations of paracetamol in healthy subjects peaked within 1 h after ingestion of 0.5 or 1 g but continued to rise up to 2 h after oral intake of 2 g (Rawlins *et al.*, 1977). Intramuscular administration of 600 mg paracetamol to healthy male volunteers resulted in a maximal average blood concentration of 7.5 μg/mL 1.7 h after dosing (Macheras *et al.*, 1989).

A comparison of dogs and humans indicated that in humans paracetamol is rapidly and relatively uniformly distributed throughout the body fluids (Gwilt *et al.*, 1963). After normal therapeutic doses of paracetamol, binding to plasma proteins is considered insignificant (Gazzard *et al.*, 1973). The apparent volume of distribution of paracetamol in humans is about 0.9 L/kg bw (Forrest *et al.*, 1982). The decrease in paracetamol concentrations in plasma is multiphasic after both intravenous injection and oral dosing with 500 or 1000 mg. When the data for six healthy volunteers were interpreted according to a two-compartment open model, the half-life of the first exponential ranged from 0.15 to 0.53 h and that of the second exponential from 2.2 to 3.3 h. The latter value was in agreement with that found after oral dosing. The mean clearance (± SEM) after intravenous administration of 1000 mg was 350 (± 40) mL/min (Rawlins *et al.*, 1977). Renal excretion of paracetamol involves glomerular filtration and passive reabsorption, and the sulfate conjugate is subject to active renal tubular secretion (Morris & Levy, 1984). Both glucuronide and sulfate metabolites have been shown to accumulate in the plasma of patients with renal failure who are taking paracetamol (Lowenthal *et al.*, 1976). Paracetamol crossed the placenta in an unconjugated form and was excreted in the urine of an exposed neonate in a similar composition to that found in the urine of a two- to three-day-old infant who had received an oral dose (Collins, 1981). During lactation, paracetamol passes rapidly into milk, and the milk:plasma concentration ratio increased from 0.9 to 1.3 between 45 min and 6 h after ingestion (Berlin *et al.*, 1980; Notarianni *et al.*, 1987).

Paracetamol is metabolized predominantly to the 4-glucuronide and 4-sulfate conjugates in human liver. In young healthy subjects, about 55 and 30% of a therapeutic dose of 20 mg/kg bw was excreted in the urine as the glucuronide and sulfate conjugates, respectively; the sum of cysteine conjugate and mercapturic acid resulting from glutathione conjugation was found to be 8% of the dose (Forrest *et al.*, 1982).

Of the total radiolabel in urine of volunteers collected over 24 h after an oral dose of 1200 mg [^{3}H]paracetamol, only 2% was unchanged paracetamol, while 52 and 41% were associated with sulfate and glucuronide conjugates, respectively. About 4% of the dose was associated with a mercapturic acid conjugate, probably through conversion of paracetamol by cytochrome P450 (CYP)-dependent hepatic mixed-function oxidase to the highly reactive *N*-acetyl-*para*-benzoquinone imine, which was subsequently inactivated by reaction with reduced glutathione and excreted as the mercapturic acid conjugate. Large doses of paracetamol can deplete glutathione stores, and the excess of the highly reactive intermediate binds covalently to vital cell elements, which may result in acute hepatic necrosis (Mitchell *et al.*, 1974).

In a study to investigate the effect of inhibitors of oxidative metabolism on the bio-conversion of paracetamol, 10 healthy men (average weight, 77.6 kg) consumed 20 mg/kg bw paracetamol dissolved in 400 mL of a soft drink over 2 min on three occasions at an interval of at least a week. On one occasion, the paracetamol was taken alone, on another with cimetidine and on the third occasion with ethanol (70° proof whisky). Cimetidine and ethanol were taken before the paracetamol and as maintenance doses for 8 h after intake. The plasma and urinary concentrations of paracetamol and its metabolites and plasma ethanol were determined. Cimetidine had no effect on the metabolism of paracetamol, but ethanol caused a highly significant decrease in the recovery of mercapturic acid and cysteine conjugates (Critchley *et al.*, 1983).

NADPH-dependent oxidation of [^{14}C]paracetamol to a reactive intermediate in microsomes from human liver obtained at autopsy was inferred from measurement of protein-bound radiolabel. The extent of inhibition of protein binding by 48 mmol/L ethanol was only one-fourth to one-half that found *in vivo* by Critchley *et al.* (1983) (Thummel *et al.*, 1989).

Liver microsomes from seven subjects converted 1 mmol/L paracetamol to a reactive intermediate detected as the paracetamol–cysteine conjugate. Antibody inhibition studies showed that two P450 isozymes, namely CYP2E1 and CYP1A1, catalyse nearly all of the paracetamol activation in human liver microsomes (Raucy *et al.*, 1989).

Microsomes isolated from four human livers were used to investigate the cytochrome P450 enzymes involved in paracetamol activation. The kinetics of the conversions of paracetamol to its glutathione conjugate suggests multiple K_m values, consistent with the involvement of several cytochrome P450s. Human cytochrome P450 enzymes expressed in HepG2 cells, CYP 2E1, CYP 1A2 and CYP 3A4, were all found to metabolize paracetamol to an activated metabolite identified as a glutathione conjugate. Because of the higher K_m of CYP 1A2, the authors proposed that CYP 3A4 and CYP 2E1 were of greater significance in the activation of paracetamol to *N*-acetyl-*para*-benzoquinone imine, and that this highly reactive intermediate is trapped by conjugation with glutathione (Patten *et al.*, 1993).

Purified human CYP 2E1 selectively oxidized paracetamol to the toxic metabolite *N*-acetyl-*para*-benzoquinone imine, whereas human CYP 2A6 selectively oxidized paracetamol to 3-hydroxyparacetamol. However, both isoforms of cytochrome P450 were capable of catalysing both reactions and the investigators concluded from their kinetic analysis that, at toxic doses of paracetamol, CYP 2A6 could contribute to formation of the toxic metabolite, although CYP 2E1 would be more efficient (Chen *et al.*, 1998).

4.1.2 *Experimental systems*

The proposed metabolic pathways of paracetamol are summarized in Figure 1. The major urinary metabolites (the glucuronide, sulfate and 3-mercapto derivatives) are observed in most species, although the percentages of these conjugates excreted in urine vary widely among species (Davis *et al.*, 1974). In rats, the proportion of biliary excretion due to the various metabolites of paracetamol increased from 20 to 49% as the intravenous doses were increased from 37.5 to 600 mg/kg bw. The glucuronide conjugate was the major metabolite recovered in bile at all doses (Hjelle & Klaassen, 1984). First-pass

Figure 1. Major pathways for the metabolism of paracetamol

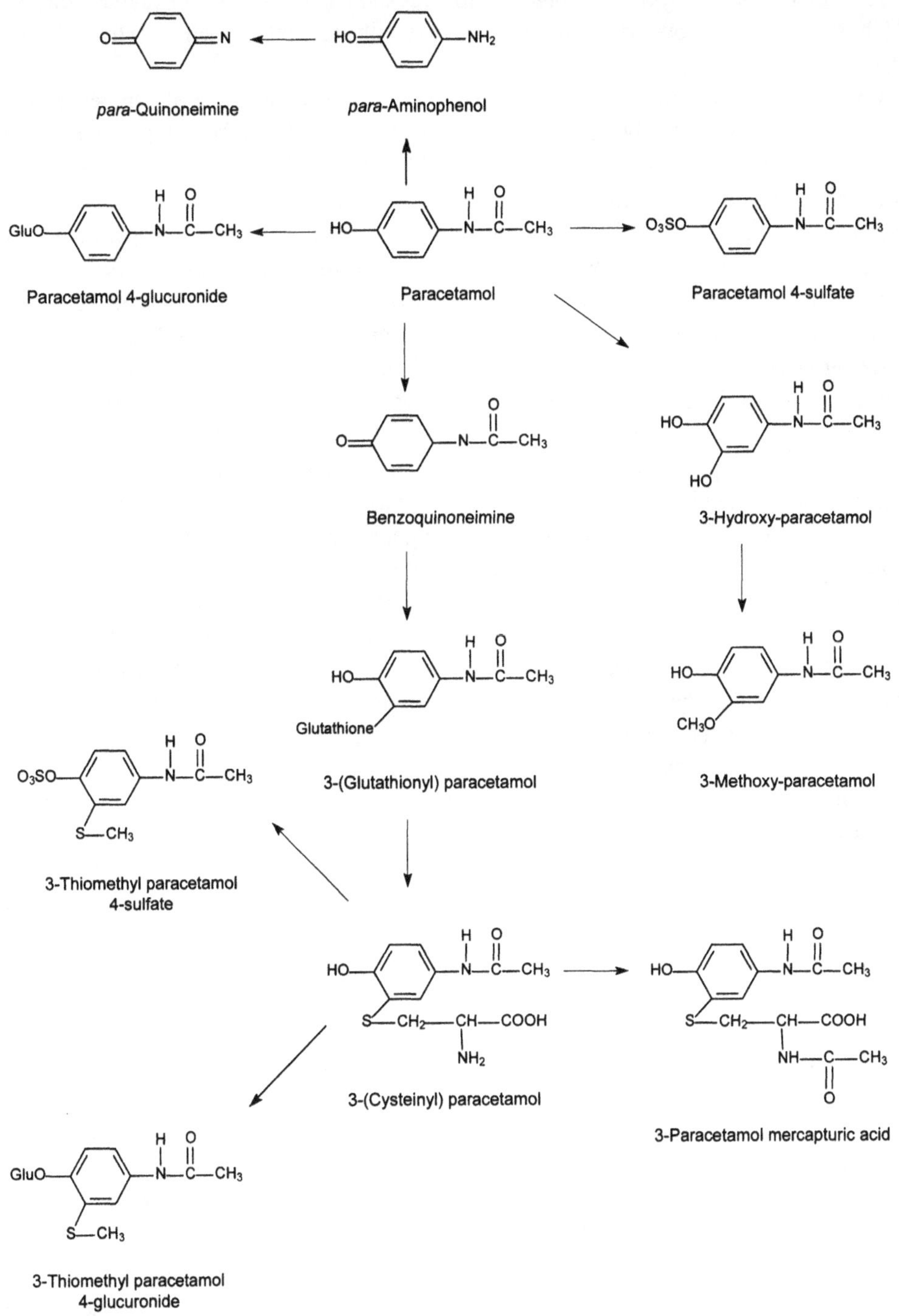
para-Quinoneimine
para-Aminophenol
Paracetamol 4-glucuronide
Paracetamol
Paracetamol 4-sulfate
Benzoquinoneimine
3-Hydroxy-paracetamol
Glutathione
3-(Glutathionyl) paracetamol
3-Methoxy-paracetamol
3-Thiomethyl paracetamol 4-sulfate
3-(Cysteinyl) paracetamol
3-Paracetamol mercapturic acid
3-Thiomethyl paracetamol 4-glucuronide

Modified from National Toxicology Program (1993)

metabolism by the intestine was reported to predominate, and saturation of paracetamol sulfate formation in the liver was suggested to be responsible for lower clearance at doses of 150 and 300 mg/kg bw administered intra-arterially and intravenously (Hirate *et al.*, 1990).

A minor but important metabolic pathway involves the conversion of paracetamol to a reactive metabolite by the hepatic cytochrome P450-dependent mixed-function oxidase system (Mitchell *et al.*, 1973; Potter *et al.*, 1973). *N*-Acetyl-*para*-benzoquinone imine was found to be formed as an oxidation product of paracetamol by purified P450 and cumene hydroperoxide. The reactive product was rapidly reduced back to paracetamol by a variety of reductants. Attempts to produce *N*-acetyl-*para*-benzoquinone imine from NADPH and microsomes were not successful owing to this rapid reduction; however, both purified *N*-acetyl-*para*-benzoquinone imine and paracetamol with an NADPH-generating system bound covalently to mouse liver microsomal protein. A subsequent reaction of *N*-acetyl-*para*-benzoquinone imine was found to be conjugation to glutathione, resulting in 3-*S*-glutathionylparacetamol (Dahlin *et al.*, 1984).

Adult male Sprague-Dawley rats received an intravenous injection of 15, 30, 150 or 300 mg/kg paracetamol, and plasma and urine were assayed during 6–7 h after dosing for paracetamol and its glucuronide and sulfate conjugates. At each dose, the plasma concentrations of paracetamol decreased exponentially with time, but at the two higher doses total clearance and the fraction excreted as sulfate conjugate decreased. Both paracetamol glucuronide and paracetamol sulfate formation appeared to be capacity-limited (Galinsky & Levy, 1981). A correlation has been found between species sensitivity to the hepatotoxicity of paracetamol and the balance between two pathways: (i) formation of glutathione conjugates and the corresponding hydrolysis products (indicative of the 'toxic' pathway) and (ii) metabolism via formation of glucuronide and sulfate esters (the 'detoxification pathway'). The susceptible species (hamsters, mice) excreted 27–42% of the dose as metabolite in the toxication pathway, whereas the more resistant species (rats, rabbits, guinea-pigs) excreted only 5–7% of the dose via this route (Gregus *et al.*, 1988). At sufficiently high doses of paracetamol, glutathione is depleted and the reactive metabolite binds covalently to cell macromolecules. It has also been noted that paracetamol and *N*-acetyl-*para*-benzoquinone imine may exert their cytotoxic effects via disruption of Ca^{2+} homeostasis secondary to the depletion of soluble and protein-bound thiols (Moore *et al.*, 1985).

Prostaglandin *H* synthase catalysed the arachidonic acid-dependent polymerization of paracetamol and, in the presence of glutathione, also catalysed the formation of 3-(glutathion-*S*-yl)paracetamol. These reactions involved the overall 1- and 2-electron oxidation of paracetamol via formation of *N*-acetyl-*para*-benzosemiquinone imine and *N*-acetyl-*para*-benzoquinone imine (Potter & Hinson, 1987a). The polymerization reaction was also observed when cumene hydroperoxide was added to microsomes and paracetamol (Potter & Hinson, 1987b). These data indicate that oxidative or free-radical reactions initiated by paracetamol play a role in the hepatotoxicity of this drug (Birge *et al.*, 1988).

The kinetics of the conversion of paracetamol to its glutathione conjugate suggested multiple equilibrium constants (K_m) consistent with the involvement of several P450s in microsomes from the livers of Sprague-Dawley rats. Antibodies specific for rat CYP 2E1 and CYP 1A2 each inhibited approximately 40% of this biotransformation in microsomes from control male rats, but only slight inhibition was observed with CYP 3A1/2 antibodies in male or female rat microsomes. In microsomes from female rats induced with dexamethasone, the kinetics of paracetamol activation indicated a single K_m. In this case, the active enzyme was shown to be CYP 3A1, because antibodies against this enzyme inhibited activity by 80% (Patten *et al.*, 1993).

The role of cytochrome P450 isoforms in the acute liver toxicity of paracetamol was further established by the use of *cyp2e1* knock-out C57BL/6N mice. Mice that received single doses of paracetamol up to 400 mg/kg bw intraperitoneally survived, whereas 50% of the wild-type mice died. Significantly increased activities of the liver enzymes aspartate aminotransferase and alanine aminotransferase were found in wild-type when compared with knock-out mice given 200 or 400 mg/kg bw paracetamol. At the highest dose (800 mg/kg bw), most of the mice died and the aspartate aminotransferase activity was elevated in both wild-type and knock-out mice, suggesting a role of another cytochrome P450 such as CYP 1A2 (Lee *et al.*, 1996).

Paracetamol is activated in the kidney by an NADPH-dependent cytochrome P450 to an arylating agent, which can bind covalently to cellular macromolecules (McMurtry *et al.*, 1978). Studies in several species have suggested that formation of *para*-aminophenol may be of importance in the nephrotoxicity of paracetamol. In a study in hamsters, *para*-aminophenol was identified as a urinary metabolite (Gemborys & Mudge, 1981). When [*acetyl*-^{14}C]paracetamol and [*ring*-^{14}C]paracetamol were compared in binding studies with renal cortex protein, the amount of covalent binding of radiolabel from [*ring*-^{14}C]paracetamol was four times higher in Fischer rats, which are sensitive to paracetamol nephrotoxicity. This suggests that deacetylation to *para*-aminophenol is the primary pathway of bioactivation. In contrast, binding of ring- and acetyl-labelled paracetamol to renal protein was similar in non-susceptible Sprague-Dawley rats, suggesting that oxidation may be an important metabolic route (Newton *et al.*, 1985). These data indicate that *para*-aminophenol may be responsible for paracetamol-induced renal necrosis in Fischer 344 rats (Newton *et al.*, 1982). Studies *in vitro* with microsomes from Sprague-Dawley rats and *in vivo* with Sprague-Dawley rats that received a 1100-mg/kg bw intraperitoneal dose of paracetamol in combination with specific inhibitors of deacetylation and oxidation suggested that both oxidative metabolism and deacetylation contribute to the nephrotoxicity of paracetamol (Mugford & Tarloff, 1995, 1997).

Exposure of CD-1 male mice to either 600 mg/kg bw paracetamol orally or 500 mg/kg bw *para*-aminophenol subcutaneously resulted in nephrotoxicity; prior inhibition of paracetamol deacylation by carboxylesterase inhibitors did not alter the hepatotoxicity or nephrotoxicity. Pretreatment of animals with the mixed-function oxidase inhibitor piperonyl butoxide decreased nephrotoxicity due to paracetamol but not that due to *para*-aminophenol. Immunohistochemical studies with antibodies directed against the *N*-acetyl moiety of paracetamol showed binding to renal tissues of mice that had received a nephrotoxic dose of paracetamol, but not of those that had received a nephrotoxic dose of *para*-aminophenol. These findings led the investigators to conclude that in these mice deacylation was not required for P450-mediated activation of paracetamol-induced nephrotoxicity (Emeigh Hart *et al.*, 1991). The activity of CYP 2E1 in kidney microsomes isolated from male C3H/HeJ mice was 50-fold higher than that in females. An important role for activation of paracetamol by CYP 2E1 in the kidney was suggested by fact that renal damage by paracetamol was restricted to those areas in which the enzyme was localized, i.e. the proximal convoluted tubule. The extent of renal glutathione depletion in the male mice was significantly greater than that in the females, but the glutathione levels were restored much faster in males. Further studies in this strain indicated that paracetamol was nephrotoxic in female mice only when they were pretreated with testosterone, which resulted in induction of renal CYP 2E1 (Hu *et al.*, 1993). These effects were confirmed in a study with CD1 mice, which showed that renal rather than hepatic biotransformation of paracetamol is central to paracetamol-induced nephrotoxicity in the mouse (Hoivik *et al.*, 1995). Further studies in which toxicity was completely prevented by inhibition of organic-anion transport suggested that a paracetamol–glutathione conjugate may contribute to the observed nephrotoxicity (Emeigh Hart *et al.*, 1996).

Immunohistochemical analysis after exposure of male CD-1 mice to an oral dose of 600 mg/kg bw paracetamol showed correspondence between the location of bound paracetamol and CYP 2E1, and both corresponded to tissue damage in centrilobular hepatocytes, renal proximal tubules, lung Clara cells and Bowman gland and sustentacular cells in the olfactory epithelium. This suggests that toxicity in the major target tissues of mice is mediated by bioactivation of paracetamol *in situ* (Emeigh Hart *et al.*, 1995).

4.1.3 *Comparison of data for humans and rodents*

The experimental data on paracetamol point to similar pathways of liver biotransformation in humans and rodents. Although none of the rodent species studied resembled humans with respect to all of the urinary metabolites of paracetamol, the hamster was judged to be the best model with respect to the metabolites formed and susceptibility towards this compound. At therapeutic doses (up to 4 mg/kg), the glucuronidation and sulfation pathways predominate in humans, but the sulfation pathway becomes saturated at higher doses. In mice, the glucuronide pathway also predominates, but in rats at doses below 400 mg/kg, the sulfation pathway predominates and becomes saturated at higher doses. A minor pathway in both humans and rodents involves formation of the reactive intermediate *N*-acetyl-*para*-benzoquinone imine via CYP 2E1, CYP 1A2—and other isoforms including CYP 2A6 in humans—and prostaglandin *H* synthase. High doses of paracetamol deplete liver glutathione, which is protective at lower doses since it conjugates with the reactive intermediate *N*-acetyl-*para*-benzoquinone imine.

Three possible mechanisms for paracetamol-induced nephrotoxicity have been investigated. Paracetamol may be converted by cytochrome P450 in the kidney to the reactive intermediate *N*-acetyl-*para*-benzoquinone imine, which then forms the glutathione conjugate 3-(glutathionyl)paracetamol, or the metabolite may be formed in the liver and transported to the kidney. Alternatively, paracetamol may be deacetylated to *para*-aminophenol, which has been shown to be nephrotoxic. Various species-, strain- and sex-related differences in these pathways in rodents have been investigated, but the pathway in humans has not been established (reviewed by Savides & Oehme, 1983).

4.2 Toxic effects

4.2.1 *Humans*

Reports on the acute toxicity, and in particular the hepatotoxicity, of paracetamol have continued to appear since the first two case reports in 1966 (Davidson & Eastham, 1966). The initial symptoms of overdose are nausea, vomiting, diarrhoea and abdominal pain. Clinical indications of hepatic damage become manifest within two to four days after ingestion of toxic doses; in adults, a single dose of 10–15 g (200–250 mg/kg bw) is toxic. The activities of serum transaminase and lactic dehydrogenase and bilirubin concentrations are elevated, and prothrombin time is prolonged (Koch-Weser, 1976). The severity of hepatic injury increases with the dose ingested and with previous consumption of other drugs that induce liver cytochrome P450 enzymes (Wright & Prescott, 1973). After an overdose of paracetamol, biopsy of the liver revealed a range of histological abnormalities, which varied from focal hyperplasia of Kuppfer cells and a few foci of hepatocytolytic necrosis to severe centrizonal necrosis, liver-cell loss, inflammation and features of active regeneration (James *et al.*, 1975). In non-fatal cases, the hepatic lesions are reversible over a period of months, without the development of cirrhosis (Hamlyn *et al.*, 1977).

Heavy alcohol consumption has been stated in several case reports to be related to more severe paracetamol hepatotoxicity than that in non- or moderate drinkers (for review see Black, 1984). Five cases of combined hepatocellular injury and renal tubular necrosis have been reported among patients with a history of chronic alcohol use who were receiving therapeutic doses of paracetamol (Kaysen *et al.*, 1985).

In a multicentre case-control study in North Carolina, United States, 554 adults with newly diagnosed kidney disease (serum creatinine, ≥ 130 μmol/L) and 516 matched control subjects selected randomly from the same area were included. Histories of use of paracetamol, phenacetin and aspirin were obtained by telephone interview, with response rates of 78% and 73% among patients and controls, respectively. The information was supplied by next-of-kin for 55% of cases and 10% of controls. The odds ratios for renal disease, adjusted for consumption of the two other analgesics, were 1.2 (95% CI, 0.77–1.9) in subjects who used paracetamol weekly and 3.2 (95% CI, 1.0–9.8) in subjects who used it daily, when compared with subjects with none or occasional use (Sandler *et al.*, 1989).

In a liver specimen obtained within 1 h of death from a five-year-old girl who died of paracetamol poisoning, covalent binding of paracetamol to proteins was observed. With use of ^{125}I-conjugated goat anti-rabbit immunoglobulin G and purified anti-paracetamol antisera with sodium dodecyl sulfate–polyacrylamide gel electrophoresis and western blotting, the most prominent protein arylation was found in the cytosolic fraction in bands corresponding to 58 and 130 kD, with lesser bands at 38 and 62 kD. There was no apparent selective binding in the microsomal fraction. Immunohistochemical analysis revealed that the paracetamol binding was in the centrilobular regions (Birge *et al.*, 1990).

Administration of 4 g paracetamol daily for three days to 10 healthy female volunteers was found to decrease urinary excretion of prostaglandin E_2 and sodium. This effect was presumably due to inhibition of renal medullary prostaglandin E_2 synthesis. No effects were found on the glomerular filtration rate or effective renal plasma flow (Prescott *et al.*, 1990).

A case–control study was conducted in Maryland, Virginia, West Virginia, and Washington DC, United States, of the association between regular use of paracetamol, aspirin and other non-steroidal anti-inflammatory drugs. A total of 716 patients identified through a population-based registry of end-stage renal disease and 361 controls from the population of the study area were interviewed by telephone about their past use of medications containing the above-mentioned drugs. The response rates were 95% and 90% among identified patients and controls, respectively. The odds ratios for end-stage renal disease, adjusted for use of other analgesic drugs, were 1.4 (95% CI, 0.8–2.4) and 2.1 (95% CI, 1.1–3.7) for subjects whose annual average intake of paracetamol was categorized as moderate (105–365 pills per year) and heavy (366 or more pills per year), respectively, when compared with subjects whose annual average intake was categorized as light (0–104 pills per year). Similarly, the odds ratios for renal disease were 2.0 (95% CI, 1.3–3.2) and 2.4 (95% CI, 1.2–4.8) for subjects whose cumulative lifetime intake of paracetamol was 1000–4999 pills and ≥ 5000 pills, respectively, when compared with subjects whose cumulative intake was < 1000 pills (Perneger *et al.*, 1994).

A woman with acute renal failure was admitted to hospital after exposure by self-medication to an estimated 15 g paracetamol over 3.5 days in combination with alcohol and several other pharmaceuticals. Acute renal tubular necrosis resulting from paracetamol poisoning occurs alone or in combination with hepatic necrosis. The margin of safety of paracetamol intake is lower in patients with risk factors such as starvation, chronic alcohol ingestion (which depletes glutathione) or use of medications (e.g. anticonvulsants) that activate the P450 system (Blakely & McDonald, 1995).

Acute renal failure without fulminant liver failure was reported after exposure to 7.5–10 g paracetamol over two days (case 1) and after exposure to an undetermined amount in a suicide attempt (case 2). In case 1, there was concomitant heavy use of alcohol and other drugs and pharmaceuticals, and in case 2 pharmaceuticals for treatment of schizophrenia and hypertension were also used. Other reported cases of acute renal failure without fulminant liver failure have been reviewed (Eguia & Materson, 1997).

4.2.2 *Experimental systems*

The LD_{50} of orally administered paracetamol in male rats was 3.7 g/kg bw (Boyd & Bereczky, 1966); the 100-day LD_{50} in rats was 765 mg/kg bw, and the maximal dose that caused no deaths was estimated to be 400 mg/kg bw per day over 100 days (Boyd & Hogan, 1968). Prior administration of β-carotene was found to protect mice against the acute toxicity of intraperitoneally administered paracetamol (Baranowitz & Maderson, 1995).

Hepatic necrosis after administration of paracetamol was first reported in rats (Boyd & Bereczky, 1966). The main signs are chromatolysis, hydropic vacuolation, centrilobular necrosis, macrophage infiltration and regenerative activity (Dixon *et al.*, 1971). Sensitivity to paracetamol-induced hepatotoxicity varies considerably among species, hamsters and mice being the most sensitive and rats, rabbits and guinea-pigs being more resistant (Davis *et al.*, 1974; Siegers *et al.*, 1978). The toxic effects in dogs and cats given a single oral dose of paracetamol at maximal doses of 500 and 120 mg/kg bw, respectively, included hepatic centrilobular lesions in dogs and more diffuse pathological changes in the liver in cats, which have only a limited capacity to glucuronidate exogenous compounds (Savides *et al.*, 1984).

Paracetamol was administered to CD-1(ICR)BR male mice at doses of 100, 300 or 600 mg/kg bw by gavage, and the mice were killed 2 or 18 h later. No histopathological changes or changes in glutathione concentrations were found at the lowest dose; the intermediate dose produced little necrosis but induced extensive glutathione depletion by 2 h after treatment; while 600 mg/kg bw caused both necrosis and glutathione depletion (Placke *et al.*, 1987a).

The histological effects of paracetamol in the livers of B6C3F$_1$ mice given 10 000 mg/kg of diet for 72 weeks included centrilobular hepatocytomegaly, cirrhosis, lipofuscin deposition and focal to massive hepatocyte necrosis (Hagiwara & Ward, 1986). At the same dose, macroscopically and microscopically deformed livers were observed in C57BL/6J mice, with extensive lobular collapse, foci of hepatic necrosis and lymphoid aggregation in portal tracts after 32 weeks (Ham & Calder, 1984). In these grossly enlarged livers, ultrastructural changes such as proliferation of smooth endoplasmic reticulum, intracellular lipid accumulation and glycogen depletion were found in Leeds rats given diets containing 1% paracetamol for up to 18 months (Flaks *et al.*, 1985).

Administration of butylated hydroxyanisole to female Swiss-Webster mice at a concentration of 1% in the diet for 12 days [600–800 mg/kg bw per day] prevented the hepatotoxicity of an intraperitoneal dose of 600 mg/kg bw paracetamol, as concluded from measurement of alanine aminotransferase and aspartate aminotransferase activity and histopathological examination. The rate of elimination of paracetamol from blood was 10-fold higher in the mice that had received butylated hydroxyanisole than in those that were given paracetamol only. Although the general pattern of excretion did not change, increases in the rate of formation of glucuronide, sulfate and glutathione conjugates were evident. Therefore, the protective effects of butylated hydroxyanisole were ascribed to enhanced conjugation (Hazelton, 1986).

In six-week-old male B6C3F$_1$ mice given 5000 or 10 000 mg/kg of diet paracetamol for up to 40 weeks, DNA synthesis and other parameters of cell proliferation and toxicity were evaluated in the liver and kidneys at 2, 8, 24 and 40 weeks. The high dose of paracetamol was very toxic, resulting in a 30–50% reduction in body weight and severe hepatic necrosis. The survival rates were 68% at 24 weeks and 45% at 32 weeks. The weights of the liver and kidney were statistically significantly increased in mice at 10 000 ppm in comparison with total body weights. Histopathological alterations in mice at the high dose included focal-to-lobular, massive hepatocyte necrosis, hepatocellular degeneration and hepatocytomegaly. At both doses, increased labelling indices and thymidine kinase activities were seen in the liver at two weeks, and an increased labelling index was seen at 40 weeks only in the low-dose group. No significant histopathological lesions or increased labelling indices or changes in thymidine kinase were seen in the kidney, except for a small decrease at both doses at eight weeks (Ward *et al.*, 1988).

Histopathological review of liver sections from B6C3F$_1$ mice of each sex fed paracetamol at 0.3, 0.6 or 1.25% in the diet for 41 weeks and from NIH outbred, white mice of each sex fed paracetamol at 1.1% in the diet for 48 weeks indicated severe liver injury, characterized by centrilobular necrosis, in animals receiving the highest doses. In the mice receiving lower doses, no significant compound-related liver lesions were found (Maruyama & Williams, 1988).

Paracetamol was tested in Fischer 344 rats and B6C3F$_1$ mice by dietary exposure. In a 13-week study, rats received up to 25 000 mg/kg of diet paracetamol. The body weights of animals of each sex at 12 500 and 25 000 ppm were significantly lower than those of controls, and two animals in each of these groups died. Hepatotoxicity and inflammation were observed in rats of each sex exposed to 25 000 ppm and in males exposed to 12 500 ppm. An increase in the severity of spontaneous age-related chronic progressive nephropathy was seen in animals of each sex exposed to 25 000 ppm. Testicular atrophy was reported in all male rats at the highest dose. No significant changes were seen in animals exposed to 6200 ppm. In a two-year study in which rats were exposed to 600, 3000 or 6000 ppm paracetamol, the only toxic effects reported were increased severity of the spontaneous age-related chronic progressive nephropathy and hyperplasia of the parathyroid gland in males. In mice exposed to up to 25 000 ppm paracetamol for 13 weeks, the body weights of mice of each sex at 12 500 and 25 000 ppm were depressed, with accompanying histopathological lesions of the liver in these groups and in males receiving 6200 ppm. In a two-year study in which mice were exposed to 600, 3000 or 6000 ppm paracetamol, follicular hyperplasia of the thyroid gland was the only reported finding (National Toxicology Program, 1993).

Inhibition of cellular respiration due to impairment of mitochondrial function, decreased cellular ATP and glutathione depletion were found in isolated mouse hepatocytes exposed to toxic concentrations of paracetamol, which were ≥ 0.5 mmol/L as determined by release of lactic dehydrogenase (Burcham & Harman, 1990).

Loss of genomic DNA, evidence of DNA fragmentation and an increase in nuclear Ca^{2+} concentration were found in the livers of Swiss mice after an intraperitoneal dose of 600 mg/kg bw paracetamol, indicating that activation of endonucleases may be an early event in necrosis (Ray *et al.*, 1990). This was confirmed in studies with paracetamol-treated mouse liver cells *in vitro*, which showed formation of a 'ladder' of DNA fragments characteristic of Ca^{2+}-mediated endonuclease activation prior to cytotoxicity and the development of necrosis (Shen *et al.*, 1992).

Pretreatment of male Wistar rats with the glutathione reductase inhibitor 1,3-bis(2-chloroethyl)-1-nitrosourea before paracetamol treatment was reported greatly to enhance the sensitivity of hepatocytes to paracetamol in liver subcellular fractions derived from these rats (*ex vivo*). A similar result was obtained with primary cultures of rat hepatocytes treated *in vitro* with this nitrosourea and paracetamol (Ellouk-Achard *et al.*, 1992). Pretreatment of male ICR mice with the adrenergic agonist phenylpropanolamine, which depleted glutathione by a moderate 30–50%, enhanced liver necrosis produced by intraperitoneal administration of 400 mg/kg bw paracetamol (James *et al.*, 1993).

Intraperitoneal administration of 1 g/kg bw paracetamol to male Sprague-Dawley rats had no effect on the levels of diene conjugates in liver mitochondria or microsomes but inhibited the formation of thiobarbituric acid-reactive substances (TBARS) by hepatocytes *in vitro*. It was concluded that lipid peroxidation does not necessarily correlate with paracetamol-induced hepatotoxicity in Sprague-Dawley rats (Kamiyama *et al.*, 1993).

In male BALB/c mice injected intraperitoneally with 500 mg/kg bw paracetamol, the concentration of TBARs in hepatic microsomes was decreased, and the activities of glutathione *S*-transferase and glutathione peroxidase were increased. In contrast, the concentration of TBARS was increased and the activities of glutathione and glutathione *S*-transferase were decreased in whole-liver homogenates. The authors concluded that glutathione-dependent enzyme defence mechanisms protect microsomes against oxidative stress (Özdemirler *et al.*, 1994).

In a time–course study, 375 mg/kg bw paracetamol were administered intraperitoneally to female Swiss mice, and biochemical changes in the liver were measured within 1 h. The initial changes after 15 min included increased spontaneous in-situ chemiluminescence and hydrogen peroxide concentration, decreased glutathione and increased oxidized glutathione levels and decreased non-Se-glutathione peroxidase activity. At 60 min, which was the last time at which measurements were made, the changes included decreased reduced and oxidized glutathione, decreased non-Se-glutathione peroxidase and decreased Se-glutathione peroxidase. Over the 60-min period, histopathological evidence of liver damage and the activity of marker enzymes for hepatic damage (lactate dehydrogenase, alanine aminotransferase and aspartate aminotransferase) increased (Arnaiz *et al.*, 1995).

In a 6-h study, 400 mg/kg bw paracetamol were administered intraperitoneally to male ICR mice. The hepatic concentrations of glutathione had decreased to 7% of baseline levels by 1 h, the concentrations of TBARS started to increase at 1 h and reached maximal values at 3 h, and the endogenous concentrations of reduced coenzyme Q_9 and Q_{10} decreased steadily over the 6-h period. Plasma alanine aminotransferase activity increased during the course of the experiment. Pretreatment with the lipid-soluble antioxidants coenzyme Q_{10} and α-tocopherol protected against lipid peroxidation but did not completely prevent hepatic injury (Amimoto *et al.*, 1995).

When male Wistar rats were injected intraperitoneally with 500 mg/kg bw paracetamol, 24-day-old animals formed 24 times more liver glutathione conjugates than three- to four-month-old animals. The younger animals also showed greater glutathione depletion and had somewhat lower initial glutathione concentrations. The investigators suggested that the increased rate of glutathione conjugation in young rats is due to more rapid saturation of competing elimination pathways, such as glucuronidation and sulfation (Allameh *et al.*, 1997).

Radiolabel was bound covalently to hepatocellular proteins after incubation of mouse, rat, hamster, rabbit or guinea-pig liver microsomes with [^{3}H]paracetamol; the degree of binding correlated with the susceptibility of the species to paracetamol-induced hepatotoxicity *in vivo* (Davis *et al.*, 1974). Similarly, covalent binding of radiolabel to liver proteins of rats 48 h after administration by gavage of [ring-^{14}C]paracetamol was proportional to the extent of liver damage (Davis *et al.*, 1976). Covalent binding of radiolabel to liver plasma membranes and microsomes was demonstrated 2.5 h after oral administration of [^{3}H]paracetamol at 2.5 g/kg bw to rats (Tsokos-Kuhn *et al.*, 1988).

Binding of paracetamol to liver proteins in three-month-old male Crl:CD-1(CR)BR mice was demonstrated 4 h after oral administration of 600 mg/kg bw paracetamol. With use of ^{125}I-conjugated goat anti-rabbit immunoglobulin G and purified anti-paracetamol antisera with sodium dodecyl sulfate–polyacrylamide gel electrophoresis and western blotting, the most prominent protein arylation was found in the cytosolic fraction in bands corresponding to 44, 58 and 130 kD. There was also selective binding to a 44-kD protein in the microsomal fraction (Birge *et al.*, 1990). Several specific proteins have now been identified as paracetamol-binding proteins, which could disrupt hepatic functions such as ammonia trapping, oxidative phosphorylation, mitochondrial function and—possibly—transmethylation reactions (reviewed by Cohen *et al.*, 1997). Paracetamol–protein binding has been identified by immunodetection not only in the liver but also in kidney, skeletal muscle, heart, lung, pancreas and stomach of male CD-1 and C57BL/6J mice that received an intraperitoneal injection of 600 mg/kg bw paracetamol (Bulera *et al.*, 1996).

Protein adducts were found in B6C3F$_1$ mice given 400 mg/kg bw paracetamol, but there was no evidence of oxidative protein damage as determined by protein aldehyde formation (Gibson *et al.*, 1996).

Diallyl sulfide, which inhibits CYP 2E1, protected rats treated with 750 or 2000 mg/kg bw paracetamol [route not specified] against death and hepatic and renal toxicity, as measured by serum lactate dehydrogenase activity and creatinine concentration. In liver microsomes *in vitro*, diallyl sulfide inhibited formation of the glutathione conjugate of *N*-acetyl-*para*-benzoquinone imine (Hu *et al.*, 1996).

The depletion of glutathione induced in female Fischer 344 rats by an oral dose of 600 mg/kg bw paracetamol was inhibited by guaiazulene, which inhibits lipid peroxidation by scavenging hydroxyl radicals. The investigators concluded that the significant protection conferred by guaiazulene against paracetamol-induced glutathione depletion and hepatic damage could be ascribed to its antioxidant activity (Kourounakis *et al.*, 1997).

In male ICR mice given doses of 10, 50, 100 or 400 mg/kg bw [^{3}H]paracetamol, the substance showed apparent binding to hepatic and renal DNA 2 h after exposure. ^{32}P-Post-labelling did not show readily detectable DNA adducts after exposure to 400 mg/kg bw paracetamol, although a few faint spots were reported after 24 h. Binding of [^{3}H]*N*-acetyl-*para*-benzoquinone imine to purified DNA was greatly enhanced by lowering the pH of the reaction mixture to < 4 or by the addition of alternative nucleophiles such as cysteine (at 0.1 mol/L but not 1 mol/L) or by the presence of the proteins in isolated nuclei or nuclear chromatin. Apparent DNA binding was also generated *in vitro* by horseradish peroxidase and hydrogen peroxidase and, to a much lesser extent, by hepatic microsomes in the presence of NADPH (Rogers *et al.*, 1997).

Intraperitoneal administration of 1 g/kg bw paracetamol to male Long Evans hooded rats resulted in expression of inducible nitric oxide synthase protein that was correlated with damage to centrilobular regions of the liver and increases in serum transaminase activity. Hepatocytes isolated from rats exposed to paracetamol were found to produce more nitric oxide than those from untreated controls. Pretreatment of rats with the inducible nitric oxide synthase inhibitor aminoguanidine prevented the hepatotoxicity of paracetamol (Gardner *et al.*, 1998).

A single subcutaneous dose of 750 mg/kg bw paracetamol to male Fischer 344 rats produced renal tubular necrosis restricted to the distal portions of the proximal tubule (McMurtry *et al.*, 1978). Continuous exposure of female Fischer 344 rats to 140–210 mg/kg bw paracetamol for up to 83 weeks did not produce nephrotoxicity, as determined by light and electron microscopy. In comparison, similar doses of aspirin caused renal papillary necrosis and decreased urinary concentrating ability (Burrell *et al.*, 1991).

In C57BL/6NIA mice given an intraperitoneal dose of 375 mg/kg bw paracetamol, the glutathione and cysteine concentrations were decreased to a greater extent in 31-month-old mice than in 12- or 3-month-old mice. Older mice also lost the ability to recover from the paracetamol-induced depletion of glutathione (Richie *et al.*, 1992).

The nephrotoxic effects of a single oral dose of 1500 mg/kg bw paracetamol to adult male Wistar rats were not prevented by administration of methionine or *N*-acetylcysteine, which protect against hepatotoxicity. Depletion of glutathione was observed in the liver but not in the kidney. Diethyldithiocarbamate, which is an inhibitor of microsomal monooxygenase, protected against both nephrotoxicity and hepatotoxicity (Möller-Hartmann & Siegers, 1991).

In other experiments, it was shown that paracetamol-induced renal toxicity may be due to a direct effect or be mediated by hepatic metabolites of paracetamol. In the isolated perfused kidney of male Wistar rats, haemodynamic and tubular function were affected directly by paracetamol at concentrations of 5–10 mmol/L; however, in these rats *in vivo*, inhibition of γ-glutamyltranspeptidase, an enzyme involved in the processing of hepatically derived glutathione conjugates, was protective against the nephrotoxicity induced by an intraperitoneal dose of 1000 mg/kg bw paracetamol (Trumper *et al.*, 1992, 1995, 1996).

In fasted adult male mice given an oral dose of 600 mg/kg bw paracetamol and killed within 48 h after treatment, degenerative and necrotic changes were detected in the bronchial epithelium and in testicular and lymphoid tissue, in addition to renal and hepatic effects (Placke *et al.*, 1987b).

A study of the effects of 0.5, 1 or 1.5% paracetamol in the diet on urothelial cell proliferation in male Sprague-Dawley rats showed transient increases in the labelling index and hyperplasia of the renal pelvis and bladder at six weeks (Johansson *et al.*, 1989).

The roles of various biochemical factors in paracetamol-induced hepatotoxicity and nephrotoxicity have been investigated, including metallothionein (Waalkes & Ward, 1989), cytokines (Blazka *et al.*, 1995), lysosomal enzymes (Khandkar *et al.*, 1996), the nuclear transcription factors NF-κB and NF-IL6 (Blazka *et al.*, 1996a), tumour necrosis factor α and interleukin 1α (Blazka *et al.*, 1996b) and AP-1 transcription factors (Blazka *et al.*, 1996c). Knock-out mice in which the gene coding for tumour necrosis factor α was inactivated were found to respond to paracetamol no differently from wild-type mice (Boess *et al.*, 1998).

4.3 Reproductive and developmental effects

4.3.1 *Humans*

The teratogenicity of paracetamol in humans has been reviewed and reported to be non-existent, on the basis of the frequency of congenital anomalies reported in multiple large cohort and case–control studies. The risk for adverse reproductive outcomes (e.g. spontaneous abortions, a variety of malformations, fetal distress and hepatic and renal toxicity in infants) was, however, considered to be significant in situations of paracetamol overdose during pregnancy (Friedman & Polifka, 1994).

In a case–control study involving 538 cases and 539 normal controls in California (United States) between 1989 and 1991, the odds ratio for neural tube defects associated with maternal use of paracetamol was 1.0 (95% confidence interval, 0.80–1.4); 144 of the patients and 141 controls had been exposed. Simultaneous adjustment for maternal race, ethnicity, age, educational level, body mass index and vitamin use did not substantially change the results (Shaw *et al.*, 1998).

In a prospective study conducted by the Teratology Information Service and the London National Poisons Information Service of the pregnancy outcomes of 300 women who took an overdose of paracetamol, either alone or in combination with other drugs, in 1984–92 fetal toxicity was not increased, even though 53% of the mothers had required treatment for the overdose. Thirty-eight per cent of the fetuses had been exposed during the first trimester. There were 219 liveborn infants with no malformations (61 of whom had been exposed in the first trimester), 11 with malformations (none with first-trimester exposure), 18 spontaneous abortions, two late fetal deaths and 54 elective terminations (McElhatton *et al.*, 1997).

4.3.2 *Experimental systems*

Paracetamol was evaluated for teratogenicity in frog embryos. In the absence of bioactivation, the 96-h median lethal concentration and the concentration inducing gross malformations in 50% of the surviving embryos were 191 and 143 mg/L, respectively, to yield a teratogenic index of 1.3. In the presence of a microsomal activating system from Arochlor-induced rat liver, these concentrations decreased by 3.9- and 7.1-fold, respectively, which suggests that a reactive metabolite was involved in the developmental toxicity noted in this test system (Fort *et al.*, 1992).

As reported in an abstract, exposure of female Sprague-Dawley rats to 0, 125, 250 or 500 mg/kg paracetamol on day 10 of gestation gave rise to enhanced immunohistochemical staining of glucose-6-phosphate dehydrogenase and reduced staining of NAD-linked isocitrate dehydrogenase in frozen sections of embryos, including the decidual mass, at all doses on day 11. The authors concluded that rat embryos are sensitive to metabolic perturbation caused by maternal exposure to paracetamol (Beck *et al.*, 1997). In another abstract, it was reported that direct exposure of gestation day-11 rat embryos in culture to 500 μmol/L paracetamol resulted in a dramatic loss of intracellular glutathione histofluorescence (Harris *et al.*, 1997).

CD-1 mice were fed diets containing paracetamol (purity, 99.7%) at doses of 0, 0.25, 0.5 and 1% (equivalent to intakes of 0, 360, 720 and 1400 mg/kg bw per day). The parental generation was exposed for 14 weeks during cohabitation, and the number of litters produced was used as a primary index of reproductive capacity. Feed consumption was reduced in the females at the highest concentration. No changes were noted in the number of pups per litter, pup viability, or adjusted [for litter size] pup weight, but 6/19 pairings at the high dose did not result in a fifth litter, and this accounted for the significantly decreased number of litters per pair in this group. The fifth litter that was produced by 13 pairs at the high dose contained fewer pups. The last litter produced by the parental generation was maintained on exposure through adulthood. A reduction in body-weight gain (range, 6–18%) was seen in treated animals of each sex throughout mating. An increase in the percentage of abnormal sperm was observed in males of the F_1 generation at the high dose. In the F_2 generation, a reduction in pup weight adjusted for litter size (11%) was seen at the high dose (Reel *et al.*, 1992; National Toxicology Program, 1997).

Groups of 24–26 male B6C3F_1/BOM M mice received intraperitoneal injections of 0 or 400 mg/kg bw paracetamol daily for five consecutive days. Treated mice lost weight during the exposure, but there was no difference between control and treated animals throughout the remainder of the post-treatment period. The relative testis weights were reduced by 16–18% by paracetamol 27 and 33 days after treatment, but the only alteration in histological appearance up to 10 days was an approximately 6% reduction in the diameter of the seminiferous tubules five days after treatment. DNA synthesis in the testis (measured by [^{3}H]thymidine incorporation) was reduced for several hours immediately after the fifth dose, and this response was seen with concentrations as low as 100 mg/kg bw per day. Flow cytometric analysis of testicular ploidy 26 days after the last dose of 400 mg/kg bw per day revealed alterations in the cell types indicative of altered transit through the cell cycle, but no effect on the chromatin structure of late-maturing spermatids (Wiger *et al.*, 1995).

4.4 Genetic and related effects

The genotoxicity of paracetamol has been reviewed (Rannug *et al.*, 1995).

4.4.1 *Humans*

Ten healthy volunteers ingested three doses of 1 g paracetamol over a period of 8 h. Blood samples were taken before and 24 h after ingestion. The frequency of sister chromatid exchange was significantly increased (0.19 ± 0.03 per chromosome before, 0.21 ± 0.024 per chromosome after exposure), as was the mean frequency of chromatid breaks (from 0.33 ± 0.50 per 100 cells before to 2.2 ± 1.3 per 100 cells after exposure). Exposure of human lymphocytes *in vitro* showed that concentrations > 0.1 mmol/L paracetamol inhibited replicative DNA synthesis, while exposure to 1–10 mmol/L paracetamol for 2 h increased the frequency of sister chromatid exchange. An increased frequency of chromatid and chromosome breaks was found after exposure of lymphocytes to 0.75–1.5 mmol/L paracetamol for 24 h (Hongslo *et al.*, 1991).

The clastogenic activity of paracetamol was determined in a group of 11 volunteers who received three doses of 1000 mg of the drug during 8 h. Blood samples were taken 0, 24, 72 and 168 h after ingestion of the first dose. The frequency of aberrant cells increased from 1.7% at 0 h to 2.8% at 24 h, and the number of breaks per cell from 0.018 (control) to 0.03. These effects had disappeared by 168 h. No increase in lipid peroxidation was observed after ingestion of paracetamol, as determined in the thiobarbituric acid assay; however, simultaneous ingestion of ascorbic acid increased lipid peroxidation (Kocišová *et al.*, 1988).

In a similar study, 11 volunteers received three doses of 1000 mg paracetamol in the course of 8 h, with or without three doses of 1000 mg ascorbic acid. Blood samples and buccal mucosa cells were collected 0, 24, 72 and 168 h after ingestion of the first dose. Unscheduled DNA synthesis induced by 1-methyl-3-nitro-1-nitrosoguanidine was determined in peripheral lymphocytes by a liquid scintillation method, and micronucleus formation was determined in buccal mucosa cells by staining with Light Green. The level of nitrosoguanidine-induced unscheduled DNA synthesis was significantly decreased 24 h after ingestion of paracetamol, and simultaneous intake of ascorbic acid prolonged this effect. A significant increase in micronucleus formation in buccal mucosa cells was observed at 72 h (Topinka *et al.*, 1989). No increase in the frequency of micronucleated buccal cells was observed, however, when the cytokinesis block micronucleus method was used in a study of 12 volunteers who took three doses of 1000 mg paracetamol over an 8-h period (Kocišová & Šrám, 1990).

In a study to investigate further the clastogenicity of paracetamol in which both participants and investigators were unaware of the treatment and placebo status of individuals, volunteers were pre-screened for normal liver function; they were all nonsmokers, and their diet and environmental exposure were controlled during the study. One group of 12 volunteers received two 500-mg tablets of paracetamol three times during an 8-h time interval, and the other 12 volunteers received placebo. Blood was drawn from each volunteer on the day before and on days 1, 3 and 7 after exposure. No significant increase in the frequency of structural chromosomal aberrations was found when pre-treatment values were compared with post-treatment values or when the treated group was compared with the placebo group (Kirkland *et al.*, 1992).

The ability of paracetamol to induce chromosomal aberrations in peripheral lymphocytes was evaluated in volunteers who received a single oral dose of 3 g paracetamol, in patients who had received 2 g paracetamol by intravenous infusion every 6 h for at least seven days and in self-poisoned patients who had ingested more than 15 g paracetamol. In none of these groups did paracetamol affect chromosomes in peripheral lymphocytes (Hantson *et al.*, 1996).

4.4.2 *Experimental systems* (see Table 2 for references)

Paracetamol did not induce gene mutation in *Salmonella typhimurium* TA100, TA102, TA1535, TA1537, TA1538 or TA98 or in *Escherichia coli* with or without exogenous metabolic activation, except in one study in which a metabolic activation system from hamster was used. It induced chromosomal aberrations in *Allium cepa*. Paracetamol did not induce sex-linked recessive lethal mutation in *Drosophila melanogaster*. It gave negative or weakly positive results for the induction of DNA strand breaks in rodent cells *in vitro*. The chemical induced unscheduled DNA synthesis in mouse hepatocytes; it gave inconsistent results in rat hepatocytes and did not induce this effect in hamster or guinea-pig hepatocytes or in Chinese hamster lung cells *in vitro*. Paracetamol did not induce gene mutation in mammalian cells *in vitro*. It induced sister chromatid exchange in Chinese hamster cells and in mouse cells with and without exogenous metabolic activation *in vitro*. It induced micronuclei in a rat kidney cell line *in vitro* but not in primary rat hepatocytes without exogenous metabolic activation. It induced chromosomal aberrations in Chinese hamster and—weakly—in mouse cells *in vitro*. Paracetamol weakly induced cell transformation in mouse cells. It induced sister chromatid exchange and chromosomal aberration in human lymphocytes without exogenous metabolic activation *in vitro*.

Paracetamol inhibited DNA synthesis in several tissues of mice and rats treated *in vivo*. It induced DNA single-strand breaks in mouse liver cells but not in mouse kidney or rat liver or kidney cells *in vivo*. Paracetamol did not induce micronuclei in mice *in vivo* but did induce chromosomal aberrations in mouse bone-marrow cells. Paracetamol induced aneuploidy in rat embryo cells *in vivo*.

5. Summary of Data Reported and Evaluation

5.1 Exposure data

Paracetamol (acetaminophen) is widely used as an analgesic and antipyretic at daily doses up to 4000 mg, with minor uses as an intermediate in the chemical and pharmaceutical industries. Occupational exposure may occur during its production and its use.

5.2 Human carcinogenicity data

In the previous monograph on paracetamol, a positive association with cancer of the ureter (but not of other sites in the urinary tract) was observed in an Australian case–control study. None of the other three case–control studies showed an association with

Table 2. Genetic and related effects of paracetamol

Test system	Results[a]		Dose[b] (LED or HID)	Reference
	Without exogenous metabolic system	With exogenous metabolic system		
Salmonella typhimurium TA100, TA98, TA1535, TA1537, TA1538, reverse mutation	–	–	3624 μg/plate	King *et al.* (1979)
Salmonella typhimurium TA100, TA98, reverse mutation	–	–	1000 μg/plate	Wirth *et al.* (1980)
Salmonella typhimurium TA100, TA98, TA102, reverse mutation	NT	–	3020	Dybing *et al.* (1984)
Salmonella typhimurium TA100, TA98, TA1535, TA1537, TA1538, reverse mutation	–	–	5000 μg/plate	Oldham *et al.* (1986)
Salmonella typhimurium TA100, TA98, TA97, TA1535, TA1537, TA1538, reverse mutation	–	–	10 000 μg/plate	Jasiewicz & Richardson (1987)
Salmonella typhimurium TA100, TA98, TA1535, TA1537, reverse mutation	–	–	10 000 μg/plate	Haworth *et al.* (1983)
Salmonella typhimurium TA100, TA98, reverse mutation	–	–	755 μg/plate	Camus *et al.* (1982)
Escherichia coli K12/343/113, forward or reverse mutation	–	–	4530	King *et al.* (1979)
Allium cepa, chromosomal aberrations	+	NT	5000	Reddy & Subramanyam (1981)
Drosophila melanogaster, sex-linked recessive lethal mutation	–		6040	King *et al.* (1979)
DNA damage, Reuber H4-II-E rat hepatoma cells *in vitro*	–	NT	1510	Dybing *et al* (1984)
DNA damage, Chinese hamster lung V79 cells *in vitro*	(+)	NT	1510	Hongslo *et al.* (1988)
Gene mutation, mouse C3H 10T1/2 clone 8 cells *in vitro*	–	NT	1000	Patierno *et al.* (1989)
Sister chromatid exchange, Chinese hamster lung V79 cells *in vitro*	+	NT	151	Holme *et al.* (1988)
Sister chromatid exchange, Chinese hamster lung V79 cells *in vitro*	+	+	453	Hongslo *et al.* (1988)
Sister chromatid exchange, mouse TA_3H cells *in vitro*	+	NT	151	Hongslo *et al.* (1990)

Table 2 (contd)

Test system	Results[a]		Dose[b] (LED or HID)	Reference
	Without exogenous metabolic system	With exogenous metabolic system		
Sister chromatid exchange, Chinese hamster ovary cells *in vitro*	(+)	(+)	150	National Toxicology Program (1993)
Micronucleus formation, rat kidney cells *in vitro*	+	NT	1510	Dunn *et al.* (1987)
Micronucleus formation, rat primary hepatocytes *in vitro*	–	NT	151	Mueller-Tegethoff *et al.* (1995)
Chromosomal aberrations, Chinese hamster lung cells *in vitro*	(+)	NT	60	Ishidate *et al.* (1978)
Chromosomal aberrations, Chinese hamster Don-6 cells *in vitro*	+	NT	75.5	Sasaki *et al.* (1980)
Chromosomal aberrations, Chinese hamster cells *in vitro*	+	+	47.8	Mueller *et al.* (1991)
Chromosomal aberrations, Chinese hamster ovary cells *in vitro*	+	+	1257	National Toxicology Program (1993)
Chromosomal aberrations, mouse TA_3H cells *in vitro*	(+)	NT	151	Hongslo *et al.* (1990)
Cell transformation, C3H10T1/2 clone 8 cells	(+)	(+)	1000	Patierno *et al.* (1989)
Sister chromatid exchange, human lymphocytes *in vitro*	+	NT	151	Hongslo *et al.* (1991)
Chromosomal aberrations, human lymphocytes *in vitro*	+	NT	200	Watanabe (1982)
Chromosomal aberrations, human lymphocytes *in vitro*	+	NT	226	Hongslo *et al.* (1991)
DNA single-strand breaks, mouse liver cells *in vivo*	+		600 ip × 1	Hongslo *et al.* (1994)
DNA single-strand breaks, mouse kidney cells *in vivo*	–		600 ip × 1	Hongslo *et al.* (1994)
DNA single-strand breaks, rat liver and kidney cells *in vivo*	–		600 ip × 1	Hongslo *et al.* (1994)
Micronucleus formation, NMRI mouse bone-marrow cells *in vivo*	–		453 ip or po × 2	King *et al.* (1979)
Chromosomal aberration, Swiss mouse bone-marrow cells *in vivo*	(+)		2.5/mouse po × 3	Reddy (1984)
Chromosomal aberration, mouse bone-marrow cells *in vivo*	+		100 ip × 1	Severin & Beleuta (1995)

Table 2 (contd)

Test system	Results[a]		Dose[b] (LED or HID)	Reference
	Without exogenous metabolic system	With exogenous metabolic system		
Chromosomal aberrations, mouse testis *in vivo*	–		2.5/mouse po × 3	Reddy & Subramanyam (1985)
Aneuploidy, rat embryos *in vivo*	+		500 po × 25	Tsuruzaki *et al.* (1982)
Binding (covalent) to DNA, ICR mouse liver *in vivo*	+		300 ip × 1	Hongslo *et al.* (1994)

[a] +, positive; (+), weakly positive; –, negative; NT, not tested
[b] LED, lowest effective dose; HID, highest ineffective dose; unless otherwise stated, in-vitro test, μg/mL; in-vivo test, mg/kg bw per day; ip, intraperitoneal; po, oral

cancer in the urinary tract. Nine new—mainly population-based—case–control studies of cancers of the urinary tract have been published, many of which addressed more than one subsite.

None of six studies from Australia, Europe and North America, including a very large international study, found a consistent association between renal-cell cancer and regular intake of paracetamol at any level. In one study from the United States which included patients with renal cancer (type not specified), the risk increased with increasing cumulative intake of paracetamol, to reach statistical significance at the highest exposure; however, this result was not adjusted for intake of other analgesics.

In one study from Australia which included patients with cancer of the renal pelvis, a nonsignificant twofold increase in risk was seen among people in the highest exposure category, with no excess risk in the two lower exposure categories. Another, large case–control study of cancer of the renal pelvis and ureter from the United States showed no association with regular intake of paracetamol.

Of the three new studies that included patients with urinary bladder cancer, that conducted in Sweden showed an elevated risk without providing details. The other two (both from the United States) showed only a slight or no association.

5.3 Animal carcinogenicity data

Paracetamol was tested for carcinogenicity by oral administration in mice and rats. An early study indicated an increased incidence of liver adenomas and carcinomas at a markedly toxic dose in mice of one strain; however, this result was not corroborated in a later study in mice, also at a dose greater than the maximal tolerated dose. A more recent, well-conducted study showed no evidence of a carcinogenic effect in mice. Paracetamol had no carcinogenic effect in rats of several strains, but in rats of one inbred strain, increased incidences of liver and bladder neoplasms were recorded in males at the high dose and an increased incidence of bladder tumours in females at the low dose. A more recent, well-conducted study showed no treatment-related carcinogenic effect in rats. Paracetamol did not promote urinary bladder carcinogenesis in rats and reduced the incidence of intestinal tumours in a two-stage model of intestinal carcinogenesis in rats. It enhanced the incidence of renal adenomas induced by one renal carcinogen but not those induced by another.

5.4 Other relevant data

Activation of a relatively small percentage of paracetamol to *N*-acetyl-*para*-benzoquinone imine by cytochrome P450, predominantly CYP 2E1, has been found to be involved in the mechanism of hepatic and, perhaps, renal toxicity. Most paracetamol is metabolized by glucuronidation, sulfation and conjugation with glutathione, which protects the liver at therapeutic doses. Doses of 300 mg/kg bw per day paracetamol and higher saturate conjugation reactions, deplete glutathione and result in binding of the benzoquinone imine to cellular proteins; this has been proposed to be the mechanism of hepatocellular injury in rodents and humans. Several protein adducts have been found in humans and rodents *in vivo* after exposure to paracetamol. DNA adducts were not observed in mice.

In humans, an association was reported in two case–control studies between daily use of paracetamol and renal disease; however, a causal relationship has not been established. Humans and rodents exposed to doses of paracetamol well above the therapeutic range have experienced centrilobular hepatotoxicity and nephrotoxicity involving the proximal renal tubule. In experimental animals, hepatic, renal and testicular damage occurred only at oral doses that exceeded 300 mg/kg bw per day in rats and 900 mg/kg bw per day in mice. At lower doses, toxic effects in rodents are minimal or absent.

Paracetamol does not present a teratogenic risk to humans at doses associated with severe maternal toxicity. It did not affect reproductive performance of mice in a continuous breeding protocol, although growth and birth weights were reduced. Sperm abnormalities have been observed in mice.

The results of studies of the cytogenetic effects of paracetamol in humans are inconclusive. Paracetamol induced sister chromatid exchange in human cells *in vivo*, and it was aneugenic and induced chromosomal aberrations but not micronuclei in mammalian cells *in vivo*. It induced DNA single-strand breaks in mice treated *in vivo*. Paracetamol induced sister chromatid exchange and chromosomal aberrations in human cells *in vitro*. It weakly induced cell transformation in a mouse cell line. It induced chromosomal aberrations, micronuclei and sister chromatid exchange in mammalian cells *in vitro*. It did not induce gene mutation, and the results of tests in mammalian cells *in vitro* for unscheduled DNA synthesis and DNA damage were inconclusive. Overall, paracetamol was genotoxic in mammalian cells *in vivo* and *in vitro*. It was not mutagenic to insects but was clastogenic in plant cells. It was not mutagenic in any standard assay in bacteria.

5.5 Evaluation

There is *inadequate evidence* in humans for the carcinogenicity of paracetamol.

There is *inadequate evidence* in experimental animals for the carcinogenicity of paracetamol.

Overall evaluation

Paracetamol is *not classifiable as to its carcinogenicity to humans (Group 3)*.

6. References

Allameh, A., Vansoun, E.Y. & Zarghi, A. (1997) Role of glutathione conjugation in protection of weanling rat liver against acetaminophen-induced hepatotoxicity. *Mech. Ageing Dev.*, **95**, 71–79

Amimoto, T., Matsura, T., Koyama, S.-Y., Nakanishi, T., Yamada, K. & Kajiyama, G. (1995) Acetaminophen-induced hepatic injury in mice: The role of lipid peroxidation and effects of pretreatment with coenzyme Q_{10} and α-tocopherol. *Free Radicals Biol. Med.*, **19**, 169–176

Arnaiz, S.L., Llesuy, S., Cutrín, J.C. & Boveris, A. (1995) Oxidative stress by acute acetaminophen administration in mouse liver. *Free Radicals Biol. Med.*, **19**, 303–310

Baranowitz, S.A. & Maderson, P.F.A. (1995) Acetaminophen toxicity is substantially reduced by beta-carotene in mice. *Int. J. Vit. Nutr. Res.*, **65**, 175–180

Beck, M.J., Lightle, R.L.-F., Harris, C. & Philbert, M.A. (1997) Maternal exposure to acetaminophen induces alterations in embryonic mitochondrial enzyme activities (Abstract). *Toxicologist*, **36**, 102

Berlin, C.M., Jr, Yaffe, S.J. & Ragni, M. (1980) Disposition of acetaminophen in milk, saliva and plasma of lactating women. *Pediatr. Pharmacol.*, **1**, 135–141

Birge, R.B., Bartolone, J.B., Nishanian, E.V., Bruno, M.K., Mangold, J.B., Cohen, S.D. & Khairallah, E.A. (1988) Dissociation of covalent binding from the oxidative effects of acetaminophen. *Biochem. Pharmacol.*, **37**, 3383–3393

Birge, R.B., Bartolone, J.B., Tyson, C.A., Emeigh Hart, S.G., Cohen, S.D. & Khairallah, E.A. (1990) Selective binding of acetaminophen (APAP) to liver proteins in mice and men. In: Witmer, C.M., ed., *Biological Reactive Intermediates IV*, New York, Plenum Press, pp. 685–688

Black, M. (1984) Acetaminophen hepatotoxicity. *Ann. Rev. Med.*, **35**, 577–593

Blakely, P. & McDonald, B.R. (1995) Acute renal failure due to acetaminophen ingestion: A case report and review of the literature. *J. Am. Soc. Nephrol.*, **6**, 48–53

Blazka, M.E., Wilmer, J.L., Holladay, S.D., Wilson, R.E. & Luster, M.I. (1995) Role of proinflammatory cytokines in acetaminophen hepatotoxicity. *Toxicol. appl. Pharmacol.*, **133**, 43–52

Blazka, M.E., Germolec, D.R., Simeonova, P.P., Bruccoleri, A., Pennypacker, K.R. & Luster, M.I. (1996a) Acetaminophen-induced hepatotoxicity is associated with early changes in NF-kB and NF-IL6 DNA binding activity. *J. Inflammation*, **47**, 138–150

Blazka, M.E., Elwell, M.R., Holladay, S.D., Wilson, R.E. & Luster, M.I. (1996b) Histopathology of acetaminophen-induced liver changes: Role of interleukin 1α and tumor necrosis factor α. *Toxicol. Pathol.*, **24**, 181–189

Blazka, M.E., Bruccoleri, A., Simeonova, P.P., Germolec, D.R., Pennypacker, K.R. & Luster, M. (1996c) Acetaminophen induced hepatotoxicity is associated with early changes in AP-1 DNA binding activity. *Res. Comm. mol. Pathol. Pharmacol.*, **92**, 259–273

Boess, F., Bopst, M., Althaus, R., Polsky, S., Cohen, S.D., Eugster, H.-P. & Boelsterli, U.A. (1998) Acetaminophen hepatotoxicity in tumor necrosis factor/lymphotoxin-alpha gene knockout mice. *Hepatology*, **27**, 1021–1029

Boyd, E.M. & Bereczky, G.M. (1966) Liver necrosis from paracetamol. *Br. J. Pharmacol.*, **26**, 606–614

Boyd, E.M. & Hogan, S.E. (1968) The chronic oral toxicity of paracetamol at the range of the LD_{50} (100 days) in albino rats. *Can J. Physiol. Pharmacol.*, **46**, 239–245

Bulera, S.J., Cohen, S.D. & Khairallah, E.A. (1996) Acetaminophen-arylated proteins are detected in hepatic subcellular fractions and numerous extra-hepatic tissues in CD-1 and C57B1/6J mice. *Toxicology*, **109**, 85–99

Burcham, P.C. & Harman, A.W. (1990) Mitochondrial dysfunction in paracetamol hepatotoxicity: In vitro studies in isolated mouse hepatocytes. *Toxicol. Lett.*, **50**, 37–48

Burrell, J.H., Yong, J.L.C. & Macdonald, G.J. (1991) Analgesic nephropathy in Fischer 344 rats: Comparative effects of chronic treatment with either aspirin or paracetamol. *Pathology*, **23**, 107–114

Camus, A.M., Friesen, M., Croisy, A. & Bartsch, H. (1982) Species-specific activation of phenacetin into bacterial mutagens by hamster liver enzymes and identification of N-hydroxyphenacetin O-glucuronide as a promutagen in the urine. *Cancer Res.*, **42**, 3201–3208

Chemical Information Services (1995) *Directory of World Chemical Producers 1995/96 Standard Edition*, Dallas, TX, p. 4

Chen, W., Koenigs, L.L., Thompson, S.J., Peter, R.M., Rettie, A.E., Trager, W.F. & Nelson, S.D. (1998) Oxidation of acetaminophen to its toxic quinone imine and nontoxic catechol metabolites by baculovirus-expressed and purified human cytochromes P450 2E1 and 2A6. *Chem. Res. Toxicol.*, **11**, 295–301

Chow, W.-H., McLaughlin, J.K., Linet, M.S., Niwa, S. & Mandel, J.S. (1994) Use of analgesics and risk of renal cell cancer. *Int. J. Cancer*, **59**, 467–470

Clements, J.A., Heading, R.C., Nimmo, W.S. & Prescott, L.F. (1978) Kinetics of acetaminophen absorption and gastric emptying in man. *Clin. Pharmacol. Ther.*, **24**, 420–431

Cohen, S.D., Pumford, N.R., Khairallah, E.A., Boekelheide, K., Pohl, L.R., Amouzadeh, H.R. & Hinson, J.A. (1997) Selective protein covalent binding and target organ toxicity. *Toxicol. appl. Pharmacol.*, **143**, 1–12

Collins, E. (1981) Maternal and fetal effects of acetaminophen and salicylates in pregnancy. *Obstet. Gynecol.*, **58**, 57s–62s

Cramer, D.W., Harlow, B.L., Titus-Ernstoff, L., Bohlke, K., Welch, W.R. & Greenberg, E.R. (1998) Over-the-counter analgesics and risk of ovarian cancer. *Lancet*, **351**, 104–107

Critchley, J.A.J.H., Dyson, E.H., Scott, A.W., Jarvie, D.R. & Prescott, L.F. (1983) Is there a place for cimetidine or ethanol in the treatment of paracetamol poisoning. *Lancet*, **ii**, 1375–1376

Dahlin, D.C., Miwa, G.T., Lu, A.Y.H. & Nelson, S.D. (1984) N-Acetyl-p-benzoquinone imine: A cytochrome P-450-mediated oxidation product of acetaminophen. *Proc. natl Acad. Sci. USA*, **81**, 1327–1331

Davidson, D.G.D. & Eastham, W.N. (1966) Acute liver necrosis following overdose of paracetamol. *Br. med. J.*, **ii**, 497–499

Davis, D.C., Potter, W.Z., Jollow, D.J. & Mitchell, J.R. (1974) Species differences in hepatic glutathione depletion, covalent binding and hepatic necrosis after acetaminophen. *Life Sci.*, **14**, 2099–2109

Davis, M., Harrison, N.G., Ideo, G., Portman, B., Labadarios, D. & Williams, R. (1976) Paracetamol metabolism in the rat: relationship to covalent binding and hepatic damage. *Xenobiotica*, **6**, 249–255

Derby, L.E. & Jick, H. (1996) Acetaminophen and renal and bladder cancer. *Epidemiology*, **7**, 358–362

Dixon, M.F., Nimmo, J. & Prescott, L.F. (1971) Experimental paracetamol-induced hepatic necrosis: A histopathological study. *J. Pathol.*, **103**, 225–229

Dunn, T.L., Gardiner, R.A., Seymour, G.J. & Lavin, M.F. (1987) Genotoxicity of analgesic compounds assessed by an *in vitro* micronucleus assay. *Mutat. Res.*, **189**, 299–306

Dybing, E., Holme, J.A., Gordon, W.P., Soderlund, E.J., Dahlin, D.C. & Nelson, S.D. (1984) Genotoxicity studies with paracetamol. *Mutat. Res.*, **138**, 21–32

Eguia, L. & Materson, B.J. (1997) Acetaminophen-related acute renal failure without fulminant liver failure. *Pharmacotherapy*, **17**, 363–370

Ellouk-Achard, S., Levresse, V., Martin, C., Pham-Huy, C., Dutertre-Catella, H., Thevenin, M., Warnet, J.M. & Claude, J.R. (1992) *Ex vivo* and *in vitro* models in acetaminophen hepatotoxicity studies. Relationship between glutathione depletion, oxidative stress and disturbances in calcium homeostasis and energy metabolism. *Res. Comm. mol. Pathol. Pharmacol.*, **92**, 209–214

Emeigh Hart, S.G., Beierschmitt, W.P., Bartolone, J.B., Wyand, D.S., Khairallah, E.A. & Cohen, S.D. (1991) Evidence against deacetylation and for cytochrome P450-mediated activation in acetaminophen-induced nephrotoxicity in the CD-1 mouse. *Toxicol. appl. Pharmacol.*, **107**, 1–15

Emeigh Hart, S.G., Cartun, R.W., Wyand, D.S., Khairallah, E.A. & Cohen, S.D. (1995) Immunohistochemical localization of acetaminophen in target tissues of the CD-1 mouse: Correspondence of covalent binding with toxicity. *Fundam. appl. Toxicol.*, **24**, 260–274

Emeigh Hart, S.G., Wyand, D.S., Khairallah, E.A. & Cohen, S.D. (1996) Acetaminophen nephrotoxicity in the CD-1 mouse. II. Protection by probenecid and AT-125 without diminution of renal covalent binding. *Toxicol. appl. Pharmacol.*, **136**, 161–169

Flaks, B., Flaks, A. & Shaw, A.P.W. (1985) Induction by paracetamol of bladder and liver tumours in the rat. *Acta path. microbiol. immunol. scand. Sect. A*, **93**, 367–377

Forrest, J.A.H., Clements, J.A. & Prescott, L.F. (1982) Clinical pharmacokinetics of paracetamol. *Clin. Pharmacokinet.*, **7**, 93–107

Fort, D., Rayburn, J.R. & Bantle, J.A. (1992) Evaluation of acetaminophen-induced developmental toxicity using FETAX. *Drug chem. Toxicol.*, **15**, 329–250

Friedman, J.M. & Polifka, J.E., eds (1994) *Teratogenic Effects of Drugs: A Resource for Clinicians: TERIS*, Baltimore, The Johns Hopkins University Press, pp. 2–4

Galinsky, R.E. & Levy, G. (1981) Dose- and time-dependent elimination of acetaminophen in rats: Pharmacokinetic implications of cosubstrate depletion. *J. Pharmacol. exp. Ther.*, **219**, 14–20

Gardner, C.R., Heck, D.E., Yang, C.S., Thomas, P.E., Zhang, X.-J., DeGeorge, G.L., Laskin, J.D. & Laskin, D.L. (1998) Role of nitric oxide in acetaminophen-induced hepatotoxicity in the rat. *Hepatology*, **27**, 748–754

Gazzard, B.G., Ford-Hutchinson, A.W., Smith, M.J.H. & Williams, R. (1973) The binding of paracetamol to plasma protein of man and pig. *J. pharm. Pharmacol.*, **25**, 964–967

Gemborys, M.W. & Mudge, G.H. (1981) Formation and disposition of the minor metabolites of acetaminophen in the hamster. *Drug Metab. Disposition*, **9**, 340–351

Gibson, J.D., Pumford, N.R., Samokyszyn, V.M. & Hinson, J.A. (1996) Mechanism of acetaminophen induced hepatotoxicity: Covalent binding versus oxidative stress. *Chem. Res. Toxicol.*, **9**, 580–585

Gregus, Z., Madhu, C. & Klaassen, C.D. (1988) Species variation in toxication and detoxication of acetaminophen *in vivo*: A comparative study of biliary and urinary excretion of acetaminophen metabolites. *J. Pharmacol. exp. Ther.*, **244**, 91–99

Gwilt, J.R., Robertson, A. & McChesney, E.W. (1963) Determination of blood and other tissue concentrations of paracetamol in dog and man. *J. Pharm. Pharmacol.*, **15**, 440–444

Hagiwara, A. & Ward, J.M. (1986) The chronic hepatotoxic, tumor-promoting and carcinogenic effects of acetaminophen in male B6C3F mice. *Fundam. appl. Toxicol.*, **7**, 376–386

Ham, K.N. & Calder, I.C. (1984) Tumor formation induced by phenacetin and its metabolites. *Adv. Inflammation Res.*, **6**, 139–148

Hamlyn, A.N., Douglas, A.P., James, O.F.W., Lesna, M. & Watson, A.J. (1977) Liver function and structure in survivors of acetaminophen poisoning: A follow-up study of serum bile acids and liver histology. *Am. J. dig. Dis.*, **22**, 605–610

Hansch, C., Leo, A. & Hoekman, D. (1995) *Exploring QSAR*, Washington DC, American Chemical Society, p. 43

Hantson, P., de Saint-Georges, L., Mahieu, P., Léonard, E.D., Crutzen-Fayt, M.C. & Leonard, A. (1996) Evaluation of the ability of paracetamol to produce chromosome aberrations in man. *Mutat. Res.*, **368**, 293–300

Harris, C., Lightle, R.L.-F., Larsen, S.J.V. & Phibert, M.A. (1997) Spatial and temporal localization of glutathione (GSH) in the organogenesis-stage rat conceptus (Abstract). *Toxicologist*, **36**, 102

Haworth, S., Lawlor, T., Mortelmans, K., Speck, W. & Zeiger, E. (1983) Salmonella mutagenicity test results for 250 chemicals. *Environ. Mutag.*, **5** (Suppl. 1), 1–142

Hazelton, G.A., Hjelle, J.J. & Klaassen, C.D. (1986) Effects of butylated hydroxyanisole on acetaminophen hepatotoxicity and glucuronidation *in vivo*. *Toxicol. appl. Pharmacol.*, **83**, 474–485

Hirate, J., Zhu, C.-Y., Horikoshi, I. & Bhargava, V.O. (1990) First-pass metabolism of acetaminophen in rats after low and high doses. *Biopharm. Drug Disposition*, **11**, 245–252

Hjelle, J.J. & Klaassen, C.D. (1984) Glucuronidation and biliary excretion of acetaminophen in rats. *J. Pharmacol. exp. Ther.*, **228**, 407–413

Hoivik, D.J., Manautou, J.E., Tveit, A., Emeigh Hart, S.G., Khairallah, E.A. & Cohen, S.D. (1995) Gender-related differences in susceptibility to acetaminophen-induced protein arylation and nephrotoxicity in the CD-1 mouse. *Toxicol. appl. Pharm.*, **130**, 257–271

Holme, J.A., Hongslo, J.K., Bjornstad, C., Harvison, P.J. & Nelson, S.D. (1988) Toxic effects of paracetamol and related structures in V79 Chinese hamster cells. *Mutagenesis*, **3**, 51–56

Hongslo, J.K., Christensen, T., Brunborg, G., Bjornstad, C. & Holme, J.A. (1988) Genotoxic effects of paracetamol in V79 Chinese hamster cells. *Mutat. Res.*, **204**, 333–341

Hongslo, J.K., Bjorge, C., Schwarze, P.E., Brogger, A., Mann, G., Thelander, L. & Holme, J.A. (1990) Paracetamol inhibits replicative DNA synthesis and induces sister chromatid exchange and chromosomal aberrations by inhibition of ribonucleotide reductase. *Mutagenesis*, **5**, 475–480

Hongslo, J.K., Brøgger, A., Bjørge, C. & Holme, J.A. (1991) Increased frequency of sister-chromatid exchange and chromatid breaks in lymphocytes after treatment of human volunteers with therapeutic doses of paracetamol. *Mutat. Res.*, **261**, 1–8

Hongslo, J.K., Smith, C.V., Brunborg, G., Soderlund, E.J. & Holme, J.A. (1994) Genotoxicity of paracetamol in mice and rats. *Mutagenesis*, **9**, 93–100

Hu, J.J., Lee, M.-J., Vapiwala, M., Reuhl, K., Thomas, P.E. & Yang, C.S. (1993) Sex-related differences in mouse renal metabolism and toxicity of acetaminophen. *Toxicol. appl. Pharmacol.*, **122**, 16–26

Hu, J.J., Yoo, J.-S.H., Lin, M., Wang, E.-J. & Yang, C.S., (1996) Protective effects of diallyl sulfide on acetaminophen-induced toxicities. *Food chem. Toxicol.*, **34**, 963–969

IARC (1987) *IARC Monographs on the Evaluation of Carcinogenic Risks to Humans*, Suppl. 7, *Overall Evaluations of Carcinogenicity: An Updating of* IARC Monographs *Volumes 1 to 42*, Lyon, pp. 310–312

IARC (1990) *IARC Monographs on the Evaluation of Carcinogenic Risks to Humans*, Vol. 50, *Pharmaceutical Drugs*, Lyon, pp. 307–332

Insel, P.A. (1996) Analgesic–antipyretic and antiinflammatory agents and drugs employed in the treatment of gout. In: Hardman, J.G. & Limbird, L.E., eds, *Goodman & Gilman's, The Pharmacological Basis of Therapeutics*, 9th Ed., New York, McGraw-Hill, pp. 631–633

Ishidate, M., Jr, Hayashi, M., Sawada, M., Matsuoka, A., Yoshikawa, K., Ono, M. & Nakadate, M. (1978) Cytotoxicity test on medical drugs—Chromosome aberration tests with Chinese hamster cells *in vitro*. *Bull. natl Inst. Hyg. Sci. (Tokyo)*, **96**, 55–61

James, O., Lesna, M., Roberts, S.H., Pulman, L., Douglas, A.P., Smith, P.A. & Watson, A.J. (1975) Liver damage after paracetamol overdose: Comparison of liver function tests, fasting serum bile acids and liver histology. *Lancet*, **ii**, 579–581

James, R.C., Harbison, R.D. & Roberts, S.M. (1993) Phenylpropanolamine potentiation of acetaminophen-induced hepatotoxicity: Evidence for a glutathione-dependent mechanism. *Toxicol. appl. Pharmacol.*, **118**, 159–168

Jasiewicz, M.L. & Richardson, J.C. (1987) Absence of mutagenic activity of benorylate, paracetamol and aspirin in the *Salmonella*/mammalian microsome test. *Mutat. Res.*, **190**, 95–100

Johansson, S.L., Radio, S.J., Saidi, J. & Sakata, T. (1989) The effects of acetaminophen, antipyrine and phenacetin on rat urothelial cell proliferation. *Carcinogenesis*, **10**, 105–111

Kamiyama, T., Sato, C., Liu, J., Tajiri, K., Miyakawa, H. & Marumo, F. (1993) Role of lipid peroxidation in acetaminophen-induced hepatotoxicity: Comparison with carbon tetrachloride. *Toxicol. Lett.*, **66**, 7–12

Kaysen, G.A., Pond, S.M., Roper, M.H., Menke, D.J. & Marrama, M.A. (1985) Combined hepatic and renal injury in alcoholics during therapeutic use of acetaminophen. *Arch. intern. Med.*, **145**, 2019–2023

Khandkar, M.A., Parmar, D.V., Das, M. & Katyare, S.S. (1996) Is activation of lysosomal enzymes responsible for paracetamol-induced hepatotoxicity and nephrotoxicity? *J. Pharm. Pharmacol.*, **48**, 437–440

King, M.-T., Beikirch, H., Eckhardt, K., Gocke, E. & Wild, D. (1979) Mutagenicity studies with X-ray-contrast media, analgesics, antipyretics, antirheumatics and some other pharmaceutical drugs in bacterial, *Drosophila* and mammalian test systems. *Mutat. Res.*, **66**, 33–43

Kirkland, D.J., Dresp, J.H., Marshall, R.R., Baumeister, M., Gerloff, C. & Gocke, E. (1992) Normal chromosomal aberration frequencies in peripheral lymphocytes of healthy human volunteers exposed to a maximum daily dose of paracetamol in a double blind trial. *Mutat. Res.*, **279**, 181–194

Koch-Weser, J. (1976) Drug therapy: acetaminophen. *New Engl. J. Med.*, **295**, 1297–1300

Kocišová, J. & Šrám, R.J. (1990) Mutagenicity studies on paracetamol in human volunteers. III. Cytokinesis block micronucleus method. *Mutat. Res.*, **244**, 27–30

Kocišová, J., Rossner, P., Binková, B., Bavorová, H. & Šrám, R.J. (1988) Mutagenicity studies on paracetamol in human volunteers. I. Cytogenetic analysis of peripheral lymphocytes and lipid peroxidation in plasma. *Mutat. Res.*, **209**, 161–165

Kourounakis, A.P., Rekka, E.A. & Kourounakis, P.N. (1997) Antioxidant activity of guaiazulene and protection against paracetamol hepatotoxicity in rats. *J. pharm. Pharmacol.*, **49**, 938–942

Kreiger, N., Marrett, L.D., Dodds, L., Hilditch, S. & Darlington, G.A. (1992) Risk factors for renal cell carcinoma: Results of a population-based case–control study. *Cancer Causes Control*, **4**, 101–110

Lee, S.S.T., Buters, J.T.M., Pineau,T., Fernandez-Salguero, P. & Gonzalez, F.J. (1996) Role of CYP2E1 in the hepatotoxicity of acetaminophen. *J. biol. Chem.*, **271**, 12063–12067

Lide, D.R., ed. (1997) *CRC Handbook of Chemistry and Physics*, 78th Ed., Boca Raton, FL, CRC Press, p. 3-4

Linet, M.S., Chow, W.-H., McLaughlin, J.K., Wacholder, S., Yu, M.C., Schoenberg, J.B., Lynch, C. & Fraumeni, J.F., Jr (1995) Analgesics and cancers of the renal pelvis and ureter. *Int. J. Cancer*, **62**, 15–18

Lowenthal, D.T., Øie, S., Van Stone, J.C., Briggs, W.A. & Levy, G. (1976) Pharmacokinetics of acetaminophen elimination by anephric patients. *J. Pharmacol. exp. Ther.*, **196**, 570–578

Macheras, P., Parissi-Poulos, M. & Poulos, L. (1989) Pharmacokinetics of acetaminophen after intramuscular administration. *Biopharm. Drug Disposition*, **10**, 101–105

Maruyama, H. & Williams, G.M. (1988) Hepatotoxicity of chronic high dose administration of acetaminophen to mice. A critical review and implications for hazard assessment. *Arch. Toxicol.*, **62**, 465–469

Maruyama, H., Takashima, Y., Murata, Y., Nakae, D., Eimoto, H., Tsutsumi, M., Denda, A. & Konishi, Y. (1990) Lack of hepatocarcinogenic potential of acetaminophen in rats with liver damage associated with a choline-devoid diet. *Carcinogenesis,* **11**, 895–901

McCredie, M. & Stewart, J.H. (1988) Does paracetamol cause urothelial cancer or renal papillary necrosis? *Nephron*, **49**, 296–300

McCredie, M., Ford, J.M. & Stewart, J.H. (1988) Risk factors for cancer of the renal parenchym. *Int. J. Cancer*, **42**, 13–16

McCredie, M., Stewart, J.H. & Day, N.E. (1993) Different roles for phenacetin and paracetamol in cancer of the kidney and renal pelvis. *Int. J. Cancer*, **53**, 245–249

McCredie, M., Pommer, W., McLaughlin, J.K., Stewart, J.H., Lindblad, P., Mandel, J.S., Mellemgaard, A., Schlehofer, B. & Niwa, S. (1995) International renal-cell cancer study. II. Analgesics. *Int. J. Cancer*, **60**, 345–349

McElhatton, P.R., Sullivan, F.M. & Volans, G.N. (1997) Paracetamol overdose in pregnancy, analysis of the outcome of 300 cases referred to the Teratology Information Service. *Reprod. Toxicol.*, **11**, 85–94

McLaughlin, J.K., Blot, W.J., Mehl, E.S. & Fraumeni, J.F., Jr (1985) Relation of analgesic use to renal cancer: Population-based findings. *Natl Cancer Inst. Monogr.*, **69**, 217–222

McMurtry, R.J., Snodgrass, W.R. & Mitchell, J.R. (1978) Renal necrosis, glutathione depletion and covalent binding after acetaminophen. *Toxicol. appl. Pharmacol.*, **46**, 87–100

Mellemgaard, A., Niwa, S., Mehl, E.S., Engholm, G., McLaughlin, J.K. & Olsen, J.H. (1994) Risk factors for renal cell carcinoma in Denmark: Role of medication and medical history. *Int. J. Epidemiol.*, **23**, 923–930

Mirasol, F. (1998) Acetaminophen market sees moderate price hike. *Chem. Mark. Rep.*, **254**, 5, 12

Mitchell, J.R., Jollow, D.J., Potter, W.Z., Davis, D.C., Gillette, J.R. & Brodie, B.B. (1973) Acetaminophen-induced hepatic necrosis. I. Role of drug metabolism. *J. Pharmacol. exp. Ther.*, **187**, 185–194

Mitchell, J.R., Thorgeirsson, S.S., Potter, W.Z., Jollow, D.J. & Keiser, H. (1974) Acetaminophen-induced hepatic injury: Protective role of glutathione in man and rationale for therapy. *Clin. Pharmacol. Ther.*, **16**, 676–684

Möller-Hartmann, W. & Siegers, C.-P. (1991) Nephrotoxicity of paracetamol in the rat—Mechanistic and therapeutic aspects. *J. appl. Toxicol.*, **11**, 141–146

Moore, M., Thor, H., Moore, G., Nelson, S., Moldéus, P. & Orrenius, S. (1985) The toxicity of acetaminophen and N-acetyl-*p*-benzoquinone imine in isolated hepatocytes is associated with thiol depletion and increased cytosolic Ca^{2+}. *J. biol. Chem.*, **260**, 13035–13040

Morris, M.E. & Levy, G. (1984) Renal clearance and serum protein binding of acetaminophen and its major conjugates in humans. *J. pharm. Sci.*, **73**, 1038–1041

Mueller, L., Kasper, P. & Madle, S. (1991) Further investigations on the clastogenicity of paracetamol and acetylsalicylic acid *in vitro*. *Mutat. Res.*, **263**, 83–92

Mueller-Tegethoff, K., Kasper, P. & Mueller, L. (1995) Evaluation studies on the *in vitro* rat hepatocyte micronucleus assay. *Mutat. Res.*, **335**, 293–307

Mugford, C.A. & Tarloff, J.B. (1995) Contribution of oxidation and deacetylation to the bioactivation of acetaminophen *in vitro* in liver and kidney from male and female Sprague-Dawley rats. *Drug Metab. Disposition*, **23**, 290–294

Mugford, C.A. & Tarloff, J.B. (1997) The contribution of oxidation and deacetylation to acetaminophen nephrotoxicity in female Sprague-Dawley rats. *Toxicol. Lett.*, **93**, 15–22

National Institute for Occupational Safety and Health (1998) *National Occupational Exposure Survey (1981–1983)*, Cincinnati, OH

National Toxicology Program (1991) *NTP Chemical Repository Data Sheet: Acetaminophen (4-Hydroxyacetanilide)*, Research Triangle Park, NC

National Toxicology Program (1993) *Toxicology and Carcinogenesis Studies of Acetaminophen (CAS No. 103-90-2) in F344/N Rats and B6C3F$_1$ Mice (Feed Studies)* (Tech. Rep. Ser. No. 394; NIH Publ. No. 93-2849), Research Triangle Park, NC

National Toxicology Program (1997) Acetaminophen. *Environ. Health Perspectives*, **105** (Suppl. 1), 267–268

Newton, J.F., Kuo, C.-H., Gemborys, M.W., Mudge, G.H. & Hook, J.B. (1982) Nephrotoxicity of *p*-aminophenol, a metabolite of acetaminophen, in the Fischer 344 rat. *Toxicol. appl. Pharmacol.*, **65**, 336–344

Newton, J.F., Pasino, D.A. & Hook, J.B. (1985) Acetaminophen nephrotoxicity in the rat: Quantitation of renal metabolic activation *in vivo*. *Toxicol. appl. Pharmacol.*, **78**, 39–46

Notarianni, L.J., Oldham, H.G. & Bennet, P.N. (1987) Passage of paracetamol into breast milk and its subsequent metabolism by the neonate. *Br. J. clin. Pharmacol.*, **24**, 63–67

Oldham, J.W., Preston, R.F. & Pauson, J.D. (1986) Mutagenicity testing of selected analgesics in Ames *Salmonella* strains. *J. appl. Toxicol.*, **6**, 237–243

Özdemirler, G., Aykaç, G., Uysal, M. & Öz, H. (1994) Liver lipid peroxidation and glutathione-related defence enzyme systems in mice treated with paracetamol. *J. appl. Toxicol.*, **14**, 297–299

Patierno, S.R., Lehman, N.L., Henderson, B.E. & Landolph, J.R. (1989) Study of the ability of phenacetin, acetaminophen, and aspirin to induce cytotoxicity, mutation, and morphological transformation on C3H/10Tfi clone 8 mouse embryo cells. *Cancer Res.*, **49**, 1038–1044

Patten, C.J., Thomas, P.E., Guy, R.L., Lee, M., Gonzalez, F.J., Guengerich, F.P. & Yang, C.S. (1993) Cytochrome P450 enzymes involved in acetaminophen activation by rat and human liver microsomes and their kinetics. *Chem. Res. Toxicol.*, **6**, 511–518

Perneger, T.V., Whelton, P.K. & Klag, M.J. (1994) Risk of kidney failure associated with the use of acetaminophen, aspirin and nonsteroidal antiinflammatory drugs. *New Engl. J. Med.*, **331**, 1675–1679

Piper, J.M., Tonascia, J. & Matanoski, G.M. (1985) Heavy phenacetin use and bladder cancer in women aged 20 to 49 years. *New Engl. J. Med.*, **313**, 292–295

Placke, M.E., Ginsberg, G.L., Wyand, D.S. & Cohen, S.D. (1987a) Ultrastructural changes during acute acetaminophen-induced hepatotoxicity in the mouse: A time and dose study. *Toxicol. Pathol.*, **15**, 431–438

Placke, M.E., Wyand, D.S. & Cohen, S.D. (1987b) Extrahepatic lesions induced by acetaminophen in the mouse. *Toxicol. Pathol.*, **15**, 381–387

Potter, D.W. & Hinson, J.A. (1987a) The 1- and 2-electron oxidation of acetaminophen catalyzed by prostaglandin *H* synthase. *J. biol. Chem.*, **262**, 974–980

Potter, D.W. & Hinson, J.A. (1987b) Mechanisms of acetaminophen oxidation to N-acetyl-p-benzoquinone imine by horseradish peroxidase and cytochome P-450. *J. biol. Chem.*, **262**, 966–973

Potter, W.Z., Davis, D.C., Mitchell, J.R., Jollow, D.J., Gillette, J.R. & Brodie, B.B. (1973) Acetaminophen-induced hepatic necrosis. III. Cytochrome P-450-mediated covalent binding *in vitro*. *J. Pharmacol. exp. Ther.*, **187**, 203–210

Prescott, L.F., Mattison, P., Menzies, D.G. & Manson, L.M. (1990) The comparative effects of paracetamol and indomethacin on renal function in healthy female volunteers. *Br. J. clin. Pharmacol.*, **29**, 403–412

Rannug, U., Holme, J.A., Hongslo, J.K. & Šrám, R.J. (1995) An evalution of the genetic toxicity of paracetamol. *Mutat. Res.*, **327**, 179–200

Raucy, J.L., Lasker, J.M., Lieber, C.S. & Black, M. (1989) Acetaminophen activation by human liver cytochromes P450IIE1 and P450IA2. *Arch. Biochem. Biophys.*, **271**, 270–283

Rawlins, M.D., Henderson, D.B. & Hijab, A.R. (1977) Pharmacokinetics of paracetamol (acetaminophen) after intravenous and oral administration. *Eur. J. clin. Pharmacol.*, **11**, 283–286

Ray, S.D., Sorge, C.L., Raucy, J.L. & Corcoran, G.B. (1990) Early loss of large genomic DNA *in vivo* with accumulation of Ca^{2+} in the nucleus during acetaminophen-induced liver injury. *Toxicol. appl. Pharmacol.*, **106**, 346–351

Reddy, G.A. (1984) Effects of paracetamol on chromosomes of bone marrow. *Caryologia*, **37**, 127–132

Reddy, G.A. & Subramanyam, S. (1981) Response of mitotic cells of *Allium cepa* to paracetamol. In: Manna, G.K. & Sinha, U., eds, *Perspectives in Cytology and Genetics*, Vol. 3, Delhi, Hindasi Publishers, pp. 571–576

Reddy, G.A. & Subramanyam, S. (1985) Cytogenetic response of meiocytes of Swiss albino mice to paracetamol. *Caryologia*, **38**, 347–355

Reel, J.R., Lawton, A.D. & Lamb, J.C., IV (1992) Reproductive toxicity evaluation of acetaminophen in Swiss CD-1 mice using a continuous breeding protocol. *Fundam. appl. Toxicol.*, **18**, 233–239

Reynolds, J.E.F., ed. (1996) *Martindale: The Extra Pharmacopoeia*, 31st Ed., London, Pharmaceutical Press

Richie, J.P., Jr, Lang, C.A. & Chen, T.S. (1992) Acetaminophen-induced depletion of glutathione and cysteine in the aging mouse kidney. *Biochem. Pharmacol.*, **44**, 129–135

Rogers, L.K., Moorthy, B. & Smith, C.V. (1997) Acetaminophen binds to mouse hepatic and renal DNA at human therapeutic doses. *Chem. Res. Toxicol.*, **10**, 470–476

Rosenberg, L., Rao, R.S., Palmer, J.R., Strom, B.L., Zauber, A., Warschauer, E., Stolley, P.D. & Shapiro, S. (1998) Transitional cell cancer of the orinary tract and renal cell cancer in relation to acetaminophen use (United States). *Cancer Causes Control*, **9**, 83–88

Ross, R.K., Paganini-Hill, A., Landolph, J., Gerkins, V. & Henderson, B.E. (1989) Analgesics, cigarette smoking, and other risk factors for cancer of the renal pelvis and ureter. *Cancer Res.*, **49**, 1045–1048

Sandler, D.P., Smith, J.C., Weinberg, C.R., Buckalew, V.M., Dennis, V.W., Blythe, W.B. & Burgess, W.P. (1989) Analgesic use and chronic renal disease. *New Engl. J. Med.*, **320**, 1238–1243

Sasaki, M., Sugimura, K., Yoshida, M.A. & Abe, S. (1980) Cytogenetic effects of 60 chemicals on cultured human and Chinese hamster cells. *Kromosomo*, **II-20**, 574–584

Satge, D., Sasco, A.J. & Little, J. (1998) Antenatal therapeutic drug exposure and fetal/neonatal tumours: Review of 89 cases. *Pediatr. perinatal. Epidemiol.*, **12**, 84–117

Savides, M.C. & Oehme, F.W. (1983) Acetaminophen and its toxicity. *J. appl. Toxicol.*, **3**, 96–111

Savides, M.C., Oehme, F.W., Nash, S.L. & Leipold, H.W. (1984) The toxicity and biotransformation of single doses of acetaminophen in dogs and cats. *Toxicol. appl. Pharmacol.*, **74**, 26–34

Severin, E. & Beleuta, A. (1995) Induction of chromosome aberrations *in vivo* bone-marrow cells of mice by paracetamol. *Morphol.-Embryol.*, **XLI**, 117–120

Shaw, G.M., Todoroff, K., Velie, E.M. & Lammer, E.J. (1998) Maternal illness, including fever, and medication use as risk factors for neural tube defects. *Teratology*, **57**, 1–7

Shen, W., Kamendulis, L.M., Ray, S.D. & Corcoran, G.B. (1992) Acetaminophen-induced cytotoxicity in cultured mouse hepatocytes: Effects of Ca^{2+}-endonuclease, DNA repair and glutathione depletion inhibitors on DNA fragmentation and cell death. *Toxicol. appl. Pharmacol.*, **112**, 32–40

Shibata, M.-A., Sano, M., Hagiwara, A., Hasegawa, R. & Shirai, T. (1995) Modification by analgesics of lesion development in the urinary tract and various other organs of rats pretreated with dihydroxy-di-N-propylnitrosamine and uracil. *Jpn. J. Cancer Res.*, **86**, 160–167

Siegers, C.-P., Strubelt, O. & Schütt, A. (1978) Relationships between hepatotoxicity and pharmacokinetics of paracetamol in rats and mice. *Pharmacology*, **16**, 273–278

Spühler, O. & Zollinger, H.U. (1950) [Chronic interstitial nephritis.] *Helv. Med.*, **17**, 564–567 (in German)

Steineck, G., Wilholm, B.E. & Gerhardsson-de Verdier, M. (1995) Acetaminophen, some other drugs, some diseases and the risk of transitional cell carcinoma. A population-based case–control study. *Acta oncol.*, **34**, 741–748

Thummel, K.E., Slattery, J.T., Nelson, S.D., Lee, C.A. & Pearson, P.G. (1989) Effect of ethanol on hepatotoxicity of acetaminophen in mice and on reactive metabolite formation by mouse and human liver microsomes. *Toxicol. appl. Pharmacol.*, **100**, 391–397

Topinka, J., Šrám, R.J., Širinjan, G., Kocišová, J., Binková, B. & Fojtíková, I. (1989) Mutagenicity studies on paracetamol in human volunteers. II. Unscheduled DNA synthesis and micronucleus test. *Mutat. Res.*, **227**, 147–152

Trumper, L., Girardi, G. & Elías, M.M. (1992) Acetaminophen nephrotoxicity in male Wistar rats. *Arch. Toxicol.*, **66**, 107–111

Trumper, L., Monasterolo, L.A., Ochoa, E. & Elías, M.M. (1995) Tubular effects of acetaminophen in the isolated perfused rat kidney. *Arch. Toxicol.*, **69**, 248–252

Trumper, L., Monasterolo, L.A. & Elías, M.M. (1996) Nephrotoxicity of acetaminophen in male Wistar rats: Role of hepatically derived metabolites. *J. Pharmacol. exp. Ther.*, **279**, 548–554

Tsokos-Kuhn, J.O., Hughes, H., Smith, C.V. & Mitchell, J.R. (1988) Alkylation of the liver plasma membrane and inhibition of the Ca^{2+} ATPase by acetaminophen. *Biochem. Pharmacol.*, **37**, 2125–2131

Tsuruzaki, T., Yamamoto, M. & Watanabe, G. (1982) Maternal consumption of antipyretic analgesics produces chromosome anomalies in F_1 embryos. *Teratology*, **26**, 42A

Verschueren, K. (1996) *Handbook of Environmental Data on Organic Chemicals*, 3rd Ed., New York, Van Nostrand Reinhold Co., p. 1444

Waalkes, M.P. & Ward, J.M. (1989) Induction of hepatic metallothionein in male B6C3F1 mice exposed to hepatic tumor promoters: effects of phenobarbital, acetaminophen, sodium barbital and di(2-ethylhexyl) phthalate. *Toxicol. appl. Pharmacol.*, **100**, 217–226

Ward, J.M., Hagiwara, A., Anderson, L.M., Lindsey, K. & Diwan, B.A. (1988) The chronic hepatic or renal toxicity of di(2-ethylhexyl) phthalate, acetaminophen, sodium barbital and phenobarbital in male B6C3F1 mice: Autoradiographic, immunohistochemical and biochemical evidence for levels of DNA synthesis not associated with carcinogenesis or tumor promotion. *Toxicol. appl. Pharmacol.*, **96**, 494–506

Watanabe, M. (1982) The cytogenetic effects of aspirin and acetaminophen on *in vitro* human lymphocytes. *Jpn. J. Hyg.*, **37**, 673–685

WHO (1993) *Guidelines for Drinking Water Quality*, 2nd Ed., Vol. 1, *Recommendations*, Geneva

Wiger, R., Hongslo, J.K., Evenson, D.P., De Angelis, P., Schwartze, P.E. & Holme, J.A. (1995) Effects of acetaminophen and hydroxyurea on spermatogenesis and sperm chromatin structure in laboratory mice. *Reprod. Toxicol.*, **9**, 21–33

Williams, G.M. & Iatropoulos, M.J. (1997) Inhibition by acetaminophen of intestinal cancer in rats induced by an aromatic amine similar to food mutagens. *Eur. J. Cancer Prev.*, **6**, 357–362

Wirth, P.J., Dybing, E., von Bahr, C. & Thorgeirsson, S.S. (1980) Mechanism of N-hydroxyacetylarylamine mutagenicity in the *Salmonella* test system: Metabolic activation of N-hydroxyphenacetin by liver and kidney fractions from rat, mouse, hamster, and man. *Mol. Pharmacol.*, **18**, 117–127

Wright, N. & Prescott, L.F. (1973) Potentiation by previous drug therapy of hepatotoxicity following paracetamol overdosage. *Scott. med. J.*, **18**, 56–58

ortho-PHENYLPHENOL AND ITS SODIUM SALT

These substances were considered by previous working groups, in 1982 (IARC, 1983) and 1987 (IARC, 1987). Since that time, new data have become available, and these have been incorporated into the monograph and taken into consideration in the present evaluation.

1. Exposure Data

1.1 Chemical and physical data

1.1.1 *Nomenclature*

***ortho*-Phenylphenol**

Chem. Abstr. Serv. Reg. No.: 90-43-7
Chem. Abstr. Name: (1,1′-Biphenyl)-2-ol
IUPAC Systematic Name: 2-Biphenylol
Synonyms: *ortho*-Biphenylol; *ortho*-diphenylol; *ortho*-hydroxybiphenyl; 2-hydroxy-biphenyl; 2-hydroxy-1,1′-biphenyl; *ortho*-hydroxydiphenyl; 2-hydroxydiphenyl; 2-phenylphenol; *ortho*-xenol

Sodium *ortho*-phenylphenate

Chem. Abstr. Serv. Reg. No.: 132-27-4
Chem. Abstr. Name: (1,1′-Biphenyl)-2-ol, sodium salt
IUPAC Systematic Name: 2-Biphenylol, sodium salt
Synonyms: *ortho*-Hydroxybiphenyl sodium salt; 2-hydroxybiphenyl sodium salt; 2-hydroxydiphenyl sodium; *ortho*-phenylphenol sodium salt; 2-phenylphenol sodium salt; sodium 2-biphenylolate; sodium 2-phenylphenate; sodium 2-phenylphenoxide; sodium *ortho*-phenylphenol; sodium *ortho*-phenylphenolate; sodium *ortho*-phenylphenoxide; SOPP

1.1.2 *Structural and molecular formulae and relative molecular mass*

***ortho*-Phenylphenol**

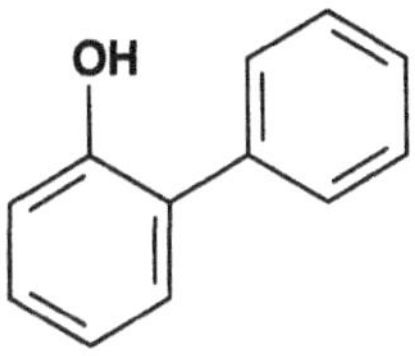

OH

$C_{12}H_{10}O$ Relative molecular mass: 170.21

Sodium *ortho*-phenylphenate

$C_{12}H_9ONa$ Relative molecular mass: 192.20

1.1.3 *Chemical and physical properties of the pure substance*

***ortho*-Phenylphenol**

(*a*) *Description*: White flaky crystals with a mild, characteristic odour (Budavari, 1996)

(*b*) *Boiling-point*: 286°C (Lide, 1997)

(*c*) *Melting-point*: 59°C (Lide, 1997)

(*d*) *Density*: 1.213 g/cm³ at 25°C (Lide, 1997)

(*e*) *Solubility*: Very slightly soluble in water (0.7 g/L at 25°C); soluble in ethanol and acetone; very soluble in diethyl ether (IARC, 1983; Lide, 1997)

(*f*) *Volatility*: Vapour pressure, 133 Pa at 100°C (National Toxicology Program, 1991a)

(*g*) *Octanol/water partition coefficient (P)*: log P, 3.09 (Hansch *et al.*, 1995)

(*h*) *Conversion factor*: mg/m³ = 6.96 × ppm

Sodium *ortho*-phenylphenate

(*a*) *Description*: White flakes (Lewis, 1993)

(*b*) *Solubility*: Soluble in water, ethanol and acetone (National Toxicology Program, 1991b; Lewis, 1993)

(*c*) *Conversion factor*: mg/m³ = 7.86 × ppm

1.2 Production and use

Information available in 1995 indicated that *ortho*-phenylphenol was produced in Germany, Japan, the United Kingdom and the United States and that sodium *ortho*-phenylphenate was produced in Germany and the United States (Chemical Information Service, 1995).

ortho-Phenylphenol and its sodium salt are used in the rubber industry, as agricultural fungicides and as disinfectants (National Toxicology Program, 1991b; Budavari, 1996). *ortho*-Phenylphenol is also used as an intermediate for dyes, resins and rubber chemicals, as a germicide, as a preservative and in food packaging. It is used as a disinfectant and fungicide for impregnation of fruit wrappers and disinfection of seed boxes and is applied during the dormant period to control apple canker. It is used as a reagent for the determination of trioses, as a household disinfectant and in dish-washing formulations (National Toxicology Program, 1991a).

1.3 Occurrence

1.3.1 *Natural occurrence*

ortho-Phenylphenol and sodium *ortho*-phenylphenate are not known to occur naturally.

1.3.2 *Occupational exposure*

According to the 1981–83 National Occupational Exposure Survey (National Institute for Occupational Safety and Health, 1998), approximately 620 000 and 56 000 workers in the United States were potentially exposed to *ortho*-phenylphenol and sodium *ortho*-phenylphenate, respectively. Occupational exposure to *ortho*-phenylphenol and/or its salt may occur during their production and use as chemical intermediates, fungicides, germicides, preservatives and disinfectants.

1.3.3 *Environmental occurrence*

According to the Environmental Protection Agency Toxic Chemical Release Inventory for 1987, 1400 kg *ortho*-phenylphenol were released into the air, 120 kg were discharged into water and 110 kg were released onto the land from manufacturing and processing facilities in the United States. By 1996, 1900 kg were released into the air and 110 kg were released onto the land (National Library of Medicine, 1998).

ortho-Phenylphenol has been found in some groundwater and drinking-water samples and in some fruits and juices (IARC, 1983).

1.4 Regulations and guidelines

No international guidelines for *ortho*-phenylphenol or for sodium *ortho*-phenylphenate in drinking-water have been established (WHO, 1993).

2. Studies of Cancer in Humans

No data were available to the Working Group.

3. Studies of Cancer in Experimental Animals

Previous evaluation

ortho-Phenylphenol was tested for carcinogenicity in mice and rats by administration in the diet. Sodium *ortho*-phenylphenate was tested in rats by administration in the diet. No evidence of carcinogenicity of *ortho*-phenylphenol was found in mice or rats, but both studies had some limitations. In rats, sodium *ortho*-phenylphenate was carcinogenic to the urinary tract, producing both benign and malignant tumours (IARC, 1983).

New studies

3.1 Oral administration

Mouse: Groups of 50 male and 50 female B6C3F$_1$ mice, six weeks of age, were fed diets containing sodium *ortho*-phenylphenate (97% pure) at concentrations of 0, 0.5, 1 or 2%; the actual concentrations achieved were 0.41, 0.82 and 1.6%. The mice were fed for 96 weeks and then continued on control diet for an additional eight weeks (total experimental period, 104 weeks). The survival rate of males but not females at the high dose was decreased, and the body weights of the males were significantly reduced throughout the experiment, while those of females were reduced from week 13. The body weights of females at 1% were reduced from week 26 and those of females at 0.5% from week 38. The mean body weight of males at 0.5% was significantly reduced in weeks 1–90. Five haemangiomas and five leiomyosarcomas of the uterus were found in female controls but only one haemangioma was found in treated females. Males given 1% had increased incidences of haemangiosarcomas of the liver, with none in controls and three, five and three in the three treated groups, respectively; and hepatocellular carcinomas were observed in 4, 9, 13 and 14 males and 4, 5, 7 and 0 females given 1 or 2%; however, the authors concluded on the basis of data for their historical controls that there was no treatment-associated carcinogenic effect (Hagiwara *et al.*, 1984).

Rat: Groups of 20–24 male F344/DuCrj rats, 38–39 days of age, were given *ortho*-phenylphenol (purity > 98%) in the diet at concentrations of 0 (control), 0.625, 1.25 or 2.5% for 91 weeks. Rats at the high dose consumed significantly less food and had a 17–24% lower weight gain compared to controls. The numbers of rats with bladder tumours were reported as: 0/24, 0/20, 23/24 ($p < 0.001$) and 4/23 in the controls and rats at the three doses, respectively. The 23 bladder tumours in rats at 1.25% were described as three papillomas, 15 non-invasive carcinomas and five invasive carcinomas (Hiraga & Fujii, 1984).

Groups of 50 male and 50 female Fischer 344/DuCrj rats, five weeks of age, were fed a pelleted diet containing 0, 0.7 or 2% (males) or 0, 0.5 or 1% (females) sodium *ortho*-phenylphenate (purity, 95.5% with 3.75% water, 0.72% free alkali as sodium hydroxide and 0.028% organic substances) for 104 weeks followed by two weeks on basal diet. Groups of 25 rats of each sex were fed the test diets containing 0, 0.25, 0.7 or 2% (males) and 0, 0.25, 0.5 or 1% (females) for 104 weeks and then basal diet until they died or were sacrificed in a moribund state. The mean body weights of males at 2% and females at 1% were lower than that of the controls throughout the first study; in the second study, males at 2% also showed lower mean body weights, but the growth of females at 1% after treatment was stopped was comparable to that of controls. The survival rate of the males but not females at the high dose decreased during weeks 50–100. The total numbers of rats with urinary bladder tumours were 0, 2 and 47 among males and 0, 1 and 4 among females treated for 106 weeks. In the second study, the numbers of rats with bladder tumours were 0, 0, 3 and 23 among males and 0, 0, 0 and 2 among females. Most of the tumours were carcinomas (Fujii & Hiraga, 1985).

3.2 Administration with known carcinogens or modifying factors

Mouse: Groups of 50 male and 50 female Swiss CD-1 mice, seven to eight weeks of age, were treated by dermal application of 55.5 mg *ortho*-phenylphenol (purity, > 99%, with water as the major impurity) in 0.1 mL acetone on three days per week for 102 weeks; with a single dermal application to the dorsal interscapular region of 0.05 mg dimethylbenz[*a*]anthracene (DMBA) in 0.1 mL acetone and then, one week later, with dermal applications at the site of DMBA application of either acetone (vehicle), *ortho*-phenylphenol (55.5 mg in 0.1 mL acetone) or 0.005 mg 12-*O*-tetradecanoylphorbol-13-acetate (TPA) in 0.1 mL acetone on three days per week for the remainder of the experiment; or dermal applications of acetone alone three times per week. All groups were treated for 103 weeks except males (85 weeks) and females (74 weeks) given DMBA plus TPA, which were killed before the end of the study because of the large number of deaths. The mean body weights of male mice receiving *ortho*-phenylphenol and those given DMBA plus *ortho*-phenylphenol were generally 5–10% lower than those receiving acetone after week 44. The mean body weights of females given DMBA plus TPA were higher than those of the other female groups during the first year of the study. The mean body weights of the remaining groups were similar to those of the corresponding controls. The survival rates of male and female mice given DMBA plus TPA were significantly lower than that of the controls, but the rates of all other groups were not significantly different from those of controls. The incidences of squamous-cell papillomas and carcinomas of the skin in males and females given DMBA plus TPA (18/50 and 31/50) were significantly greater than those of mice given DMBA (5/50 and 7/50) or DMBA plus *ortho*-phenylphenol (5/50 and 5/50). The incidence of basal-cell tumours in males given DMBA plus *ortho*-phenylphenol (4/50) was significantly greater than that in the controls (0/50) but was not significantly increased over that of mice given DMBA alone (1/50). No significant increase in the incidence of basal-cell tumours or carcinomas was observed in females given DMBA plus *ortho*-phenylphenol over that in mice given DMBA alone. No basal-cell tumours were seen in mice given either *ortho*-phenylphenol or the vehicle alone. The incidences of squamous-cell papillomas and carcinomas in mice given *ortho*-phenylphenol were not increased over those in vehicle controls, and those in mice given DMBA plus *ortho*-phenylphenol were no higher than those in mice given DMBA alone. No squamous-cell papillomas or carcinomas occurred in mice given *ortho*-phenylphenol or acetone alone. The authors concluded that *ortho*-phenylphenol is not a complete carcinogen or promoter when administered by the dermal route to mice (National Toxicology Program, 1986).

Eight groups of 20 female CD-1 mice, eight weeks of age, received dermal applications of 10 mg sodium *ortho*-phenylphenate (technical grade Dowicide A; purity, 97%) in 0.1 mL dimethyl sulfoxide (DMSO), followed by TPA (10 μg in 0.1 mL acetone); 10 mg sodium *ortho*-phenylphenate followed by acetone; 10 μg DMBA in 0.1 mL DMSO followed by 5 mg sodium *ortho*-phenylphenate in 0.1 mL acetone; DMSO followed by sodium *ortho*-phenylphenate; DMBA followed by TPA; DMBA followed by acetone; DMSO followed by TPA; or DMSO followed by acetone. The initiation treatment was given twice weekly for five weeks, and the promotion treatment twice weekly for 47 weeks. The survival rate was significantly decreased only in the group treated with DMBA plus TPA, because of the growth of skin tumours. All mice survived beyond 26 weeks of the experiment. The numbers of mice in the eight groups with skin tumours were 1, 0, 15, 0, 20, 5, 2 and 0, respectively, and the average numbers of skin tumours per mouse were 0.05, 0, 1.25, 0, 2.9, 0, 0.30, 0.15 and 0, respectively. The incidences and numbers of tumours were significantly increased ($p < 0.01$) in mice receiving DMBA plus sodium *ortho*-phenylphenate and in those receiving DMBA plus TPA, indicating that sodium *ortho*-phenylphenate can promote but not initiate skin tumours in mice (Takahashi *et al.*, 1989).

Rat: Two groups of 30 male Fischer 344 rats, five weeks of age, were given drinking-water treated with 0.01% *N*-nitrosobutyl(4-hydroxybutyl)amine (NBHBA), while a third received untreated drinking-water for four weeks. Then, one of the treated groups and the untreated group received 32 weeks of treatment with 2% sodium *ortho*-phenylphenate (purity, 97%) in the diet, and the other nitrosamine-treated group received basal diet. The only evidence of toxicity was a slight retardation in the growth of rats given sodium *ortho*-phenylphenate. The incidences of bladder carcinoma were 2/28, 1/30 and 0/29, respectively, in the groups given NBHBA plus sodium-*ortho*-phenylphenate, NBHBA alone and the phenylphenate alone, and the incidences of papillomas were 9, 8 and 5, respectively. In a second experiment, with the same overall protocol, 30 rats received NBHBA followed by 2% sodium *ortho*-phenylphenate in the diet; 30 rats received 2% *ortho*-phenylphenol (purity, 98%) in the diet; 30 rats received NBHBA followed by basal diet; 15 rats received untreated drinking-water followed by sodium *ortho*-phenylphenate; and 15 rats received untreated drinking-water followed by *ortho*-phenylphenol. The only evidence of toxicity was mild growth retardation with sodium *ortho*-phenylphenate and *ortho*-phenylphenol and brown discolouration of the external genital area due to continuous micturition. The numbers of rats with bladder carcinoma were 27, 6, 2, 1 and 0 in the five groups, respectively. The authors concluded that sodium *ortho*-phenylphenate, but not *ortho*-phenylphenol, promotes bladder tumours (Fukushima *et al.*, 1983).

Groups of 30 male Fischer 344 rats, six weeks of age, were fed diets containing 2% sodium *ortho*-phenylphenate [purity not stated] after treatment with either 0.01% NBHBA in the drinking-water or untreated drinking-water for four weeks; a group of 10 rats received NBHBA only followed by untreated diet. The experiment lasted 68 weeks. In another experiment, groups of 30 rats were fed 2% *ortho*-phenylphenol [purity not stated] in the diet after either NBHBA pretreatment or untreated water. A group of 30 rats served as controls and were treated with NBHBA only. Slight retardation of growth was seen, which was more pronounced with *ortho*-phenylphenol than with sodium *ortho*-phenylphenate. The incidences of bladder carcinoma were 15/29 with NBHBA followed by sodium *ortho*-phenylphenate, 3/10 with NBHBA alone and 6/28 with sodium *ortho*-phenylphenate alone. Following treatment with *ortho*-phenylphenol after NBHBA, 21/28 rats developed bladder cancer, whereas none developed bladder cancer without prior

NBHBA treatment; of the rats treated with NBHBA alone, 19/29 developed bladder carcinoma. The authors concluded that sodium *ortho*-phenylphenate, but not *ortho*-phenylphenol, promotes bladder carcinogenesis. In a further experiment, sodium *ortho*-phenylphenate was administered in the diet at various concentrations and tumour incidences were calculated in 10 rats at each dose at 36 weeks and in 7–9 rats at 104 weeks. The incidences of bladder carcinoma were 0/10 at 36 weeks and 2/5 at 104 weeks with 2% sodium *ortho*-phenylphenate; at 104 weeks, two rats also had papillomas. No tumours were found in groups of 10 rats given sodium *ortho*-phenylphenate at concentrations of 1, 0.5 or 0.25% in the diet or in the untreated controls (Fukushima *et al.*, 1985). [The Working Group noted the small numbers of animals in these experiments, especially in the two-year study.]

As part of a bioassay of 17 environmental chemicals, sodium *ortho*-phenylphenate [purity not stated] was fed for 20 weeks in the diet of male Fischer 344 rats which had received 0.05% NBHBA in the drinking-water for two weeks. One week after the start of administration of sodium *ortho*-phenylphenate, the lower section of the left ureter was ligated. The rats were six weeks of age at the beginning of the experiment, and the experiment lasted 24 weeks. A second group received NBHBA and one week later underwent unilateral ureteral ligation, and a third group was treated with sodium *ortho*-phenylphenate with unilateral ureteral ligation without prior NBHBA treatment. In the first group, 7/19 rats developed bladder papillomas in contrast to 1/15 in the group not pretreated with NBHBA. No bladder tumours occurred in rats given only NBHBA (Miyata *et al.*, 1985). [The Working Group noted the complexity of the experimental protocol and the short period of administration of the chemical.]

Six groups of 15 male and 15 female Fischer 344 rats, five weeks of age, were either untreated; received 0.2% thiabendazole (purity, 98.5%) in the diet; received 1% sodium *ortho*-phenylphenate (purity, 95.5% with 3.75% free water, 0.72% free sodium hydroxide and 0.028% organic substances and no detectable residues of heavy metals) in the diet; received 2% sodium *ortho*-phenylphenate alone; received 1% sodium *ortho*-phenylphenate and 0.2% thiabendazole; or received 2% sodium *ortho*-phenylphenate plus 0.2% thiabendazole. Treatment was continued for 65 weeks except for males and females receiving 1% sodium *ortho*-phenylphenate. The mean body weights of animals of each sex were significantly reduced throughout the study. The survival rates of males given 2% of the phenylphenate with or without thiabendazole and females given 1% phenylphenate and thiabendazole were slightly but not statistically significantly reduced. The incidences of bladder papillomas plus carcinomas in the six groups were 0, 1, 0, 15, 12 and 14, respectively, for males and 0, 0, 0, 2, 1 and 12, respectively, for females. The authors concluded that sodium *ortho*-phenylphenate is carcinogenic to male and female rats at 2% in the diet but not at 1% and that thiabendazole enhanced its tumorigenicity in females (Fujii *et al.*, 1986). [The Working Group noted the small numbers of animals in each group and the relatively short length of the experiment.]

Groups of 30–31 male Fischer 344/CuCrj rats, four weeks of age, received *ortho*-phenylphenol at a concentration of 1.25% in the diet; received 1.25% *ortho*-phenylphenol in the diet plus 0.4% sodium bicarbonate in the drinking-water; received 2% sodium *ortho*-phenylphenate in the diet; received 2% sodium *ortho*-phenylphenate in the diet plus ammonium chloride in the drinking-water; or were untreated. Treatment was continued for 26 weeks. The water consumption of rats given 1.25% *ortho*-phenylphenol plus sodium bicarbonate or 2% of the sodium salt plus ammonium chloride was increased in comparison with the groups receiving the phenylphenol or its salt alone, and that of rats given the sodium salt was increased as compared with the control group. Urinary pH measured at week 25 of the experiment was 6.4, 7.0, 7.0, 5.9 and 6.4 for the five groups, respectively. There was no effect on survival. A significant decrease in body weight was seen only in the group given 2% sodium salt plus ammonium chloride. The numbers of rats with bladder papillomas were 12, 20, 21, 3 and 0, respectively, in the five groups. Only one bladder carcinoma was seen in this experiment, in a rat given 2% sodium *ortho*-phenylphenate (Fujii *et al.*, 1987). [The Working Group noted the short duration of the experiment and the relatively small number of animals evaluated.]

Groups of 30–31 male Fischer 344 rats, six weeks of age, received 2% sodium *ortho*-phenylphenate (purity, 72.02%, with 26.78% water and 1.25% sodium hydroxide) in the diet; received 1.25% *ortho*-phenylphenol (purity, 99.45% with 0.55% inert ingredients) in the diet plus 0.64% sodium bicarbonate; received 1.25% *ortho*-phenylphenol plus 0.32% sodium bicarbonate; received 1.25% *ortho*-phenylphenol plus 0.16% sodium bicarbonate; received 1.25% *ortho*-phenylphenol; received 0.64% sodium bicarbonate; or served as untreated controls. The experimental period was 104 weeks. There was no significant effect on survival, but body weights were decreased by > 10% in comparison with controls at the end of the experiment, except in the group given sodium bicarbonate, which had a decrease of approximately 7%. The incidences of bladder carcinoma were 12/29, 9/29, 4/29, 4/26, 0/27, 1/28 and 0/27 in the seven groups, respectively. The incidences in the first four groups were significantly increased in comparison with controls or with rats given *ortho*-phenylphenol alone. In associated studies, increasing doses of sodium bicarbonate increased the urinary pH in the groups given *ortho*-phenylphenol plus sodium bicarbonate, so that the two highest doses of sodium bicarbonate produced a urinary pH similar to that produced by sodium *ortho*-phenylphenate (Fukushima *et al.*, 1989).

Groups of 27 male Fischer 344 rats, five weeks of age, were subjected to freeze-ulceration of the bladder, and two weeks later were given a diet containing 0.5% sodium *ortho*-phenylphenate [purity not stated] for 76 weeks; were subjected to freeze-ulceration and 12 weeks later given 0.5% sodium *ortho*-phenylphenate in the diet for 66 weeks; were subjected to freeze-ulceration and then given control diet for 78 weeks; were sham-operated and two weeks later given 0.5% sodium *ortho*-phenylphenate; or were sham-operated and given control diet for 78 weeks. There were no significant differences between the groups in terms of body-weight gain or survival. Three rats in the first group developed a bladder papilloma, and one in the second group developed a bladder carcinoma ($p < 0.24$). In a second experiment, 25 male Fischer 344 rats were subjected to freeze-ulceration of the bladder and six weeks later given 2% sodium *ortho*-

phenylphenate in the diet for 30 weeks; 25 rats underwent freeze-ulceration and six weeks later were given 1% sodium *ortho*-phenylphenate; 20 rats underwent freeze-ulceration and were given control diet for 36 weeks; and 20 rats were sham-operated and six weeks later were given 2% sodium *ortho*-phenylphenate in the diet for 30 weeks. The growth of rats that received 2% of the compound with or without freeze-ulceration was significantly decreased when compared with freeze-ulceration alone. Seven rats subjected to freeze-ulceration and given the phenylphenate developed bladder papillomas, and 12 other rats had carcinomas (total bladder tumour incidence, 76%). One rat given the compound alone had a bladder carcinoma (5%). No bladder tumours occurred in the other groups (Hasegawa *et al.*, 1989).

A group of 20 male Fischer 344 rats, six weeks of age, were given sodium *ortho*-phenylphenate [purity not stated] at a concentration of 2% in the diet for 16 weeks after pretreatment with 20 mg/kg bw *N*-methyl-*N*-nitrosourea (MNU) administered intraperitoneally (dissolved shortly before each treatment) twice a week for four weeks. A second group of 23 rats received MNU without further treatment, and a third group of 14 rats received sodium *ortho*-phenylphenate without MNU. The tumour incidences in the thyroid, forestomach, kidney and urinary bladder were enhanced in the group given MNU plus sodium *ortho*-phenylphenate when compared with those given MNU only. No tumours were observed in the thyroid, lung, liver, pancreas, oesophagus, forestomach, small intestine, kidney or urinary bladder of rats that received sodium *ortho*-phenylphenate only, but four of these rats had papillary or nodular hyperplasia of the urinary bladder (Uwagawa *et al.*, 1991). [The Working Group noted the complex treatment protocol of this experiment, the small number of animals and the short treatment period.]

3.3 Carcinogenicity of metabolites

Mouse: Ten groups of 25 female CD-1 mice, eight weeks of age, were treated as follows: the first seven groups received initiation treatment for five weeks and promotion for 34 weeks, with a one-week period of no treatment between the two phases; groups 8–10 received continuous treatment for the entire 40 weeks. Group 1 received 10 μg DMBA in 0.1 mL DMSO twice a week, followed by 2.5 μg TPA in 0.1 mL acetone twice a week; group 2 received 2 mg 2-phenyl-1,4-benzoquinone [purity unspecified] in DMSO, followed by TPA in acetone; group 3 received 20 mg 2,5-dihydroxybiphenyl in DMSO, followed by TPA in acetone; group 4 received DMSO followed by TPA in acetone; group 5 received DMBA followed by 1 mg 2-phenyl-1,4-benzoquinone; group 6 received DMBA followed by 10 mg 2,5-dihydroxybiphenyl; group 7 received DMBA followed by acetone; group 8 received 1 mg 2-phenyl-1,4-benzoquinone; group 9 received 10 mg 2,5-dihydroxybiphenyl; and group 10 received DMSO (0.1 mL). There were no differences in survival except for a reduction in group 1 due to extensive growth of skin tumours; in addition, five mice in group 1 were accidently lost during the early period of the experiment. There was no statistically significant increase in the incidence of skin tumours in any group except group 1 when compared with mice receiving DMBA only. No skin tumours were observed in group 8 or 9 (Sato *et al.*, 1990).

Rat: Seven groups of 20 female Fischer 344 rats, six weeks of age, were treated in two phases of 5 and 31 weeks. In the first phase, the chemicals were instilled intravesically twice a week for five weeks; during the second phase of 31 weeks, the animals were fed the appropriate dietary treatments. 2-Phenyl-1,4-benzoquinone (prepared fresh; purity, > 99%) was instilled into the bladders of groups 1 and 4, phenylhydroquinone [purity not specified] was instilled into those of groups 2 and 5, and saline was instilled into those of groups 3 and 6. The chemicals were dissolved as 0.1% solutions in saline, and a total volume of 0.2 mL was instilled. Sodium saccharin was fed at a concentration of 5% in the diet to groups 1–3, and untreated diet was fed to groups 4–6 in the second phase. Group 7 served as a positive control and was treated with 0.05% NBHBA in drinking-water followed by 5% sodium saccharin. The length of the entire experiment was 36 weeks. There were no significant differences in body-weight gain and no significant effect on survival. The only bladder tumours detected were two papillomas in group 7. Papillary or nodular hyperplasia occurred in 3/18 animals in group 1 and 9/20 rats in group 7, but not in the other groups (Hasegawa *et al.*, 1990a). [The Working Group noted the small number of animals, the short period of administration and the lack of tumours as an end-point.]

4. Other Data Relevant to an Evaluation of Carcinogenicity and its Mechanisms

4.1 Absorption, distribution, metabolism and excretion

[^{14}C]*ortho*-Phenylphenol was applied onto the skin of the forearm of six volunteers for 8 h at a dose of 0.4 mg/person (0.006 mg/kg bw). Urine was collected 24 and 48 h after exposure. By 48 h, 99% of the dose had been recovered in urine. Sulfation was the major metabolic pathway, accounting for 69% of the metabolites, while conjugates of 2-phenylhydroquinone accounted for 15%. Little or no free *ortho*-phenylphenol was present in the urine, and no free 2-phenylhydroquinone or 2-phenyl-1,4-benzoquinone was detected (Bartels *et al.*, 1998).

4.1.2 *Experimental systems*

[^{14}C]*ortho*-Phenylphenol was administered by gavage to 10 male B6C3F$_1$ mice at a dose of 15 or 800 mg/kg bw in 0.5% aqueous Methocel® and to two male and two female Fischer 344 rats at a dose of 28 or 27 mg/kg bw. Urine was collected at 12-h intervals for 24 h (rats) and 48 h (mice) after exposure. After administration of 15 or 800 mg/kg bw, 84 and 98% of the administered *ortho*-phenylphenol was recovered in the urine of mice and 86 and 89% in that of male and female rats. Sulfation of *ortho*-phenylphenol was the major metabolic pathway at low doses, accounting for 57 and 82% of the urinary metabolites in male mice dosed with 15 mg/kg bw and rats dosed with 28 mg/kg bw, respectively. Conjugates of 2-phenylhydroquinone accounted for 12 and 5%, respectively. Little or no free *ortho*-phenylphenol was present in the urine, and no free 2-phenylhydroquinone or 2-phenyl-1,4-benzoquinone was detected in either species. Dose-dependent shifts in metabolism were observed in mice for conjugation of *ortho*-phenylphenol, suggesting saturation of the sulfation pathway. Dose-dependent increases in total 2-phenylhydroquinone were observed in mice. The authors noted that their findings did not provide a metabolic explanation for the difference in carcinogenicity in rats and in mice (Bartels *et al.*, 1998).

The metabolism of the sodium salt of *ortho*-phenylphenol was investigated in male and female Fischer 344 rats dosed at 2% in the feed from the age of five weeks for 136 days. Urinary metabolites accounted for 55% of the dose in males and 40% of the dose in females. The main metabolites were *ortho*-phenylphenol-glucuronide and 2,5-dihydroxybiphenyl-glucuronide. Male rats excreted 1.8 times as much *ortho*-phenylphenol-glucuronide and nearly eight times as much 2,5-dihydroxybiphenyl-glucuronide as the females (Nakao *et al.*, 1983).

The free metabolites phenylhydroquinone and phenylbenzoquinone were also identified as minor urinary metabolites of sodium *ortho*-phenylphenate administered at 0.5, 1 or 2% in the diet to male and female Fischer 344/DuCrj rats. The concentration of phenylhydroquinone represented 1/60 of the 2% dose (93 μmol/g diet), while phenylbenzoquinone was excreted only in traces (10–100-fold lower amounts than phenylhydroquinone). The concentration of phenylhydroquinone in the urine of male rats was approximately 25 times greater than that in the urine of female rats (1500 versus 62 nmol/mL) (Morimoto *et al.*, 1989). Metabolism was investigated in the fifth month of this five-month study, mainly to investigate induction of DNA strand breaks (see section 4.5).

Male Fischer 344 rats were given *ortho*-phenylphenol at doses of 0, 1000, 4000, 8000 or 12 500 ppm (0, 140, 580, 1100 and 1800 mg/m^3) in the diet for 13 weeks and placed in urine collection cages overnight. The urinary volume of rats at the two highest doses was increased, with corresponding decreases in osmolality and the concentrations of creatinine and other solutes. The total urinary excretion of *ortho*-phenylphenol metabolites increased with dose, and the metabolites consisted almost entirely of conjugates of *ortho*-phenylphenol and 2-phenylhydroquinone; free *ortho*-phenylphenol and its metabolites accounted for less than 2% of the total excreted metabolites (Smith *et al.*, 1998).

ortho-Phenylphenol was converted to phenylhydroquinone by microsomal cytochrome P450 *in vitro*. Phenylhydroquinone was oxidized to phenylquinone by cumene hydroperoxide-supported microsomal cytochrome P450, and phenylquinone was reduced back to phenylhydroquinone by cytochrome P450 reductase, providing direct evidence of redox cycling of *ortho*-phenylphenol (Roy, 1990).

Male rats were given 1000 mg/kg bw *ortho*-phenylphenol orally, and their bile was collected for 6 h. In addition to the glucuronide conjugates of *ortho*-phenylphenol and phenylhydroquinone, phenylbenzoquinone and the glutathione conjugate of phenylhydroquinone were identified in the bile, the latter amounting to 4% of the administered dose (Nakagawa & Tayama, 1989).

ortho-Phenylphenol was shown to be converted to phenylhydroquinone by mixed-function oxidases *in vitro*, and conversion of phenylhydroquinone to phenylbenzoquinone was shown to be mediated by prostaglandin (H) synthetase in the presence of arachidonic acid and hydrogen peroxide as cofactors (Kolachana *et al.*, 1991). The authors suggested that this pathway may play an important role in *ortho*-phenylphenol-induced bladder and kidney carcinogenesis in rats, since the activity of prostaglandin (H) synthetase is high in the kidney and bladder, the target organs of *ortho*-phenylphenol.

Over the pH range 6.3–7.6 observed in the urine, phenylhydroquinone was shown to be auto-oxidized to phenylbenzoquinone *in vitro*, with an average yield of 0.92 ± 0.02. The rate of phenylhydroquinone auto-oxidation increased rapidly at pH above 7 (Kwok & Eastmond, 1997).

4.2 Toxic effects

4.2.1 *Humans*

No data were available to the Working Group.

4.2.2 *Experimental systems*

ortho-Phenylphenol and sodium *ortho*-phenylphenate induced similar levels of macromolecular binding in the bladder (and also in the liver and kidney) when administered by gavage at a dose of 500 mg/kg bw to groups of four male Fischer 344 rats. The experiment was terminated 17 h after gavage, and macromolecular binding was detected in all tissues, with a marked, non-linear dose–response relationship. Administration of 200 mg/kg bw of *ortho*-phenylphenol or sodium *ortho*-phenylphenate did not increase macromolecular binding in the bladder significantly above control values, while *ortho*-phenylphenol and sodium *ortho*-phenylphenate at 500 mg/kg bw induced 130-fold and 210-fold increases, respectively (Reitz *et al.*, 1984).

The effects of *ortho*-phenylphenol and sodium *ortho*-phenylphenate were investigated in Fischer 344 rats after administration in the diet over 8–24 weeks at a concentration of 2%. Urinary pH and sodium concentrations were increased only by sodium *ortho*-phenylphenate, which also consistently induced simple (diffuse thickening of the epithelium with four to eight cell layers) and nodular or papillary hyperplasia of the bladder epithelium at all times investigated (8, 16 and 24 weeks) (Fukushima *et al.*, 1986).

Sodium *ortho*-phenylphenate and *ortho*-phenylphenol were administered in the diet at a concentration of 2% for four or eight weeks to groups of 10 male Fischer 344 rats. DNA synthesis in the bladder (assessed after four weeks), urinary pH, sodium content, volume and crystalluria were all increased by sodium *ortho*-phenylphenate but not by *ortho*-phenylphenol. Furthermore, sodium *ortho*-phenylphenate but not *ortho*-phenylphenol induced morphological changes in the urothelium characteristic of those induced by other genotoxic and non-genotoxic bladder carcinogens, including formation of pleomorphic or short, uniform microvilli and ropy or leafy microridges. [The Working Group noted that similar alterations were induced by the bladder tumour promoter sodium-L-ascorbate but not by the parent compound L-ascorbic acid which lacks tumour promoting activity in the bladder.] Sodium *ortho*-phenylphenate but not *ortho*-phenylphenol induced hyperplasia in the renal pelvis of rats treated for four weeks. The authors commented that the observed differences might be due to changes in urinary Na^+ and pH, since sodium *ortho*-phenylphenate induced natriuresis and urinary alkalinization but *ortho*-phenylphenol did not (Shibata *et al.*, 1989a,b).

Administration of *ortho*-phenylphenol at concentrations of 0, 1000, 4000, 8000 or 12 500 mg/kg of diet (ppm) to male Fischer 344 rats for 13 weeks slightly increased the urinary volume and correspondingly decreased its osmolality and creatinine concentration at the two highest doses. Increased urinary solids (precipitate, crystals or calculi) or abnormal crystals were not detected at any dose. At 8000 and 12 500 ppm, increased urothelial hyperplasia of the bladder was seen, with an increased bromodeoxyuridine labelling index and features of increased proliferation, as detected by scanning electron microscopy. In addition, superficial cell necrosis and exfoliation were observed at these doses, indicating that *ortho*-phenylphenol induced cytotoxicity with subsequent regenerative hyperplasia (Smith *et al.*, 1998).

Species differences in urinary bladder hyperplasia induced by sodium *ortho*-phenylphenate were investigated in groups of 30 male Fischer 344 rats, $B6C3F_1$ mice, Syrian golden hamsters and Hartley guinea-pigs. The compound was administered in the diet at a concentration of 2% for 4, 8, 12, 24, 36 or 48 weeks. Simple and nodular or papillary hyperplasia was observed by light microscopy, and pleomorphic microvilli were seen by scanning electron microscopy only in rats, the lesions becoming more marked over time. In mice, guinea-pigs and hamsters, no proliferative lesions were observed. The urinary pH of treated rats was elevated at 12 weeks in comparison with controls, but there was virtually no difference at week 48. The treatment did not affect the urinary pH of animals of the other species, which is normally higher than that of the rat (Hasegawa *et al.*, 1990b).

Male and female Fischer 344 rats were given diets containing 1.25% *ortho*-phenylphenol or 2% sodium *ortho*-phenylphenate alone or in combination with 3% sodium bicarbonate or 1% ammonium chloride for eight weeks. Administration of *ortho*-phenylphenol alone did not cause proliferative effects, but combination with 3% sodium bicarbonate induced marked urothelial hyperplasia in the urinary bladders of both male and female rats, the response being more severe in males. Sodium bicarbonate alone induced only a borderline effect. Sodium *ortho*-phenylphenate alone significantly increased the incidence of hyperplasia only in males, which was less pronounced than that seen after concomitant treatment with *ortho*-phenylphenol and sodium bicarbonate. The hyperplastic effect of sodium *ortho*-phenylphenate in male rat bladders was completely prevented by co-administration of ammonium chloride, indicating the involvement of alkalinization of the urine in the induction of the observed cell proliferation and hyperplasia. Increased urinary pH and sodium concentrations were positively associated with the induction of hyperplasia in males. There was no significant difference between the sexes in terms of pH, but the sodium concentration was elevated only in males treated with sodium *ortho*-phenylphenate alone. The urinary concentrations of non-conjugated *ortho*-phenylphenol metabolites (phenylhydroquinone and phenylbenzoquinone) did not correlate with the development of hyperplasia, suggesting that these metabolites are not important for urinary bladder carcinogenesis induced by sodium *ortho*-phenylphenate (Hasegawa *et al.*, 1991).

Groups of BALB/c mice were given intraperitoneal injections of 600 mg/kg bw sodium *ortho*-phenylphenate or 100 mg/kg bw phenylbenzoquinone, a metabolite of *ortho*-phenylphenol. Maximal decreases in the concentrations of protein and non-protein reduced thiols were observed in the bladder to 66–76% of the control values, in the kidney to 26–72% of control values and in the liver, only by phenylbenzoquinone, to 25–44% that of controls. The concentrations of non-protein disulfide and protein disulfide were increased in a similar manner. Increased contents of both protein and non-protein disulfides after administration of sodium *ortho*-phenylphenate acounted for only 33% of the entire loss of non-protein reduced thiol, so that direct reaction of a metabolite (probably phenyl-2,5-*para*-benzoquinone) with glutathione probably contributed to the decrease (Narayan & Roy, 1992).

4.3 Reproductive and developmental effects

4.3.1 *Humans*

No data were available to the Working Group.

4.3.2 *Experimental systems*

Groups of 25–35 Sprague-Dawley rats received 0, 100, 300 or 700 mg/kg bw *ortho*-phenylphenol (commercial-grade Dowicide® containing 99.69% *ortho*-phenylphenol) per day orally in cottonseed oil on days 6–15 of gestation. The fetuses were examined on day 21 of gestation. One female at the high dose died, and the body-weight gain of dams was reduced on days 6–9 and maternal liver weight on day 21. There were no effects on the numbers of implantation sites, live fetuses or resorptions or on litter size or fetal development. Significant increases were seen in the incidence of delayed ossification of the sternebrae, foramina and the bones of the skull in fetuses at the high dose (John *et al.*, 1981).

4.4 Genetic and related effects

4.4.1 *Humans*

No data were available to the Working Group

4.4.2 *Experimental systems* (see Tables 1–3 for references)

Incubation of supercoiled pUC18 DNA with phenylhydroquinone, the proximate metabolite of *ortho*-phenylphenol, produced a strand scission to the linear form that was dose-dependent; in contrast, DNA cleavage by *ortho*-phenylphenol and its ultimate metabolite phenylbenzoquinone was barely detectable. The hypothesis that oxygen radicals generated in the process of oxidation of phenylhydroquinone are responsible for the DNA cleavage is supported by the finding of inhibition of DNA strand scission by superoxide dismutase, catalase and several oxygen radical scavengers.

ortho-Phenylphenol induced DNA repair in various strains of *Escherichia coli*, but did not cause DNA cleavage in plasmid DNA. The compound did not induce differential

Table 1. Genetic and related effects of *ortho*-phenylphenol and sodium *ortho*-phenylphenate

Test system	Result[a]		Dose[b] (LED or HID)	Reference
	Without exogenous metabolic system	With exogenous metabolic system		
Escherichia coli pUC18, DNA strand scission	–	NT	6800	Nagai *et al.* (1990)
Bacillus subtilis rec strains, differential toxicity	–	–	NR	Kawachi *et al.* (1980)
Salmonella typhimurium TA100, TA98, TA1535, TA1537, TA1538, reverse mutation	–	–	NR	Cline & McMahon (1977)
Salmonella typhimurium TA100, TA98, TA1535, TA1537, TA1538, reverse mutation	–	–	NR	Kawachi *et al.* (1980)
Salmonella typhimurium TA100, TA98, TA1535, TA1537, TA1538, reverse mutation	–	–	250 μg/plate[c]	Reitz *et al.* (1983)
Salmonella typhimurium TA100, TA98, TA1535, TA1537, TA1538, reverse mutation	–	–	5000 μg/plate	Moriya *et al.* (1983)
Salmonella typhimurium TA100, TA98, TA1535, TA1537, reverse mutation	–	–	200 μg/plate	National Toxicology Program (1986)
Escherichia coli WP2, *uvr*A, reverse mutation	–	–	NR	Cline & McMahon (1977)
Escherichia coli WP2, reverse mutation	–	–	NR	Cline & McMahon (1977)
Escherichia coli WP2 *hcr*, reverse mutation	–	–	5000 μg/plate	Moriya *et al.* (1983)
Drosophila melonogaster, sex-linked recessive lethal mutations	–		500 ppm feed	National Toxicology Program (1986)
DNA damage (8-OH-dGua), calf thymus DNA *in vitro*	–	NT	1700	Nagai *et al.* (1995)
Unscheduled DNA synthesis, rat primary hepatocytes *in vitro*	–	NT	17	Probst *et al.* (1981)
Unscheduled DNA synthesis, rat primary hepatocytes *in vitro*	–	NT	17[c]	Reitz *et al.* (1983)
Gene mutation, mouse lymphoma L5178Y cells, *tk* locus *in vitro*	(+)	(+)	5	National Toxicology Program (1986)
Sister chromatid exchange, Chinese hamster ovary CHO-K1 cells *in vitro*	–	NT	75	Nawai *et al.* (1979)
Sister chromatid exchange, Chinese hamster ovary CHO-K1 cells *in vitro*	+	NT	100	Tayama-Nawai *et al.* (1984)

Table 1 (contd)

Test system	Result[a]		Dose[b] (LED or HID)	Reference
	Without exogenous metabolic system	With exogenous metabolic system		
Sister chromatid exchange, Chinese hamster ovary cells *in vitro*	–	–	75.4	National Toxicology Program (1986)
Sister chromatid exchange, Chinese hamster ovary CHO-K1 cells *in vitro*	–	+	25	Tayama *et al.* (1989)
Sister chromatid exchange, Chinese hamster ovary CHO-K1 cells *in vitro*	+	+	100	Tayama & Nakagawa (1991)
Sister chromatid exchange, Chinese hamster ovary CHO-K1 cells *in vitro*	NT	+	50	Tayama & Nakagawa (1994)
Chromosomal aberrations, Chinese hamster ovary CHO-K1 cells *in vitro*	–	NT	NR[c]	Yoshida *et al.* (1979)
Chromosomal aberrations, Chinese hamster ovary CHO-K1 cells *in vitro*	+	NT	100	Tayama-Nawai *et al.* (1984)
Chromosomal aberrations, Chinese hamster ovary cells *in vitro*	(+)	(+)	90	National Toxicology Program (1986)
Chromosomal aberrations, Chinese hamster ovary CHO-K1 cells *in vitro*	–	+	25	Tayama *et al.* (1989)
Chromosomal aberrations, Chinese hamster ovary CHO-K1 cells *in vitro*	+	+	100	Tayama & Nakagawa (1991)
Gene mutation, human RSa cells, Na^+/K^+ ATPase locus *in vitro*	+	NT	15	Suzuki *et al.* (1985)
Host-mediated assay, *Salmonella typhimurium* G46 in mouse peritoneal cavity	–		600 po × 5	Shirasu *et al.* (1978) [abst]
DNA strand breaks, cross-links or related damage, Fischer 344 rat urinary bladder epithelium *in vivo*	–		0.05% ives × 1	Morimoto *et al.* (1987)
DNA strand breaks, cross-links or related damage, Fischer 344 rat urinary bladder epithelium *in vivo*	+		2% diet 3–5 mo[c]	Morimoto *et al.* (1989)
DNA strand breaks, cross-links or related damage, Comet assay, CD-1 mouse cells (five organs) *in vivo*	+		2000 po × 1	Sasaki *et al.* (1997)

Table 1 (contd)

Test system	Result[a]		Dose[b] (LED or HID)	Reference
	Without exogenous metabolic system	With exogenous metabolic system		
Chromosomal aberrations, Wistar rat bone-marrow cells *in vivo*	–		800 po × 5 or 4000 po × 1	Shirasu *et al.* (1978) [abst]
Dominant lethal mutation, mice	–		500 po × 1	Kaneda *et al.* (1978)
Dominant lethal mutation, C3H mice	–		500 po × 5	Shirasu *et al.* (1978) [abst]
Dominant lethal mutation, mice	–		4% diet × 2 mo[c]	Ogata *et al.* (1978)
Dominant lethal mutation, rats	–		4% diet × 3 mo[c]	Ogata *et al.* (1980)
Binding (covalent) to DNA *in vitro*	NT	+	17	Pathak & Roy (1992)
Binding (covalent) to calf thymus DNA *in vitro*	–	+	4	Ushiyama *et al.* (1992)
Binding (covalent) to DNA *in vitro*	NT	+	170	Pathak & Roy (1993)
Binding (covalent) to DNA, Fischer 344 rat urinary bladder cells *in vivo*	–		500 po × 1	Reitz *et al.* (1983)
Binding (covalent) to DNA, Fischer 344 rat urinary bladder cells *in vivo*	+		2% diet × 13 w	Ushiyama *et al.* (1992)
Binding (covalent) to DNA, CD-1 mouse skin cells *in vivo*	+		10 mg/mouse (skin) × 1	Pathak & Roy (1993)
Binding (covalent) to DNA, Fischer 344 rat urothelium *in vivo*	–		12 500 ppm diet × 13 w	Smith *et al.* (1998)

abst, abstract; 8-OH-dGua, 8-hydroxydeoxyguanosine

[a] +, positive; (+), weakly positive; –, negative; NT, not tested

[b] LED, lowest effective dose; HID, highest ineffective dose; unless otherwise stated, *in-vitro* tests, μg/mL; *in-vivo* tests, mg/kg bw per day; NR, not reported; po, oral; ives, intravesical; mo, months; w, week

[c] Sodium *ortho*-phenylphenate

Table 2. Genetic and related effects of phenylhydroquinone

Test system	Result[a]		Dose[b] (LED or HID)	Reference
	Without exogenous metabolic system	With exogenous metabolic system		
Escherichia coli pUC18 DNA strand breaks	(+)	NT	744	Nagai *et al.* (1990)
DNA damage (8-OH-dGua), calf thymus DNA *in vitro*	+	NT	18.6	Nagai *et al.* (1995)
DNA damage (8-OH-dGua), Chinese hamster ovary CHO-K1 cells *in vitro*	–[c]	NT	9.3	Nakagawa & Tayama (1996)
Gene mutation, Chinese hamster lung V79 cells, *hprt* locus *in vitro*	–	NT	NR	Lambert & Eastmond (1994)
Sister chromatid exchange, Chinese hamster ovary CHO-K1 cells *in vitro*	+	+	5	Tayama *et al.* (1989)
Sister chromatid exchange, Chinese hamster ovary CHO-K1 cells *in vitro*	+	+	25	Tayama & Nakagawa (1991)
Sister chromatid exchange, Chinese hamster ovary CHO-K1 cells *in vitro*	+	NT	2.5	Tayama & Nakagawa (1994)
Micronucleus formation, Chinese hamster lung V79 cells *in vitro*	–[d]	NT	35	Lambert & Eastmond (1994)
Chromosomal aberrations, Chinese hamster ovary CHO-K1 cells *in vitro*	–	+	50	Tayama *et al.* (1989)
Chromosomal aberrations, Chinese hamster ovary CHO-K1 cells *in vitro*	–	+	100	Tayama & Nakagawa (1991)
Binding (covalent) to DNA *in vitro*	NT	+	18.6	Pathak & Roy (1992, 1993)
Binding (covalent) to calf thymus DNA *in vitro*	+	NT	7440	Ushiyama *et al.* (1992)
Binding (covalent) to DNA, human HL-60 cells *in vitro*	+	NT	4.7	Horvath *et al.* (1992)

Table 2 (contd)

Test system	Result[a]		Dose[b] (LED or HID)	Reference
	Without exogenous metabolic system	With exogenous metabolic system		
DNA strand breakage, Fischer 344 rat urinary bladder cells *in vivo*	+		200 µg bladder inj × 1 (10 min)	Morimoto *et al.* (1987)
Binding (covalent) to female CD1 mouse skin DNA *in vivo*	+		5 mg/mouse, skin	Pathak & Roy (1993)

8-OH-dGua, 8-hydroxydeoxyguanosine

[a] +, positive; (+), weakly positive; –, negative; NT, not tested

[b] LED, lowest effective dose; HID, highest ineffective dose; unless otherwise stated, *in-vitro* tests, µg/mL; *in-vivo* tests, mg/kg bw per day; NR, not reported; inj, injection

[c] Weakly positive after inhibition of catalase activity

[d] Positive with arachidonic acid supplement (LED = 125 µmol/L)

Table 3. Genetic and related effects of phenylbenzoquinone

Test system	Result [a]		Dose[b] (LED or HID)	Reference
	Without exogenous metabolic system	With exogenous metabolic system		
Escherichia coli pUC18, DNA strand breaks	–	NT	7360	Nagai *et al.* (1990)
DNA damage (8-OH-dGua), calf thymus DNA *in vitro*	–	NT	1840	Nagai *et al.* (1995)
Gene mutation, Chinese hamster lung V79 cells, *hprt* locus *in vitro*	–	NT	NR	Lambert & Eastmond (1994)
Sister chromatid exchange, Chinese hamster ovary CHO-K1 cells *in vitro*	+	+	5	Tayama & Nakagawa (1991)
Micronucleus formation, Chinese hamster lung V79 cells *in vitro*	?	NT	9.3	Lambert & Eastmond (1994)
Chromosomal aberrations, Chinese hamster ovary CHO-K1 cells *in vitro*	+	+	5	Tayama & Nakagawa (1991)
Cell transformation, BALB/c3T3 mouse cells (with TPA post-treatment)	+	NT	0.6	Sakai *et al.* (1995)
Binding (covalent) to DNA and dGMP *in vitro*	+	NT	450	Pathak & Roy (1992)
Binding (covalent) to DNA *in vitro*	+	NT	7360	Ushiyama *et al.* (1992)
Binding (covalent) to calf thymus DNA *in vitro*	+	NT	500	Horvath *et al.* (1992)
Binding (covalent) to DNA, human HL-60 cells *in vitro*	+	NT	4.6	Horvath *et al.* (1992)
DNA strand breakage, Fischer 344 rat urinary bladder cells *in vivo*	+		200 μg bladder inj × 1 (10 min)	Morimoto *et al.* (1987)

TPA, 12-*O*-tetradecanoylphorbol-13-acetate; 8-OH-dGua, 8-hydroxydeoxyguanosine

[a] +, positive; –, negative; NT, not tested; ?, inconclusive

[b] LED, lowest effective dose; HID, highest ineffective dose; unless otherwise stated, in-vitro tests, μg/mL; in-vivo tests, mg/kg bw per day; NR, not reported; inj, injection

toxicity in *Bacillus subtilis*. *ortho*-Phenylphenol was consistently non-mutagenic in tests for reversion in five strains (TA100, TA1535, TA1537, TA1538 and TA98) of *Salmonella typhimurium* and a strain (WP2 *hcr*) of *Escherichia coli* in the presence and absence of metabolic activation; the only exception was a weakly positive response in strain TA1535 in the absence of exogenous metabolic activation, but the addition of metabolic activation from rat and hamster liver eliminated this effect.

It was reported in an abstract that sodium *ortho*-phenylphenate induced aneuploidy in *Aspergillus* (Kappas & Georgopoulos, 1975).

ortho-Phenylphenol did not induce sex-linked recessive lethal mutations in *Drosophila*. It did not induce unscheduled DNA synthesis in cultured rat hepatocytes in the absence of an exogenous metabolic system.

At cytotoxic concentrations, *ortho*-phenylphenol was weakly mutagenic in mouse lymphoma L5178Y/$tk^{+/-}$ cells, both in the absence and presence of exogenous metabolic activation from rat liver.

Studies on the ability of *ortho*-phenylphenol to induce sister chromatid exchange and chromosomal aberrations in Chinese hamster ovary cells provided contradictory results. In one study performed in the absence of metabolic activation, dose-dependent increases in the incidence of both chromosomal aberrations and sister chromatid exchange were detected after a 27-h post-treatment incubation; the presence of only chromosomal aberrations after 42-h suggested that DNA damage resulting in sister chromatid exchange can be repaired during the longer incubation time. In a second study, a borderline increase in the frequency of chromosomal aberrations occurred in both the presence and absence of exogenous metabolic activation from rat liver, but no sister chromatid exchange was seen. In a third study in the presence of metabolic activation, an increased frequency of sister chromatid exchange occurred, which was not inhibited by several scavengers of oxygen reactive species. Finally, in the presence of 15% metabolic activation, *ortho*-phenylphenol increased the incidences of both chromosomal aberrations and sister chromatid exchange; both these cytogenetic effects were inhibited by cysteine and glutathione, and the frequency of sister chromatid exchange was found to correlate with the formation of the reactive metabolite phenylhydroquinone.

Phenylhydroquinone and phenylbenzoquinone caused sister chromatid exchange in Chinese hamster ovary cells, but the activity of the latter metabolite was lower in the presence of an exogenous metabolic activating system. Both metabolites also caused chromosomal aberrations in the same cell type, phenylhydroquinone requiring metabolic activation.

ortho-Phenylphenol caused a dose-dependent increase in the number of ouabain-resistant mutants in an ultra-violet-sensitive human RSa cell strain in the absence of metabolic activation. Gene mutation was not induced in a host-mediated assay in which mice were injected intraperitoneally with *S. typhimurium* and then given oral doses of *ortho*-phenylphenol.

In the urinary bladder epithelium of male rats, no DNA damage was detectable by the alkaline elution assay after intravesicular injection of *ortho*-phenylphenol, but it was present in rats of each sex injected with solutions of phenylhydroquinone or phenylbenzoquinone. DNA damage was observed in the urinary bladder epithelium of male rats fed 2% sodium *ortho*-phenylphenate in the diet for three to five months. In male CD-1 mice given a single oral dose of *ortho*-phenylphenol, DNA damage, as detected by the Comet assay, was present in stomach, liver, lung kidney and bladder but absent from brain and bone marrow.

ortho-Phenylphenol did not induce chromosomal aberrations in rat bone marrow after exposure *in vivo* and did not give rise to dominant lethal mutations in mice or rats.

Several studies were carried out *in vitro* and *in vivo* to investigate the covalent binding of *ortho*-phenylphenol to DNA. Reaction of DNA with *ortho*-phenylphenol or its hydroxylated metabolite phenylhydroquinone produced four major adducts when carried out in the presence of rat liver microsomes and NADPH. The formation of adducts was drastically decreased by cytochrome P450 inhibitors and did not occur in the absence of microsomes, except at high doses. The same major adducts were detected by the ^{32}P-postlabelling technique in deoxyguanosine-3′-phosphate or DNA reacted with the reactive metabolite of *ortho*-phenylphenol, phenylbenzoquinone. [^{14}C]*ortho*-Phenylphenol was found to bind covalently to calf thymus DNA in the presence but not in the absence of microsomes, indicating that its conversion to an activated metabolite is essential; this was confirmed by the formation of adducts, detected by ^{32}P-postlabelling analysis, in calf thymus DNA incubated with phenylhydroquinone and phenylbenzoquinone. ^{32}P-Postlabelling analysis revealed one major adduct in whole urinary bladder DNA of rats fed a diet containing *ortho*-phenylphenol for 13 weeks, but the presence of DNA adducts was not confirmed in a subsequent study, in which only the bladder epithelium was evaluated. Topical application to female CD-1 mice of sodium *ortho*-phenylphenol or phenylhydroquinone produced adducts in skin DNA, as detected by ^{32}P-postlabelling; the levels of these adducts were reduced in mice pretreated with inhibitors of cytochrome P450 or of prostaglandin synthase. The dose of sodium *ortho*-phenylphenate applied to the mouse skin was far in excess of the concentrations attained in urine by feeding it to mice or rats at high doses. Incubation of DNA with *ortho*-phenylphenol or phenylhydroquinone in the presence of cytochrome P450 activation or prostaglandin synthase activation systems *in vitro* produced adducts similar to those detected *in vivo*.

Formation of 8-hydroxyguanosine, which reflects oxidative DNA damage, occurred in calf thymus DNA incubated with phenylhydroquinone, the major metabolite formed from *ortho*-phenylphenol by P450 monooxygenase, but was absent after incubation with *ortho*-phenylphenol and minimal after incubation with the ultimate metabolite phenylbenzoquinone; these findings indicate that DNA damage is likely to be due to the production of oxygen radicals during the conversion of phenylhydroquinone to phenylbenzoquinone.

2,5-Dihydroxybiphenyl, an intermediate of *ortho*-phenylphenol metabolism, was found to alkylate calf thymus DNA in the absence of metabolic activation (Grether *et al.*, 1989).

In the presence of Cu(II)$^{++}$, *ortho*-phenylphenol did not induce damage in DNA fragments from the protooncogene c-Ha-*ras*-1, whereas DNA lesions were observed under the same experimental conditions with the two *ortho*-phenylphenol metabolites 2,5-dihydroxybiphenyl and 2-phenyl-1,4-benzoquinone (Inoue *et al.*, 1990).

Dose-dependent formation of DNA adducts, as detected by ^{32}P-postlabelling, was observed in human HL-60 cells exposed to *ortho*-phenylhydroquinone and *ortho*-phenylbenzoquinone at 25–250 µmol/L; reaction of calf thymus DNA with *ortho*-phenylbenzoquinone resulted in the formation of one DNA adduct, which did not correspond to the major adduct produced in HL-60 cells.

Phenylhydroquinone at 31–187 µmol/L induced the formation of CREST-positive micronuclei (which represent whole chromosomes that fail to segregate during mitosis) in an arachidonic acid-supplemented prostaglandin H synthase-containing V79 Chinese hamster cell line. Treatment with phenylbenzoquinone had only a minor effect on micronucleus formation in unsupplemented cells. Neither phenylhydroquinone nor phenylbenzoquinone increased the frequency of mutation at the *hprt* locus in the same cells. The results suggest that phenylhydroquinone is oxidized to phenylbenzoquinone by prostaglandin H synthase.

Phenylbenzoquinone was found to act as initiatior in the two-stage transformation of BALB/c 3T3 cells, in which the cells were subsequently treated with TPA.

Induction of 8-hydroxy-2-deoxyguanosine, an index of oxidative DNA modification, was not observed in Chinese hamster ovary CHO-K1 cells exposed to phenylhydroquinone. Weakly positive results were observed after inhibition of catalase activity.

4.5 Mechanistic considerations

Sodium *ortho*-phenylphenate and *ortho*-phenylphenol induce urinary bladder tumours predominantly in male rats, the sodium salt being more potent. Urothelial toxicity and increased cell proliferation in the bladder epithelium are induced by sodium *ortho*-phenylphenate in male rats only at high doses (Shibata *et al.*, 1989a,b; Hasegawa *et al.*, 1991; Smith *et al.*, 1998). Urothelial hyperplasia was not observed in male or female rats treated with *ortho*-phenylphenol but was observed in male rats when the compound was administered with sodium bicarbonate.

The urothelial toxicity of *ortho*-phenylphenol does not appear to be related to the formation of urinary precipitates, microcrystals or calculi, whereas precipitates or crystals may contribute to the greater effects observed with high doses of sodium *ortho*-phenylphenol.

DNA adducts have been found in several test systems including the urinary bladder after administration of *ortho*-phenylphenol but not in urinary bladder epithelium, appears to be oxidized to phenylhydroquinone and subsequently to phenylbenzoquinone, which may damage DNA.

5. Summary of Data Reported and Evaluation

5.1 Exposure data

Exposure to *ortho*-phenylphenol and its sodium salt may occur during their production and use as industrial and agricultural fungicides, germicides and disinfectants, and as chemical intermediates. *ortho*-Phenylphenol has been detected in some groundwater and drinking-water samples as well as in some fruits and juices.

5.2 Human carcinogenicity data

No data were available to the Working Group.

5.3 Animal carcinogenicity data

ortho-Phenylphenol was tested for carcinogenicity in one experiment in mice and two experiments in rats by administration in the diet. Benign and malignant bladder tumours were induced at significant incidence in male rats in one study. Sodium *ortho*-phenylphenate was tested in mice in one study and in rats in two studies. It induced tumours of the bladder and renal pelvis in male rats in both studies and a marginal increase in the incidence of bladder tumours in female rats in one of the studies. There was no evidence of carcinogenicity in mice.

Bladder carcinogenesis induced in male rats by administration of *N*-nitrosobutyl-(4-hydroxybutyl)amine was enhanced by sodium *ortho*-phenylphenate but not by *ortho*-phenylphenol. In one study, dermal application of sodium *ortho*-phenylphenate enhanced skin tumorigenesis in mice given 7,12-dimethylbenz[*a*]anthracene.

5.4 Other relevant data

The major urinary metabolites of sodium *ortho*-phenylphenate are the glucuronide and sulfate conjugates of *ortho*-phenylphenol and phenylhydroquinone. The capacity of male rats to metabolize sodium *ortho*-phenylphenate is several times greater than that of females.

Urothelial toxic effects and increased regenerative cell proliferation in the bladder epithelium are induced in rats. Although the mechanism of toxicity is unknown, the higher pH induced by the sodium salt may enhance the toxic effect of sodium *ortho*-phenylphenate in comparison with that of *ortho*-phenylphenol.

In a study of rats exposed to *ortho*-phenylphenol by oral gavage during gestation, the high dose resulted in delayed skeletal maturation of pups but had no effect on their viability, growth or morphological appearance.

No data were available on the genetic and related effects of *ortho*-phenylphenol and its sodium salt in humans. Mixed results were found in assays with *ortho*-phenylphenol for genotoxicity in rodents *in vivo* and in cultured mammalian cells *in vitro*. It induced gene mutation in mammalian cells *in vitro*. It was not mutagenic to bacteria or *Drosophila* but induced aneuploidy in fungi.

5.5 Evaluation

There is *inadequate evidence* in humans for the carcinogenicity of *ortho*-phenylphenol and sodium *ortho*-phenylphenate.

There is *limited evidence* in experimental animals for the carcinogenicity of *ortho*-phenylphenol.

There is *sufficient evidence* in experimental animals for the carcinogenicity of sodium *ortho*-phenylphenate.

Overall evaluation

ortho-Phenylphenol is *not classifiable as to its carcinogenicity to humans (Group 3).*

Sodium *ortho*-phenylphenate is *possibly carcinogenic to humans (Group 2B).*

6. References

Bartels, M.J., McNett, D.A., Timchalk, C., Mendrala, A.L., Christenson, W.R., Sangha, G.K., Brzak, K.A. & Shabrang, S.N. (1998) Comparative metabolism of *ortho*-phenylphenol in mouse, rat and man. *Xenobiotica*, **28**, 579–594

Budavari, S., ed. (1996) *The Merck Index*, 12th Ed., Whitehouse Station, NJ, Merck & Co., Inc., p. 1257

Chemical Information Services (1995) *Directory of World Chemical Producers 1995/96 Standard Edition*, Dallas, TX, p. 402

Cline, J.C. & McMahon, R.E. (1977) Detection of chemical mutagens: Use of concentration gradient plates in a high capacity screen. *Res. Commun. Chem. Pathol. Pharmacol.*, **16**, 523–533

Fujii, T. & Hiraga, K. (1985) Carcinogenicity testing of sodium orthophenylphenate in F344 rats. *J. Saitama med. School*, **12**, 277–287

Fujii, T., Mikuriya, H., Kamiya, N. & Hiraga, K. (1986) Enhancing effect of thiabendazole on urinary bladder carcinogenesis induced by sodium *o*-phenylphenate in F344 rats. *Food chem. Toxicol.*, **24**, 207–211

Fujii, T., Nakamura, K. & Hiraga, K. (1987) Effect of pH on the carcinogenicity of *o*-phenylphenol and sodium *o*-phenylphenate in the rat urinary bladder. *Food chem. Toxicol.*, **25**, 359–362

Fukushima, S., Kurata, Y., Shibata, M., Ikawa, E. & Ito, N. (1983) Promoting effect of sodium *o*-phenylphenate and *o*-phenylphenol on two-stage urinary bladder carcinogenesis in rats. *Gann*, **74**, 625–632

Fukushima, S., Kurata, Y., Ogiso, T., Okuda, M., Miyata, Y. & Ito, N. (1985) Pathological analysis of the carcinogenicity of sodium *o*-phenylphenate and *o*-phenylphenol. *Oncology*, **42**, 304–311

Fukushima, S., Shibata, M.-A., Kurata, Y., Tamano, S. & Masui, T. (1986) Changes in the urine and scanning electron microscopically observed appearance of the rat bladder following treatment with tumor promoters. *Jpn. J. Cancer Res.*, **77**, 1074–1082

Fukushima, S., Inoue, T., Uwagawa, S., Shibata, M.-A. & Ito, N. (1989) Co-carcinogenic effects of $NaHCO_3$ on *o*-phenylphenol-induced rat bladder carcinogenesis. *Carcinogenesis*, **10**, 1635–1640

Grether T., Brunn, H. & Laib, R.J. (1989) ^{32}P-Postlabelling method as a sensitive indicator for analysis of genotoxicity of biphenyl derivatives. *Arch. Toxicol.*, **63**, 423–424

Hagiwara, A., Shibata, M., Hirose, M., Fukushima, S. & Ito, N. (1984) Long-term toxicity and carcinogenicity study of sodium *o*-phenylphenate in $B6C3F_1$ mice. *Food chem. Toxicol.*, **22**, 809–814

Hansch, C., Leo, A. & Hoekman, D. (1995) *Exploring QSAR*, Washington DC, American Chemical Society, p. 97

Hasegawa, R., Furukawa, F., Toyoda, K., Sato, H., Shimoji, N., Takahashi, M. & Hayashi, Y. (1989) *In situ* freezing of the urinary bladder: A trigger of rapid development of sodium *o*-phenylphenate-induced urinary bladder tumors in the rat. *Carcinogenesis*, **10**, 571–575

Hasegawa, R., Furukawa, F., Toyoda, K., Sato, H., Takahashi, M. & Hayashi, Y. (1990a) Urothelial damage and tumor initiation by urinary metabolites of sodium *o*-phenylphenate in the urinary bladder of female rats. *Jpn. J. Cancer Res.*, **81**, 483–488

Hasegawa, R., Takahashi, S., Asamoto, M., Shirai, T. & Fukushima, S. (1990b) Species differences in sodium *o*-phenylphenate induction of urinary bladder lesions. *Cancer Lett.*, **50**, 87–91

Hasegawa, R., Fukuoka, M., Takahashi, T., Yamamoto, A., Yamaguchi, S., Shibata, M.-A., Tanaka, A. & Fukushima, S. (1991) Sex differences in *o*-phenylphenol and sodium *o*-phenylphenate rat urinary bladder carcinogenesis: Urinary metabolites and electrolytes under conditions of aciduria and alkalinuria. *Jpn. J. Cancer Res.*, **82**, 657–664

Hiraga, K. & Fujii, T. (1984) Induction of tumours of the urinary bladder in F344 rats by dietary administration of *o*-phenylphenol. *Food chem. Toxicol.*, **22**, 865–870

Horvath, E., Levay, G., Pongracz, K. & Bodell, W.J. (1992) Peroxidative activation of *o*-phenylhydroquinone leads to the formation of DNA adducts in HL-60 cells. *Carcinogenesis*, **13**, 1937–1939

IARC (1983) *IARC Monographs on the Evaluation of the Carcinogenic Risk of Chemicals to Humans*, Vol. 30, *Miscellaneous Pesticides*, Lyon, pp. 329–344

IARC (1987) *IARC Monographs on the Evaluation of Carcinogenic Risks to Humans*, Suppl. 7, *Overall Evaluations of Carcinogenicity: An Updating of* IARC Monographs *Volumes 1 to 42*, Lyon, p. 70

Inoue, S., Yamamoto, K. & Kawanishi, S. (1990) DNA damage induced by metabolites of *o*-phenylphenol in the presence of copper (II) ion. *Chem. Res. Toxicol.*, **3**, 144–149

John, J.A., Murray, F.J., Rao, K.S. & Schwetz, B.A. (1981) Teratological evaluation of ortho-phenylphenol in rats. *Fundam. appl. Toxicol.*, **1**, 282–285

Kaneda, M., Teramoto, S., Shingu, A. & Shirasu, Y. (1978) Teratogenicity and dominant lethal studies with *o*-phenylphenol. *J. Pestic. Sci.*, **3**, 365–370

Kappas, A. & Georgopoulos, S.D. (1975) Fungicides causing mitotic segregation in *Aspergillus* diploids (Abstract No. 31). *Mutat. Res.*, **29**, 236

Kawachi, T., Yahagi, T., Kada, T., Tazima, Y., Ishidate, M., Sasaki, M. & Sugiyama, T. (1980) Cooperative programme on short-term assays for carcinogenicity in Japan. In: Montesano, R., Bartsch, H. & Tomatis, L., eds, *Molecular and Cellular Aspects of Carcinogen Screening Tests* (IARC Scientific Publications No. 27), Lyon, IARC, pp. 323–330

Kolachana, P., Subrahmnyam, V.V., Eastmond, D.A. & Smith, M.T. (1991) Metabolism of phenylhydroquinone by prostaglandin (H) synthase: Possible implications in *o*-phenylphenol carcinogenesis. *Carcinogenesis*, **12**, 183–191

Kwok, E.S.C. & Eastmond, D.A. (1997) Effects of pH on nonenzymatic oxidation of phenylhydroquinone: Potential role in urinary bladder carcinogenesis induced by *o*-phenylphenol in Fischer 344 rats. *Chem. Res. Toxicol.*, **10**, 742–749

Lambert, A.C. & Eastmond, D.A (1994) Genotoxic effects of the *o*-phenylphenol metabolites phenylhydroquinone and phenylbenzoquinone in V79 cells. *Mutat. Res.*, **322**, 243–256

Lewis, R.J., Jr (1993) *Hawley's Condensed Chemical Dictionary*, 12th Ed., New York, Van Nostrand Reinhold Co., p. 1065

Lide, D.R., ed. (1997) *CRC Handbook of Chemistry and Physics*, 78th Ed., Boca Raton, FL, CRC Press, p. 3-86

Miyata, Y., Fukushima, S., Hirose, M., Masui, T. & Ito, N. (1985) Short-term screening of promoters of bladder carcinogenesis in *N*-butyl-*N*-(4-hydroxybutyl)nitrosamine-initiated unilaterally ureter-ligated rats. *Jpn. J. Cancer Res.*, **76**, 828–834

Morimoto, K., Fukuoka, M., Hasegawa, R., Tanaka, A., Takahashi, A. & Hayashi, Y. (1987) DNA damage in urinary bladder epithelium of male F344 rats treated with 2-phenyl-1,4-benzoquinone, one of the non-conjugated urinary metabolites of sodium phenylphenate *Jpn. J. Cancer. Res. (Gann)*, **78**, 1027–1030

Morimoto, K., Sato, M., Fukuoka, M., Hasegawa, R., Takahashi, T., Tsuchiya, T., Tanaka, A., Takahashi, A. & Hayashi, Y. (1989) Correlation between the DNA damage in urinary bladder epithelium and the urinary 2-phenyl-1,4-benzoquinone levels from F344 rats fed sodium *o*-phenylphenate in the diet. *Carcinogenesis*, **10**, 1823–1827

Moriya, M., Ohta, T., Watanabe, K., Miyazawa, T., Kato, K. & Shirasu, Y. (1983) Further mutagenicity studies on pesticides in bacterial reversion assay systems. *Mutat. Res.*, **116**, 185–216

Nagai, F., Ushiyama, K., Satoh, K. & Kano, I. (1990) DNA cleavage by phenylhydroquinone: The major metabolite of a fungicide *o*-phenylphenol. *Chem.-biol. Interactions*, **76**, 163–179

Nagai, F., Ushiyama, K., Satoh, K., Kasai, H. & Kano, I. (1995) Formation of 8-hydroxydeoxyguanosine in calf thymus DNA treated *in vitro* with phenylhydroquinone the major metabolite of *o*-phenylphenol. *Carcinogenesis*, **16**, 837–840

Nakagawa, Y. & Tayama, S. (1989) Formation of ortho-phenylphenol glutathione conjugates in the rat liver. *Xenobiotica*, **19**, 499–507

Nakagawa, Y. & Tayama, S. (1996) Induction of 8-hydroxy-2′-deoxyguanosine in CHO-K1 cells exposed to phenyl-hydroquinone, a metabolite of *ortho*-phenylphenol. *Cancer Lett.*, **101**, 227–232

Nakao, T., Ushiyama, K., Kabashima, J., Nagai, F., Nakagawa, A., Ohno, T., Ichikawa, H., Kobayashi, H. & Hiraga, K. (1983) The metabolic profile of sodium *o*-phenylphenate after subchronic oral administration to rats. *Food chem. Toxicol.*, **21**, 325–329

Narayan, S. & Roy, D. (1992) Changes in protein and nonprotein thiol contents in bladder, kidney and liver of mice by the pesticide sodium-o-phenylphenol and their possible role in cellular toxicity. *Biochem. int.*, **26**, 191–198

National Institute for Occupational Safety and Health (1998) *National Occupational Exposure Survey (1981–1983)*, Cincinnati, OH

National Library of Medicine (1998) *Toxic Chemical Release Inventory 1987 & 1996* (TRI87 & TRI96), Bethesda, MD

National Toxicology Program (1986) *Toxicology and Carcinogenesis Studies of* ortho-*Phenylphenol (CAS No. 93-43-7) Alone and with 7,12-Dimethylbenz[a]anthracene (CAS No. 57-97-6) in Swiss CD-1 Mice (Dermal Studies)* (Tech. Rep. Ser. No. 301; NIH Publ. No. 86-2557), Research Triangle Park, NC

National Toxicology Program (1991a) *NTP Chemical Repository Data Sheet: o-Phenylphenol*, Research Triangle Park, NC

National Toxicology Program (1991b) *NTP Chemical Repository Data Sheet: 2-Biphenylol, Sodium Salt*, Research Triangle Park, NC

Nawai, S., Yoshida, S., Nakao, T. & Hiraga, K. (1979) [Examination of mutagens by induced sister chromatid exchange (SCE). II. Test of two fungicides by induced SCE *in vitro*.] *Tokyo-toritsu Eisei Kenkyusho Nempo*, **30**, 51–53 [*Chem. Abstr.*, **94**, 25909g] (in Japanese)

Nishioka, J. & Ogasawara, H. (1978) Mutagenicity testing for diphenyl derivatives in bacterial systems (Abstract No. 22). *Mutat. Res.*, **54**, 248–249

Ogata, A., Yoshida, S., Nawai, S., Ando, H., Kubo, Y., Hiraga, K. & Masubuchi, M. (1978) [Dominant lethal tests of long-term administration with sodium *ortho*-phenylphenol in mice.] *Tokyo-toritsu Eisei Kenkyusho Kenkyu Nempo*, **29**, 99–103 (in Japanese)

Ogato, A., Ando, H., Kubo, Y. & Hiraga, K. (1980) [Dominant lethal tests of long-tem administration with sodium *o*-phenylphenol in rats.] *Tokyo-toritsu Eisei Kenkyusho Kenkyu Nempo*, **31**, 17–19 (in Japanese)

Pathak, D.N. & Roy, D. (1992) Examination of microsomal cytochrome P450-catalyzed *in vitro* activation of *o*-phenylphenol to DNA binding metabolite(s) by ^{32}P-postlabeling technique. *Carcinogenesis*, **13**, 1593–1597

Pathak, D.N. & Roy, D. (1993) In vivo genotoxicity of sodium *ortho*-phenylphenol: Phenylbenzoquinone is one of the DNA-binding metabolite(s) of sodium *ortho*-phenylphenol. *Mutat. Res.*, **286**, 309–319

Probst, G.S., McMahon, R.E., Hill, L.E., Thompson, C.Z., Epp, J.K. & Neal, S.B. (1981) Chemically-induced unscheduled DNA synthesis in primary rat hepatocyte cultures: A comparison with bacterial mutagenicity using 218 compounds. *Environ. Mutag.*, **3**, 11–32

Reitz, R.H., Fox, T.R., Quast, J.F., Hermann, E.A. & Watanabe, P.G. (1983) Molecular mechanisms involved in the toxicity and carcinogenicity of orthophenylphenol and its sodium salt. *Chem.-biol. Interactions*, **43**, 99–119

Reitz, R.H., Fox, T.R., Quast, J.F., Hermann, E.A. & Watanabe, P.G. (1984) Biochemical factors involved in the effects of orthophenylphenol (OPP) and sodium orthophenylphenate (SOPP) on the urinary tract of male F344 rats. *Toxicol. appl. Pharmacol.*, **73**, 345–349

Roy, D. (1990) Cytochrome P-450 catalyzed redox cycling of orthophenylphenol. *Biochem. int.*, **22**, 849–857

Sakai, A., Miyata, N. & Takahashi, A. (1995) Initiating activity of quinones in the two-stage transformation of BALB/3T3 cells. *Carcinogenesis*, **16**, 477–481

Sasaki, Y.F., Saga, A., Akasaka, M., Yoshida, K., Nishidata, E., Su, Y.Q., Matsusaka, N. & Tsuda, S. (1997) In vivo genotoxicity of *ortho*-phenylphenol, biphenyl, and thiabendazole detected in multiple mouse organs by the alkaline single cell gel electrophoresis assay. *Mutat. Res.*, **395**, 189–198

Sato, H., Toyoda, K., Takamura, N., Furukawa, F., Hasegawa, R., Fukuoka, M., Imaida, K., Takahashi, M. & Hayashi, Y. (1990) Effects of 2-phenyl-1,4-benzoquinone and 2,5-dihydroxybiphenyl on two-stage mouse skin carcinogenesis. *Cancer Lett.*, **55**, 233–238

Shibata, M.-A., Tanaka, H., Yamada, M., Tamano, S. & Fukushima, S. (1989a) Proliferative response of renal pelvic epithelium in rats to oral administration of *ortho*-phenylphenol, sodium *ortho*-phenylphenate and diphenyl. *Cancer Lett.*, **48**, 19–28

Shibata, M.-A., Yamada, M., Tanaka, H., Kagawa, M. & Fukushima, S. (1989b) Changes in urine composition, bladder epithelial morphology, and DNA synthesis in male F344 rats in response to ingestion of bladder tumor promoters. *Toxicol. appl. Pharmacol.*, **99**, 37–49

Shirasu, Y., Moriya, M., Kato, K., Tezuka, H., Henmi, R., Shingu, A., Kaneda, M. & Teamoto, S. (1978) Mutagenicity testing on *o*-phenylphenol (Abstract No. 31). *Mutat. Res.*, **54**, 227

Smith, R.A., Christenson, W.R., Bartels, M.J., Arnold, L.L., St John, M.K., Cano, M., Garland, E.M., Lake, S.G., Wahle, B.S., McNett, D.A. & Cohen, S.M. (1998) Urinary physiologic and chemical metabolic effects on the urothelial cytotoxicity and potential DNA adducts of *o*-phenylphenol in male rats. *Toxicol. appl. Pharmacol.*, **150**, 402–413

Suzuki, H., Suzuki, N., Sasaki, M. & Hiraga, K. (1985) Orthophenylphenol mutagenicity in a human cell strain. *Mutat. Res.*, **156**, 123–127

Takahashi, M., Sato, H., Toyoda, K., Furukawa, F., Imaida, K., Hasegawa, R. & Hayashi, Y. (1989) Sodium *o*-phenylphenate (OPP-Na) promotes skin carcinogenesis in CD-1 female mice initiated with 7,12-dimethylbenz[*a*]anthracene. *Carcinogenesis*, **10**, 1163–1167

Tayama, S. & Nakagawa, Y. (1991) Sulfhydryl compounds inhibit the cyto- and genotoxicity of *o*-phenylphenol metabolites in CHO-K1 cells. *Mutat. Res.*, **259**, 1–12

Tayama, S. & Nakagawa, Y. (1994) Effect of scavengers of active oxygen species on cell damage caused in CHO-K1 cells by phenylhydroquinone, an *o*-phenylphenol metabolite. *Mutat. Res.*, **324**, 121–131

Tayama, S., Kamiya, N. & Nakagawa, Y. (1989) Genotoxic effects of *o*-phenylphenol metabolites in CHO-K1 cells. *Mutat Res.*, **223**, 23–33

Tayama-Nawai, S., Yoshida, S., Nakao, T. & Hiraga, K. (1984) Induction of chromosome aberrations and sister-chromatid exchanges in CHO-K1 cells by *o*-phenylphenol. *Mutat. Res.*, **141**, 95–99

Ushiyama, K., Nagai, F., Nakagawa, A. & Kano, I. (1992) DNA adduct formation by *o*-phenylphenol metabolite *in vivo* and *in vitro*. *Carcinogenesis*, **13**, 1469–1473

Uwagawa, S., Tsuda, H., Inoue, T., Tagawa, Y., Aoki, T., Kawaga, M., Ogiso, T. & Ito, N. (1991) Enhancing potential of 6 different carcinogens on multi-organ tumorigenesis after initial treatment with *N*-methyl-*N*-nitrosourea in rats. *Jpn. J. Cancer Res.*, **82**, 1397–1405

WHO (1993) *Guidelines for Drinking Water Quality*, 2nd Ed., Vol. 1, *Recommendations*, Geneva

Yoshida, S., Nawai, S. & Hiraga, K. (1979) [Cytogenetic studies of sodium *o*-phenylphenate.] *Tokyo-toritsu Eisei Kenkyusho Nempo*, **33**, 44–47 (in Japanese)

POTASSIUM BROMATE

This substance was considered by previous working groups, in 1985 (IARC, 1986) and 1987 (IARC, 1987). Since that time, new data have become available and these have been incorporated into the monograph and taken into consideration in the present evaluation.

1. Exposure Data

1.1 Chemical and physical data

1.1.1 *Nomenclature*

Chem. Abstr. Serv. Reg. No.: 7758-01-2
Chem. Abstr. Name: Bromic acid, potassium salt
IUPAC Systematic Name: Potassium bromate

1.1.2 *Structural and molecular formulae and relative molecular mass*

$KBrO_3$ Relative molecular mass: 167.01

1.1.3 *Chemical and physical properties of the pure substance*

From Budavari (1996)

(*a*) *Description*: White crystals or granules
(*b*) *Melting-point*: About 350°C; decomposes at about 370°C with evolution of oxygen
(*c*) *Density*: 3.27 g/cm^3
(*d*) *Solubility*: Soluble in water; slightly soluble in acetone, dimethyl sulfoxide, ethanol, methanol and toluene (National Toxicology Program, 1991)

1.2 Production and use

Information available in 1995 indicated that potassium bromate was produced in Argentina, Brazil, China, Germany, India, Israel, Italy, Japan and Spain (Chemical Information Services, 1995).

Potassium bromate is used primarily as a maturing agent for flour and as a dough conditioner. It is also used as a laboratory reagent and oxidizing agent, in permanent-wave compounds, as a food additive and in explosives (National Toxicology Program, 1991; Budavari, 1996).

1.3 Occurrence

1.3.1 *Natural occurrence*

Potassium bromate is not known to occur naturally.

1.3.2 *Occupational exposure*

According to the 1981–83 National Occupational Exposure Survey (National Institute for Occupational Safety and Health, 1998), approximately 27 000 workers in the United States were potentially exposed to potassium bromate. Occupational exposure to potassium bromate may occur during its production and during its use as a dough conditioner and food additive.

1.3.3 *Dietary exposure*

In a survey of retail bread samples in the United Kingdom in 1989, potassium bromate was found in all six unwrapped breads analysed, with a median concentration of 35 μg/kg (range, 17–317 μg/kg), and in seven of 22 wrapped breads, with a median concentration of < 12 μg/kg (range, < 12–238 μg/kg). In a second survey of the same brands in 1992, all samples contained less than the detection limit of 12 μg/kg flour (Dennis *et al.*, 1994).

1.3.4 *Water*

Ozonization of surface waters containing bromide ion can result in the formation of bromate (Glaze, 1986).

1.4 Regulations and guidelines

No international guidelines for potassium bromate in drinking-water have been established (WHO, 1993).

2. Studies of Cancer in Humans

No data were available to the Working Group.

3. Studies of Cancer in Experimental Animals

Previous evaluation

Potassium bromate was tested for carcinogenicity in one experiment in rats by oral administration. It produced a high incidence of renal tubular tumours (adenomas and/or carcinomas) in animals of each sex, an increased incidence of mesotheliomas of the peritoneum of males and tumours of the thyroid in female rats. Experiments in mice and rats fed diets containing bread baked from flour containing potassium bromate were inadequate for evaluation. In two experiments with rats, potassium bromate exerted an enhancing effect on the induction by *N*-nitrosoethylhydroxyethylamine of kidney tumours and dysplastic foci (IARC, 1986).

New studies

3.1 Oral administration

Mouse: Groups of 50 male B6C3F$_1$ mice, 28–30 days of age, were given potassium bromate (purity, > 99%) in their drinking-water at target concentrations of 0, 0.08, 0.4 or 0.8 g/L (ppm) for up to 100 weeks, when all surving mice were killed. The mean daily dose was calculated to be 0, 9.1, 42 and 98 mg/kg bw per day for the four groups, respectively. The survival rate ranged from 82% in the group at the high dose to approximately 69% in that at the low dose, with controls intermediate at 75%. There were also no significant differences between groups in body-weight gain. A statistically significant ($p < 0.05$) increased incidence of renal-cell tumours (adenomas and carcinomas) occurred at the low dose, but the incidences at the higher doses were not statistically significant. The incidences were 0/40 (controls), 5/38 (low dose), 3/41 (intermediate dose) and 1/44 (high dose) (De Angelo *et al*., 1998).

Rat: Groups of 20 or 24 male Fischer 344 rats, seven weeks of age, were given potassium bromate (food-additive grade) in their drinking-water at concentrations of 0, 15, 30, 60, 125, 250 or 500 mg/L (ppm) for 104 weeks. When water intake and body weight were accounted for, the intakes represented doses of 0, 0.9, 1.7, 3.3, 7.3, 16 and 43 mg/kg bw per day. Because the group receiving 500 mg/L had lower body weights and higher water consumption than other groups, their total intake of potassium bromate was approximately three times greater than that of the group given 250 ppm. The survival of rats receiving 500 ppm was significantly shorter ($p < 0.01$) at 83 ± 12 weeks than that of controls at 100 ± 3.3 weeks, but the lengths of survival of controls and other treated groups were comparable. As shown in Table 1, the incidences of renal tubular tumours (adenomas and adenocarcinomas) were significantly increased at doses of 125, 250 and 500 ppm, and the incidences of tubules with atypical hyperplasia were significantly increased at 30 ppm and higher. The incidences of thyroid follicular tumours and mesotheliomas of the peritoneum were also increased at the high dose of 500 ppm (Kurokawa *et al*., 1986).

Groups of 50 male Fischer rats, 28–30 days of age, were given potassium bromate (purity, > 99%) in the drinking-water at target concentrations of 0, 0.02 0.08, 0.4 or 0.8 g/L (ppm) for up to 100 weeks, when all surviving rats were killed. The mean daily doses were calculated to be 0, 1.5, 7.9, 17 and 38 mg/kg bw per day for the five groups, respectively. The survival rates ranged from 44% at the high dose to approximately 72% at the low dose, with 65% in the controls. Animals at the high dose also had a significant decrease in body-weight gain. There were statistically significant increases in the incidences of mesotheliomas of the testicular tunica vaginalis, renal-cell tumours and thyroid follicular adenomas and carcinomas. The incidences of mesotheliomas were 0/47, 4/49, 5/49 ($p < 0.05$), 10/47 ($p < 0.002$) and 27/43 ($p < 0.002$); those of renal tumours were 1, 1, 6, 3 and 12 ($p < 0.002$); and those of thyroid tumours (adenomas and carcinomas

Table 1. Incidences of primary tumours in male Fischer 344 rats exposed to potassium bromate

Treatment (ppm)	Animals with tumours		
	Renal tubular adenoma or carcinoma	Peritoneal mesothelioma	Follicular cell adenoma or carcinoma of the thyroid
Control	0/19	0/19	0/16
15	0/19	0/20	0/19
30	0/20	3/20	0/20
60	1/24	4/24	1/24
125	5/24*	2/24	0/24
250	5/20**	3/20	3/20
500	9/20*	15/20**	7/19*

From Kurokawa *et al.* (1986)
*Significantly different from controls at $p < 0.05$; **at $p < 0.001$

combined) were 0, 4, 1, 4 and 14 ($p < 0.002$) at the five doses, respectively (De Angelo *et al.*, 1998).

Hamster: Groups of 20 male Syrian golden hamsters, six weeks of age, were given potassium bromate (purity, 99.5%) in the drinking-water at concentrations of 0, 125, 250, 500 or 2000 mg/L (ppm) for 89 weeks. These concentrations represented total intakes of potassium bromate of 0, 5.6, 12, 20 and 84 g/kg bw, respectively. There was no difference in survival rate between groups. The incidence of renal tubular tumours was increased but not in a statistically significant or dose-related manner (0 in controls compared with 0, 1, 4 and 2 in the respective dose groups) (Takamura *et al.*, 1985).

3.2 Subcutaneous injection

Mouse: Groups of newborn male and female ICR mice [initial numbers not specified] were injected subcutaneously at one day of age or once a week for four weeks until weaning, with potassium bromate (food-additive grade) in olive oil at doses of 0, 12.5, 25, 50, 100 or 200 mg/kg bw. The high dose of 200 mg/kg bw had been determined to be the maximally tolerated dose. Animals that survived beyond 52 weeks were included as effective numbers, which ranged from 7 to 20. The combined incidence of lymphomas and leukaemias was increased ($p < 0.05$) in male mice receiving cumulative total doses of 400–800 mg/kg bw (8/20) when compared with controls (1/15) (Matsushima *et al.*, 1986).

Rat: Groups of newborn male and female Fischer 344 rats [initial number not specified] were injected subcutaneously at one day of age or once a week for four weeks until weaning, with potassium bromate (food-additive grade) in olive oil at doses of 0, 12.5, 25,

50 or 100 mg/kg bw. The high dose of 100 mg/kg bw had been determined to be the maximally tolerated dose. Animals that survived beyond 52 weeks were included as effective numbers, which ranged from 6 to 21. There were no significant differences in tumour incidence between treated and control rats of either sex (Matsushima *et al.*, 1986).

3.3 Administration with known carcinogens or modifying factors

Rat: Potassium bromate was tested for promoting activity in a model of renal tubular carcinogenesis. Groups of 15 male Wistar rats, six weeks old, were fed a diet containing *N*-nitrosoethylhydroxyethylamine (NEHEA) for two weeks and were then unilaterally nephrectomized by removal of the left kidney at week 3; subsequently, potassium bromate [purity unspecified] was administered in the diet at a concentration of 500 mg/kg (ppm), or the rats received basal diet alone. Five rats per group were killed at weeks 8, 12 and 20. The incidence of preneoplastic renal tubular lesions, diagnosed as adenomatous hyperplasia, was increased at weeks 12 and 20 (2/5 and 2/5 and 3/5) over that in the group given NEHEA plus basal diet (0/5 and 0/5) (Hiasa *et al.*, 1991).

Potassium bromate was tested for initiating activity in a model of renal tubular carcinogenesis. Groups of 39 male Fischer 344/NCr rats, six weeks of age, were given a single intragastric dose of 300 mg/kg bw potassium bromate in distilled water, followed two weeks later by either a basal diet or a diet containing 4000 mg/kg diet (ppm) sodium barbital as a promoting agent until termination of the study at week 104. Other groups of 29 rats received basal diet alone or sodium barbital in the diet from week 2. There was no difference in the incidence of renal tubular tumours or atypical tubular hyperplasia between the group exposed to both potassium bromate and sodium barbital and the group exposed only to sodium barbital, indicating no renal tumour initiating activity (Kurata *et al.*, 1992).

4. Other Data Relevant to an Evaluation of Carcinogenicity and its Mechanisms

The Working Group noted that in experiments in which animals were fed bread made from flour treated with potassium bromate, bromate at the concentrations tested would have been converted to bromide during bread-making.

4.1 Absorption, distribution, metabolism and excretion

4.1.1 *Humans*

No data were available to the Working Group.

4.1.2 *Experimental systems*

After mice (Theiller's original strain) received diets containing 79% bread crumbs made from flour treated with 50 or 75 mg/kg (ppm) potassium bromate, concentrations of

1 and 2 mg/kg bromine, respectively, were detected in adipose tissue (Ginocchio *et al.*, 1979).

Bromine did not accumulate in the adipose tissue of Wistar-derived Porton rats fed for 104 weeks on diets composed of 79% bread crumbs made from flour treated with 75 mg/kg potassium bromide (Fisher *et al.*, 1979). In a further study, male Wistar rats, six to eight weeks of age, were given 100 mg/kg bw potassium bromate by gavage in an aqueous solution as bromate. Animals were killed at various times after treatment, and bromate was assayed in the stomach, small intestinal contents, plasma and bladder urine. Bromate was found to be rapidly absorbed and eliminated (or degraded): 2 h after administration, bromate was no longer detected in plasma, and 4 h after treatment, bromate was no longer detected in bladder urine or small intestine. Twenty-four hours after administration of potassium bromate at a dose ≤ 2.5 mg/kg bw, bromate was not detected in urine. At doses of 5–100 mg/kg bw, the concentrations of bromate in urine after 24 h increased proportionally with dose (Fujii *et al.*, 1984).

4.2 Toxic effects

4.2.1 *Humans*

A number of case reports of acute poisoning by potassium bromate solutions have been reviewed (Norris, 1965). In children 1.5–3 years of age, ingestion of 2–4 oz (57–133 g) of a 2% solution of potassium bromate caused nausea and vomiting, usually with epigastric and/or abdominal pain; diarrhoea and haematemesis occurred in some cases (Parker & Barr, 1951; Gosselin *et al.*, 1976). In both children and adults, oliguria and death from renal failure have been observed (Dunsky, 1947; Ohashi *et al.*, 1971; Gradus *et al.*, 1984). Partial hearing loss and complete deafness have also been reported (Matsumoto, 1973; Quick *et al.*, 1975; Gradus *et al.*, 1984). The toxic or lethal dose of potassium bromate in humans has not been accurately established (Kurokawa *et al.*, 1990), but a dose of 500 mg caused serious symptoms in a 15-month-old child (Quick *et al.*, 1975).

De Vriese *et al.* (1997) described the clinical symptoms of a patient who ingested 300 mL of a cold-wave neutralizer consisting of 10% potassium bromate. They also reviewed 49 other cases of human exposure published since 1947. The characteristic symptoms after ingestion of various solutions containing bromate include nausea, vomiting, abdominal pain and diarrhoea shortly after ingestion. Acute renal failure varying from mild to severe anuric forms have been reported in both children and adults. Nine cases of adult poisoning (33%) resulted in death. Severe irreversible sensorineural hearing loss within 4–16 h of ingestion was recorded in almost all of the adults but in only a few children.

4.2.2 *Experimental systems*

The oral LD_{50} of potassium bromate in Fischer 344 rats was 400–500 mg/kg bw. A dose of ≥ 700 mg/kg bw potassium bromate given as a single intragastric administration was lethal to rats, mice and hamsters (Kurokawa *et al.*, 1990).

The acute hypotensive effects of potassium bromate in rabbits are due to both the potassium and the bromate ions. Rabbits did not survive single intravenous injections of

0.2 g potassium bromate solution for longer than 4 min, and did not survive six intravenous injections (total dose, 1 g) longer than 43 min. The resulting gastric damage was ascribed to the bromate ion. Renal and gastric damage were seen in guinea-pigs and dogs treated with sodium bromate (Santesson & Wickberg, 1913).

In guinea-pigs, subcutaneous injections of 100 mg/kg bw sodium bromate produced cochlear damage—i.e. degenerative changes of the outer hair cells—by 24 h. Animals killed at that time revealed hyaline degeneration, cloudy swelling and necrosis of the epithelial cells in renal tubules, which were most severe in the proximal convoluted tubules. After injection of 200 mg/kg bw, there was more rapid onset of similar effects (Matsumoto, 1973).

Mice (Theiller's original strain) fed for 80 weeks on diets containing 79% bread crumbs prepared from flour treated with 50 or 75 mg/kg potassium bromate showed no significant alteration in blood chemistry, renal function or histopathological parameters, except for a transient reduction in red blood cell counts at three months (Ginocchio *et al.*, 1979). No adverse effect was detected in Wistar rats fed similar diets for 104 weeks (Fisher *et al.*, 1979).

Dogs (greyhounds, red Irish setters and spaniels) of each sex fed diets containing flour treated with 200 mg/kg potassium bromate for 17 months showed no adverse effect (Impey *et al.*, 1961).

Potassium bromate administered intragastrically at a dose of 400 mg/kg bw increased the concentration of 8-hydroxydeoxyguanosine, a DNA lesion formed by oxygen radicals, in kidneys but not the liver of male Fischer 344 rats (Kasai *et al.*, 1987). An active oxygen species—probably singlet oxygen—was formed *in vitro* from the interaction of potassium bromate with cells or homogenates prepared from male Fischer 344 rat kidney, but not liver. 8-Hydroxydeoxyguanosine concentrations were also elevated when potassium bromate was incubated with renal proximal tubules or renal nuclei (Sai *et al.*, 1992).

Potassium bromate given as a single intravenous dose of 77–150 mg/kg bw increased lipid peroxidation in the kidneys of male Fischer 344 rats, but no significant increases were detected in the kidneys of male BDF_1, CDF_1 or $B6C3F_1$ mice or male Syrian golden hamsters. Dose- and time-dependent increases in serum non-protein nitrogen, blood urea nitrogen and creatinine concentrations and in the absolute and relative weights of the kidneys of male rats were seen. Eosinophilic droplets were observed in the cytoplasm of the proximal tubular epithelium of potassium bromate-treated rats. Treatment of rats given potassium bromate with cysteine and glutathione had a protective effect against the lethality and the other changes reported (Kurokawa *et al.*, 1987).

Male Fischer 344 rats were given a single intragastric dose of potassium bromate at 0, 50, 300, 600 or 1200 mg/kg bw and were observed for four weeks for deaths, kidney:body weight ratios and histological appearance of the kidneys. The maximal tolerated dose was 300 mg/kg bw, since most of the animals died after administration of higher doses. Basophilic regenerative tubules and focal accumulation of eosinophilic droplets in the proximal tubules were observed in rats that survived the 300 mg/kg bw dose (Kurata *et al.*, 1992).

Male and female Fischer 344 rats, six weeks of age, were exposed to potassium bromate, potassium bromide (males only) or sodium bromate (males only) at concentrations of 500, 1750 or 500 mg/L (ppm), respectively, in their drinking-water for two weeks to assess protein droplet accumulation and immunohistochemical staining for α_{2u}-globulin in their kidneys. [As the consumption of drinking-water was not given, the Working Group could not convert the doses to milligrams per kilogram of body weight.] A separate group of rats was exposed to the same concentrations of chemicals for two, four and eight weeks to assess renal cell proliferation. Protein droplets were observed in male rat kidneys after administration of potassium bromate or sodium bromate, and these droplets stained for α_{2u}-globulin. Cell proliferation in the proximal tubules was increased only in male rats exposed to potassium bromate or sodium bromate, but not potassium bromide, at two, four and eight weeks of treatment (Umemura *et al.*, 1993).

No treatment-related increase in the frequency of non-neoplastic lesions in liver, kidney or thyroid and no alterations in serum chemical measurements were seen in male B6C3F$_1$ mice and Fischer 344 rats given drinking-water containing 0, 0.08, 0.4 or 0.8 g/L potassium bromate [0, 9.1, 42 or 78 mg/kg per day] or 0, 0.02, 0.1, 0.2 or 0.4 g/L potassium bromate [0, 1.5, 7.9, 17 or 38 mg/kg bw per day], respectively, for up to 100 weeks (De Angelo *et al.*, 1998).

4.3 Reproductive and developmental effects

4.3.1 *Humans*

No data were available to the Working Group.

4.3.2 *Experimental systems*

The reproductive toxicity of sodium bromate in Sprague-Dawley rats was evaluated in a short-term test for reproductive and developmental toxicity (Kaiser *et al.*, 1996; National Toxicology Program, 1996). The compound was administered in drinking-water at concentrations of 0, 25, 80 or 250 mg/L (ppm) over 35 days to one group of 10 male rats and two groups of 10 and 13 female rats. The overall average daily consumption was 2.6, 9.1 and 26 mg/kg bw sodium bromate, respectively. The first group of females was exposed during conception and early gestation, while the second group was exposed from gestation day 6 until parturition. The reproductive outcomes measured included the numbers of ovulations, implantations and viable fetuses, growth and clinical and histological assessment and sperm analysis in the adults. No changes were observed in the reproductive function of the females. There were no changes in body weights, feed consumption, clinical observations, gross findings or relative organ weights (males only). Males showed no treatment-related histological changes in the kidneys, liver, spleen, testis or epididymis, but the activity of serum alanine aminotransferase was decreased by 14% at the two higher doses. There was a significant (18%) decrease in epididymal sperm density in males at the high dose.

4.4 Genetic and related effects

4.4.1 *Humans*

No data were available to the Working Group.

4.4.2 *Experimental systems* (see Table 2 for references)

Potassium bromate did not induce DNA repair in *Bacillus subtilis*. It induced gene mutation in *Salmonella typhimurium* TA100 in the presence of exogenous metabolic activation but not in TA98. It induced 8-hydroxydeoxyguanosine in isolated Fischer 344 rat renal proximal tubules *in vitro*. In several studies, potassium bromate was clastogenic in Chinese hamster and rat cells *in vitro*. It inhibited gap-junctional intercellular communication in Madin-Darby canine kidney epithelial cells. It induced 8-hydroxydeoxyguanosine in the DNA of rat kidney cells *in vivo* in several studies; only a weak or no response was observed in two studies in rat liver cells *in vivo*. Potassium bromate induced micronucleus formation in mice in five studies and in rats in one study. It also induced chromosomal aberrations in the bone-marrow cells of rats treated *in vivo* by intraperitoneal or oral administration.

4.5 Mechanistic considerations

Potassium bromate is highly toxic. It produces lipid peroxidation and oxidative DNA damage in rat kidney; there is also evidence that it increases the concentration of α_{2u}-globulin in male rat kidneys. The available data, including evidence of genetic toxicity, suggest, however, that potassium bromate causes renal tumours through a mechanism that involves oxidative damage to DNA.

Potassium bromate induced 8-hydroxydeoxyguanosine in rat kidney, which is the target organ of carcinogenesis in that species, but the response in liver was questionable. In contrast, the activity of 8-hydroxyguanine glycosylase, which removes 8-hydroxyguanine residues from DNA strands as a free base, was increased in the kidney but not in the liver of potassium bromate-treated rats (Lee *et al.*, 1996). Therefore, the contribution of 8-hydroxydeoxyguanosine to gene mutation is not clear.

5. Summary of Data Reported and Evaluation

5.1 Exposure data

Exposure to potassium bromate may occur during its production and use as a dough conditioner and food additive. Bromate may also be found in some drinking-water samples as a by-product of ozone disinfection.

5.2 Human carcinogenicity data

No data were available to the Working Group.

Table 2. Genetic and related effects of potassium bromate

Test system	Results[a]		Dose[b] (LED or HID)	Reference
	Without exogenous metabolic system	With exogenous metabolic system		
Bacillus subtilis rec strains, differential toxicity	–	–	NR	Kawachi *et al.* (1980)
Salmonella typhimurium TA100, reverse mutation	–	+	NR	Kawachi *et al.* (1980)
Salmonella typhimurium TA100, reverse mutation	NT	+	3000 μg/plate	Ishidate *et al.* (1984)
Salmonella typhimurium TA98, reverse mutation	–	–	NR	Kawachi *et al.* (1980)
Salmonella typhimurium TA98, reverse mutation	NT	–	3000 μg/plate	Ishidate *et al.* (1984)
DNA damage (8-OH-dGua formation), rat kidney cells *in vitro*	+	NT	334	Sai *et al.* (1994)
Chromosomal aberrations, Chinese hamster Don-6 cells *in vitro*	+	NT	84	Sasaki *et al.* (1980)
Chromosomal aberrations, Chinese hamster lung cells *in vitro*	+	+	63	Ishidate *et al.* (1984)
Chromosomal aberrations, Chinese hamster lung fibroblasts *in vitro*	+	NT	NR	Kawachi *et al.* (1980)
Inhibition of gap-junctional intercellular communication, canine kidney cells *in vitro*	+	NT	84	Noguchi *et al.* (1998)
DNA damage (8-OH-dGua formation), Fischer 344 rat kidney *in vivo*	+		400 po × 1	Kasai *et al.* (1987)
DNA damage (8-OH-dGua formation), Fischer 344 rat liver *in vivo*	–		400 po × 1	Kasai *et al.* (1987)
DNA damage (8-OH-dGua formation), Fischer 344 rat kidney *in vivo*	+		80 ip × 1	Sai *et al.* (1992a)
DNA damage (8-OH-dGua formation), Sprague-Dawley rat kidney *in vivo*	+		500 ip × 1	Cho *et al.* (1993)
DNA damage (8-OH-dGua formation), Sprague-Dawley rat liver *in vivo*	(+)		500 ip × 1	Cho *et al.* (1993)
DNA damage (8-OH-dGua formation), Sprague-Dawley rat kidney *in vivo*	+		100 ip × 1	Chipman *et al.* (1998)
DNA damage (8-OH-dGua formation), Fischer 344 rat kidney *in vivo*	+		500 ppm (drinking-water; 1 w)	Umemura *et al.* (1998)
Micronucleus formation, MS and ddY mouse bone-marrow cells *in vivo*	+		25 ip × 1	Hayashi *et al.* (1982)
Micronucleus formation, ddY mouse bone-marrow cells *in vivo*	+		100 po × 2	Hayashi *et al.* (1988)
Micronucleus formation, MS/Ae and CD-1 mouse bone-marrow cells *vivo*	+		37.5 ip or po × 1	Nakajima *et al.* (1989)
Micronucleus formation, CD-1 mouse peripheral blood reticulocytes *in vivo*	+		37.5 ip × 1	Awogi *et al.* (1992)

Table 2 (contd)

Test system	Results[a]		Dose[b] (LED or HID)	Reference
	Without exogenous metabolic system	With exogenous metabolic system		
Micronucleus formation, ddY mouse peripheral blood reticulocytes *in vivo*	+		50 ip × 1	Suzuki *et al.* (1995)
Micronucleus formation, Fischer 344 rat peripheral blood reticulocytes *in vivo*	+		40 ip × 1	Sai *et al.* (1992b)
Chromosomal aberrations, rat bone-marrow cells *in vivo*	+		NR	Kawachi *et al.* (1980)
Chromosomal aberrations, male Long-Evans rat bone-marrow cells *in vivo*	+		167 ip × 1	Fujie *et al.* (1988)
Chromosomal aberrations, male Long-Evans rat bone-marrow cells *in vivo*	+		344 po × 1	Fujie *et al.* (1988)

8-OH-dGua, 8-hydroxydeoxyguanosine

[a] +, positive; (+), weakly positive; –, negative; NT, not tested

[b] LED, lowest effective dose; HID, highest ineffective dose; unless otherwise stated, in-vitro test, μg/mL; in-vivo test, mg/kg bw per day; NR, not reported; po, oral; ip, intraperitoneal; w, week

5.3 Animal carcinogenicity data

Potassium bromate has been tested by oral administration in several studies in rats and in one study each in mice and hamsters. In rats, it produced renal tubular tumours (adenomas and carcinomas) and thyroid follicular tumours in animals of each sex and peritoneal mesotheliomas in males. In mice, it produced a low incidence of renal tubular tumours in males. In hamsters, the incidence of renal tubular tumours was marginally increased. Potassium bromate did not increase tumour incidence in bioassays in newborn rats and mice, but it enhanced the induction of kidney tumours by *N*-nitrosoethylhydroxyethylamine in several experiments.

5.4 Other relevant data

No data were available on the absorption, distribution, metabolism or excretion of potassium bromate in humans, and limited information was available on rats. Bromate was found to be rapidly absorbed in rats and eliminated (or degraded).

A number of case reports of acute poisoning by potassium bromate have been reported. Potassium bromate is highly toxic. It produces lipid peroxidation and oxidative DNA damage in rat kidney. There is also evidence that it increases the amount of α_{2u}-globulin in male rat kidney. The available data, including evidence of genetic toxicity, indicate, however, that potassium bromate causes renal tumours through a mechanism involving oxidative damage.

No data were available on the developmental and reproductive effects of potassium bromate. However, in a single, short-term assay to screen for reproductive toxicity, involving exposure of male and female rats to sodium bromate before and during gestation, no developmental toxicity was observed. A decrease in epididymal sperm concentration was found in males.

No data were available on the genetic and related effects of potassium bromate in humans. It is genotoxic in experimental systems *in vivo* and in rodent cells *in vitro*. No conclusion could be drawn with respect to its mutagenicity to bacteria.

5.5 Evaluation

There is *inadequate evidence* in humans for the carcinogenicity of potassium bromate.

There is *sufficient evidence* in experimental animals for the carcinogenicity of potassium bromate.

Overall evaluation

Potassium bromate is *possibly carcinogenic to humans (Group 2B)*.

6. References

Awogi, T., Murata, K., Uejima, M., Kuwahara, T., Asanami, S., Shimono, K. & Morita, T. (1992) Induction of micronucleated reticulocytes by potassium bromate and potassium chromate in CD-1 male mice. *Mutat. Res.*, **278**, 181–185

Budavari, S., ed. (1996) *The Merck Index*, 12th Ed., Whitehouse Station, NJ, Merck & Co., p. 1313

Chemical Information Services (1995) *Directory of World Chemical Producers 1995/96 Standard Edition*, Dallas, TX, p. 587

Chipman, J.K., Davies, J.E., Parsons, J.L., Nair, J., O'Neill, G. & Fawell, J.K. (1998) DNA oxidation by potassium bromate; a direct mechanism or linked to lipid peroxidation? *Toxicol.*, **126**, 93–102

Cho, D.H., Hong, J.T., Chin, K., Cho, T.S. & Lee, B.M. (1993) Organotropic formation and disappearance of 8-hydroxydeoxyguanosine in the kidney of Sprague-Dawley rats exposed to adriamycin and $KBrO_3$. *Cancer Lett.*, **74**, 141–145

De Angelo, A.B., George, M.H., Kilburn, S.R., Moore, T.M. & Wolf, D.C. (1998) Carcinogenicity of potassium bromate administered in drinking water to male B6C3F1 mice and Fischer 344/N rats. *Toxicol. Pathol.*, **26**, 587–594

Dennis, M.J., Burrell, A., Mathieson, K., Willetts, P. & Massey, R.C. (1994) The determination of the flour improver potassium bromate in bread by gas chromatography and ICP-MS methods. *Food Addit. Contam.*, **11**, 633–639

De Vriese, A., Vanholder, R. & Lameire, N. (1997) Severe acute renal failure due to bromate intoxication: Report of a case and discussion of management guidelines based on a review of the literature. *Nephrol. Dialysis Transplant*, **12**, 204–209

Dunsky, I. (1947) Potassium bromate poisoning. *Am. J. Dis. Child.*, **74**, 730–734

Fisher, N., Hutchinson, J.B., Berry, R., Hardy, J., Ginocchio, A.V. & Waite, V. (1979) Long-term toxicity and carcinogenicity studies of the bread improver potassium bromate. 1. Studies in rats. *Food Cosmet. Toxicol.*, **17**, 33–39

Fujie, K., Shimazu, H., Matsuda, M. & Sugiyama, T. (1988) Acute cytogenetic effects of potassium bromate on rat bone marrow cells *in vivo*. *Mutat. Res.*, **206**, 455–458

Fujii, M., Oikawa, K., Saito, H., Fukuhara, C., Onosaka, S. & Tanaka, K. (1984) Metabolism of potassium bromate in rats. I. In vivo studies. *Chemosphere*, **13**, 1207–1212

Ginocchio, A.V., Waite, V., Hardy, J., Fisher, N., Hutchinson, J.B. & Berry, R. (1979) Long-term toxicity and carcinogenicity studies of the bread improver potassium bromate. 2. Studies in mice. *Food Cosmet. Toxicol.*, **17**, 41–47

Glaze, W.H. (1986) Reaction products of ozone: A review. *Environ. Health Perspectives*, **69**, 151–157

Gosselin, R.E., Hodge, H.C., Smith, R.P. & Gleason, M.N. (1976) *Clinical Toxicology of Commercial Products: Acute Poisoning,* 4th Ed., Baltimore, MD, Williams & Wilkins, p. 66

Gradus (Ben-Ezer), D., Rhoads, M., Bergstrom, L.B. & Jordan, S.C. (1984) Acute bromate poisoning associated with renal failure and deafness presenting as hemolytic uremic syndrome. *Am. J. Nephrol.*, **4**, 188–191

Hayashi, M., Sofuni, T. & Ishidate, M., Jr (1982) High-sensitivity in micronucleus induction of a mouse strain (MS). *Mutat. Res.*, **105**, 253–256

Hayashi, M., Kishi, M., Sofuni, T. & Ishidate, M., Jr (1988) Micronucleus tests in mice on 39 food additives and eight miscellaneous chemicals. *Food chem. Toxicol.*, **26**, 487–500

Hiasa, Y., Konishi, N., Nakaoka, S., Nakamura, M., Nishii, S., Kitahori, Y. & Ohshima, M. (1991) Possible application to medium-term organ bioassays for renal carcinogenesis modifiers in rats treated with *N*-ethyl-*N*-hydroxyethylnitrosamine and unilateral nephrectomy. *Jpn. J. Cancer Res.*, **82,** 1385–1390

IARC (1986) *IARC Monographs on the Evaluation of the Carcinogenic Risk of Chemicals to Humans*, Vol. 40, *Some Naturally Occurring and Synthetic Food Components, Furocoumarins and Ultraviolet Radiation*, Lyon, pp. 207–220

IARC (1987) *IARC Monographs on the Evaluation of Carcinogenic Risks to Humans*, Suppl. 7, *Overall Evaluations of Carcinogenicity: An Updating of* IARC Monographs *Volumes 1 to 42*, Lyon, p. 70

Impey, S.G., Moore, T. & Sharman, I.M. (1961) Effects of flour treatment on the suitability of bread as food for dogs. *J. Sci. Food Agric.*, **11**, 729–732

Ishidate, M., Jr, Sofuni, T., Yoshikawa, K., Hayashi, M., Nohmi, T., Sawada, M. & Matsuoka, A. (1984) Primary mutagenicity screening of food additives currently used in Japan. *Food chem. Toxicol.*, **22**, 623–636

Kaiser, L.B., Wolfe, G.W., Lanning, L., Chapin, R.E., Klinefelter, G. & Hunter, E.S. (1996) Short term reproductive and developmental effects of sodium bromate in S-D rats when administered in the drinking water (Abstract). *Toxicologist*, **30**, 121–122

Kasai, H., Nishimura, S., Kurokawa, Y. & Hayashi, Y. (1987) Oral administration of the renal carcinogen, potassium bromate, specifically produces 8-hydroxydeoxyguanosine in rat target organ DNA. *Carcinogenesis*, **8**, 1959–1961

Kawachi, T., Yahagi, T., Kada, T., Tazima, Y., Ishidate, M., Sasaki, M. & Sugimura, T. (1980) Cooperative programme on short-term assays for carcinogenicity in Japan. In: Montesano, R., Bartsch, H. & Tomatis, L., eds, *Molecular and Cellular Aspects of Carcinogen Screening Tests* (IARC Scientific Publications No. 27), Lyon, IARC, pp. 323–330

Kurata, Y., Diwan, B.A. & Ward, J.M. (1992) Lack of renal tumor-initiating activity of a single dose of potassium bromate, a genotoxic renal carcinogen in male Fischer 344/NCr rats. *Food chem. Toxicol.*, **30**, 251–259

Kurokawa, Y., Aoki, S., Matsushima, Y., Takamura, N., Imazawa, T. & Hayashi, Y. (1986) Dose-response studies on the carcinogenicity of potassium bromate in F344 rats after long-tem oral administration. *J. natl Cancer Inst.*, **77,** 977–982

Kurokawa, Y., Takamura, N., Matsuoka, C., Imazawa, T., Matsushima, Y., Onodera, H. & Hayashi, Y. (1987) Comparative studies on lipid peroxidation in the kidney of rats, mice and hamsters and on the effect of cysteine, glutathione and diethyl maleate treatment on mortality and nephrotoxicity after administration of potassium bromate. *J. Am. Coll. Toxicol.*, **6**, 489–501

Kurokawa, Y., Maekawa, A., Takahashi, M. & Hayashi, Y. (1990) Toxicity and carcinogenicity of potassium bromate—A new renal carcinogen. *Environ. Health Perspectives*, **87**, 309–335

Lee, Y.-S., Choi, J.-Y., Park, M.-K., Choi, E.-M., Kasai, H. & Chung, M.-H. (1996) Induction of OH^8Gua glycosylase in rat kidneys by potassium bromate ($KBrO_3$), a renal oxidative carcinogen. *Mutat. Res.*, **364**, 227–233

Matsumoto, I. (1973) [Clinical and experimental studies on the ototoxicity of bromate.] *Otol. Fukuoka*, **19**, 220–236 (in Japanese)

Matsushima, Y., Takamura, N., Imazawa, T., Kurokawa, Y. & Hayashi, Y. (1986) Lack of carcinogenicity of potassium bromate after subcutaneous injection to newborn mice and newborn rats. *Sci. Rep. Res. Inst. Tohoku Univ.*, **33**, 22–26

Nakajima, M., Kitazawa, M., Oba, K., Kitagawa, Y. & Toyoda, Y. (1989) Effect of route of administration in the micronucleus test with potassium bromate. *Mutat. Res.*, **223**, 399–402

National Institute for Occupational Safety and Health (1998) *National Occupational Exposure Survey (1981–1983)*, Cincinnati, OH

National Toxicology Program (1991) *NTP Chemical Repository Data Sheet: Potassium Bromate*, Research Triangle Park, NC

National Toxicology Program (1996) *Final Report: Sodium Bromate: Short Term Reproductive and Developmental Toxicology Study When Administered to Sprague-Dawley Rats in the Drinking Water* (NTP/NIEHS No. NOI-ES-15323; NTP-RDGT No. 94-007), Research Triangle Park, NC

Noguchi, M., Nomata, K., Watanabe, J., Kanetake, H. & Saito, Y. (1998) Changes in the gap junctional intercellular communication in renal tubular epithelial cells *in vitro* treated with renal carcinogens. *Cancer Lett.*, **122**, 77–84

Norris, J.A. (1965) Toxicity of home permanent waving and neutralizer solutions. *Food Cosmet. Toxicol.*, **3**, 93–97

Ohashi, N., Shiba, T., Kamiya, K. & Takamura, T. (1971) [Acute renal failure following potassium bromate ('cold wave' neutralizer) poisoning (recovery from prolonged oliguria).] *Jpn. J. Urol.*, **62**, 639–646 (in Japanese)

Parker, W.A. & Barr, J.R. (1951) Potassium bromate poisoning. *Br. med. J.*, **i**, 1363–1364

Quick, C.A., Chole, R.A. & Mauer, S.M. (1975) Deafness and renal failure due to potassium bromate poisoning. *Arch. otolaryngol.*, **101**, 494–495

Sai, K., Uchiyama, S., Ohmo, Y., Hasegawa, R. & Kurokawa, Y. (1992) Generation of active oxygen species *in vitro* by the interaction of potassium bromate with rat kidney cell. *Carcinogenesis*, **13**, 333–339

Sai, K., Umemura, T., Takagi, A. , Hasegawa, R. & Kurokawa, Y. (1992a) The protective role of glutathione, cysteine and vitamin C against oxidative DNA damage induced in rat kidney by potassium bromate. *Jpn. J. Cancer Res.*, **83**, 45–51

Sai, K., Hayashi, M., Takagi, A., Hasegawa, R. Sofuni, T. & Kurokawa, Y. (1992b) Effects of antioxidants on induction of micronuclei in rat peripheral blood reticulocytes by potassium bromate. *Mutat. Res.*, **269**, 113–118

Sai, K., Tyson, C.A., Thomas, D.W., Dabbs, J.E., Hasegawa, R. & Kurokawa, Y. (1994) Oxidative DNA damage induced by potassium bromate in isolated rat renal proximal tubules and renal nuclei. *Cancer Lett.*, **87**, 1–7

Santesson, C.G. & Wickberg, G. (1913) [On the action of sodium bromate.] *Scand. Arch. Physiol.*, **30**, 337–374 (in German)

Sasaki, M., Sugimura, K., Yoshida, M.A. & Abe, S. (1980) Cytogenetic effects of 60 chemicals on cultured human and Chinese hamster cells. *Kromosomo*, **II-20**, 574–584

Suzuki, T., Hayashi, M., Hakura, A., Asita, O.A., Kodama, Y., Honma, M. & Sofuni, T. (1995) Combination effects of clastogens in the mouse peripheral blood micronucleus assay. *Mutagenesis*, **10**, 31–36

Takamura, N., Kurokawa, Y., Matsushima, Y., Imazawa, T., Onodera, H. & Hayashi, Y. (1985) Long-term oral administration of potassium bromate in male Syrian golden hamsters. *Sci. Rep. Res. Inst. Tohoku Univ.,* **32,** 43–46

Umemura, T., Sai, K., Takagi, A., Hasegawa, R. & Kurokawa, Y. (1993) A possible role for cell proliferation in potassium bromate ($KBrO_3$) carcinogenesis. *J. Cancer Res. clin. Oncol.*, **119**, 463–469

Umemura, T., Takagi, A., Sai, K., Hasegawa, R. & Kurokawa, Y. (1998) Oxidative DNA damage and cell proliferation in kidneys of male and female rats during 13-weeks exposure to potassium bromate ($KBrO_3$). *Arch. Toxicol.*, **72**, 264–269

WHO (1993) *Guidelines for Drinking Water Quality*, 2nd Ed., Vol. 1, *Recommendations*, Geneva

QUERCETIN

This substance was considered by previous working groups, in 1982 (IARC, 1983) and 1987 (IARC, 1987). Since that time, new data have become available, and these have been incorporated into the monograph and taken into consideration in the present evaluation.

1. Exposure Data

1.1 Chemical and physical data

1.1.1 *Nomenclature*

Chem. Abstr. Serv. Reg. No.: 117-39-5
Deleted CAS Reg. No.: 73123-10-1; 74893-81-5
Chem. Abstr. Name: 2-(3,4-Dihydroxyphenyl)-3,5,7-trihydroxy-4*H*-1-benzopyran-4-one
IUPAC Systematic Name: 3,3′,4′,5,7-Pentahydroxyflavone
Synonyms: CI 75670; CI Natural Yellow 10; 3,3′,4′,5,7-pentahydroxyflavone; 3,4′,5,5′,7-pentahydroxyflavone; 3,5,7,3′,4′-pentahydroxyflavone; quercetine

1.1.2 *Structural and molecular formulae and relative molecular mass*

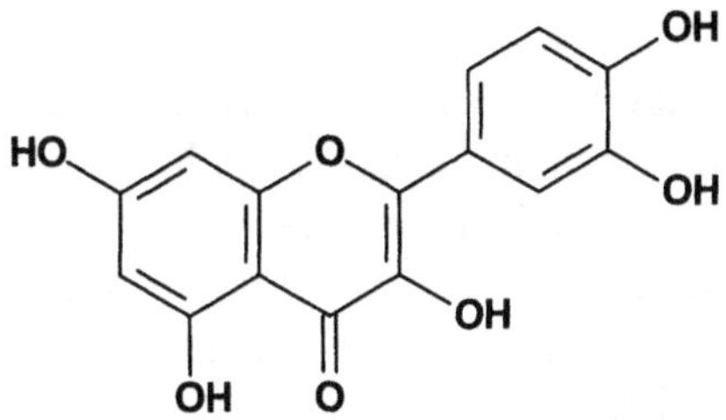

$C_{15}H_{10}O_7$ Relative molecular mass: 302.24

1.1.3 *Chemical and physical properties of the pure substance*

(*a*) *Description*: Pale-yellow needles (dihydrate) (Budavari, 1996)
(*b*) *Boiling-point*: Sublimes (Lide, 1997)
(*c*) *Melting-point*: 316.5°C (Lide, 1997)
(*d*) *Solubility*: Slightly soluble in water and diethyl ether; soluble in ethanol and acetone (Lide, 1997)
(*e*) *Conversion factor*: mg/m^3 = 12.36 × ppm

1.2 Production and use

Information available in 1995 indicated that quercetin was produced in Brazil, Germany, Japan, Spain, Switzerland, the United Kingdom and the United States (Chemical Information Services, 1995).

Quercetin has been used in medicine to decrease capillary fragility. It has also been used in dyes and as a veterinary drug (National Toxicology Program, 1991).

1.3 Occurrence

Quercetin is widely distributed, usually as a glycoside, especially in the peels and leaves of many fruits and vegetables (Budavari, 1996). No data were available on occupational exposure to or the environmental occurrence of quercetin.

1.4 Regulations and guidelines

No international guidelines for quercetin in drinking-water have been established (WHO, 1993).

2. Studies of Cancer in Humans

No data were available to the Working Group.

3. Studies of Cancer in Experimental Animals

Previous evaluation

Quercetin was tested for carcinogenicity in three experiments in rats, two in mice and one in hamsters by oral administration. Negative results were obtained in all but one of the studies in rats; intestinal and bladder tumours were produced in the one study with positive results. Quercetin was also tested by skin application in one study in mice, with a negative outcome for skin tumours. In one study in mice that received implantations of cholesterol pellets in the bladder, bladder carcinomas were produced in both treated and control groups. Rutin, the 3-rhamno-glucoside of quercetin, was tested by oral administration in one study in rats and one study in hamsters. No significant difference in tumour incidence from that in controls was observed (IARC, 1983).

New studies

3.1 Oral administration

Rat: Groups of 15 male and 15 female Fischer 344 rats, six weeks of age, were given quercetin (purity, 99%) in the diet at a concentration of 0.1% for 540 days. All of the treated animals survived. The incidence of tumours in the treated groups was not statistically different from that in controls (Takanashi *et al.*, 1983). [The Working Group noted the small numbers of animals, which made the study inadequate for evaluation.]

Groups of 50 male and 50 female Fischer 344/DuCrj rats, six weeks of age, were fed quercetin (purity, at least 99.4%) in the diet at concentrations of 0 (control), 1.25 or 5% for 104 weeks and were maintained for a further eight weeks without quercetin. The high dose was the maximum tolerated. At the end of the 112-week study, the survival rates for males were 56, 66 and 68% and those for females were 66, 62 and 72% for the three groups, respectively. No statistically significant increase in incidence of tumours was seen, but males at the high dose showed a significant increase in the incidence of non-neoplastic hyperplastic polyps of the caecum, and one adenoma and two adenocarcinomas of the caecum were found in males at this dose and two adenomas of the colon occurred in females (Ito *et al.*, 1989).

Groups of 70 male and 70 female Fischer 344/N rats, seven weeks of age, were given quercetin (purity, > 95%; ellagic acid was the predominant impurity at 1.1–2.6%) in the diet at concentrations of 0, 1000, 10 000 or 40 000 mg/kg (ppm) for 104 weeks. Ten animals per group were killed at 6 and 15 months. The high dose approached the maximum tolerated. Treatment did not affect the survival of either male or female rats, but the decreased body-weight gain of animals at the high dose was attributed to quercetin. As shown in Table 1, males at the high-dose had an increased incidence of renal tubular tumours (three adenomas and one adenocarcinoma) with none in control males, but the increase did not achieve statistical significance. After step-sectioning, a total of nine renal tubular tumours were found in these animals, and the increase was statistically significant. The severity of spontaneous progressive nephropathy was exacerbated in male rats by exposure to quercetin (Dunnick & Hailey, 1992; National Toxicology Program, 1992).

Table 1. Incidences of primary renal tubular adenomas or carcinomas in Fischer 344 rats exposed to quercetin

Treatment (ppm)	Animals with tumours			
	Males		Females	
	Initial evaluation	Single plus step-section	Initial evaluation	Single plus step section
Control	0/50	1/50	0/49	1/49
1 000	0/50	2/50	0/49	–
10 000	0/50	7/50[a]	1/50	–
40 000	4/50[b]	9/50[c]	0/50	0/50

From National Toxicology Program (1992)
–, not determined
[a] $p < 0.0032$
[b] $p = 0.064$
[c] $p = 0.01$

3.2 Administration with known carcinogens

Many new studies have been conducted in which quercetin was tested in various initiation–promotion regimens with various carcinogens, with variable results. Both enhancing and inhibiting activity were found.

Mouse: In a study of skin carcinogenesis in groups of 30 CD-1 mice, prior treatment with quercetin had no effect on initiation of tumours by benzo[*a*]pyrene (Chang *et al.*, 1985). Quercetin given by intramuscular injection or in the diet was reported to enhance the carcinogenicity of 3-methylcholanthrene in C57BL/6 mice by significantly shortening the latency of sarcomas at the site of intramuscular injection of 3-methylcholanthrene (Ishikawa *et al.*, 1985). When quercetin was tested as a potential initiator in a two-stage model of mouse skin carcinogenesis with 12-*O*-tetradecanoylphorbol 13-acetate (TPA) as the promoting agent, local application twice a week for five weeks induced two skin tumours in 1/21 mice after 47 weeks of TPA treatment. No skin tumour was produced with quercetin alone or with dimethyl sulfoxide plus TPA (Sato *et al.*, 1987).

Dietary administration of quercetin has been shown in some studies to inhibit tumours, including azoxymethane-induced colonic tumours in mice (Deschner *et al.*, 1991) and skin tumour formation in three models of skin carcinogenesis in mice when administered by topical application (Nishino *et al.*, 1984; Khan *et al.*, 1988, Mukhtar *et al.*, 1988).

Rat: In a model of pancreatic carcinogenesis with *N*-methyl-*N*-nitrosourea as the carcinogen, quercetin significantly enhanced focal acinar-cell hyperplasia in rats of each sex and produced a non-significant increase in the incidence of carcinomas *in situ* (Barotto *et al.*, 1998).

Quercetin did not enhance the bladder tumour incidence induced in rats by *N*-nitrosobutyl-*N*-(4-hydroxybutyl)amine (Fukushima *et al.*, 1983; Hirose *et al.*, 1983), mammary gland, ear-duct and forestomach tumours induced in rats by 7,12-dimethylbenz[*a*]anthracene (DMBA) (Hirose *et al.*, 1988) or intestinal carcinogenesis induced in rats by methylazoxymethanol acetate (Kato *et al.*, 1984). In models of colon and mammary carcinogenesis, quercetin inhibited the development of aberrant crypt foci in rat colon (Matsukawa *et al.*, 1997) and the incidence of DMBA- and *N*-methyl-*N*-nitrosourea-induced mammary cancer (Verma *et al.*, 1988).

Hamster: Administration of 3% quercetin in the diet of male Syrian hamsters increased the mean number of renal tumour masses and the incidence of metastases after subcutaneous implants of oestradiol (Zhu & Liehr, 1994). Quercetin inhibited DMBA-induced buccal pouch carcinogenesis in hamsters (Balasubramanian & Govindasamy, 1996).

4. Other Data Relevant to an Evaluation of Carcinogenicity and its Mechanisms

4.1 Absorption, distribution, metabolism and excretion

4.1.1 *Humans*

After oral administration of a single dose of 4 g quercetin to four male and two female volunteers, neither quercetin nor its conjugates was detected in the blood or urine during the first 24 h; 53% of the dose was recovered in the faeces within 72 h. After a single intravenous injection of 100 mg quercetin to six volunteers, the blood plasma levels declined biphasically, with half-lives of 8.8 min and 2.4 h; protein binding exceeded 98%. In the urine, 0.65% of the intravenous dose was excreted as unchanged quercetin and 7.4% as a conjugate within 9 h; no further excretion occurred up to 24 h (Gugler *et al.*, 1975).

One male and one female volunteer were given a diet containing quercetin glucosides (64.2 mg expressed as the aglycone). The mean peak plasma concentration of quercetin was 196 ng/mL which was reached 2.9 h after ingestion. The time-course of the plasma concentration of quercetin was biphasic, with half-lives of 3.8 h for the distribution phase and 16.8 h for the elimination phase. Quercetin was still present in plasma 48 h after ingestion (Hollman *et al.*, 1996). Similar findings were made for nine other human subjects (Hollman *et al.*, 1997). The authors suggested that this slow elimination rate would lead to accumulation in plasma with repeated ingestion.

The metabolites of quercetin flavonols identified in urine samples collected from two male volunteers who consumed their habitual diets for three days were 3,4-dihydroxyphenylacetic acid, *meta*-hydroxyphenylacetic acid, and 4-hydroxy-3-methoxyphenylacetic acid (Gross *et al.*, 1996).

4.1.2 *Experimental systems*

Autoradiographic analysis of a fasted rat 3 h after administration of a single oral dose of 2.3 mg/kg bw [4-^{14}C]quercetin showed that although most of the radiolabel remained in the digestive tract it also occurred in blood, liver, kidney, lung and ribs. After oral administration of 630 mg/kg bw of the labelled compound to rats, 34% of the radiolabel excreted within 24 h, expressed as a proportion of the dose, was expired carbon dioxide, 12% in bile and 9% in urine; within 48 h, 45% was recovered in the faeces. Approximately 60% of the radiolabel in the faeces was identified as unmetabolized quercetin. Sulfate and glucuronide conjugates of quercetin and of an unidentified flavonoid were found in bile and urine. Incubation of [4-^{14}C]quercetin with rat caecal and colon contents *in vitro* under conditions that were probably anaerobic resulted in the release of 6% of the radiolabel as carbon dioxide (Ueno *et al.*, 1983).

After oral administration of 0.5 g/kg bw quercetin to rabbits, the main urinary metabolites were 3,4-dihydroxyphenylacetic acid, 3-methoxy-4-hydroxyphenylacetic acid and 3-hydroxyphenylacetic acid (Booth *et al.*, 1956).

Quercetin was rapidly metabolized by *O*-methylation in male Syrian hamsters (Harlan Sprague-Dawley) two to four months of age given an intraperitoneal injection of 50 or 500 mg/kg bw quercetin mixed in 50% glycerol:water. The major metabolite of quercetin in the ether extract of urine was identified as 3′-*O*-methylquercetin. A major portion of the 3′-*O*-methylquercetin eliminated in urine was conjugated by glucuronidation or sulfation. Only 2% of the total flavonoid content of the extract was unmetabolized quercetin. The rates of *O*-methylation of quercetin *in vitro* catalysed by porcine liver catechol-*O*-methyltransferase or cytosolic fractions of Syrian hamster kidney were about three orders of magnitude higher than the rates for endogenous catechols, such as catechol oestrogens and catecholamines (Zhu *et al.*, 1994).

4.2 Toxic effects

4.2.1 *Humans*

No data were available to the Working Group.

4.2.2 *Experimental systems*

The acute oral and subcutaneous LD_{50} values of quercetin in the mouse are 160 and 100 mg/kg bw (Sullivan *et al.*, 1951). Rabbits were unaffected by intravenous administration of 100 mg/kg bw or by diets containing 1% quercetin for 410 days (Ambrose *et al.*, 1952).

Male and female Fischer 344 rats were given a diet containing 0, 1.25 or 5% quercetin for 104 weeks and then a normal diet for a further eight weeks (see section 3 for details), with average intakes for males and females, respectively, of 427 and 497 mg/kg bw per day for those consuming the 1.25% quercetin diet and 1926 and 2372 mg/kg bw per day for rats consuming the 5% diet. With 5% quercetin, the body weights of males and females at the high dose were decreased throughout the study. There were no treatment-ascribed effects on clinical signs, deaths or the results of urinalysis or haematology. Decreases in serum glucose concentration and increases in some relative organ weights were observed at the high dose, the latter being attributed to growth retardation. A higher incidence of hyperplastic polyps of the caecum was observed at the high dose in comparison with controls. No significant increase in adverse changes was observed in other organs (Ito *et al.*, 1989).

Male and female Fischer 344 rats, seven weeks of age, were given quercetin in the diet at concentrations of 0, 1000, 10 000 or 40 000 mg/kg of diet (ppm) for two years (to provide estimated doses of approximately 40, 410 and 1900 mg/kg bw per day during the second year). Rats were necropsied after 6 and 15 months of treatment for interim evaluations. The body weights of animals at the high dose were reduced relative to those of controls during the last year of the study. The only treatment-related toxic lesions were detected microscopically at the 6- and 15-month evaluations and consisted of pigmentation of the superficial epithelium of the glandular stomach and the distal segments of the small intestine, the latter also being seen at two years. The authors noted that quercetin is a yellow compound, and adsorption of this chemical or a metabolite was probably the cause of the tissue pigmentation. After two years of quercetin administration, the incidence of hyperplasia of the renal tubular epithelium was increased, with mild exacerbation of chronic nephropathy in male rats (see section 3 for neoplastic effects). Male rats also had dose-related increases in the incidence of renal pelvic epithelial hyperplasia and of parathyroid gland hyperplasia, which are commonly observed in male rats with advanced nephropathy (Dunnick & Hailey, 1992).

Quercetin inhibits Na^+-K^+ ATPase in both plasma and mitochondrial membranes (Lang & Racker, 1974; Suolinna *et al.*, 1975). Inhibition of glucose oxidation in neutrophils via the hexose monophosphate pathway and inhibition of uptake of 2-deoxyglucose were also reported (Long *et al.*, 1981). Quercetin inhibited glycolysis in Erhlich ascites tumour cells, due probably to a lowering of the intracellular pH by inhibition of lactate efflux (Belt *et al.*, 1979). Administration of 5–20 μg/mL quercetin caused pronounced inhibition of the growth of several cell lines (Suolinna *et al.*, 1975). Liposome-encapsulated quercetin inhibited DNA synthesis in Ehrlich ascites tumour cells (Podhajcer *et al.*, 1980).

Quercetin inhibited ethoxyresofurin *O*-deethylation by liver microsomes prepared from β-naphthoflavone-treated Long Evans rats, by 15% at a concentration of 10 nmol/L to 80% at 250 nmol/L (Sousa & Marletta, 1985); and it had a similar effect in microsomes prepared from 3-methylcholanthrene-treated Sprague-Dawley rats, causing 50% inhibition at a concentration of 15 μmol/L (Moon *et al.*, 1998). Quercetin also inhibited ethoxyresorufin *O*-deethylase activity in human microsomes, causing 50% inhibition at 12 ± 6 μmol/L (Siess *et al.*, 1995). Quercetin also inhibited *para*-nitroanisole demethylation and benzo[*a*]pyrene hydroxylation reactions of β-naphthoflavone-treated Long Evans rat microsomes, by 26% at a concentration of 0.25 μmol/L, 78% at 5 μmol/L, 32% at 0.1 μmol/L and 95% at 500 μmol/L (Sousa & Marletta, 1985). Hydroxylation of benzo[*a*]pyrene by a sample of human liver microsomes was also inhibited by quercetin, by 14% at a concentration of 0.005 mmol/L and 81% at 1 mmol/L (Buening *et al.*, 1981). Quercetin was a potent uncoupler of P450 reactions, acting by dissociation of the reduced P450–oxygen complex, and increased the rate of hydrogen peroxide formation by almost twofold (Sousa & Marletta, 1985).

In liver nuclei isolated from male Sprague-Dawley rats, quercetin caused a concentration-dependent increase in DNA damage and lipid peroxidation and a concentration-dependent decrease in nuclear glutathione content and glutathione *S*-transferase activity (Sahu & Washington, 1991; Sahu & Gary, 1996).

Quercetin was reported to have 1% of the oestrogenic activity of oestradiol in HeLa cells transfected with the human oestrogen receptor and the pERE-TK-CAT reporter plasmid (Santti *et al.*, 1997).

4.3 Reproductive and developmental effects

4.3.1 *Humans*

No data were available to the Working Group.

4.3.2 *Experimental systems*

Groups of 8–12 pregnant rats received 0, 2, 20, 200 or 2000 mg/kg bw quercetin on day 9 or on days 6–15 of gestation by oral gavage. No overt signs of toxicity were observed in the dams at any dose. Quercetin did not affect embryonic viability or morphology but fetal growth retardation was seen after exposure to 200 or 2000 mg/kg bw on day 9 and to 2 or 2000 mg/kg bw on days 9–15 (Wilhite, 1982).

4.4 Genetic and related effects

The genotoxicity of quercetin has been reviewed (Brown, 1980).

4.4.1 *Humans*

No data were available to the Working Group.

4.4.2 *Experimental systems* (see Table 2 for references)

Quercetin induced DNA damage and SOS repair in bacterial cells. It did not induce differential toxicity in DNA repair-deficient strains of *Samonella.* It was mutagenic in several strains of *Salmonella typhimurium* and *Escherichia coli* in the absence of exogenous metabolic activation. In single studies, quercetin induced gene conversion but not gene mutation in *Saccharomyces cerevisiae* and induced sex-linked recessive lethal mutation in *Drosophila melanogaster. In vitro*, it caused DNA unwinding in rat liver nuclei and induced DNA single-strand breaks in mouse lymphoma L5178Y cells, but it did not induce unscheduled DNA synthesis in rat hepatocytes. Quercetin consistently induced gene mutation at the *tk* locus in mammalian cells *in vitro*, but *hprt* locus mutants were induced in only one of four studies. Sister chromatid exchange was induced in three of four studies in Chinese hamster cells *in vitro*, and chromosomal aberrations were induced in several Chinese hamster cell lines and in a human cell line *in vitro*. It induced cell transformation in mammalian cells. It induced sister chromatid exchange, micronuclei and chromosomal aberrations in human lymphocytes *in vitro* with and without exogenous metabolic activation. Urine and faecal extracts of rats treated with quercetin were mutagenic to *Salmonella typhimurium* TA98. Micronuclei were not induced by quercetin administered *in vivo*, either in bone-marrow cells of mice in four studies, in peripheral blood cells of mice in one study or in bone-marrow cells of rats in one study. Chromosomal aberrations were not induced in bone-marrow cells of rats treated *in vivo* in one study. Dominant lethal effects were not induced in either male mice or male rats in a single study.

5. Summary of Data Reported and Evaluation

5.1 Exposure data

Exposure to quercetin may occur during its production and use in dyes and from its presence in a variety of fruits and vegetables.

Table 2. Genetic and related effects of quercetin

Test system	Results[a]		Dose[b] (LED or HID)	Reference
	Without exogenous metabolic system	With exogenous metabolic system		
SOS chromotest, *Escherichia coli* PQ37	+	+	2.7	Rueff *et al.* (1986)
SOS chromotest, *Escherichia coli* PQ37	+	+	16	Dayan *et al.* (1987)
SOS chromotest, *Escherichia coli* PQ37	(+)	(+)	10	Czeczot & Kusztelak (1993)
Salmonella typhimurium, DNA repair-deficient strains, differential toxicity	–	–	200 µg/plate	Czeczot & Kusztelak (1993)
Salmonella typhimurium TA100, reverse mutation	+	+	5 µg/plate	Stoewsand *et al.* (1984)
Salmonella typhimurium TA100, TA98, TA97, TA102, TA1538, reverse mutation	+	+	10 µg/plate	Czeczot *et al.* (1990)
Salmonella typhimurium TA100, TA98, TA1537, reverse mutation	+	+	25 µg/plate	Hardigree & Epler (1978)
Salmonella typhimurium TA100, TA98, reverse mutation	+	+	3 µg/plate	National Toxicology Program (1992)
Salmonella typhimurium TA100, TA102, reverse mutation	–	NT	100 µg/plate	Cross *et al.* (1996)
Salmonella typhimurium TA98, TA102, reverse mutation	+	+	5 µg/plate	Crebelli *et al.* (1987)
Salmonella typhimurium TA1538, TA1534, TA1978, TA94, D3052, reverse mutation	–	NT	150 µg/plate	Crebelli *et al.* (1987)
Salmonella typhimurium TA97, TA1537, reverse mutation	+	NT	5 µg/plate	Busch *et al.* (1986)
Salmonella typhimurium TA1535, reverse mutation	–	–	500 µg/plate	Hardigree & Epler (1978)
Salmonella typhimurium TA1535, reverse mutation	–	NT	100 µg/plate	Czeczot *et al.* (1990)
Salmonella typhimurium TA98, reverse mutation	+	NT	3 µg/plate	Cross *et al.* (1996)
Salmonella typhimurium TA98, reverse mutation	+	+	25 µg/plate	Ochiai *et al.* (1984)
Salmonella typhimurium TA98, reverse mutation	+	+	10 µg/plate	Hatcher & Bryan (1985)
Salmonella typhimurium TA98, reverse mutation	+	+	5.4 µg/plate	Rueff *et al.* (1986)
Salmonella typhimurium TA98, reverse mutation	+	+	2.5 µg/plate	Nguyen *et al.* (1989)

Table 2 (contd)

Test system	Results[a]		Dose[b] (LED or HID)	Reference
	Without exogenous metabolic system	With exogenous metabolic system		
Salmonella typhimurium TA98, reverse mutation	+	+	15 μg/plate	Vrijsen *et al.* (1990)
Escherichia coli K-12 343/113, reverse mutation, *nad* locus	+	NT	1000	Hardigree & Epler (1978)
Escherichia coli K-12 343/113, forward or reverse mutation, *gal* or *arg* loci	–	–	NR	Hardigree & Epler (1978)
Saccharomyces cerevisiae D4, gene conversion	+	NT	2000	Hardigree & Epler (1978)
Saccharomyces cerevisiae, XΛ4-8Cp^- forward mutation, CAN^R	–	–	10 000	Hardigree & Epler (1978)
Saccharomyces cerevisiae D4, reverse mutation	–	–	10 000	Hardigree & Epler (1978)
Drosophila melanogaster, sex-linked recessive lethal mutations	+		25 000	Watson (1982)
DNA single-strand breaks, mouse lymphoma L5178Y cells *in vitro*	+	NT	10	Meltz & MacGregor (1981)
DNA damage, rat liver nuclei *in vitro* (unwinding assay)	+	NT	6	Sahu & Washington (1991)
Unscheduled DNA synthesis, rat primary hepatocytes *in vitro*	–	NT	6	Cross *et al.* (1996)
Gene mutation, Chinese hamster ovary CHO-AT3-2 cells, *tk* locus *in vitro*	+	NT	9	Carver *et al.* (1983)
Gene mutation, Chinese hamster ovary CHO-AT3-2 cells, *hprt* locus *in vitro*	–	NT	15	Carver *et al.* (1983)
Gene mutation, Chinese hamster ovary CHO-AT3-2 cells, *hprt* locus *in vitro*	–	NT	15	Carver *et al.* (1983)
Gene mutation, Chinese hamster ovary cells, Na^+/K^+ ATPase locus *in vitro*	–	NT	15	Carver *et al.* (1983)
Gene mutation, Chinese hamster lung V79 cells, *hprt* locus *in vitro*	+	+	20	Maruta *et al.* (1979)

Table 2 (contd)

Test system	Results[a]		Dose[b] (LED or HID)	Reference
	Without exogenous metabolic system	With exogenous metabolic system		
Gene mutation, Chinese hamster lung V79 cells, *hprt* locus *in vitro*	–	–	89.4	van der Hoeven *et al.* (1984)
Gene mutation, mouse lymphoma L5178Y cells, *tk* locus *in vitro*	+	+	10	Meltz & MacGregor (1981)
Gene mutation, mouse lymphoma L5178Y cells, *tk* locus *in vitro*	(+)	–	17.8	van der Hoeven *et al.* (1984)
Gene mutation, mouse lymphoma L5178Y cells, *hprt* locus *in vitro*	–	–	44.7	van der Hoeven *et al.* (1984)
Gene mutation (recombination by DNA fingerprinting), other animal cells *in vitro*	+	NT	16.6	Suzuki *et al.* (1991)
Gene mutation, Chinese hamster lung cells, DT^R *in vitro*	+	NT	100	Nakayasu *et al.* (1986)
Sister chromatid exchange, Chinese hamster cells *in vitro*	(+)	NT	2.5	Kubiak & Rudek (1990)
Sister chromatid exchange, Chinese hamster ovary CHO-AT3-2 cells *in vitro*	+	?	15	Carver *et al.* (1983)
Sister chromatid exchange, Chinese hamster lung V79 cells *in vitro*	–	–	22.3	van der Hoeven *et al.* (1984)
Sister chromatid exchange, Chinese hamster ovary cells *in vitro*	+	+	0.67	National Toxicology Program (1992)
Micronucleus formation, Chinese hamster lung V79 cells *in vitro*	+	+	3	Caria *et al.* (1995)
Chromosomal aberrations, Chinese hamster Don-6 and B-131 fibroblasts *in vitro*	+	NT	5	Yoshida *et al.* (1980)
Chromosomal aberrations, Chinese hamster ovary cells *in vitro*	+	NT	10	Kubiak & Rudek (1990)

Table 2 (contd)

Test system	Results[a]		Dose[b] (LED or HID)	Reference
	Without exogenous metabolic system	With exogenous metabolic system		
Chromosomal aberrations, Chinese hamster lung V79 cells *in vitro*	+	+	9.8	Gaspar *et al.* (1994)
Chromosomal aberrations, Chinese hamster CHO-AT3-2 cells *in vitro*	+	NT	6	Carver *et al.* (1983)
Chromosomal aberrations, Chinese hamster ovary cells *in vitro*	+	+	10.1	National Toxicology Program (1992)
Cell transformation, BALB/c 3T3 mouse cells	(+)	NT	15	Meltz & MacGregor (1981)
Cell transformation, BALB/c 3T3 mouse cells	(+)	NT	10	Tanaka *et al.* (1987)
Cell transformation, Syrian hamster embryo cells, focus assay	+	NT	5	Umezawa *et al.* (1977)
Sister chromatid exchange, human lymphocytes *in vitro*	+	+	10	Rueff *et al.* (1986)
Micronucleus formation, human lymphocytes *in vitro*	+[c]	+[c]	3	Caria *et al.* (1995)
Chromosomal aberrations, human lymphocytes *in vitro*	+	NT	8	Yoshida *et al.* (1980)
Chromosomal aberrations, human HE2144 fibroblasts *in vitro*	+	NT	1	Yoshida *et al.* (1980)
Urine from Fischer 344 rats in *Salmonella typhimurium* TA100	–	(+)	0.2% in diet, 9 w	Stoewsand *et al.* (1984)
Urine and faeces from Sprague-Dawley rats in *Salmonella typhimurium* TA98	+	+	500 ip or po × 1	Crebelli *et al.* (1987)
Micronucleus formation, mouse bone-marrow cells *in vivo*	–		1000 po or ip	MacGregor (1979) [abst]
Micronucleus formation, mouse bone-marrow cells *in vivo*	–		1000 po × 2	Aeschbacher (1982)
Micronucleus formation, CD-1 mouse bone marrow cells *in vivo*	–		558 ip × 1	Caria *et al.* (1995)
Micronucleus formation, mouse bone-marrow cells and peripheral blood erythrocytes *in vivo*	–		400 ip × 1	Ngomuo & Jones (1996)
Micronucleus formation, Wistar rat bone-marrow cells *in vivo*	–		0.1% diet × 1 w	Taj & Nagarajan (1996)

Table 2 (contd)

Test system	Results[a]		Dose[b] (LED or HID)	Reference
	Without exogenous metabolic system	With exogenous metabolic system		
Chromosomal aberrations, Wistar rat bone-marrow cells *in vivo*	–		0.1% diet × 1 w	Taj & Nagarajan (1996)
Dominant lethal mutation, inbred Swiss mice	–		400 ip × 2	Aravindakshan *et al.* (1985)
Dominant lethal mutation, Wistar rats	–		300 ip × 2	Aravindakshan *et al.* (1985)

[a] +, positive; (+), weakly positive; –, negative; NT, not tested
[b] LED, lowest effective dose; HID, highest ineffective dose; unless otherwise stated, in-vitro test, μg/mL; in-vivo test, mg/kg bw per day; NR, not reported; w, week; ip, intraperitoneal; po, oral
[c] Increased CREST-negative micronuclei

5.2 Human carcinogenicity data

No data were available to the Working Group.

5.3 Animal carcinogenicity data

Quercetin was tested in several studies in rats by oral administration in the diet and by topical application in mice. Carcinogenicity was seen in only two studies in rats. Quercetin increased the incidences of intestinal and urinary bladder tumours in one study, but this effect was not seen in subsequent studies. Quercetin produced a low but significant increase in the incidence of renal tubular neoplasms, primarily adenomas in male rats, which was observed only after step-sectioning of renal tissue. When tested in several two-stage models of organ carcinogenesis, quercetin did not significantly enhance tumour incidence, except that of renal tumours induced by oestradiol in a model in hamsters.

5.4 Other relevant data

Although the metabolism of quercetin appears to be similar in humans and rabbits (the same three metabolites were identified in urine), no information on rats or mice was available for comparison. No information was available on the toxicity of quercetin in humans.

Quercetin increased the frequency of DNA damage and lipid peroxidation in liver nuclei of rats *in vitro*. In long-term studies in rats, there were no treatment-related clinical signs of toxicity, but renal hyperplasia occurred in males.

Quercetin inhibited cytochrome P450 enzymes in both human and rodent microsomes *in vitro*.

Fetal growth retardation was observed in a study in rats exposed to quercetin by oral gavage.

No data were available on the genetic and related effects of quercetin in humans. It was not genotoxic in experimental systems *in vivo*. It produced cytogenetic damage in human and rodent cells *in vitro*, but conflicting results were obtained in assays for gene mutation. It was mutagenic to *Drosophila*.

5.5 Evaluation

There is *inadequate evidence* in humans for the carcinogenicity of quercetin.

There is *limited evidence* in experimental animals for the carcinogenicity of quercetin.

Overall evaluation

Quercetin is *not classifiable as to its carcinogenicity to humans (Group 3)*.

6. References

Aeschbacher, H.U. (1982) The significance of mutagens in food. In: Sorsa, M. & Vainio, H., eds, *Mutagens in Our Environment*, New York, Alan R. Liss, pp. 349–362

Ambrose, A.M., Robbins, D.J. & DeEds, F. (1952) Comparative toxicities of quercetin and quercitrin. *J. Am. pharm. Assoc.*, **41**, 119–122

Aravindakshan, M., Chauhan, P.S. & Sundaram, K. (1985) Studies on germinal effects of quercetin, a naturally occurring flavonoid. *Mutat. Res.*, **144**, 99–106

Balasubramanian S. & Govindasamy, S. (1996) Inhibitory effect of dietary flavonol quercetin on 7,12-dimenthylbenz[a]anthracene-induced hamster buccal pouch carcinogenesis. *Carcinogenesis*, **17**, 877–879

Barotto, N.N., López, C.B., Eymard, A.R., Fernández Zapico, M.E. & Valentich, M.A. (1998) Quercetin enhances pretumorous lesions in the NMU model of rat pancreatic carcinogenesis. *Cancer Lett.*, **129**, 1–6

Belt, J.A., Thomas, J.A., Buchsbaum, R.N. & Racker, E. (1979) Inhibition of lactate transport and glycolysis in Ehrlich ascites tumor cells by bioflavonoids. *Biochemistry*, **18**, 3506–3511

Booth, A.N., Murray, C.W., Jones, F.T. & DeEds, F. (1956) The metabolic fate of rutin and quercetin in the animal body. *J. biol. Chem.*, **223**, 251–257

Brown, J.P. (1980) A review of the genetic effects of naturally occurring flavonoids, anthraquinone and related compounds. *Mutat. Res.*, **75**, 243–277

Budavari, S., ed. (1996) *The Merck Index*, 12th Ed., Whitehouse Station, NJ, Merck & Co., p. 1381

Buening, M.K., Chang, R.L., Huang, M.-T., Fortner, J.G., Wood, A.W. & Conney, A.H. (1981) Activation and inhibition of benzo(*a*)pyrene and aflatoxin B_1 metabolism in human liver microsomes by naturally occurring flavonoids. *Cancer Res.*, **41**, 67–72

Busch, D.B., Hatcher, J.F. & Bryan, G.T. (1986) Urine recovery experiments with quercetin and other mutagens using the Ames test. *Environ. Mutag.*, **8**, 393–399

Caria, H., Chaveca, T., Laires, A. & Rueff, J. (1995) Genotoxicity of quercetin in the micronucleus assay in mouse bone marrow erythrocytes, human lymphocytes, V79 cell line and identification of kinetochore-containing (CREST staining) micronuclei in human lymphocytes. *Mutat. Res.*, **343**, 85–94

Carver, J.H., Carrano, A.G. & MacGregor, J.T. (1983) Genetic effects of the flavonols quercetin, kampherol, and galangin in Chinese hamster ovary cells *in vitro*. *Mutat. Res.*, **113**, 45–60

Chang, R.L., Huang, M.-T., Wood, A.W., Wong, C.-Q., Newmark, H.L., Haruhiko, Y., Sayer, J.M., Jerina, D.M. & Conney, A.H. (1985) Effect of ellagic acid and hydroxylated flavonoids on the tumorigenicity of benzo[a]pyrene and (±)-7β,8α-dihydroxy-9α,10α-epoxy-7,8,9,10-tetrahydrobenzo[a]pyrene on mouse skin and in the newborn mouse. *Carcinogenesis*, **6**, 1127–1133

Chemical Information Services (1995) *Directory of World Chemical Producers 1995/96 Standard Edition*, Dallas, TX, p. 608

Crebelli, R., Aquilina, G., Falcone, E. & Carere, A. (1987) Urinary and faecal mutagenicity in Sprague-Dawley rats dosed with the food mutagens quercetin and rutin. *Food chem. Toxicol.*, **25**, 9–15

Cross, H.J., Tilby, M., Chipman, K., Fery, D.R. & Gescher, A. (1996) Effect of quercetin on the genotoxic potential of cisplatin. *Int. J. Cancer*, **66**, 404–408

Czeczot, H. & Kusztelak, J. (1993) A study of the genotoxic potential of flavonoids using short-term bacterial assays. *Acta biochim. pol.*, **40**, 549–554

Czeczot, H., Tudek, B., Kusztelak, J., Szymczyk, T., Dobrowolska, B., Glinkowska, G., Malinowski, J. & Strzelecka, H. (1990) Isolation and studies of the mutagenic activity in the Ames test of flavonoids naturally occurring in medical herbs. *Mutat. Res.*, **240**, 209–216

Dayan, J., Deguingand, S., Truzman, C. & Chevron, M. (1987) Application of the SOS chromotest to 10 pharmaceutical agents. *Mutat. Res.*, **187**, 55–66

Deschner, E.E., Ruperto, J., Wong, G. & Newmark, H.L. (1991) Quercetin and rutin as inhibitors of azoxymethanol-induced colonic neoplasia. *Carcinogenesis*, **12**, 1193–1196

Dunnick, J.K. & Hailey, J.R. (1992) Toxicity and carcinogenicity studies of quercetin, a natural component of foods. *Fundam. appl. Toxicol.*, **19**, 423–431

Fukushima, S., Hagiwara, A., Ogiso, T., Shibata, M. & Ito, N. (1983) Promoting effects of various chemicals in rat urinary bladder carcinogenesis initiated by *N*-nitroso-*n*-butyl-(4-hydroxybutyl)amine. *Food chem. Toxicol.*, **21**, 59–68

Gaspar, J., Rodrigues, A., Laires, A., Silva, F., Costa, S., Monteiro, M.J., Monteiro, C. & Rueff, J. (1994) On the mechanisms of genotoxicity and metabolism of quercetin. *Mutagenesis*, **9**, 445–449

Gross, M., Pfeiffer, M., Martini, M., Cambell, D., Slavin, J. & Potter, J. (1996) The quantitation of metabolites of quercetin flavonols in human urine. *Cancer Epidemiol. Biomarkers Prev.*, **5**, 711–720

Gugler, R., Leschik, M. & Dengler, H.J. (1975) Disposition of quercetin in man after single oral and intravenous doses. *Eur. J. clin. Pharmacol.*, **9**, 229–234

Hardigree, A.A. & Epler, L.L. (1978) Comparative mutagenesis of plant flavonoids in microbial systems. *Mutat. Res.*, **58**, 231–239

Hatcher, J.F. & Bryan, G.T. (1985) Factors affecting the mutagenic activity of quercetin for *Salmonella typhimurium* TA98: Metal ions, antioxidants and pH. *Mutat. Res.*, **148**, 13–23

Hirose, M., Fukushima, S., Sakata, T., Inui, M. & Ito, N. (1983) Effect of quercetin on two-stage carcinogenesis of the rat urinary bladder. *Cancer Lett.*, **21**, 23–27

Hirose, M., Masuda, A., Fukashima, S. & Ito, N. (1988) Effects of subsequent antioxidant treatment on 7,12-dimethylbenz[a]anthracene-initiated carcinogenesis of the mammary gland, ear duct and forestomach in Sprague Dawley rats. *Carcinogenesis*, **9**, 101–104

van der Hoeven, J.C.M., Bruggeman, I.M. & Debets, F.M.H. (1984) Genotoxicity of quercetin in cultured mammalian cells. *Mutat. Res.*, **136**, 9–21

Hollman, P.C.H., Gaag, M.V.D., Mengelers, M.J.B., van Trijp, J.M.P., deVries, J.H.M. & Katan, M.B. (1996) Absorption and disposition kinetics of the dietary antioxidant quercetin in man. *Free Rad. Biol. Med.*, **21**, 703–707

Hollman, P.C.H., van Trijp, J.M.P., Mengelers, M.J.B., deVries, J.H.M. & Katan, M.B. (1997) Bioavailability of the dietary antioxidant flavonol quercetin in man. *Cancer Lett.*, **114**, 139–140

IARC (1983) *IARC Monographs on the Evaluation of the Carcinogenic Risks of Chemicals to Humans*, Vol. 31, *Some Food Additives, Feed Additives and Naturally Occurring Substances*, Lyon, pp. 213–229

IARC (1987) *IARC Monographs on the Evaluation of Carcinogenic Risks to Humans*, Suppl. 7, *Overall Evaluations of Carcinogenicity: An Updating of* IARC Monographs *Volumes 1 to 42*, Lyon, p. 71

Ishikawa, M., Oikawa, T., Hosokawa, M., Hamada, J., Morikawa, K. & Kobayashi, H. (1985) Enhancing effect of quercetin on 3-methylcholanthrene carcinogenesis in C57BL/6 mice. *Neoplasma*, **32**, 435–441

Ito, N., Hagiwara, A., Tamano, S., Kagawa, M., Shibata, M.-A., Kurata, Y. & Fukushima, S. (1989) Lack of carcinogenicity of quercetin in F344/DuCrj rats. *Jpn. J. Cancer Res.*, **80**, 317–325

Kato, K., Mori, H., Fujii, M., Bunai, Y., Nishikawa, A., Shima, H., Takahashi, M., Kawai, T. & Hirono, I. (1984) Lack of promotive effect of quercetin on methylazoxymethanol acetate carcinogenesis in rats. *J. toxicol. Sci.*, **9**, 319–325

Khan, W.A., Wang, Z.Y., Athar, M., Bickers, D.R. & Mukhtar H. (1988) Inhibition of the skin tumorigenicity of (±)-7β,8α-dihydroxy-9α,10α-epoxy-7,8,9,10-tetrahydrobenzo[a]pyrene by tannic acid, green tea polyhenols and quercetin in Sencar mice. *Cancer Lett.*, **42**, 7–12

Kubiak, R. & Rudek, Z. (1990) SCEs and chromosome aberrations in mammalian cells in vitro treated with quercetin. *Acta biol. hung.*, **41**, 121–124

Lang, D.R. & Racker, E. (1974) Effects of quercetin and F_1 inhibitor on mitochondrial ATPase and energy-linked reactions in submitochondrial particles. *Biochim. biophys. Acta*, **333**, 180–186

Lide, D.R., ed. (1997) *CRC Handbook of Chemistry and Physics*, 78th Ed., Boca Raton, FL, CRC Press, p. 3-78

Long, G.D., DeChatelet, L.R., O'Flaherty, J.T., McCall, C.E., Bass, D.A., Shirley, P.S. & Parce, J.W. (1981) Effects of quercetin on magnesium-dependent adenosine triphosphatase and the metabolism of human polymorphonuclear leukocytes. *Blood*, **57**, 561–566

MacGregor, J.T. (1979) Mutagenicity studies of flavonoids *in vivo* and *in vitro* (Abstract No. 94). *Toxicol. appl. Pharmacol.*, **48**, A47

Maruta, A., Enaka, K. & Umeda, M. (1979) Mutagenicity of quercetin and kaempferol on cultured mammalian cells. *Gann*, **70**, 273–276

Matsukawa, Y., Nishino, H., Okuyama, Y., Matsui, T., Matsumoto, T., Matsumura, S., Shimizu, Y., Sowa, Y. & Sakai, T. (1997) Effects of quercetin and/or restraint stress on formation of aberrant crypt foci induced by azoxymethane in rat colons. *Oncology*, **54**, 118–121

Meltz, M.L. & MacGregor, J.T. (1981) Activity of the plant flavonol quercetin in the mouse lymphoma L5178Y $TK^{+/-}$ mutation, DNA single-strand break, and Balb/c 3T3 chemical transformation assays. *Mutat. Res.*, **88**, 317–324

Moon, J.-Y., Lee, D.-W. & Park, K.-H. (1998) Inhibition of 7-ethoxycoumarin *O*-deethylase activity in rat liver microsomes by naturally occurring flavonoids: Structure–activity relationships. *Xenobiotica*, **28**, 117–126

Mukhtar, H., Das, M., Khan, W. A., Wang, Z. Y., Bik, D. P. & Bickers, D. R. (1988) Exceptional activity of tannic acid among naturally occurring plant phenols in protecting against 7,12-dimethylbenz(*a*)anthracene-, benzo(*a*)pyrene-, 3-methylcholanthrene-, and *N*-methyl-*N*-nitrosourea-induced skin tumorigenesis in mice. *Cancer Res.*, **48**, 2361–2365

Nakayasu, M., Sakamoto, H., Terada, M., Nagao, M. & Sugimura, T. (1986) Mutagenicity of quercetin in Chinese hamster lung cells in culture. *Mutat. Res.*, **174**, 79–83

National Toxicology Program (1991) *NTP Chemical Repository Data Sheet: Quercetin*, Research Triangle Park, NC

National Toxicology Program (1992) *Toxicology and Carcinogenesis Studies of Quercetin (CAS No. 117-39-5) in F344/N Rats (Feed Studies)* (Tech. Rep. Ser. No. 409; NIH Publ. No. 92-3140), Research Triangle Park, NC

Ngomuo, A.J. & Jones, R.S. (1996) Genotoxicity studies of quercetin and shikimate *in vivo* in the bone marrow of mice and gastric mucosal cells of rats. *Vet. hum. Toxicol.*, **38**, 176–180

Nguyen, T., Fluss, L., Madej, R., Ginther, C. & Leighton, T. (1989) The distribution of mutagenic activity in red, rose and white wines. *Mutat. Res.*, **223**, 205–212

Nishino, H., Iwashima, A., Fujiki, H. & Sugimura, T. (1984) Inhibition by quercetin of the promoting effect of teleocidin on skin papilloma formation in mice initiated with 7,12-dimethylbenz[*a*]anthracene. *Gann*, **75**, 113–116

Ochiai, M., Nagao, M., Wakabayashi, K. & Sugimura, T. (1984) Superoxide dismutase acts as an enhancing factor for quercetin mutagenesis in rat-liver cytosol by preventing its decomposition. *Mutat. Res.*, **129**, 19–24

Podhajcer, O.L., Friedlander, M. & Graziani, Y. (1980) Effect of liposome-encapsulated quercetin on DNA synthesis, lactate production, and cyclic adenosine 3′:5′-monophosphate level in Ehrlich ascites tumor cells. *Cancer Res.*, **40**, 1344–1350

Rueff, J., Laires, A., Borba, H., Chaveca, T., Gomes, M.I. & Halpern, M. (1986) Genetic toxicology of flavonoids: The role of metabolic conditions in the induction of reverse mutation, SOS functions and sister chromatid exchanges. *Mutagenesis*, **1**, 179–183

Sahu, S.C. & Gray, G.C. (1996) Pro-oxidant activity of flavonoids: effects on glutathione and glutathione *S*-transferase in isolated rat liver nuclei. *Cancer Lett.*, **104**, 193–196

Sahu, S.C. & Washington, M.C. (1991) Quercetin-induced lipid peroxidation and DNA damage in isolated rat-liver nuclei. *Cancer Lett.*, **58**, 75–79

Santti, R., Makela, S., Strauss, L., Korkman, J. & Kostian, M. (1997) Phytoestrogens: Potential endocrine disruptors in males. *Toxicol. ind. Health*, **14**, 233–237

Sato, H., Takahashi, M., Furukawa, F., Miyakawa, Y., Hasegawa, R., Toyoda, K. & Hayashi, Y. (1987) Initiating potential of 2-(2-furyl)-3-(5-nitro-2-furyl)acrylamide (AF-2), butylated hydroxyanisole (BHA), butylated hydroxytoluene (BHT) and 3,3′,4′,5,7-pentahydroxyflavone (quercetin) in two-stage mouse skin carcinogenesis. *Cancer Lett.*, **38**, 49–56

Siess, M.-H., Leclerc, J., Canivenc-Lavier, M.-C., Rat, P. & Suschetet, M. (1995) Heterogenous effects of natural flavonoids on monooxygenase activities in human and rat liver microsomes. *Toxicol. appl. Pharmacol.*, **130**, 73–78

Sousa, R.L. & Marletta, M.A. (1985) Inhibition of cytochrome *P*-450 activity in rat liver microsomes by the naturally occurring flavonoid, quercetin. *Arch. Biochem. Biophys.*, **240**, 345–357

Stoewsand, G.S., Andeerson, J.L., Boyd, J.N. & Hrazdina, G. (1984) Quercetin: A mutagen, not a carcinogen, in Fischer rats. *J. Toxicol. environ. Health*, **14**, 105–114

Sullivan, M., Follis, R.H., Jr & Hilgartner, M. (1951) Toxicology of podophyllin. *Proc. Soc. exp. Biol. Med.*, **77**, 269–272

Suolinna, E.-M., Buchsbaum, R.N. & Racker, E. (1975) The effect of flavonoids on aerobic glycolysis and growth of tumor cells. *Cancer Res.*, **35**, 1865–1872

Suzuki, S., Takada, T., Sugawara, Y., Muto, T. & Kominami, R. (1991) Quercetin induces recombinational mutations in cultured cells as detected by DNA fingerprinting. *Jpn. J. Cancer Res.*, **82**, 1061–1064

Taj, S. & Nagarajan, B. (1996) Inhibition by quercetin and luteolin of chromosomal aberrations induced by salted, deep-fried fish and mutton in rats. *Mutat. Res.*, **369**, 97–106

Takanashi, H., Aiso, S. & Hirono, I. (1983) Carcinogenicity test of quercetin and kaempferol in rats by oral administration. *J. Food Saf.*, **5**, 55–60

Tanaka, K., Ono, T. & Umeda, M. (1987) Pleiotropic effects of quercetin on the transformation of BALB 3T3 cells. *Jpn. J. Cancer Res.*, **78**, 819–825

Ueno, I., Nakano, N. & Hirono, I. (1983) Metabolic fate of [^{14}C]quercetin in the ACI rat. *Jpn. J. exp. Med.*, **53**, 41–50

Umezawa, K., Matsushima, T., Sugimura, T., Hirakawa, T., Tanaka, M., Katoh, Y. & Takayama, S. (1977) *In vitro* transformation of hamster embryo cells by quercetin. *Toxicol. Lett.*, **1**, 175–178

Verma, A.K., Johnson, J.A., Gould, M.N. & Tanner M.A. (1988) Inhibition of 7,12-dimethylbenz(*a*)anthracene- and *N*-nitrosomethylurea-induced rat mammary cancer by dietary flavonol quercetin. *Cancer Res.*, **48**, 5754–5758

Vrijsen, R., Michotte, Y. & Boeye, A. (1990) Metabolic activation of quercetin mutagenicity. *Mutat. Res.*, **232**, 243–248

Watson, W.A.F. (1982) The mutagenic activity of quercetin and kaempferol in *Drosophila melanogaster. Mutat. Res.*, **103**, 145–147

WHO (1993) *Guidelines for Drinking Water Quality*, 2nd Ed., Vol. 1, *Recommendations*, Geneva

Wilhite, C.C. (1982) Teratogenic potential of quercetin in the rat. *Food Cosmet. Toxicol.*, **20**, 75–79

Yoshida, M.A., Sasaki, M., Sugimura, K. & Kawachi, T. (1980) Cytogenetic effects of quercetin on cultured mammalian cells. *Proc. Jpn. Acad. Ser. B*, **56**, 443–447

Zhu, B.T. & Liehr, J.G. (1994) Quercetin increases the severity of estradiol-induced tumorigenesis in hamster kidney. *Toxicol. appl. Pharmacol.*, **125**, 149–158

Zhu, B.T., Ezell, E.L. & Liehr, J.G. (1994) Catechol-*O*-methyltransferse-catalyzed rapid *O*-methylation of mutagenic flavonoids. *J. biol. Chem.*, **269**, 292–299

SACCHARIN AND ITS SALTS

These substances were considered by previous working groups, in 1979 (IARC, 1980) and 1987 (IARC, 1987). Since that time, new data have become available, and these have been incorportated into the monograph and taken into consideration in the present evaluation.

1. Exposure Data

1.1 Chemical and physical data

1.1.1 *Nomenclature*

In the literature characterizing exposure to saccharin and its salts, the term 'saccharin' is sometimes used in a generic sense to encompass both saccharin and its salts. It is therefore not always possible to identify clearly the form of saccharin being described.

Saccharin

Chem. Abstr. Serv. Reg. No.: 81-07-2

Deleted CAS Reg. Nos: 474-91-9; 61255-27-4; 126987-83-5

Chem. Abstr. Name: 1,2-Benzisothiazol-3(2*H*)-one, 1,1-dioxide

IUPAC Systematic Name: 1,2-Benzisothiazolin-3-one, 1,1-dioxide

Synonyms: Acid saccharin; anhydro-*ortho*-sulfaminebenzoic acid; 3-benzisothiazolinone 1,1-dioxide; benzoic sulfimide; benzoic sulphinide; benzosulfimide; benzosulfinide; *ortho*-benzoic acid sulfimide; *ortho*-benzoic sulfimide; *ortho*-benzosulfimide; *ortho*-benzoyl sulfimide; 1,2-dihydro-2-ketobenzisosulfonazole; 2,3-dihydro-3-oxobenzisosulfonazole; 1,1-dioxo-1,2-benzisothiazol-3(2*H*)-one; 3-hydroxybenzisothiazole-*S,S*-dioxide; saccharimide; saccharin acid; saccharin insoluble; saccharine; saccharinol; saccharinose; saccharol; *ortho*-sulfobenzimide; *ortho*-sulfobenzoic acid imide

Sodium saccharin

Chem. Abstr. Serv. Reg. No.: 128-44-9

Deleted CAS Reg. No.: 38279-26-4

Chem. Abstr. Name: 1,2-Benzisothiazol-3(2*H*)-one, 1,1-dioxide, sodium salt

IUPAC Systematic Name: 1,2-Benzisothiazolin-3-one, 1,1-dioxide, sodium salt

Synonyms: *ortho*-Benzoylsulfimide sodium salt; saccharin sodium; saccharin sodium salt; saccharin soluble; sodium *ortho*-benzosulfimide; sodium saccharide; sodium saccharinate; sodium saccharine; soluble saccharin

Calcium saccharin

Chem. Abstr. Serv. Reg. No.: 6485-34-3
Deleted CAS Reg. No.: 17105-05-4
Chem. Abstr. Name: 1,2-Benzisothiazol-3(2*H*)-one, 1,1-dioxide, calcium salt
IUPAC Systematic Name: 1,2-Benzisothiazolin-3-one, 1,1-dioxide, calcium salt
Synonyms: Calcium *ortho*-benzosulfimide; calcium saccharinate

1.1.2 *Structural and molecular formulae and relative molecular mass*

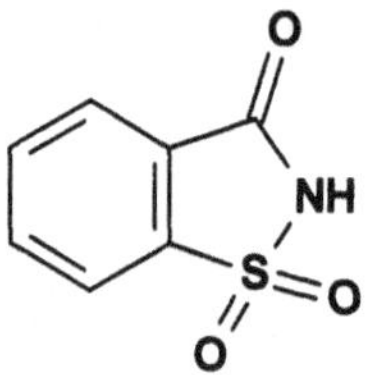

Saccharin

$C_7H_5NO_3S$ Relative molecular mass: 183.19

Sodium saccharin

$C_7H_4NO_3S.Na$ Relative molecular mass: 205.18

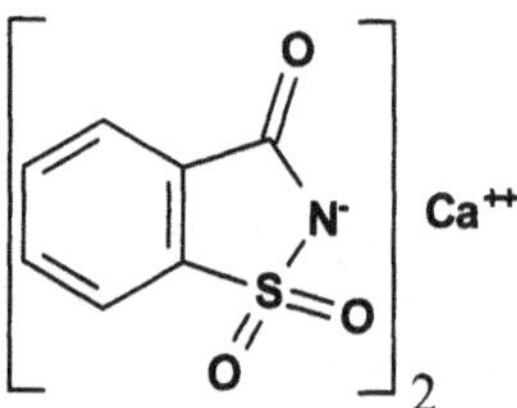

Calcium saccharin

$(C_7H_4NO_3S)_2.Ca$ Relative molecular mass: 404.46

1.1.3 *Chemical and physical properties of the pure substance*

(*a*) *Description*: Monoclinic crystals (Budavari, 1996); white crystalline powder [all forms] (Mitchell & Pearson, 1991); exceedingly sweet taste (300 times that of sucrose) [acid] (Bizzari *et al.*, 1996)

(*b*) *Boiling-point*: Acid sublimes (Lide, 1997)

(*c*) *Melting-point*: decomposes at 228°C [acid] (Lide, 1997); > 300°C [sodium and calcium salts] (Mitchell & Pearson, 1991)

(*d*) *Density*: d_4^{25} 0.828 [acid] (Lide, 1997)

(*e*) *Spectroscopy data*: Infrared (prism [322], grating [110]), ultraviolet [15734] and nuclear magnetic resonance (proton [6667], C-13 [4010]) spectral data have been reported [acid] (Sadtler Research Laboratories, 1980).

(*f*) *Solubility*: Acid slightly soluble in water (2 g/L at 20°C) and diethyl ether; soluble in ethanol and acetone; freely soluble in solutions of alkali carbonates (Mitchell & Pearson, 1991; Budavari, 1996; Lide, 1997). Sodium salt soluble in water (1 kg/L at 20°C). Calcium salt soluble in water (370 g/L at 20°C) (Mitchell & Pearson, 1991).

(*g*) *Acid ionization constant*: pK_a, 1.3 (Mitchell & Pearson, 1991)

(*h*) *Stability*: Saccharin solutions buffered at pHs ranging from 3.3 to 8.0 were essentially unchanged after heating for 1 h at 150°C (Mitchell & Pearson, 1991).

(*i*) *Conversion factor*: Saccharin: $mg/m^3 = 7.49 \times ppm$

1.1.4 *Technical products and impurities*

Saccharin is available commercially in three forms: the acid and the sodium (typically the dihydrate [6155-57-3]) and calcium (typically the 3.5 hydrate [6381-91-5]) salts (von Rymon Lipinski, 1995). All are manufactured to meet Food Chemicals Codex specifications, which include: heavy metals (as Pb), not more than 10 ppm (mg/kg); loss on drying, not more than 1%; residue on ignition, not more than 0.2%; selenium, not more than 0.003% [30 mg/kg]; and toluenesulfonamides, not more than 0.0025% [25 mg/kg] (National Academy of Sciences, 1996). Several additional salts of saccharin have been reported, including silver, ammonium, cupric, lithium, magnesium, zinc and potassium salts; although all of these are intensely sweet, none is available commercially. X-ray crystallography has shown that the acid form of saccharin exists as dimers, formed by hydrogen bonding between the imide hydrogen and the keto oxygen (Mitchell & Pearson, 1991).

More than 30 impurities have been reported to occur in saccharin or sodium saccharin produced by either the Remsen or the Maumee process (National Research Council/ National Academy of Sciences, 1978; Riggin *et al.*, 1978). These include in decreasing concentrations: *ortho*- and *para*-toluenesulfonamide, 1,2-benzisothiazol-1,1-dioxide, 1,2-benzisothiazoline-1,1-dioxide, 3-aminobenzisothiazol-1,1-dioxide, 5-chlorosaccharin, 6-chlorosaccharin, methyl saccharin, diphenyl sulfone, ditolylsulfone (various isomers), sulfamoylbenzoic acid, *ortho*-chlorobenzoic acid, *ortho*-sulfobenzoic acid and its ammonium salt, *n*-tetracosane, bis(4-carboxyphenyl) sulfone, toluene-2,4-disulfonamide, saccharin-6-sulfonamide, *N*-methyl-*ortho*-toluenesulfonamide, 4,4′-dibenzoylsulfone, 2- or 3-carboxythiaxanthone-5-dioxide, *ortho*-sulfobenzamide, methyl-*ortho*-sulfamoylbenzoate, methyl-*N*-methylsulfamoyl benzoate and saccharin-*ortho*-toluenesulfoxylimide.

Trade names for saccharin include [Azucaretas], Dulcibona, Garantose, Glucid, Gluside, Hollandia, Maca, Necta Sweet, Sakarin, Saxin, Slim & Sweet, Sucredulcor, [Sucrettes], Sucrosa, Suita, Sukrettine, Suktar-Maro, Sweeta, Sweetex and Syncal. Trade names for sodium saccharin include Cristallose, Cristalosetas, Crystallose, Dagutan,

[Edulcorant Pege], [Gaosucryl], Hermesetas, Kristallose, [Luetta], [Oda], Ril-Sweet, Saccharin Sodium Oral Solution USP 23, Saccharin Sodium Tablets USP 23, [Sanix], Saxin, [Sucromat], Sugarina, Suita Presta, [Sun-Suc], Sweeta, Sykose, Willosetten and Zero. [Names in brackets are for formerly manufactured products] (American Chemical Society, 1998; Reynolds, 1998; Swiss Pharmaceutical Society, 1998).

1.1.5 *Analysis*

Several international pharmacopoeias specify colorimetry and infrared absorption spectrophotometry as the methods for identification, and titration with sodium hydroxide or perchloric acid as methods for assaying the purity of saccharin, sodium saccharin and calcium saccharin. Sodium saccharin in tablets is assayed by ultraviolet spectrophotometry, and sodium saccharin in oral solutions is assayed by liquid chromatography with ultraviolet detection (British Pharmacopoeial Commission, 1993; Council of Europe, 1994; United States Pharmacopeial Convention, 1994; British Pharmacopoeial Commission, 1995; Society of Japanese Pharmacopoeia, 1996; Council of Europe, 1997).

The Food Chemicals Codex specifies titration with sodium hydroxide as the method for assaying the purity of saccharin and its sodium and calcium salts (National Academy of Sciences, 1996).

Gravimetric [method 973.29] and differential pulse polarographic [method 980.18] methods have been described for the determination of saccharin in food, including fruit juices and syrups, alcoholic liquids and solid or semisolid preparations; a colorimetric method [method 934.04] is described for the determination of saccharin in non-alcoholic beverages (Association of Official Analytical Chemists International, 1995). Although several analytical methods for the quantitative determination of saccharin and sodium saccharin in foods and other products are available, high-performance liquid chromatography, which allows simultaneous determination of saccharin, sodium saccharin and other sweeteners, is often preferred (von Rymon Lipinski, 1995).

1.2 Production and use

1.2.1 *Production*

Saccharin was discovered by the chemists Ira Remsen and Constantine Fahlberg in 1878. In 1900, the annual production of saccharin in Germany was reported to be 190 tonnes. In 1902, partly at the insistence of beet sugar producers, saccharin production in Germany was brought under strict control, and saccharin was made available only through pharmacies. Saccharin use increased during the First World War and immediately thereafter as a result of sugar rationing, particularly in Europe. By 1917, saccharin was a common tabletop sweetener in America and Europe; it was introduced to the Far East in 1923. The consumption of saccharin continued between the Wars, with an increase in the number of products in which it was used. The shortage of sugar during the Second World War again produced a significant increase in saccharin usage. In the early 1950s, calcium saccharin was introduced as an alternative soluble form (Mitchell & Pearson, 1991).

A number of companies around the world manufacture saccharin. Most manufacturers use the basic synthetic route described by Remsen and Fahlberg in which toluene is treated with chlorosulfonic acid to produce *ortho*- and *para*-toluenesulfonyl chloride. Subsequent treatment with ammonia forms the corresponding toluenesulfonamides. *ortho*-Toluenesulfonamide is separated from the *para*-isomer (this separation is alternatively performed on the sulfonyl chlorides), and *ortho*-toluenesulfonamide is then oxidized to *ortho*-sulfamoylbenzoic acid, which on heating is cyclized to saccharin (Mitchell & Pearson, 1991). *ortho*-Toluenesulfonamide can occur as a contaminant in saccharin produced by this process, but not in that produced by the Maumee process, described below (Arnold *et al.*, 1980; Cohen, 1999).

The only producer in the United States currently uses the Maumee process, in which saccharin is produced from purified methyl anthranilate, a substance occurring naturally in grapes. In this process, methyl anthranilate is first diazotized to form 2-carbomethoxybenzenediazonium chloride. Sulfonation followed by oxidation yields 2-carbomethoxybenzenesulfonyl chloride. Amidation of this sulfonyl chloride, followed by acidification, forms insoluble acid saccharin. Subsequent addition of sodium hydroxide or calcium hydroxide produces the soluble sodium or calcium salt (Mitchell & Pearson, 1991).

China is the world's largest producer of saccharin, accounting for 30–40% of world production, with an annual production of approximately 18 000 tonnes in recent years; its exports amounted to approximately 8000 tonnes. In 1995, the United States produced approximately 3400 tonnes of saccharin and its salts, and Japan produced approximately 1900 tonnes. In the past, several western European companies produced sodium saccharin; however, by 1995, western European production had nearly ceased due to increasing imports of lower-priced saccharin from Asia (Bizzari *et al.*, 1996).

Information available in 1995 indicated that saccharin was produced in 20 countries, calcium saccharin was produced in five countries, and sodium saccharin was produced in 22 countries (Chemical Information Services, 1995).

1.2.2 *Use*

Over the last century, saccharin and its salts have been used in a variety of beverages, foods, cosmetics and pharmaceuticals. Its primary function is to provide sweetness without adding calories, and it is used in the following foods and beverages: soft drinks, fruit juices, other beverages and other beverage bases or mixes; table-top sweeteners in tablet, powder or liquid form; processed fruits, chewing-gum and confections; gelatin desserts, jams and toppings; and sauces and dressings. Lesser amounts of saccharin are used in a variety of non-food applications, as a nickel electroplating brightener, chemical intermediate, animal feed sweetener and anaerobic adhesive accelerator (Mitchell & Pearson, 1991).

Worldwide consumption of saccharin and its salts in 1995 was approximately 28 000 tonnes. The consumption pattern of saccharin and its salts in the United States in 1995 (4500 tonnes) was: beverages and table-top sweeteners, 40%; personal-care products (primarily toothpaste and mouthwash), 30%; industrial, 18%; and pharmaceuticals, food, animal feed and tobacco, 12%. In Canada, approximately 142 tonnes of saccharin and its salts were consumed in 1995 (Bizzari *et al.*, 1996). Western European consumption of saccharin and its salts in 1995 was approximately 4100 tonnes as high-intensity sweeteners and 300–500 tonnes for industrial applications, mainly in electroplating and feed additives.

The largest and only growing application for saccharin in Japan (2510 tonnes in 1995) is as an intermediate in production of the rice fungicide, probenazole. Consumption as a feed additive has been at 140–150 tonnes annually. Japanese consumption of saccharin as a high-intensity sweetener has been limited and has decreased in recent years. Consumption for all uses in 1995 was 2800 tonnes.

1.3 Occurrence

1.3.1 *Natural occurrence*

Saccharin and its salts are not known to occur naturally.

1.3.2 *Occupational exposure*

According to the 1981–83 National Occupational Exposure Survey (National Institute for Occupational Safety and Health, 1998), approximately 225 000, 68 000 and 1000 workers in the United States were potentially exposed to saccharin, sodium saccharin and calcium saccharin, respectively. Occupational exposure to saccharin and its salts may occur during its production and during its use as an intensive sweetener in foods, beverages and pharmaceuticals.

1.3.3 *Dietary intake*

An acceptable daily intake (ADI) of 5 mg/kg bw for saccharin (including its sodium, calcium and potassium salts) was established in 1993 by the WHO/FAO Joint Expert Committee on Food Additives (WHO, 1993a) and in 1995 by the Scientific Committee for Food of the European Union (International Sweeteners Association, 1998). Before these dates, the ADI was 2.5 mg/kg bw (see also section 1.4).

The probable daily intakes of saccharin and its salts in the United States in the early 1980s were estimated from data on food intake derived from a survey in which respondents were asked to record each food consumed at each eating occasion over 14 consecutive days. The results showed that saccharin-sweetened carbonated and non-carbonated soft drinks accounted for a high proportion of the saccharin intake, and table-top and kitchen uses of saccharin as a sugar substitute were also important sources of saccharin in the diet. Other foods did not represent significant sources. The highest average daily intakes of saccharin per kilogram body weight (for saccharin consumers only) were those of men and women aged 18–54 (0.39 mg/kg bw), women in this age group (0.46 mg/kg bw), children aged 2–5 years (0.44 mg/kg bw) and children under two years of age (0.40 mg/kg bw). The average daily intakes for other groups were: 0.36 mg/kg bw for boys and girls aged 6–12; 0.26 mg/kg bw for boys and girls aged 13–17 (0.24 mg/kg bw for boys in this age group) and 0.38 mg/kg bw for men and women aged ≥ 55 years (Calorie Control Council, 1996a).

A survey of intense sweetener consumption in Australia in 1994 consisted of a seven-day survey of high consumers of the main sources of sweeteners, carbonated drinks, cordials and table-top, with allowance for body weight. Mean intake (expressed as % ADI of 5 mg/kg bw) of saccharin and its salts was 9% for all consumers aged 12–39 (men, 11%; women, 8%); 16% for all consumers aged 12–17; 3% for all consumers aged 18–24; and 9% for consumers aged 25–39 (National Food Authority, 1995).

In a study of the potential intake of intense sweeteners in Brazil in 1990–91, it was found that 72% of the studied population consumed saccharin. The main reasons given for use of intense sweeteners were weight control diet (36%), diabetes (35%) and obesity (23%). Table-top sweeteners were the major source of sweeteners, followed by soft drinks. The median daily intake of saccharin was approximately 16% of the ADI of 5 mg/kg bw (Toledo & Ioshi, 1995).

The use of table-top sweeteners and diet soft drinks and the intake of saccharin were assessed on the basis of the second Dutch National Food Consumption Survey, conducted in 1992. The median daily intake of saccharin by users of intense sweeteners, evaluated from two-day records and a food frequency questionnaire, was 0.2 mg/kg bw. Less than 0.5% of the total population had an intake above the ADI of 2.5 mg/kg bw (Hulshof *et al.*, 1995).

The dietary intake of intense sweeteners was evaluated in Germany in 1988-89. In the first part of the study, sweetener intake was evaluated in a representative sample of the population from complete 24-h records of the amounts and types of all foods and drinks consumed by 2291 individuals; 36% of the participants had ingested one or more sweeteners on the examination day. The mean intake of saccharin by users of intense sweeteners was 0.25 mg/kg bw per day; at the 90th percentile of intake, the ingestion of saccharin was about 2.5 times higher. Table-top sweeteners and beverages were the most important sources of sweeteners, contributing more than 80% to the total intake. In the second part of the study, the sweetener intake of the 41 subjects in the one-day study who had ingested any of the sweeteners at levels in excess of 75% of the ADI was further evaluated during a seven-day period. The mean intake of saccharin of this group was 0.42 mg/kg bw per day, which corresponded to 17% of the corresponding ADI value of 2.5 mg/kg bw in the European Union at that time (Bär & Biermann, 1992).

A survey of the intake of food additives in Finland in 1980 included an assessment of the intake of saccharin. The report gave few details of the study design or method and indicated only that the average per-capita daily intake (calculated from consumption figures for various foods and drinks) of saccharin was 5.9 mg/person per day. The ADI at that time was 2.5 mg/kg bw (Penttilä *et al.*, 1988). These figures are considerably lower than those found in more recent studies (Renwick, 1995).

1.4 Regulations and guidelines

No national or international occupational exposure limits have been proposed or established for exposure to saccharin in workplace air, and no international guidelines for saccharin in drinking-water have been established (WHO, 1993b).

European Commission regulations and standards stipulate that: (1) saccharin, sodium saccharin or calcium saccharin is allowed for use in non-alcoholic drinks (maximum useable dose, 80–100 mg/L), in desserts and similar products (100 mg/kg), in confectionery (80–1200 mg/kg) and in vitamins and dietary preparations (1200 mg/kg) (European Commission, 1994a); (2) saccharin, sodium saccharin or calcium saccharin may be added as an aromatic and appetizing substance to animal feedstuffs (European Commission, 1970, 1994b). The Scientific Committee for Food of the European Commission increased the ADI for saccharin from 2.5 mg/kg bw to 5 mg/kg bw in June 1995 (International Sweeteners Association, 1998); however, it has been recommended that intake of saccharin by children should be minimized, and use of saccharin in infant foods should be prohibited (European Commission, 1978; United Nations Environment Programme, 1998).

The Joint FAO/WHO Expert Committee on Food Additives in 1993 re-allocated a group ADI of 5 mg/kg bw for saccharin, sodium saccharin, potassium saccharin and calcium saccharin, singly or in combination (WHO, 1993a). In 1977, it had changed the unconditional ADI for humans of 5 mg/kg bw established for saccharin and its potassium and calcium salts to a temporary ADI of 2.5 mg/kg bw (WHO, 1978).

The regulatory status of saccharin in foods, beverages and table-top and pharmaceutical preparations in a number of countries is presented in Table 1. These data were collected over a period of years and do not necessarily represent the current situation (Calorie Control Council, 1996b).

Regulations and standards in the United Kingdom stipulate that saccharin, sodium saccharin or calcium saccharin is a permitted sweetener for food intended for human consumption. The sale, importation, supply and advertisement of any sweetener, of any food containing a sweetener or of the use of any sweetener as an ingredient in the preparation of foods other than as a permitted sweetener is prohibited. The sale of food for babies and young children which contains an added sweetener is restricted. The use of all permitted sweeteners in jam and similar products intended for diabetic patients and in soft drinks is permitted (Her Majesty's Stationery Office, 1983; United Nations Environment Programme, 1998).

In India, sodium saccharin is permitted in carbonated water up to 100 ppm [mg/L] (as saccharin) and may be sold as a table-top sweetener (Anon., 1981, 1988; United Nations Environment Programme, 1998).

Regulations and standards in Kenya stipulate that saccharin or sodium saccharin is a food additive permitted as a non-nutritive sweetening agent. The food products in or upon which it is permitted and maximum levels of use are listed (Anon., 1978; United Nations Environment Programme, 1998).

In the Russian Federation, regulations and standards stipulate a preliminary safety level for saccharin in ambient air of 0.02 mg/m^3 (Anon., 1983; United Nations Environment Programme, 1998).

In the United States, saccharin is currently approved for use under an interim food additive regulation permitting use for special dietary purposes and in special dietary foods. The food additives saccharin, ammonium saccharin, calcium saccharin and sodium saccharin may be safely used as sweetening agents in food in accordance with the following conditions: if the substitution for nutritive sweeteners is for a valid, special dietary purpose and

Table 1. Regulatory status of saccharin

Country or region	Food[a]	Beverage	Table-top	Pharmaceutical
Afghanistan		+		
Algeria	–	–	–	–
Antigua and Barbuda		+		
Argentina	+	+	+	+
Australia	+	+	+	+
Austria	+	+	+	+
Bahamas	+	+		
Barbados		+		
Belgium	+	+	+	
Bermuda		+		
Bolivia	–	–	+	–
Brazil	+	+	+	
Bulgaria	+	+		
Burundi		+		
Canada	–	–	+	+
Caribbean	+	+	+	
Chile		+	+	+
China	+	+		
Colombia	+	+	+	
Costa Rica	+	+	+	
Cyprus	+	+	+	+
Czech Republic	+	–	+	
Denmark	+	+	+	+
Dominica	+	+	+	
Ecuador	+	+	+	+
Egypt		+		
El Salvador	+	+	+	
Ethiopia		+	+	
Fiji	+	–	–	–
Finland	+	+	+	+
France	+	+	+	+
Germany	+	+	+	+
Greece	+	+	+	
Guam	+	+		
Guatemala	+	+	+	
Guyana	+	+		
Haiti		+	+	
Honduras	+	+		
Hong Kong	+	+	+	
Hungary	+	+	+	
Iceland	+	+	+	–
India		+	+	+
Indonesia	+	+	+	
Iran	+	–	–	–

Table 1 (contd)

Country or region	Food[a]	Beverage	Table-top	Pharmaceutical
Ireland	+	+	+	+
Israel	+	+	+	+
Italy	+	+	+	+
Japan	+	+	+	+
Korea, Republic of	+	+	+	+
Kenya	+	+	+	
Kuwait	+	+	+	
Lebanon	+	+	+	
Luxembourg	+	+	+	–
Malaysia	+	+	+	+
Malta	+	+	+	
Mexico	+	+	+	
Monserrat		+		
Morocco	+	+	+	–
Nassau		+		
Netherlands	+	+	+	+
New Zealand	+	+	+	+
Nicaragua	+	+	+	
Nigeria	+	+	+	
Norway	+	+	+	+
Oman	–	–	+	+
Pakistan	+	+	+	
Panama	+	+	+	
Papua New Guinea	+	+	+	
Paraguay	+	–	+	
Peru	+	+	+	–
Philippines	+	+	+	+
Poland	+		+	
Portugal	+	+	+	+
Puerto Rico	+	+		
Qatar			+	
Russian Federation	+	–	+	+
Rwanda		+		
Samoa	+	+		
Saudi Arabia	+	–	+	
Sierra Leone	+		+	
Singapore	+	+	+	+
Slovakia	+	–	+	
South Africa	+	+	+	
Spain	+	+	+	+
Sri Lanka		+	+	
Surinam	+	+	+	
Sweden	+	+	+	
Switzerland	+	+	+	

Table 1 (contd)

Country or region	Food[a]	Beverage	Table-top	Pharmaceutical
Taiwan	+	+	+	–
Thailand	+	+	+	
Trinidad	+	+		
Tunisia	–	–	–	–
Turkey	+	+	+	+
United Arab Emirates			+	
United Kingdom	+	+	+	+
United States	+	+	+	+
United States Virgin Islands	+	+		
Uruguay	+	+	+	
Venezuela	+	+	+	
Yugoslavia	+	+		
Zaire		+		
Zambia		+		

From Calorie Control Council (1996b); abbreviations: +, permitted; –, prohibited
[a] May not apply to all food categories

is in accord with current special dietary food regulations and policies or if the use or intended use is for an authorized technological purpose other than calorie reduction. The additives are authorized for use as sweetening agents only in special dietary foods, as follows: (1) in beverages, fruit juices and bases or mixes when prepared for consumption in accordance with directions, in amounts not to exceed 12 mg of the additive, calculated as saccharin, per fluid ounce; (2) as a sugar substitute for cooking or table use, in amounts not to exceed 20 mg of the additive, calculated as saccharin, for each expressed teaspoonful of sugar sweetening equivalence; and (3) in processed foods, in amounts not to exceed 30 mg of the additive, calculated as saccharin, per serving of designated size. The additives are authorized for use only for the following technological purposes: to reduce bulk and enhance flavours in chewable vitamin tablets, chewable mineral tablets or combinations thereof; to retain the flavour and physical properties of chewing-gum; and to enhance the flavour of flavour chips used in non-standardized bakery products (Food and Drug Administration, 1998).

2. Studies of Cancer in Humans

2.1 Observational study

The risk for cancer of the urinary bladder was studied among persons in Denmark born in 1941–45, at a time when the use of saccharin had increased by four- to fivefold as a result of a scarcity of sugar. The risk was compared with that of persons born one decade earlier. For people up to age 34, the relative risks were 1.0 (based on 22 observed cases; 95% confidence interval [CI], 0.7–1.6) for men and 0.3 (3 observed cases; 95% CI, 0.1–1.0) for women (Jensen & Kamby, 1982).

2.2 Case–control studies

Case–control studies of the use of saccharin and other sources of sweeteners and cancer of the urinary bladder are summarized in Table 2. About half of the studies described below involved controls who were hospitalized patients. Use of hospital controls in studies of artificial sweeteners can lead to underestimates of cancer risk, as pointed out by Silverman *et al.* (1983), as hospital controls are more likely than population controls to have a condition that requires them to use artificial sweeteners.

A hospital-based Canadian study included 158 male and 74 female cases of urinary bladder cancer and as many age- and sex-matched controls, who were men with benign prostatic hypertrophy and women with stress incontinence. Patients and controls were interviewed by mail; the response rates were 69% for the patients and 57% for the controls. Despite age-matching, the average age of both female and male controls was two to three years lower than that of cases. There was no difference in the intake of artificial sweeteners between patients and controls when analysed by their smoking history. Use of table-top artificial sweeteners for more than one year was reported by 30 men and 13 women among the patients and 30 men and 28 women among controls. Matched analysis resulted in odds ratios of 1.0 for men and 0.4 ($p < 0.01$) for women (Morgan & Jain, 1974).

A study in 10 hospitals in urban areas of Massachusetts and Rhode Island, United States, addressed the consumption of coffee, tea, artificial sweeteners and other coffee additives by white women, on the basis of previous findings that had suggested an association of a lower incidence of urinary-tract cancer with coffee consumption, which was particularly strong in white women. Two-hundred-and-sixteen histologically verified cases newly diagnosed during 1965 and 1971 were retrospectively identified from clinical records, excluding those reported as dead. Three controls per case were drawn from the discharge registers of the same hospitals and matched to the cases by age, area of residence and hospital; those with urinary tract problems were excluded. Of the 216 eligible cases, 40 had died and 41 did not respond to the questionnaire; the corresponding figures among controls were 110 and 148. The analysis was based on 135 cases and 390 controls. Cases and controls were sent a questionnaire which included separate questions on use of cyclamates and saccharin in coffee and in tea. All of the relevant odds ratios were between 1.0 and 1.2, and their 95% confidence intervals included unity (Simon *et al.*, 1975). [The Working Group noted the high proportion of non-participants.]

A hospital-based case–control study carried out during 1969–74 in 17 hospitals in six cities in the United States included 574 male and 138 female cases of urinary bladder cancer and equal numbers of controls matched for age, sex, race and hospital status (private, semiprivate, ward), excluding people with previous or current tobacco-related conditions. Cases and controls were selected from a larger pool assembled for studies on the effects of tobacco and alcohol and were interviewed in hospital. Diabetic patients

Table 2. Case–control studies of the use of saccharin and other sources of sweeteners and cancer of the urinary bladder

Reference	Study type	Sex	No. of cases	No. of controls	Type of sweetener	No. of exposed cases/ no. of exposed controls	Odds ratio	95% CI or p value	Additional estimates and comments
Morgan & Jain (1974)	H	M	158	158	SW	30/30	1.0		Not significant
		F	74	74		13/28	0.4	$p < 0.01$	
Simon *et al.* (1975)	H	F	135	390	SA		1.0	0.5–1.7	
Wynder & Goldsmith (1977)	H	M	132	124	SW	13/16	[0.8]	NR	Crude odds ratio
		F	31	29	SW	4/5	[0.8]	NR	
Howe *et al.* (1977, 1980); Howe & Burch (1981)	P	M	480	480	SW	73/47	1.6	1.1–2.4	Dose–response relationship
		F	152	152	SW	18/30	0.6	NR	Risk ratio for 2500 tablets/year
		M	466	469	SA	55/33	1.7	$p < 0.05$	≥ 3 years, 5.3 (10 cases, 2 controls)
Kessler & Clark (1978)	P	M	365	365	TA	85/83	0.9	0.6–1.4	Adjusted odds ratio = 2.6 in non-smoking men; adjusted for confounders
					DB	78/77	1.0	0.6–1.4	
		F	154	154	TA	48/48	0.9	0.5–1.6	
					DB	49/42	1.0	0.6–1.6	
Morrison & Buring (1980)	P	M	469	461	TA	101/113	0.8	0.5–1.1	Adjusted for confounders
					DB	144/155	0.7	0.6–1.1	Adjusted for confounders
					DB ≥ 5 years	44/55	0.7	[0.4–1.2]	
		F	197	165	TA	54/39	1.5	0.9–2.6	Adjusted for confounders
					DB	69/46	1.6	0.9–2.7	Adjusted for confounders
					DB ≥ 5 years	22/6	3.7		
		M NS	44	74	TA	18/31	1.1	NR	Adjusted for confounders
		F NS	39	84	TA	15/28	2.1	NR	Adjusted for confounders
		M NS	47	87	DB	21/44	0.9	NR	Adjusted for confounders
		F NS	43	83	DB	19/27	2.6	NR	

Table 2 (contd)

Reference	Study type	Sex	No. of cases	No. of controls	Type of sweetener	No. of exposed cases/ no. of exposed controls	Odds ratio	95% CI or p value	Additional estimates and comments
Wynder & Stellmann (1980)	H	M	302	302	TA	76/80	0.9	0.7–1.3	Current long-term smokers: odds ratio, 0.6 (95% CI, 0.3–1.1)
					DB	45/52	0.9	0.6–1.2	
		F	65	65	TA	14/19	0.6	0.3–1.4	Current long-term smokers: odds ratio, 1.0 (95% CI, 0.2–5.1)
					DB	10/16	0.6	0.3–1.3	
Hoover & Harge-Strasser (1980)	P	M	2258	4277	TA	592/1066	1.0	0.9–1.2	Odds ratio 1.5 for ≥ 3 servings TA and ≥ 2 DB daily or equivalent. All odds ratios adjusted for confounders
					DB	607/1204	1.0	0.8–1.1	
		F	742	1499	TA	236/474	1.0	0.8–1.3	
					DB	262/504	1.0	0.8–1.3	
		F LR	130	402	TA	82/210	1.2	NR	Dose– and duration–response relationships. Odds ratio = 2.7 for ≥ 2 servings for ≥ 10 years (16 cases, 18 controls)
					DB	71/219	1.1	NR	Dose– and duration–response relationships. Odds ratio, 3.0 for ≥ 2 servings for ≥ 10 years (6 cases, 7 controls). Non-smoking men reported to show significantly decreased odds ratios with increasing daily doses.
		M HR	166	226	TA	62/59	[1.7]	$p = 0.01$	Dose–response relationship
						69/81	[1.4]	$p = 0.01$	Dose–response relationship
									Among heavy female smokers, heavier users of TA and DB reported to give higher odds ratios than no use of AS

Table 2 (contd)

Reference	Study type	Sex	No. of cases	No. of controls	Type of sweetener	No. of exposed cases/ no. of exposed controls	Odds ratio	95% CI or p value	Additional estimates and comments
Cartwright (1981)	H	M NS	216	362	SA	33/27	2.2	$p < 0.05$	All adjusted for confounders
		M S	415	427		71/81	0.9		
		F NS	112	181		16/19	1.6		
		F S	99	90		17/14	1.2		
Najem (1982)	H	M/F	65/10	123/19	SA	12/19	1.3	0.6–2.8	
Morrison *et al.* (1982) Manchester	P	M	382	470	SW	140/183	0.9	0.7–1.2	No dose–response relationship. Odds ratio for ≥ 10 TA per day, 2.3 for women (9 cases, 8 controls) and 0.6 for men (10 cases, 19 controls). All adjusted for confounders
		F	142	220		50/87	0.9	0.6–1.4	
		M NS	30	68		11/22	1.6	NR	
		F NS	63	102		24/44	1.2	NR	
Nagoya		M	223	432	SW	100/238	0.7	0.5–0.9	
		F	66	144		26/83	0.5	0.3–0.8	
		M NS	24	76		9/41	0.5	NR	
		F NS	44	129		16/76	0.4	NR	
Møller Jensen *et al.* (1983)	P	M	284	592	SW	54/152	0.7	0.5–1.0	No dose–response relationship; adjusted for confounders; analyses broken down by TA and DB did not alter estimates
		F	98	195		26/50	1.1	0.6–1.9	
		M NS	9	68		4/5	1.9	0.5–7.8	
		M S	267	506		51/127	[0.7]	[0.5–1.0]	
Mommsen *et al.* (1983)	H	F	47	94	SA	6/2	6.7	1.5–30	Adjusted for confounders
Piper *et al.* (1986)	P	F	173	173	SW	77/74	1.1	0.7–1.7	Adjusted for confounders

Table 2 (contd)

Reference	Study type	Sex	No. of cases	No. of controls	Type of sweetener	No. of exposed cases/ no. of exposed controls	Odds ratio	95% CI or *p* value	Additional estimates and comments
Risch *et al.* (1988)	P	M	835	792	TA		1.0	0.7–1.2	No difference between smokers and non-smokers; adjusted for confounders
		F					1.1	0.7–1.8	
		M			SA		1.0	0.9–1.2	No dose–response relationship for either sex; adjusted for confounders
		F					1.0	0.8–1.2	
		M			DB		1.0	0.8–1.3	No dose-response relationship
		F					1.8	0.8–3.9	TA: ever versus never; SA and DB: total lifetime intake as continuous variable
Akdas *et al.* (1990)	H	M	168	168	SW	19/8	[2.5]	$p < 0.05$	
		F	26	26					

H, hospital-based; P, population-based; M, male; F, female; NR, not reported; NS, nonsmoker; S, smoker; SW, sweeteners (unspecified); TA, tablets; DB, dietetic beverage; SA, saccharin; LR, low risk; HR, high risk represented a slightly higher proportion of cases than controls. Data on use of artificial sweeteners were available only for 132 male cases, 124 male controls, 31 female cases and 29 female controls, as this question was added to the questionnaire only in 1973. Table-top artificial sweeteners were never used by 90% of male cases, 87% of male controls, 87% of female cases and 83% of female controls. The relative risks for three strata of duration of use were all lower than 1.0. The authors noted that the results do not refer to cyclamates, which had entered the United States market too recently to allow any carcinogenic effect to be recognizable (Wynder & Goldsmith, 1977).

A population-based study was carried out in three provinces of Canada (British Columbia, Newfoundland and Nova Scotia) of cases of urinary bladder cancer newly diagnosed during 1974–76 and identified through cancer registries. Of 821 eligible patients, 632 were interviewed (among those excluded, 43% were not interviewed because they were too ill or dead), i.e. 401 in British Columbia, 101 in Newfoundland and 230 in Nova Scotia. Each interviewed patient was matched by sex and age to a randomly selected control living in the same neighbourhood. The percentages of participating controls were 80% of those originally identified in British Columbia, 96% of those in Newfoundland and 100% of those in Nova Scotia. Participants answered a detailed questionnaire on use of a variety of sources of artificial sweeteners. Of the controls, 47/480 men and 30/152 women reported any use of artificial sweeteners. Through matched-pair analysis, relative risks associated with any use of any type of artificial sweeteners of 1.6 (lower limit of 95% CI, 1.1) and 0.6 (not significant) were estimated for men and women, respectively. In men, the relative risks adjusted for level of education, occupational exposures, history of urological diseases, smoking and use of instant coffee were between 1.5 and 1.8. The relative risks for bladder cancer among diabetic patients were 1.0 in men and 0.8 in women. Among diabetic men, the relative risk associated with use of artificial sweeteners was 1.7, based on 20 exposed cases. Of the male users, 82% reported use of brands of table-top artificial sweeteners known to have always contained saccharin only and 94% reported use of one brand only. Thus, for saccharin consumption, men were divided into three categories for both consumption (never, < 2500 and > 2500 tablets per year) and duration (never, ≤ 3 and > 3 years). Relative to people who had never used the preparations, the risks for the two increasing categories of consumption were 1.5 (based on 42 exposed cases; lower 95% CI, 1.0) and 2.1 (16 exposed cases; lower 95% CI, 0.9), respectively. The corresponding findings for duration were 1.4 (based on 30 exposed cases; lower 95% CI, 0.9) and 2.0 (28 exposed cases; lower 95% CI, 1.2). In the highest category of consumption (> 2500 tablets per year for more than three years), the risk relative to that of non-users was 5.3, based on 10 exposed cases and two exposed controls (Howe *et al.*, 1977). [The Working Group noted that it is not clearly stated whether the relative risks for consumption and duration were adjusted for potential confounding.] The risks associated with consumption of table-top sweeteners were also estimated in a multivariate analysis, with similar results (Howe *et al.*, 1980).

In a study in Baltimore (United States), 519 of 634 surviving patients in whom urinary bladder cancer had been diagnosed in 1972–75 agreed to participate in a study.

Controls, individually matched to each case by sex, age, race and marital status, were randomly chosen from lists in the same hospitals and periods as the patients, but those with diagnoses of cancer or urological conditions were excluded; 75% of the controls were selected at the first sampling. Both male and female patients had a higher level of education than their controls. The study included 365 male and 154 female cases and the same numbers of controls. All were interviewed about smoking habits, occupation and consumption of artificial sweeteners, including table-top sweeteners, dietetic beverages, dietetic foods and total intake in all forms. Artificial sweeteners in any form had been used by 129 male patients and 126 controls and by 77 female patients and 79 controls. The average duration of consumption of various forms of artificial sweeteners was between 3.4 and 8.3 years for male patients, between 5.8 and 7.7 years for male controls, between 2.9 and 7.8 years for female cases and between 5.4 and 8.3 for female controls, depending on the specific type. Any consumption of dietetic beverages was reported by 78 male patients and 77 controls and 49 female patients and 42 controls; and any consumption of dietetic foods by 54 male patients, 39 male controls, 34 female patients and 41 female controls. The odds ratios, adjusted for a series of potential confounders, showed no consistent trend by level of exposure. The relative risks for use of saccharin ranged between 0.7 and 1.1. In matched-pair analyses for 'more than occasional' use of non-nutritive sweeteners (powders, tablets, drops and any table-top sweetener), six types of dietetic beverage plus any dietetic beverage, 10 types of dietetic food plus any dietetic food, the only 95% confidence interval of the estimated odds ratios that excluded unity was that for consumption of dietetic ice cream by women (odds ratio, 3.5; 95% CI, 1.1–11). Stratification by smoking status showed non-significant relative risks associated with consumption of artificial sweeteners of 0.84 for smokers and 1.4 for nonsmokers. In nonsmoking men, the odds ratio was 1.7, which increased to 2.6 (95% CI, 1.2–5.7) after adjustment for a number of confounding factors (Kessler, 1976; Kessler & Clark, 1978). [The Working Group noted the potential bias of including only surviving patients and the possible selection bias represented by the higher level of education of patients than controls.]

The database of a population-based study in the Boston (United States) metropolitan area included 741 histologically confirmed incident cases of benign or malignant cancer of the lower urinary tract diagnosed over 16 months (identified in 65/66 hospitals of the area). A random sample of 677 residents of similar age and sex distribution in the same area during the same period were used as controls. The participation rates were 81% for cases and 80% for controls, leaving 597 cases and 544 controls for the analysis; 98 cases and 15 controls did not participate because they were too ill, dead or their physician declined permission for an interview. A questionnaire and a personal interview addressed a variety of lifetime exposures. In men, any use of dietetic beverages and sugar substitutes was associated with odds ratios of 0.8 (based on 144 exposed cases; 95% CI, 0.6–1.1) and 0.8 (101 exposed cases; 95% CI, 0.5–1.1). The corresponding odds ratios for women were 1.6 (69 exposed cases; 95% CI, 0.9–2.7) and 1.5 (54 exposed cases; 95% CI, 0.9–2.6). Multivariate analyses of the data for men, with adjustment for age, education, marital status, religion and tobacco consumption, led to a summary estimated relative risk of 0.7 for use of artificially sweetened beverages and 0.8 for use of sugar substitutes. [The Working Group noted that no corresponding multivariate analysis was reported for women.] The frequency or duration of use of either dietetic beverages (four strata), sugar substitutes or dietetic foods was analysed separately for the two sexes. The odds ratios were not consistently associated with increasing use, except for women reporting use of dietetic beverages for longer than five years, with an odds ratio of 3.7 [95% CI, 1.3–10] based on 22 exposed cases. In analyses by smoking status, the odds ratios for women who never smoked were 2.6 for consumption of dietetic drinks (based on 19 exposed cases) and 2.1 for consumption of non-nutritive sweeteners (15 exposed cases). Among men, the odds ratios were no higher among those who had never smoked than in the other groups (Morrison & Buring, 1980).

In a hospital-based study similar to that of Wynder and Goldsmith (1977), 302 male and 65 female bladder cancer patients and equal numbers of controls were interviewed during 1977–79 about lifetime use of table-top artificial sweeteners (mainly saccharin) and of dietetic beverages. Men who had never consumed artificial sweeteners represented 75% of cases and 74% of controls, and the corresponding proportions of women were 79% and 71%; 85% of male patients, 83% of male controls, 85% of female patients and 75% of female controls reported never having drunk dietetic beverages. In a matched analysis, the odds ratios for any use of either artificial sweeteners or dietetic beverages were all lower than 1.0 and all of the 95% confidence intervals included unity. Analyses limited to current long-term (≥ 10 years) cigarette smokers gave relative risks for consumption of sweeteners or dietetic beverages of about 0.6 (95% CI, 0.3–1.1) in men and 1.0 (95% CI, 0.2–5.1) in women (Wynder & Stellman, 1980).

A large population-based case–control study on bladder cancer was specifically designed to address the hypothesis of a role of artificial sweeteners. Newly diagnosed, histologically confirmed cases were identified in 10 areas in the United States; cases of benign papilloma were excluded. Controls represented an age- and sex-matched random sample from the same areas. The participation rates were 87% of eligible cases and 86% of eligible controls, resulting in 2258 male patients, 4277 male controls, 742 female patients and 1499 female controls, who were interviewed at home about a variety of risk factors, including use of table-top sweeteners, dietetic beverages and dietetic foods. All of the odds ratios reported below, unless otherwise specified, were adjusted for age, race, cigarette smoking, coffee drinking and occupational exposure. Any use of any type of artificial sweetener was reported by 909 male patients, 1723 male controls, 384 female patients and 732 female controls, corresponding to odds ratios of 1.0 (95% CI, 0.1–1.1) for men and 1.1 (95% CI, 0.1–1.3) for women. Analyses of consumption were based on six strata of average daily use of table-top sweeteners and five strata of average daily consumption of dietetic drinks. The trend for average daily use of table-top sweeteners by women was statistically significant (p = 0.03, one-tailed), and the highest consumption (six or more daily uses of table-top sweeteners) corresponded to an odds ratio of 1.4, based on 16 exposed cases. In the logistic regression analysis (with adjustment for sex, region, education and the other variables mentioned above) of combined consumption of dietetic drinks and table-top artificial sweeteners, an odds ratio of 1.5 (95% CI, 1.0–2.1) was estimated for heavy consumers (either at least three servings of table-top artificial sweeteners and at least two dietetic drinks daily or at least some dietetic drinks and six or more servings of table-top artificial sweeteners), with no difference by sex. Individuals considered to be at low and high risk for bladder cancer were analysed separately, as it was hypothesized that an effect of a weak carcinogen would be easier to detect in a population not exposed to bladder carcinogens, and analysis of a high-risk group would reveal any co-carcinogenic effect. The group considered to be at low risk comprised 283 female patients and 831 female controls who were white, did not smoke and were not exposed occupationally to bladder carcinogens. The group considered to be at high risk comprised 235 male patients and 307 male controls who were white and smoked > 40 cigarettes per day. In the low-risk stratum, 130 patients and 402 controls were unexposed, 82 patients and 210 controls used table-top artificial sweeteners, and 71 patients and 219 controls used dietetic drinks. The risk increased with level of intake: for consumption of table-top sweeteners, the odds ratios increased from 0.9 (based on 15 exposed cases) for less than one daily use to 1.8 (based on 22 exposed cases) for three or more daily uses (p for trend < 0.01); for duration of consumption among women reporting two or more daily uses, the odds ratios were 1.3 (based on 14 exposed cases), 1.8 (13 exposed cases) and 2.7 (16 exposed cases) for consumption lasting ≤ 5, 5–9 and ≥ 10 years, respectively (p for trend, < 0.01); for consumption of dietetic drinks, the odds ratios increased from 0.9 (based on 36 exposed cases) for less than one daily use to 1.6 (based on 3 exposed cases) for three or more daily uses (p for trend, not significant); for duration of consumption among women reporting two or more daily uses, the odds ratios were 0.5 (based on 1 exposed case), 1.4 (3 exposed cases) and 3.0 (6 exposed cases) for consumption lasting ≤ 5, 5–9 and ≥ 10 years, respectively (p for trend, < 0.05). In the high-risk stratum, 104 patients and 167 controls were unexposed, 62 patients and 59 controls used table-top artificial sweeteners and 69 patients and 81 controls used dietetic drinks. The odds ratios for the highest consumers were 1.9 (based on 7 exposed cases) for six or more daily uses of table-top artificial sweeteners and 2.6 (based on 6 exposed cases) for three or more daily servings of dietetic drinks (Hoover & Harge-Strasser, 1980). [The Working Group noted that estimates of risk by strata corresponding to duration of consumption were not included for the high-risk population.] An independent analysis gave similar risk estimates (Walker *et al.*, 1982).

More recently, the same data were analysed by strata corresponding to tumour stage and histological grade in logistic regression models including the following variables: age, race, education, sex, cigarette smoking, exposures in the workplace, bladder stones, urinary infections, coffee consumption, family history of bladder cancer, use of artificial sweeteners and geographical region. Risks were estimated for persons consuming more than 1680 mg/day of artificial sweeteners in comparison with a group consuming less than that amount. A significantly increased risk was seen only for tumours of histological grade III/IV (odds ratio, 2.2; 95%, CI 1.3–3.6; based on 23 exposed cases) (Sturgeon *et al.*, 1994). [The Working Group noted that the cut-off for consumption corresponded to a very high level and the reason for its choice was not given.]

A large hospital-based case–control study carried out in the United Kingdom in the 1970s included questions on consumption of saccharin as a food additive; a preliminary analysis was reported. The study included 161 newly diagnosed cases in men and 58 in women and 470 prevalent cases in men and 152 in women. Controls were matched by age and sex, with two controls for each newly diagnosed case and one for each prevalent case. Smokers who had quit five years or more previously were considered to be non-smokers; people who had regularly consumed saccharin for at least one year, five or more years before diagnosis or interview were considered to be saccharin consumers. Of the 631 male patients, 33 were nonsmokers and saccharin consumers, 183 were non-smokers and did not consume saccharin (reference group), 71 were smokers and saccharin consumers, and 344 were smokers and did not consume saccharin. Among the female cases, the corresponding figures were 16, 96, 17 and 81. The odds ratios for non-smokers who consumed saccharin were 2.2 (95% CI, 1.3–3.8) for men and 1.6 (95% CI, 0.8–3.2) for women. The other odds ratios ranged between 0.9 and 1.2, and their confidence intervals included unity (Cartwright *et al.*, 1981). [The Working Group noted that use of prevalent cases might be associated with bias in the recall of previous exposures and selection bias in relation to survival.]

A hospital-based study among white persons in New Jersey (United States) included 75 cases (65 male) and 142 controls (123 male) matched by age, sex, place of birth, place of residence and hospital. Twelve cases and 19 controls had ever used saccharin (crude odds ratio, 1.3; 95% CI, 0.6–2.8). The average consumption was 3.6 tablets per day among patients versus 2.5 among controls; the average duration of use was 6.3–6.4 years in both groups (Najem *et al.*, 1982).

In parallel studies in Manchester, United Kingdom, and Nagoya, Japan, use of artificial sweeteners was compared for patients with newly diagnosed cancer of the lower urinary tract, reported to be all cases in each population, and for a sample of residents in each area. The database included 555 patients and 735 controls in Manchester and 293 patients and 589 controls in Nagoya who were interviewed, out of 577, 817, 348 and 735 subjects, respectively. Questions about consumption of dietetic beverages and foods were more limited in Japan than in the United Kingdom, because product labels used in Japan do not allow assessment of the content of artificial sweeteners. No association between cancer of the lower urinary tract and consumption of artificial sweeteners was detected in either area. Whereas the overall odds ratio in Manchester was 0.9 (95% CI, 0.7–1.2, based on 140 exposed cases) in people of each sex, in Nagoya, the odds ratios for a history of use of sugar substitutes were 0.7 (based on 100 exposed cases; 95% CI, 0.5–0.9) in men and 0.5 (based on 26 exposed cases; 95% CI, 0.3–0.8) in women. The odds ratios estimated by duration of use or current frequency did not suggest a dose–response relationship, except that an odds ratio of 2.3 (based on nine exposed cases) was found for women in Manchester consuming more than 10 tablets per day; the corresponding odds ratio in men was 0.6. Stratum-specific odds ratios by category of tobacco smoking did not suggest an association, although the age-adjusted odds ratio for use of sugar substitutes by nonsmoking men in Manchester was 1.6 (based on 11 exposed cases) (Morrison *et al.*, 1982).

A population-based study of bladder cancer carried out in Copenhagen (Denmark) included 290 male patients, 592 male controls, 98 female patients and 195 female controls aged up to 75. A comparison with data in the Cancer Registry showed that the cases represented two-thirds of those originally eligible, but there were no differences in age, sex, area of residence or occupation between included and excluded cases. Some 99% of the cases had been verified histologically as either invasive or non-invasive. Controls were drawn randomly from among residents in the same municipalities as the cases, and 75% of those originally approached agreed to participate in the study. Any use of artificial sweeteners in coffee, tea or foods was reported by 19% of male patients and 26% of controls and 27% of female patients and 26% of controls. These proportions corresponded to age-adjusted odds ratios of 0.7 (95% CI, 0.5–1.0) for men and 1.1 (95% CI, 0.6–1.9) for women. Analyses restricted to any use of table-top artificial sweeteners or current use in coffee or in tea led to almost identical estimates. For men, analyses by strata corresponding to number of daily uses gave odds ratios lower than 1.0 in all strata; corresponding analyses in women showed no trend in odds ratios, and none of the 95% confidence intervals excluded unity. Analyses restricted to consumption of artificial sweeteners for more than 15 years gave nonsignificant odds ratios of 0.5 (95% CI, 0.2–1.0) for men and 0.8 (95% CI, 0.3–2.5) for women (based on 10 and five exposed cases, respectively). No consistent association emerged from analyses stratified by sex and clinical stage at diagnosis or by sex and histological grade of bladder cancer. The odds ratio for use of artificial sweeteners by men who had never smoked was 1.9 (95% CI, 0.5–7.8, based on four exposed cases), and the odds ratios decreased with increasing average number of cigarettes smoked daily throughout life down to 0.2 (95% CI, 0.1–0.5) among smokers of ≥ 25 cigarettes daily. The corresponding estimates for women were based on small absolute numbers and showed no consistent finding. An analysis restricted to the 70% of users who reported exclusive use of saccharin throughout life gave nonsignificant odds ratios of 0.7 for men and 1.0 for women (Møller Jensen *et al.*, 1983).

A study in Aarhus (Denmark) included 47 women with newly diagnosed histologically confirmed bladder cancer attending one hospital and twice as many controls matched by age and area of residence. Six patients and two controls reported saccharin consumption, corresponding to an odds ratio (adjusted for a variety of potential confounders) of 6.7 (95% CI, 1.5–30). The odds ratio for women who had never smoked and were saccharin users was 3.3 (95% CI, 1.4–7.8) [the corresponding odds ratio for women who had ever smoked was not given] (Mommsen *et al.*, 1983). [The Working Group noted that the terms 'artificial sweetener' and 'saccharin' appeared to be used synonymously.]

A study in New York (United States) was intended to explore the possible exposure to bladder carcinogens of women aged 20–49, who are commonly considered to be at low risk for bladder cancer. A total of 259 cases diagnosed in 1975–80 were identified through the cancer registry; 40 were excluded because the diagnosing physician refused to grant permission for the patient to be contacted, and an additional 42 did not participate in a telephone interview for unspecified reasons. Controls identified through random-digit dialling were matched to cases by age and telephone area code. A total of 173 pairs were formed, for eight of which some were data missing. Associations were estimated by analyses of matched pairs with the test of McNemar. Regular use (i.e. 100 or more times used) of table-top artificial sweeteners and/or artificially sweetened beverages was reported by 77 cases and 74 controls, corresponding to an odds ratio of 1.1 (95% CI, 0.7–1.7). It was reported that there was 'no suggestion of a dose–response relationship for the cases', but details were not given (Piper *et al.*, 1986). [The Working Group noted that the high proportion of non-participating patients might have biased the selection of study subjects.]

A population-based study was carried out in Alberta and Ontario (Canada) during 1979–82, after saccharin had been banned in Canada in 1978. Patients with newly diagnosed urinary bladder cancer (any degree of histological malignancy) and who were resident in urban centres in the two provinces were individually matched to controls by age, sex and area of residence, identified from a list of residents (some errors in recording demographic data for cases led to an excess of eligible controls). Those interviewed were 835 out of 1251 cases and 792 out of 1483 controls; 32% of cases and 9% of controls were not interviewed because of severe illness or death. The questionnaire included questions on regular consumption of table-top artificial sweeteners and low-calorie foods and drinks. The reported sweeteners were classified as saccharin, cyclamate or both on the basis of brand name and period of use. Conditional logistic regression techniques were used to estimate associations. The odds ratio for a history of and treatment for diabetes mellitus was 1.6 (95% CI, 1.1–2.4, based on 131 subjects with diabetes mellitus) and did not change when variables for sweeteners were included in the model. Twelve series of odds ratios were estimated for people of each sex, i.e. any regular use of table-top artificial sweeteners in all subjects, in nonsmokers only and excluding use in the last 10 years; use of saccharin stratified on three doses and total lifetime intake; use of cyclamate stratified on two doses and total lifetime intake; low-calorie foods stratified on two doses and total lifetime intake; low-calorie foods excluding use within the last 10 years; dietetic soft drinks on two doses and total lifetime intake. Among the 34 odds ratios (17 for each sex), the only one for which the 95% confidence interval excluded unity was that for total lifetime intake of low-calorie foods (odds ratio, 1.5; 95% CI, 1.0 –2.3) by women; the corresponding odds ratio for men was 1.0 (95% CI, 0.8–1.2). No consistent dose-related trend was seen for use of saccharin (Risch *et al.*, 1988).

A hospital-based study in Turkey included 168 male and 26 female newly diagnosed or prevalent cases of histologically confirmed bladder cancer and equal numbers of age- and sex-matched hospital controls. Nineteen patients and eight controls reported use of artificial sweeteners ($p < 0.05$) [odds ratio not presented] (Akdas *et al.*, 1990). [The

Working Group noted that the conditions from which the controls were suffering were not reported, but that a large proportion had undergone urological examinations.]

2.3 Cancer occurrence among diabetic patients

Patients with diabetes are known to use artificial sweeteners extensively. They also differ from the general population with regard to a number of lifestyle factors, including smoking habits. The Working Group considered that epidemiological studies of cancer in this population are uninformative with regard to the carcinogenicity of saccharin, since individual data on the use of artificial sweeteners and confounders are not provided. In addition, estimates of the risk for smoking-related cancers, such as those of the urinary bladder and kidney, can be expected to be negatively confounded because of the low smoking rates among diabetic patients.

3. Studies of Cancer in Experimental Animals

Saccharin

3.1 Oral administration

3.1.1 *Single-generation exposure*

Mouse: Groups of 50 female Swiss mice, 9–14 weeks of age, were given 0 or 5% saccharin made by the Remsen-Fahlberg method in the diet for 18 months, at which time the survivors were killed. The average survival rates were not affected, and the tumour incidences were similar in tested and control animals. No pathological alterations were observed macroscopically in the urinary bladder (Roe *et al.*, 1970). [The Working Group noted that the urinary bladders were not examined histologically.]

As part of a multigeneration study, two groups of 50 male and 50 female Swiss SPF mice [age unspecified] were fed diets containing 0.5 or 0.2% saccharin (free acid) made by the Remsen-Fahlberg method (containing 0.5% *ortho*-toluenesulfonamide) for up to 21 months. A concurrent control group of 50 males and 50 females received a standard diet. At 18 months, 62, 64 and 66 animals were still alive in the groups receiving 0.5 and 0.2% saccharin and in the control group, respectively. One control female developed an anaplastic carcinoma of the bladder, and one male fed 0.2% saccharin had a noninvasive transitional-cell carcinoma of the bladder (Kroes *et al.*, 1977) (see also section 3.1.2).

Groups of 25 male and 25 female Charles River CD mice, eight weeks of age, received diets containing sodium saccharin (containing 345 mg/kg (ppm) *ortho*-toluenesulfonamide) at concentrations of 0, 1 or 5% for up to two years. Animals that died before six months were not examined, and the survival times were not reported. Animals were killed when obvious tumours were seen or when they were moribund; all survivors were killed at two years. All animals that survived six months or longer were examined grossly, and any tissues with abnormal changes were examined histologically; in addition, all vital organs from at least 12 animals in each group were examined histologically. In high-dose males, two cases of papillary hyperplasia of the bladder and two small papillomas were found. One transitional-cell carcinoma of the bladder associated with a stone was found in male controls. Vascular tumours were seen at increased frequency in male mice at the high dose, while lung tumours, hepatomas and lymphomas occurred with apparently equal incidence in control and treated groups. Any differences in the incidence of tumours were considered not to be significant, and none were found in a duplicate experiment for which no data were given (Homburger, 1978). [The Working Group noted the inadequate reporting of the experiment.]

Fifty male B6C3F$_1$ mice, six weeks of age, were fed sodium saccharin (purity, 99.5%; with 7 ppm *ortho*-toluenesulfonamide) at a dose of 5% in Oriental M diet for 52 weeks with interim kills of five mice at 0, 4, 8, 16 and 20 weeks after the beginning of the experiment; 20 mice were still alive at the end of the experiment. A control group of 35 mice was fed Oriental MF diet only. There was no effect on growth or survival, and no bladder lesions were detected by autoradiography, histology or scanning electron microscopy (Fukushima *et al.*, 1983a). [The Working Group noted the small number of animals and the short duration of the experiment.]

Groups of 10 male and 10 female inbred ICR Swiss mice, six weeks of age, received 0, 0.5, 1 or 1.5 g/kg bw per day saccharin dissolved in 1 mL distilled water by oral gavage for one year, at which time all remaining mice were killed. No deaths occurred in any of the treated groups. The mice fed 1.5 g/kg bw per day showed slight weight loss when compared with controls (48 versus 55 g); both groups consumed 10 g of food per day per mouse. Five males and three females at the high dose had papillary adenocarcinomas of the thyroid. No thyroid tumours were reported in the other groups, and no tumours of other sites were reported (Prasad & Rai, 1986). [The Working Group noted the inadequate number of mice and the incomplete reporting of this experiment. It also noted that the finding of thyroid tumours has not been replicated in any other study in mice or in other species.]

As part of study of two-stage carcinogenesis, female BALB/c StCrlfC3H/Nctr mice were randomly divided into five groups of 192, 192, 192, 144 and 96 mice and were fed 0, 0.1, 0.5, 1, or 5 sodium saccharin, respectively, in Purina Lab Chow beginning at 19 weeks of age and continuing until 135 weeks of age. A slight but nonsignificant statistically increase in the length of survival was observed in treated mice. No bladder neoplasms were observed in any of the groups, and the incidence of bladder hyperplasia was similar: 8/164 (5%), 10/162 (6%), 9/161 (5%), 7/130 (5%) and 3/79 (4%), respectively. The incidences of Harderian gland neoplasms were 27/163 (17%), 32/172 (19%), 29/160 (18%), 22/132 (17%) and 22/84 (26%), respectively ($p < 0.04$, test for trend). A significant, dose-related reduction in the time to onset of lymphomas was observed, although the incidences were similar among groups (Frederick *et al.*, 1989; see also section 3.4). [The Working Group noted that Harderian gland tumours are common age-related, spontaneous neoplasms, the variable percentage of Harderian glands examined, the variability of the incidence of these tumours in control animals, the unequal numbers of animals per group and the long survival time.]

Rat: Groups of 10 male and 10 female Osborne-Mendel rats, 21 days of age, received diets containing 0, 1 or 5% saccharin [source and purity unspecified] for up to two years. The mortality rate in pooled controls was 14% at one year and 68% at two years; at one year, seven males and nine females in the control group, 10 males and 10 females in the group receiving 1% and nine males and nine females at 5% were still alive; the two-year survival rates were not given. It was reported that 7/18 rats [sex unspecified] at 5% had abdominal lymphosarcomas, and that four of the seven also had thoracic lymphosarcomas. The urinary bladders were not examined (Fitzhugh *et al.*, 1951). [The Working Group noted the multiple inadequacies of this study, including the small number of animals in each group.]

Groups of 20 male and 20 female Boots-Wistar rats [age unspecified] were fed 0, 0.005, 0.05 or 5% saccharin made by the Remsen-Fahlberg method [purity unspecified] for two years. At 18 months, 15 male and 14 female controls and 10 male and 10 female rats at the highest dose level were still alive. No statistically significant differences in tumour incidence were found between treated and control animals. Only five bladders, all from animals at the highest dose, were examined histologically. Urothelial hyperplasia was found in one male and one female, and a bladder papilloma was found in another female. Bladder parasites were not found. Bladder calculi were found in four male and one female rats fed 5% saccharin (Lessel, 1971).

Groups of 52 male and 52 female BD rats [age unspecified] were fed 0 (control), 0.2 or 0.5% sodium saccharin made by the Remsen-Fahlberg method [purity unspecified] for up to 30 months starting between 70 and 90 days of age, providing average total doses of 0, 83 and 210 g/kg bw. The survival rates at 18 months were 55/104 controls, 50/104 at the low dose and 41/104 at the high dose; at 24 months, the survival rates were 6/104, 3/104 and 5/104, respectively. Sixteen percent of all animals had parasites (*Strongyloides capillaria*) in the urinary tract. Benign and malignant mesenchymal tumours were found with similar frequency in all groups. No bladder tumours were observed (Schmähl, 1973).

In a study reported in an abstract, groups of Charles River CD male and female rats [number and age unspecified] received saccharin [source and purity unspecified] by an unspecified route (in the diet or by gastric intubation thrice weekly) for 18 months, followed by a six-month period of observation. A high incidence of benign tumours of the pituitary and mammary glands was found in surviving controls and experimental animals. The survival times, types of pathological examination, tumour types and other important experimental details were not reported (Ulland *et al.*, 1973). [The Working Group noted the inadequacy of this experiment.]

In a study reported in an abstract, groups of 54–56 male Wistar rats [age unspecified] were fed 0 or 2.5 g/kg bw per day sodium saccharin [source and purity unspecified] for up to 28 months. Ten to 16 rats from each group were killed at 12 months, 11 from each group at 24 months and all survivors [number unspecified] at 28 months. No urinary bladder tumours were observed (Furuya *et al.*, 1975). [The Working Group noted the incomplete reporting of this experiment.]

Groups of 60 male and 60 female Charles River CD rats [age unspecified] were fed diets containing sodium saccharin made by the Remsen-Fahlberg method (purity conformed to United States Pharmacopoeia, British Pharmacopoeia and Food Chemicals Codex specifications) for 26 months, to give daily intakes of 0, 0.09, 0.27, 0.81 or 2.4 g/kg bw. Saccharin treatment did not affect the survival of female rats: at 18 months, approximately 50% of the original animals were alive. The survival of male rats was affected in a dose-related manner: thus, at 18 months, about 80% of male control rats but only about 50% of those at the highest dose were still alive. By 24 months, about 10% of the animals in all groups were alive. Four transitional-cell tumours of the bladder were found, one in a male and one in a female given 0.09 g/kg bw and two in males fed 0.81 g/kg bw; an angiosarcoma of the bladder was found in a male control. Bladder calculi were recorded, but there was no association between the presence of calculi, saccharin treatment and/or bladder tumours. The animals were free from bladder parasites. The combined incidences of lymphomas and leukaemias were 7/54 in males at the highest dose of saccharin and 2/57 in untreated male controls (Munro *et al.*, 1975).

Groups of 25 male Charles River CD-1 rats [age unspecified] received sodium saccharin (containing 345 mg/kg (ppm) *ortho*-toluenesulfonamide) in the diet at concentrations of 0, 1 or 5% for up to two years. Animals that died before six months were not examined, and the survival times were not reported. Animals were killed when obvious tumours were seen or when they were moribund; all survivors were killed at two years. All animals that survived six months or longer were examined grossly, and any tissues with abnormal changes were examined histologically; in addition, all vital organs from at least 12 animals in each group were examined histologically. Tumours of the urinary bladder, pituitary, breast and subcutaneous tissue were seen with equal incidence in all groups (Homburger, 1978). [The Working Group noted the inadequate reporting of the experiment].

A group of 75 male and 50 female Wistar SPF rats, eight weeks of age, received sodium saccharin made by the Remsen-Fahlberg method (containing 698 mg/kg (ppm) *ortho*-toluenesulfonamide) in the drinking-water, to give a daily intake of 2 g/kg bw saccharin. Another group of 75 males and 75 females received 4 g/kg bw per day saccharin in the diet. A group of 55 males and 50 females served as controls. The males receiving saccharin in the drinking-water were also given 1% ammonium chloride for four weeks and then 0.5% for life, in order to correct a treatment-associated rise in urinary pH. Of the male controls, 25 were given ammonium chloride at the same concentrations. No treatment-associated change in urinary pH occurred in either of the treated groups of females or in males receiving saccharin in the diet. The experiment was terminated after two years. Survival at 18 months was 49/55 male and 43/50 female untreated controls, 65/75 males and 44/50 females that received saccharin in the drinking-water and 55/75 males and 52/75 females fed saccharin in the diet. At 100 weeks, 37/55 male and 13/50 female controls, 49/75 males and 29/50 females receiving saccharin in the drinking-water and 12/75 males and 16/75 females fed saccharin in the diet were still alive. In control animals, the total tumour incidence was 1/52 males and 9/46 females. In rats receiving saccharin in the drinking-water at 2 g/kg bw per day, the incidence was 11/71 in males and 10/44 in females; while in rats fed saccharin at 4 g/kg bw per day it was 10/70 in males and 7/68 in females. Transitional-cell carcinomas of the urothelium were not seen in male or female controls, but accounted for 1/71 in males (in the ureter) and 1/44 in females (in the renal pelvis) in rats receiving saccharin in the drinking-water and 3/70 in males (all in the bladder) and 0/68 in females fed saccharin. The incidence of lymphosarcomas and/or leukaemia was 0/52 in male and 0/46 in female controls, 4/71 in males and 1/44 in females given saccharin in the drinking-water, and 2/70 in male and 1/68 in female saccharin-fed rats. One Leydig-cell tumour was found in each of the saccharin-treated groups of males, but none occurred in the testes of untreated male controls. There was a treatment-associated increase in the number of microcalculi within the renal tubules of male (but not female) saccharin-treated rats, with an incidence of 2/52 in controls, 30/71 in males given saccharin in the drinking-water and 16/70 in saccharin-fed males. The animals were free from bladder parasites (Chowaniec & Hicks, 1979). [The Working Group noted the incomplete histopathological examination and the lack of lymphomas and/or leukaemia, a common neoplasm in controls.]

As part of a two-generation study (see section 3.1.2), groups of 50 male and 50 female Charles-River CD (Sprague-Dawley) rats, 30 days of age, were fed either a control diet or a diet containing 5% sodium saccharin prepared by the Maumee process and free of *ortho*-toluenesulfonamide. Survival was not affected by treatment. Bladder tumours (benign and malignant) were observed in 1/36 control males and in 7/38 male rats ($p < 0.03$) fed saccharin which survived 87 weeks or more (the time at which the first tumour was observed). In addition, one treated male and two treated females had urothelial tumours of the renal pelvis, and one treated male had a urethral tumour; no other urothelial tumours were observed in controls. The incidence of bladder calculi was not related to treatment or to tumour incidence. The animals were free of bladder parasites (Arnold *et al.*, 1980).

As part of a two-generation study, 50 female Wistar rats [age unspecified] were given 2 g/kg bw per day sodium saccharin made by the Maumee process in the diet for two years. A group of 63 animals served as controls. At week 84, 50/63 controls and 37/50 saccharin-fed rats were still alive. The overall tumour incidences were similar in the two groups, and no bladder neoplasm occurred. Mild focal urothelial hyperplasia was seen in one rat fed saccharin. The animals were free from bladder parasites (Hooson *et al.*, 1980). [The Working Group noted that the animals were not started on the test at weaning but had been fed a normal diet for several weeks before the start of the study.]

Groups of 40–48 male ACI, Wistar, Fischer 344 and Sprague-Dawley rats, six weeks of age, were fed 5% sodium saccharin (food additive grade; purity, 99.5%, with 7 ppm *ortho*-toluenesulfonamide) in powdered diet, and surviving rats were killed at the end of 52 weeks of treatment. Interim sacrifices were also performed on five rats of each strain at 12, 24 and 36 weeks. Corresponding control groups of 40–45 rats were fed untreated diet. The treated groups had significant growth retardation, with average body weights at week 52 of treated versus control groups as follows: ACI, 299 versus 327 g; Wistar, 400 versus 447 g; Fischer 344, 403 versus 427 g; and Sprague-Dawley, 593 versus 716 g. There was no apparent effect on survival. At the end of 52 weeks, no urinary bladder lesions were seen in the Wistar, Fischer 344 or Sprague-Dawley rats; of the ACI rats, 1/28 controls had simple hyperplasia and 25/32 (78%) rats treated with sodium saccharin had simple hyperplasia, 20 (62.5%) had papillary/nodular hyperplasia, nine (28.1%) had papillomas and three (9.4%) had carcinomas. It was also reported that one of the ACI rats had a bladder calculus, but more than half of the control and test ACI rats bore the bladder nematode, *Trichosomoides crassicauda* (Fukushima *et al.*, 1983a). [The Working Group noted the limited duration of treatment.]

A group of 68 male Fischer 344 rats, seven weeks of age, were fed 5% sodium saccharin in Oriental MF diet; a control group of 31 rats were fed the basal diet alone. Interim sacrifices were carried out during the course of the experiment, and the remaining rats were killed at the end of 112 weeks of treatment. The body-weight gain was similar in the two groups up to 15 weeks, whereas after 20 weeks the body weight increased more slowly in treated rats than in controls. Simple hyperplasia was seen in the bladders of about two-thirds of treated rats at all timepoints, and was occasionally seen in control rats: 2/6 rats at four weeks, 1/5 at 20 weeks, and 1/7 at 100 weeks. Papillary or nodular hyperplasia was observed in the bladders of approximately one-third of rats killed after 8, 12, 20, 80 and 112 weeks of treatment, althought at 4, 16, 60, 90 and 100 weeks, no papillary or nodular hyperplasia was observed. No papillary or nodular hyperplasia was seen in the control group, and no papilloma or transitional-cell carcinoma was seen in either group. *Trichosomoides crassicauda* were not present in the bladders. When the stomachs of 20 treated and 11 control rats killed after 80 weeks were examined, all of the sodium saccharin-treated rats had hyperkeratosis at the limiting ridge of the forestomach, and five papillomas of the limiting ridge of the forestomach were reported.Ulcers were seen in the glandular stomach in four animals. No squamous-cell carcinomas or adenocarcinomas were observed in either group (Hibino *et al.*, 1985). [The Working Group noted the incomplete sampling of the stomach between groups. The Group could not agree on the diagnosis of papillomas from the illustrations provided.]

A group of 36 male Sprague-Dawley and 35 male analbuminaemic (a mutant strain derived from Sprague-Dawley rats) rats, six weeks of age, were fed 5% sodium saccharin in powdered CE-2 diet for 80 weeks. Fourteen Sprague-Dawley and 12 analbuminaemic rats served as controls. There was no apparent effect on body weight or on survival. No bladder tumours were present in any of the rats. Simple hyperplasia of the urinary bladder was observed in 2/35 analbuminaemic and 2/36 Sprague-Dawley rats given sodium saccharin (Homma *et al.*, 1991). [The Working Group noted that the treatment period was less than two years.]

Hamster: Groups of 30 male and 30 female random-bred Syrian golden hamsters, eight weeks of age, received saccharin made by the Maumee process at concentrations of 0, 0.156, 0.312, 0.625 or 1.25% in the drinking-water for their natural lifespan. The highest dose used in this study was the maximum tolerated, as determined in an eight-week study. The average daily consumption ranged from 44 mg/animal given 0.156% to 353 mg/animal given 1.25%. The mean survival time was 50–60 weeks in all groups. The pathological changes observed and the distribution and histological types of neoplasms were within the range of tumours that occur commonly in hamsters in this colony (Althoff *et al.*, 1975).

Fifty male Syrian golden hamsters, six weeks of age, were fed 5% sodium saccharin (purity, 99.5%, with 7 ppm *ortho*-toluenesulfonamide) in the diet for 52 weeks. Five animals were killed at 0, 4, 8, 16 or 20 weeks after the beginning of the experiment; 20 hamsters were available at the terminal sacrifice. A group of 35 hamsters served as untreated controls. There was no effect on growth or survival, and no bladder lesions were detected by autoradiography, histology or scanning electron microscopy (Fukushima *et al.*, 1983a). [The Working Group noted the small number of animals and the short duration of the experiment.]

Guinea-pig: A group of 30 male Hartley guinea-pigs, six weeks of age, were fed 5% sodium saccharin (purity, 99.5%, with 7 ppm *ortho*-toluenesulfonamide) in Oriental RC diet for 52 weeks with interim sacrifices of three guinea-pigs at 0, 4, 12, 16 or 20 weeks from the beginning of the experiment; 12 guinea-pigs were available at the terminal sacrifice. A group of 20 guinea-pigs served as untreated controls. Treated guinea-pigs had lower body-weight gain than the controls, but no bladder lesions were detected by autoradiography, histology or scanning electron microscopy (Fukushima *et al.*, 1983a). [The Working Group noted the small number of animals and the short duration of the experiment.]

Monkey: In a study reported in an abstract, one of two batches of sodium saccharin made by the Remsen-Fahlberg method (containing 2.4 and 3.2 mg/kg *ortho*-toluene-sulfonamide) (Coulston *et al.*, 1975) was given orally at doses of 20, 100 or 500 mg/kg bw per day on six days a week to groups of two, two and three *Macaca mulatta* (rhesus) monkeys of each sex, respectively. Three animals of each sex served as controls. After 79 months on this regimen, 11 monkeys remained in the treated groups, and all monkeys were killed and autopsied. Histopathological examination revealed no abnormal lesions in the urinary bladder, kidneys or testis in monkeys that survived the treatment or in those that died during the test (McChesney *et al.*, 1977).

Groups of five female and one male African green (*Cercopithecus aethiops*), two female and five male rhesus (*Macaca mulatta*), three female and three male cynomolgus (*Macaca fascicularis*) and one hybrid (rhesus male cross cynomolgus female) monkey, 0–10 days of age, were given 25 mg/kg bw sodium saccharin (purity, > 99%) in the diet on five days a week for up to 283 months. Eight monkeys died during the course of the experiment, after 103, 128, 157, 168, 170, 192, 214 and 282 months of feeding. The remainder were killed at the end of the experiment, after 207–283 months. Five male and four female cynomolgus and five male and two females rhesus monkeys were available for comparison and were killed at 206–301 months of age. No bladder tumours were detected, and there was no evidence of hyperplasia by light or scanning electron microscopy (Takayama *et al.*, 1998). (Preliminary reports of this experiment were published by

Sieber & Adamson, 1978; Thorgeirsson *et al.*, 1994). [The Working Group noted the relatively small dose of saccharin administered, the relatively small number of monkeys used and the multiplicity of species.]

3.1.2 *Multigeneration exposure*

In these studies, animals of each sex of the parent (F_0) generation were fed saccharin or sodium saccharin from weaning (or very soon after weaning) throughout both pregnancy and before weaning of their offspring. As the offspring were then placed on the same diet as their parents for their lifespan, their exposure to saccharin was greater than that of the F_0 generation by the length of the gestation and suckling periods.

Mouse: Saccharin containing 0.5% *ortho*-toluenesulfonamide was fed to groups of Swiss mice in a multigeneration study for life at concentrations of 0, 0.2 or 0.5% in the diet. The F_0, F_{3b} and F_{6a} generations, consisting of 50 males and 50 females, were used to test the compound for carcinogenicity. The experiments were terminated at 21 months. The survival rates at 18 months were 66, 62, 64 (F_0), 61, 54, 53 (F_{3b}) and 67, 48, 54 (F_{6a}) at 0, 0.2 and 0.5% respectively. Histopathological examination showed that lesions were equally distributed in the control and experimental groups. Two male mice, one of the F_0 generation receiving 0.2% saccharin and one of the F_{3b} generation receiving 0.5% saccharin, developed transitional-cell carcinomas of the bladder at 20.5 months. One female control of the F_0 generation had an anaplastic carcinoma of the bladder at 20.5 months (Kroes *et al.*, 1977).

Rat: Groups of 20 male and 20 female weanling Sprague-Dawley rats of the F_1 generation were fed sodium saccharin made by the Remsen-Fahlberg method [purity unspecified] at concentrations of 0, 0.05, 0.5 or 5% of the basal diet for up to 100 weeks. Of the F_1 animals, 12, 10, 11 and 15 males and 16, 14, 14 and 19 females, respectively, survived to 80 weeks. Seven transitional-cell carcinomas of the urinary bladder developed, all in F_1 males on the 5% saccharin diet ($p = 0.001$). The presence or absence of bladder parasites was not recorded. The total numbers of tumour-bearing animals were two males and eight females at 0%, one male and six females at 0.05%, one male and five females at 0.5%, and seven males and 13 females at 5% (Tisdel *et al.*, 1974).

Groups of 50 male and 50 female Charles River CD (Sprague-Dawley) rats, 30 days of age, were fed either a control diet or a diet containing 5% sodium saccharin continuously for life. The saccharin was prepared by the Maumee process and was free of *ortho*-toluenesulfonamide. After three months on test, the animals were mated on a one-to-one basis. All litters were culled to eight pups (four males and four females) four days *post partum* in a random manner. The pups were weaned onto their parents' diet, and 50 males and 50 females from each group were randomly selected to constitute the second generation. The survival of the offspring (F_1 generation) was not affected by treatment. Of the F_1 animals surviving 67 weeks or longer, at which time the first tumour was observed, none of the 42 male controls but eight of the 45 saccharin-treated males had developed transitional-cell carcinomas of the bladder [$p = 0.002$], and four had transitional-cell papillomas; two of the 49 surviving females fed 5% sodium saccharin also had bladder cancers. Although urinary bladder calculi were noted occasionally, their incidence was not related to treatment, nor were they associated with the tumours. The animals were free of bladder parasites (Arnold *et al.*, 1980).

Groups of five to seven female Sprague-Dawley were treated by oral gavage with saccharin [form not specified] (containing < 10 ppm *ortho*-toluenesulfonamide) at doses of 0.2, 1 or 5 g/kg bw on days 14, 17 and 20 of pregnancy. Solutions containing 2.5 g/mL of the test compound were given by gavage to the rats, which had received no food or drinking-water overnight. A control group consisted of the offspring of five untreated rats. The numbers of offspring at the low, intermediate and high doses which survived to 28 days of age were 24 males and 27 females, 35 males and 23 females and 32 males and 25 females, respectively; the untreated controls had 25 male and 33 female offspring. Nine of 69 of the offspring of dams treated with the highest dose of saccharin died within the first four days after birth. The F_1 generation offspring were observed for life [time not specified] or killed when found moribund. The mean survival times of males tended to be higher with the higher doses of saccharin but were lower than those of controls. No significant differences in survival were found between groups. There were no lesions of the bladders in any of the treated groups, and there was no increase in the incidence of tumours at other sites. The tumours seen in the treated groups were the same as those seen in controls (Schmähl & Habs, 1980). [The Working Group noted the incomplete reporting of this experiment.]

Groups of 48 male and 48 female Charles River CD (Sprague-Dawley) rats of the F_1 generation were fed dietary levels of 0, 0.01, 0.1, 1, 5 or 7.5% sodium saccharin [method of production and purity unspecified] for 28 months after their parents had been fed the same diet from weaning. There were no significant differences in survival between treated and control animals. Although no difference in bladder tumour incidence was found between F_1 males fed 5% saccharin (1/21) and the F_1 controls (1/25) that survived beyond 18 months, 6/23 F_1 male rats fed 7.5% saccharin developed transitional-cell papillomas or carcinomas of the bladder. This result was significantly different from that in controls. There was no apparent correlation between tumour incidence and presence of bladder stones. The bladders were reported to be 'free of visible parasites' (Taylor *et al.*, 1980).

Male Charles River CD rats of the F_1 generation were treated as follows: group 1 (350 rats), untreated controls; group 2 (700 rats), 1% sodium saccharin (produced by the Maumee process; purity, > 99%) in the diet; group 3 (500 rats), 3% sodium saccharin in the diet; group 4 (200 rats), 4% sodium saccharin in the diet; group 5 (125 rats), 5% sodium saccharin in the diet; group 6 (125 rats), 6.25% sodium saccharin in the diet; group 7 (125 rats), 7.5% sodium saccharin in the diet; group 8 (125 rats), 5% sodium saccharin administered through gestation period and then the F_1 rats fed control diet from birth until the end of the experiment; group 9 (125 rats), 5% sodium saccharin in the diet from the time of birth and continuing until the end of the experiment; group 10 (125 rats), 5% sodium hippurate (purity > 98%) in the diet until the age of eight weeks and then as 3% of the diet until the end of the experiment. The parents (the F_0 generation) were given the same diets from six weeks of age and continuing for nine weeks before the beginning of mating; they were then given the same diets through gestation and lactation (except as noted for groups 8 and 9). Group 8 received sodium saccharin throughout gestation and then received control diet. In group 9, the F_0 generation was given control diet until the birth of the F_1 generation, at which time the dams were given 5% sodium saccharin. There was significant growth retardation in all groups given sodium saccharin at doses of greater than 3% of the diet, including group 9. There were minimal changes in the growth of the rats in group 8, given sodium saccharin until parturition. Survival was comparable in the nine groups, except for a significant increase in survival in groups 5 and 7. The numbers of survivors of the F_1 generation in the nine groups at the time of killing at 30 months of age were: 80/350 (23%), 172/700 (25%), 114/500 (23%), 38/200 (19%), 46/125 (37%), 33/125 (26%), 42/125 (34%), 25/125 (20%), 33/125 (26%) and 38/125 (30%), respectively. The effective numbers of rats were those alive at 15 months of age when the first bladder tumour was detected. The incidences of transitional-cell papillomas were 0/324, 4/658 (0.6%), 4/472 (0.8%), 4/189 (2.1%), 4/120 (3.3%), 12/120 (10%), 18/118 (15%), 0/122, 4/120 (3.3%) and 0/118, respectively. The incidences of transitional-cell carcinomas were 0, 1 (0.2%), 4 (0.8%), 8 (4.2%), 11 (9.2%), 8 (6.7%), 19 (16%), 0, 8 (6.7%) and 0, respectively. It was noted that the background incidence of bladder neoplasia at the study laboratory was 0.8%. In this study, the incidences of bladder neoplasia were significantly increased in groups 3–7 and in group 9. The tumour incidences when 1% sodium saccharin and 5% were fed throughout gestation were not significantly greater than those of controls. There was no difference in the incidence of bladder neoplasms between groups 5 and 9 (5% sodium saccharin throughout gestation and after parturition and 5% sodium saccharin after parturition only) (Schoenig *et al.*, 1985). [The Working Group noted that re-examination of the histopathology of the bladders was performed by Squire (1985), who found a significant increase in the incidence of bladder tumours only at doses of 4, 5, 6.25 and 7.25% sodium saccharin. There were no compound-related effects at 1%, and there was no statistically significant increase in the incidence of transitional-cell carcinomas ($p = 0.25$) at the 3% dose.]

3.2 Intraperitoneal administration

Mouse: In a screening assay of 41 food additives and 22 chemotherapeutic agents in the primary lung tumour bioassay in A/St mice, groups of 20 female mice, six to eight weeks of age, received intraperitoneal injections of sodium saccharin three times a week for the first eight weeks of the experiment (total doses, 15.6 and 78 g/kg bw) followed by an additional 13 weeks of observation. All of the mice were killed at the end of 21 weeks. Fifteen mice at each dose survived until the end of experiment. Lung adenomas were observed in four and eight mice treated with the two doses of saccharin, respectively, and the numbers of lung tumours per mouse were 0.27 ± 0.07 and 0.67 ± 0.17, respectively. Of a group of 30 female mice that received only water, 28 survived until the end of the experiment; 37% developed lung adenomas and the number of tumours per mouse was 0.37 ± 0.07. There was no significant difference between these groups (Stoner *et al.*, 1973). [The Working Group noted that this bioassay is no longer considered a valid screen for the carcinogenic activity of chemicals.]

3.3 Other experimental systems

3.3.1 *Skin application*

A total dose of 0.24 g saccharin [form not specified], made by the Remson-Fahlberg method, was applied as an 8% solution in acetone thrice weekly to the skin of 'S' strain mice. Twenty-five days after the start of the treatment, the animals were given 18 weekly applications of 0.17% croton oil in acetone. At the end of the croton oil treatment, 15 skin papillomas were observed in seven of the 20 saccharin-treated animals, by comparison with four papillomas in four of 19 controls treated with croton oil only. The increase was not statistically significant (Salaman & Roe, 1956).

3.3.2 *Bladder insertion (implantation)*

Saccharin [source and purity unspecified] was mixed with four times its weight of cholesterol, and pellets (9–11 mg) containing 2 mg saccharin were then inserted into the urinary bladder lumina of 20 'stock' mice [sex and age unspecified]. An identical group composed of 28 mice received 9–11-mg pellets of cholesterol. The experiment lasted 52 weeks. Of mice that lived 30 weeks, 4/13 saccharin-treated and 1/24 control animals developed bladder tumours ($p = 0.01$) (Allen *et al.*, 1957). [The Working Group noted serious difficulties in interpreting the results of studies conducted with pellet implantation in the bladder because of the significant carcinogenic effect of the pellet itself (Clayson, 1974; Jull, 1979; DeSesso, 1989).]

Sodium saccharin (analytically pure) was mixed at 4–5 mg with four times its weight of cholesterol; pellets weighing 20–24 mg containing sodium saccharin were then inserted into the urinary bladder lumina in two trials with groups each composed of 100 female Swiss mice aged 60–90 days. Ninety-nine percent of the sodium saccharin had disappeared from the pellet within 1.5 days. Identical groups received 20–24 mg pellets of pure cholesterol for 56 weeks. Only the bladders of animals surviving more than 25 weeks were examined microscopically. The first urinary bladder carcinoma was seen in a saccharin-treated animal 42 weeks after surgical insertion. The overall incidences of bladder carcinomas were 31/66 (trial 1) and 33/64 (trial 2) in saccharin-treated mice as compared with 8/63 (trial 1) and 5/43 (trial 2) in animals exposed to pure cholesterol pellets ($p < 0.001$). The carcinomas in saccharin-exposed mice were more frequently multiple and invasive ($p < 0.009$). They were composed of cells with a high mitotic index and exhibited more squamous or glandular metaplasia than was found in tumours in control animals. The incidence of tumours in other tissues were not different from those in control mice (Bryan *et al.*, 1970). [The Working Group noted the paucity of details regarding this experiment and the difficulty in interpreting the results of studies involving pellet implantation technique in mice (Clayson, 1974; Jull, 1979; DeSesso, 1989)].

3.4 Administration with known carcinogens

3.4.1 *Benzo[a]pyrene*

Groups of 50 female Swiss mice, 9–14 weeks of age, received an initial single gastric instillation of 0.2 mL polyethylene glycol either alone or containing 50 µg benzo[*a*]pyrene [purities unspecified]. Seven days later, the test diet containing 5% saccharin [purity unspecified] was fed for 72 weeks. The average survival rates were not different from those of controls. Although mice treated with benzo[*a*]pyrene had an increased incidence of squamous papillomas of the forestomach (20/61), saccharin did not enhance the occurrence (10/32). Hepatocellular adenomas, pulmonary neoplasms and malignant lymphomas occurred at similar frequencies in all groups. No pathological alterations were observed macroscopically in the urinary bladder (Roe *et al.*, 1970). [The Working Group noted that benzo[*a*]pyrene is not organotropic for the bladder and that the urinary bladders were not examined histologically.]

3.4.2 *2-Acetylaminofluorene*

Two groups of 12 female Horton Sprague-Dawley rats [age unspecified] were fed a diet supplemented with 300 mg/kg 2-acetylaminofluorene (AAF) for 40 weeks and/or 5% sodium saccharin. Eleven of the controls given AAF and 6/12 rats fed AAF plus saccharin developed palpable mammary and ear-duct tumours. Liver tumours were observed in both groups, but they were smaller and less malignant in the saccharin-fed animals. Microscopic examination of the urinary bladders indicated that the mucosal lining was hyperplastic in all rats fed AAF but more particularly so in those fed AAF plus saccharin; one animal fed AAF plus saccharin had squamous metaplasia and precancerous changes of the mucosal epithelium. No malignant lesions of the urinary bladder were observed (Ershoff & Bajwa, 1974). [The Working Group noted the inadequate number of animals and that the intake of AAF and saccharin could not be assessed since food consumption was not measured.]

Ten groups of weanling female BALB/c StCrlfCrlfC3H/Nctr mice, 21–26 days old, were fed control diet (groups 1–5) or were pretreated with 200 mg/kg diet (ppm) AAF (purity > 97%) (groups 6–10) for 13 weeks, followed by two weeks of control diet, and were then fed 0 (groups 1 and 6), 0.1% (groups 2 and 7), 0.5% (groups 3 and 8), 1% (groups 4 and 9) or 5% (groups 5 and 10) sodium saccharin (purity, > 98%). The saccharin was administered when the mice were 19–135 weeks old. There were 192 mice in each of groups 1–3 and 6–8, 144 mice in each of groups 4 and 9, and 96 mice in each of groups 5 and 10. The mortality rate of mice pretreated with AAF followed by control diet was significantly higher than that of mice that received only the control diet. Addition of sodium saccharin to the diet of AAF-pretreated animals increased their longevity in a dose-related fashion ($p = 0.011$). A less pronounced effect was observed in non-pretreated mice ($p = 0.099$). The incidences of bladder tumours were 2/164 (1%) for the group given AAF plus control diet and 3/165 (2%) for the groups given AAF plus 0.1% saccharin, respectively; no bladder tumours were seen in any of the other groups. The incidences of bladder hyperplasia were similar in the five groups pretreated with AAF and in the groups not pretreated with AAF. There was no dose–related increase in the incidence of neoplasms in any other tissues, including the Harderian gland, but a decreased incidence of lymphomas was seen in the group pretreated with AAF and given 5% saccharin (50% versus 62% in the controls). There was a statistically significant, dose-related reduction in the time to onset of lymphomas in AAF-pretreated and non-pretreated mice, correlated with the decreased mortality rate observed in saccharin-treated mice. An increase in the incidence of liver neoplasms was seen in AAF-pretreated when compared with non-pretreated mice, but there were no differences between the incidences at the different doses of saccharin and the corresponding controls (Frederick *et al.*, 1989; see also section 3.1.1).

3.4.3 N-*Methyl*-N-*nitrosourea*

A group of 50 female Wistar SPF rats, six to eight weeks of age, were pretreated with a preparation of 1.5 mg *N*-methyl-*N*-nitrosourea (MNU) dissolved in 0.9% sodium chloride (pH 7.0) and instilled into the bladder, and then two days later received 4 g/kg bw per day sodium saccharin (Remsen-Fahlberg, containing an average of 698 mg/kg (ppm) *ortho*-toluenesulfonamide) in the diet for life or up to two years; a further group of 50 females was pretreated with 2 mg MNU and then given 2 g/kg bw sodium saccharin per day in the drinking-water. The control groups consisted of 55 male and 50 female untreated rats, 75 males and 50 females given 2 g/kg bw sodium saccharin per day in drinking-water, 75 males and 75 females fed 4 g/kg bw sodium saccharin per day in the diet, 85 males and females given 1.5 mg MNU, and 50 given 2 mg MNU and maintained on a saccharin-free diet for two years. The incidences of transitional-cell neoplasms of the bladder in surviving animals whose bladders were examined histologically were: 0/52 male and 0/46 female untreated controls, 0/71 males and 0/44 females at 2 g/kg bw per day sodium saccharin in drinking-water, 3/70 males and 0/68 females at 4 g/kg bw day sodium saccharin in the diet, 0/124 in MNU-treated animals, 23/49 females (47%; $p < 0.0005$) given MNU followed by 2 g/kg bw per day of sodium saccharin in drinking-water and 27/47 females (52%; $p < 0.0005$) given MNU followed by 4 g/kg bw per day sodium saccharin in the diet. The first bladder tumour was seen after 95 weeks in the saccharin-fed control group and after eight weeks in the MNU-initiated and sodium saccharin-treated test groups. The animals were free from bladder parasites (Hicks *et al.*, 1978; Chowaniec & Hicks, 1979). [The Working Group noted the difficulty in determining the actual dose of MNU because of possible decay in solution over time.]

A single dose of 2 mg MNU was instilled into the urinary bladders of female Wistar rats (AF-Han strain) weighing 195 g. Thereafter, 50 animals were given 2% saccharin [purity unspecified] in the diet, the dose being increased after 10 weeks to 4%, for life, resulting in doses of 1.4–2.5 g/kg bw per day. The control groups consisted of 100 untreated female rats, 50 females receiving MNU alone and 50 females receiving distilled water. A further group of 50 female rats treated with MNU were given 3% calcium carbonate in the diet instead of saccharin. The survival rates at two years were 59/100 untreated controls, 28/50 water controls, 13/50 MNU-treated animals, 15/50 receiving MNU plus calcium and 14/50 given MNU plus saccharin. In the MNU-treated groups, the first tumour of the urinary bladder was found after 14 weeks. Benign and malignant urothelial neoplasms occurred in the renal pelvis, ureter and urinary bladder, the overall incidences of urinary tract tumours being 57% with MNU only (survival, 76 ± 29 weeks), 65% with MNU plus saccharin (survival, 78 ± 25 weeks) and 65% with

MNU plus calcium carbonate (survival, 86 ± 23 weeks). The frequencies were 28, 57 and 43% in the renal pelvis, 17, 12 and 11% in the ureter and 39, 31 and 39% in the urinary bladder, respectively. The frequency of calcification in the urinary tract, including stone formation, was similar in all treated groups, including controls receiving water, and the occurrence did not correlate with that of tumours. One tumour of the urinary tract was found in an untreated control and one in a control receiving a water instillation into the urinary bladder. The presence or absence of bladder parasites was not reported (Mohr *et al.*, 1978). [The Working Group noted that many bladder tumours were found and that the animals were heavier than those used in the experiment by Hicks *et al.* (1978).]

Groups of 50 female Wistar/AF-Han rats, average body weight 195 g, were treated with a single intravesicular instillation of water, a single intravesicular instillation of 2 mg MNU in 0.5 mL water with no further treatment, a single intravesicular instillation of 2 mg MNU followed by treatment with 3% calcium carbonate in the diet, a single intravesicular instillation of 2 mg MNU followed by 2% sodium saccharin in the diet for 10 weeks and then increased to 4% of the diet for the remainder of the experiment or a single intravesicular instillation of 2 mg MNU followed by 2% sodium cyclamate in the diet for 10 weeks and then increased to 4% of the diet for the remainder of the experiment. Satellite groups of 12, 15 and 12 rats for the last three groups, respectively, received the same treatments as the other rats in the group but were examined periodically by radiography for the presence of stones. A group of 100 rats was untreated. The incidences of bladder tumours were 0/100 in untreated controls, 1/50 in water controls, 19/49 with MNU, 24/49 with MNU plus calcium carbonate and 25/50 with MNU plus sodium saccharin, indicating no significant increase in tumorigenic activity due to saccharin. Bladder stones were noted in 0, 0, 6, 3 and 10 rats, respectively. No correlation between the presence of stones and the induction of bladder tumours was found (Green & Rippel, 1979). [The Working Group noted the incomplete reporting of this experiment.]

Three groups of 63 female Wistar rats [age unspecified] were pretreated with 0.15 mL of a saturated solution of MNU in saline (10 mg/mL) instilled into the bladder. Two weeks later, rats were given 0 or 2 g/kg bw per day sodium saccharin in the drinking-water for two years; one group received saccharin prepared by the Maumee process and the second group received saccharin prepared by the Remsen-Fahlberg method (containing 40 mg/kg (ppm) *ortho*-toluenesulfonamide). By week 84, 22 controls, 43 animals given 'Maumee' sodium saccharin and 37 rats given 'Remsen-Fahlberg' sodium saccharin had died. An increase in the number of proliferative bladder lesions occurred in animals treated with MNU plus saccharin. The incidence of bladder neoplasia was not significantly different in the saccharin-treated groups, but the mean latent period was shorter (55 and 52 weeks versus 87 weeks). The animals were free from bladder parasites (Hooson *et al.*, 1980). [The Working Group noted that the animals were not started on the test at weaning but had been fed a normal diet for several weeks before the start of the study.]

Male Fischer 344 rats weighing 130 g were kept for one week on basal diet and then given twice weekly intraperitoneal injections of 20 mg/kg bw MNU for four weeks followed by either 32 weeks of 0.05% phenobarbital or 5% sodium saccharin in the diet; given the same four-week treatment with MNU followed by 32 weeks of control diet; or given twice weekly injections of 5 mg/kg bw citrate buffer for four weeks and then either 0.05% phenobarbital or 5% sodium saccharin in the diet. The rats were killed at the end of 36 weeks. No information was provided on growth or survival. MNU followed by sodium saccharin produced papillary or nodular hyperplasia of the bladder in 9/19 (47%) rats, whereas no hyperplasia was seen in the bladders of other animals. Sodium saccharin did not increase the incidences of adenoma or adenocarcinoma of the thyroid, γ-glutamyl transferase-positive foci in the liver or lesions of the forestomach or glandular stomach when administered alone or after MNU. Phenobarbital increased the incidences of thyroid tumours and liver hyperplastic foci but not of neoplasia in the bladder. MNU by itself induced a high incidence of forestomach and glandular stomach foci and tumours and thyroid adenomas (Tsuda *et al.*, 1983). [The Working Group noted the relatively short period of administration and lack of bladder tumour induction with this protocol.]

Female Sprague-Dawley rats, eight weeks of age, were treated with a single intravesicular instillation of 0.5 mg MNU (synthesized at the institute and quantified on the day of use) in 300 μL saline or with an intravesicular instillation of 300 μL of saline. Two days after dosing, the rats were fed diets containing either 0 (120 rats), 0.1% (150 rats), 0.5% (120 rats), 1% (90 rats), 2.5% (60 rats) or 5% (60 rats) sodium saccharin in the diet. Groups of 60 rats were also given 5% saccharin in the diet or sodium saccharin in the drinking-water at a concentration of 2, 3 or 4% to achieve maximum consumption and yet preserve the animals' health. The 2% dose was then used for the remainder of the study. An additional group of 60 rats received four doses of MNU at weekly intervals and were then fed untreated diet for the remainder of the experiment. The experiment was terminated at the end of two years. Administration of MNU did not affect body weight. The average weight of rats receiving saccharin was lower than that of control animals, but the decrease exceeded 10% of the control weight only with 5% sodium saccharin and 5% saccharin in the diet and with 2% sodium saccharin in water. The mortality rates in these groups were not significantly different from each other or from those of the controls. Animals not treated with MNU lived longer than did those treated with MNU, and saccharin appeared to lower the mortality rate substantially throughout much of the study. Animals receiving sodium saccharin in the drinking-water had high, early morbidity and mortality. Two of the 233 rats given sodium saccharin in the diet but not pretreated with MNU developed bladder tumours [specific groups not specified]. The incidences in the group receiving sodium saccharin in the diet after MNU pretreatment were 17/106 (16%) with no sodium saccharin, 15/140 (11%) with 0.1%, 21/107 (20%) with 0.5%, 15/78 (19%) with 1%, 20/50 (40%) with 2.5% and 8/49 (16%) with 5%. The incidence in the group given sodium saccharin in the drinking-water was 9/46 (20%), that in the group given saccharin was 8/49 (16%), and that in the group given four intravesicular instillations of MNU was 24/57 (42%). A significantly increased incidence was seen only in the group given 2.5% sodium saccharin after MNU pretreatment (West *et al.*, 1986). [The Working Group noted the unconventional statistical analysis of the incidence of bladder tumours, whereby animals dying during the course of the experiment were analysed separately from those killed at the end. The Working Group also noted the lack of an increased incidence of bladder tumours with 5% sodium saccharin, in contrast to other reports with the MNU model. The authors attributed the lack of activity at the highest dose to toxicity, but the degree of toxicity was similar to that seen in other experiments with MNU at a dose of 5% sodium saccharin.]

Groups of 60 female Sprague-Dawley rats, eight weeks of age, were treated with a single instillation of 0.5 mg MNU in 300 μL saline or with 300 μL of saline alone. The MNU was synthesized freshly and quantified on the day of use. Sodium saccharin was administered in the diet by a variety of schedules: 0, 1, 2.5 or 5% was administered in the diet either four weeks immediately preceding, following or on the day of bladder instillation with MNU, and the animals were then maintained on control diet until the end of the experiment at 106 weeks of age; additionally, one group of rats were exposed neonatally through the milk of their mothers, which were given sodium saccharin in the diet for the three weeks of lactation, starting on the day of parturition, and were then fed control diet from weaning until the end of the experiment. An interim sacrifice was conducted at approximately 85 weeks of age, and the experiment was terminated when the rats were 112 weeks of age (106 weeks for the neonatal treatment). There was no apparent effect on body weight or on survival, and deaths were due primarily to the development of mammary tumours. The mortality rate was significantly lower than that of controls for animals given MNU and 1% sodium saccharin at 4–8 and 6–10 weeks, 2.5% sodium saccharin at 8–12 weeks or 5% sodium saccharin at 4–8 and 6–10 weeks. In the groups not given MNU, there were no deaths due to sodium saccharin treatment. Transitional-cell neoplasms of the urinary bladder were diagnosed only in animals treated with MNU; the incidences of bladder tumours ranged from 20 to 41% in the various groups, but there was no statistically significant increase in the incidence of bladder tumours between groups for any treatment period or for any dose of sodium saccharin (West *et al.*, 1994).

3.4.4 N-*[4-(5-Nitro-2-furyl)-2-thiazolyl]formamide*

Groups of 20 male Fischer rats, four weeks of age received 0.2% *N*-[4-(5-nitro-2-furyl)-2-thiazolyl]formamide (FANFT) in powdered diet for six weeks, followed immediately by 5% sodium saccharin (containing < 0.03 mg/kg *ortho*-toluenesulfonamide) in powdered diet for up to 83 weeks, then standard diet up to 104 weeks; pretreatment with FANFT as above, followed by six weeks on standard diet, 5% sodium saccharin in the diet for 77 weeks, then standard diet up to 104 weeks; normal diet for six weeks, followed by 5% sodium saccharin in the diet for 83 weeks, then standard diet up to 104 weeks; or pretreatment with FANFT, followed by standard diet for 98 weeks. Forty-two untreated controls received standard diet for 104 weeks. The experiment was terminated after 104 weeks, at which time 6/20, 9/20, 19/20, 16/20 and 27/42 animals were still alive. The incidences of urothelial carcinomas were 18/19 and 13/18 in the groups given FANFT plus saccharin, 0/20 in the group receiving saccharin alone, 4/20 in the group receiving FANFT alone and 0/42 in the untreated controls. In addition, 1/19 and 1/18 animals given FANFT plus saccharin had urinary bladder sarcomas, and 1/20 given FANFT only had a bladder papilloma. The presence or absence of bladder parasites was not reported (Cohen *et al.*, 1979).

Male Fischer rats, five weeks of age, were given 0.2% FANFT in the diet for four weeks followed by 5% sodium saccharin in the diet for 100 weeks; control diet for four weeks followed by sodium saccharin for 100 weeks; FANFT followed by 2% L-tryptophan; control diet followed by L-tryptophan; FANFT followed by control diet; FANFT for the entire course of the experiment; or control diet for the entire experiment. The incidences of bladder carcinoma were 5/26, 0/26, 2/26, 0/26, 0/25, 8/8 and 0/27, respectively, and the incidences of bladder papilloma were 2, 0, 3, 0, 1, 0 and 0, respectively (Fukushima *et al.*, 1981).

Male Fischer 344 rats, five weeks of age, were treated as follows: 5% sodium saccharin plus 2% L-tryptophan in the diet (13 rats); 5% sodium saccharin plus 0.005% FANFT in the diet (16 rats); 5% sodium saccharin in the diet (20 rats); 2% L-tryptophan in the diet (16 rats); FANFT in the diet (11 rats); or were untreated (23 rats). The respective diets were fed for two years, at which time the remaining rats were killed. A significant decrease in weight gain was seen only in the group given sodium saccharin plus L-tryptophan. Bladder tumours were seen only in the group given sodium saccharin plus FANFT, in which three papillomas and two carcinomas were observed; five rats had nodular or papillary hyperplasia of the bladder. Two of 11 rats in the group given FANFT alone also had nodular or papillary hyperplasia (Murasaki & Cohen, 1983a). [The Working Group noted the small numbers of animals.]

Groups of 30 male Fischer rats, five weeks of age, were treated in two phases, the first lasting for six weeks and the second for 61 weeks with a one-week interval between them. The treatments were as follows: 0.5% aspirin for two days, 0.2% FANFT and 0.5% aspirin in the diet for six weeks, one week of aspirin followed by 5% sodium saccharin up to 68 weeks; 0.2% FANFT, one week of control diet followed by aspirin plus sodium saccharin; 0.2% FANFT, one week of control diet followed by sodium saccharin; 0.5% aspirin for two days, 0.2% FANFT plus aspirin, one week of aspirin followed by control diet; 0.2% FANFT followed by control diet; control diet for seven weeks followed by aspirin plus sodium saccharin; control diet for seven weeks followed by sodium saccharin; aspirin for the entire course of the experiment; or control diet for the entire course of the experiment (40 rats). The experiment was terminated at the end of 68 weeks. The incidences of transitional-cell carcinoma of the urinary bladder were 6 (20%), 8 (28%), 24 (83%), 3 (10%) and 3 (10%) in the five groups given FANFT, respectively, with none in the other groups. The incidences of papillomas were 1, 2, 1, 0 and 3 in the groups given FANFT, respectively, and 1 in the group given only aspirin. The total bladder tumour incidence was significantly lower in the groups given aspirin with FANFT when compared with that given sodium saccharin and FANFT, indicating inhibition by aspirin of the bladder tumorigenic effects of both FANFT and sodium saccharin (Sakata *et al.*, 1986). Johansson *et al.* (1986) reported the effects on the kidneys of the rats in this study separately. The lesions reported included renal pelvic hyperplasia, metaplasia and atypia, calcification, renal papillary necrosis, vascular changes and rat nephropathy. It was noted that administration of sodium saccharin significantly inhibited the incidence and severity of nephropathy due to ageing but significantly increased the incidence and severity of hyperplasia and calcification in the renal pelvis. Aspirin was noted to increase the incidence and severity of renal papillary necrosis and vascular changes. [The Working Group noted the short period of administration of sodium saccharin.]

Groups of weanling male Fischer rats were treated for five-week pretreatment periods as follows: groups 1–4 (42 rats per group) were fed untreated diet and untreated water; groups 5–8 (42 rats per group) were given 0.2% FANFT in the diet with untreated drinking-water; and groups 9–12 (43, 41, 42 and 42 rats per group) were given untreated diet with 0.005% *N*-nitrosodibutylamine (NDBA) in the drinking-water. For the remaining 95 weeks of the experiment, the rats were all given untreated drinking-water and fed diets containing either no additional chemical (groups 1, 5 and 9), 0.05% phenobarbital (groups 2, 6, and 10), 0.15% phenobarbital (groups 3, 7 and 11) or 5% sodium saccharin (groups 4, 8 and 12). Body-weight gain was decreased by ≥ 10% in groups 3, 4, 5, 6, 7, 11 and 12 relative to their respective controls. There was slightly decreased survival in rats given phenobarbital, but survival was not affected by treatment with FANFT, NDBA or sodium saccharin. The incidences of bladder carcinoma were 0, 0, 0, 0, 8/40 (20%), 15/40 (38%), 19/39 (49%), 15/39 (38%), 5/43 (12%), 2/37 (5%), 9/40 (23%) and 27/40 (18%) for the 12 respective groups. The only group that showed a statistically significant increase in the incidence of bladder carcinomas relative to the respective controls was the group given FANFT followed by 0.15% phenobarbital. Benign papillomas were seen in 0, 0, 0, 0, 10, 10, 6, 3, 2, 2, 2 and 4 rats in the 12 respective groups; again, the only group that showed a significantly increased incidence of papillomas plus carcinomas when compared with the respective controls was group 7. Hepatocellular carcinomas were found in 0, 0, 0, 0, 0, 0, 2.5%, 2.6%, 0, 7%, 27%, 43% and 2.5%, respectively, and oesophageal squamous-cell carcinomas were observed in no animals in groups 1–8 and in 46, 32, 45 and 45% of the rats in groups 9–12, respectively (Imaida & Wang, 1986).

In a later report (Masui *et al.*, 1990), all rats given 5 or 7.5% sodium saccharin in the diet were reported to have squamous-cell hyperplasia and hyperkeratosis at the limiting ridge of the forestomach. Further experiments indicated that administration of saccharin in various diets (AIN-76, Prolab, Purina and NIH-07), either as the acid or the sodium or calcium salt, nearly always produced squamous-cell hyperplasia at the limiting ridge but without progression to papilloma or carcinoma in both Fischer 344 and Sprague-Dawley rats. Control diets, in particular AIN-76 diet, also caused some hyperplasia of the limiting ridge.

Groups of 30 male Fischer 344 rats, five weeks of age, were treated as follows: 0.2% FANFT in pelleted AIN-76A diet (prepared on site) was fed for four weeks followed by an interval of one week of control diet, followed by 5% sodium saccharin in AIN-76A diet up to 104 weeks; 0.2% in AIN-76A diet for four weeks followed by AIN-76A diet up to 104 weeks; group 3 (only 25 rats), AIN-76A control diet for five weeks followed by 5% sodium saccharin in AIN-76A diet up to 104 weeks; group 4, 0.2% FANFT in Prolab 3200 diet for four weeks followed by one week of control Prolab diet followed by 5% sodium saccharin in Prolab diet up to 104 weeks; group 5, 0.2% FANFT in Prolab diet for four weeks followed by control Prolab diet up to 104 weeks; group 6, 0.2% FANFT in AIN-76A diet for four weeks followed by one week of Prolab control diet followed by 5% sodium saccharin in Prolab diet up to 104 weeks; group 7, 0.2% FANFT in AIN-76A diet for four weeks followed by Prolab control diet up to 104 weeks; group 8, AIN-76A control diet for four weeks followed by one week of Prolab control diet followed by 5% sodium saccharin in Prolab diet up to 104 weeks; group 9, 0.2% FANFT in AIN-76A diet for two weeks followed by one week of control Prolab diet followed by 5% sodium saccharin in Prolab diet up to 104 weeks; group 10, 0.2% FANFT in AIN-76A diet for one week followed by one week of control Prolab diet followed by 5% sodium saccharin in Prolab diet up to 104 weeks; group 11, 0.2% FANFT in AIN-76A diet for two weeks followed by one week of control Prolab diet followed by control Prolab diet up to 104 weeks; group 12, 0.1% FANFT in AIN-76A diet for two weeks followed by one week of Prolab control diet followed by 5% sodium saccharin in Prolab diet up to 104 weeks; group 13, 0.1% FANFT in AIN-76A diet for one week followed by one week of control Prolab diet followed by 5% sodium saccharin in Prolab diet up to 104 weeks; and group 14, 0.1% FANFT in AIN-76A diet for two weeks followed by control Prolab diet up to 104 weeks. The number of rats alive after 50 weeks of the experiment, when the first bladder tumour was detected, was considered to be the effective number of rats. A significant decrease in body weight and a significant effect on survival were seen only in group 3. Transitional-cell carcinomas of the urinary bladder were observed in 2/27 (7.4%), 5/30 (17%), 0/22, 9/30 (30%), 3/30 (10%), 9/30 (30%), 3/29 (10%), 1/30 (3.3%), 0/30, 0/29, 0/30, 2/30 (6.7%), 0 and 1/29 (3.5%) rats, respectively. In addition, papillomas were observed in 1, 2, 0, 3, 2, 1, 0, 1, 0, 0, 1, 0, 0 and 1 rats, respectively. The authors concluded that sodium saccharin promotes bladder cancer when administered to male rats in Prolab diet but not when administered in AIN-76A diet (Okamura *et al.*, 1991). [The Working Group noted the absence of a group administered AIN-76A diet only throughout the experiment. They also noted the lack of bladder tumours in rats given sodium saccharin in AIN-76A diet (group 3), whereas two rats given sodium saccharin in Prolab diet (group 8) had one papilloma and one carcinoma of the bladder.]

Groups of 40 male Fischer 344 rats, six weeks of age, were treated in two phases, the first phase lasting six weeks and the second phase the subsequent 72 weeks. Chemicals were administered in Prolab 3200 diet in groups 1–18 and in NIH-07 diet in groups 19–20. Groups 1–14, 19 and 20 were treated with 0.2% FANFT in the diet and groups 15–18 with control diet in the first phase. The dietary treatments in the second phase were as follows: group 1, 5% sodium saccharin; group 2, 3% sodium saccharin; group 3, 5.2% calcium saccharin; group 4, 3.12% calcium saccharin; group 5, 4.21% saccharin; group 6, 2.53% saccharin; group 7, 5% sodium ascorbate; group 8, 4.4% ascorbic acid; group

9, 5% sodium saccharin plus 1.15% calcium carbonate; group 10, 5.2% calcium saccharin plus 1.34% sodium chloride; group 11, 5% sodium saccharin plus 1.23% ammonium chloride; group 12, 1.15% calcium carbonate; group 13, 1.34% sodium chloride; group 14, control diet; group 15, 5% sodium saccharin; group 16, 5.2% calcium saccharin; group 17, 4.21% acid saccharin; group 18, control diet (untreated controls); group 19, 5% sodium saccharin; and group 20, control diet. The experiment was terminated at the end of 78 weeks. The effective number of rats in each group was considered to be 40, but there were 39 in groups 1, 14, 16 and 18. In comparison with the untreated controls (group 18), all groups except groups 12, 14 and 20 showed decreased body-weight gain. The numbers of rats with urothelial bladder carcinomas were 38, 29, 21, 20, 19, 13, 30, 16, 37, 34, 11, 16, 27, 12, 1, 0, 0, 2, 38 and 21, respectively. The numbers of rats with carcinomas plus papillomas in the various groups were 39, 34, 27, 22, 24, 19, 32, 21, 38, 37, 16, 21, 32, 17, 1, 0, 0, 2, 38 and 26, respectively. Statistically significant enhancement of the incidence of bladder cancer was seen with sodium saccharin, calcium saccharin, sodium ascorbate, sodium saccharin plus calcium carbonate, calcium saccharin plus sodium chloride and sodium chloride. Sodium saccharin enhanced the bladder tumour incidence when given in either the Prolab or the NIH-07 diet. The authors noted that the increased urinary pH resulting from the administration of 0.2% FANFT in the diet remained after FANFT treatment was discontinued. Sodium saccharin, calcium saccharin and acid saccharin by themselves did not significantly increase the incidence of bladder tumours or other lesions, except for simple hyperplasia in the group given sodium saccharin (Cohen *et al.*, 1991a). [The Working Group noted the limited period of administration of the test compound for evaluating single-generation carcinogenic effects.]

3.4.5 *Combinations of* N-*[4-(5-nitro-2-furyl)-2-thiazolyl]formamide, cyclophosphamide, freeze-ulceration and sodium saccharin*

Male Fischer 344 rats, five weeks of age, were treated as follows: group 1 (23 rats), freeze-ulceration of the urinary bladder on day 0, followed immediately by administration of 0.2% FANFT in powdered diet for two weeks and then 5% sodium saccharin for 102 weeks; group 2 (23 rats), freeze-ulceration of the urinary bladder on day 0, followed immediately by 0.2% FANFT in powdered diet for two weeks and then control diet for 102 weeks; group 3 (23 rats), freeze-ulceration of the urinary bladder on day 0, two weeks of control diet and then 5% sodium saccharin in the diet for 102 weeks; group 4 (23 rats), freeze-ulceration on day 0 followed by 104 weeks of control diet; group 5 (21 rats), 0.2% FANFT in powdered diet for two weeks followed by 102 weeks of 5% sodium saccharin in the diet; group 6 (22 rats), 0.2% FANFT in powdered diet for two weeks followed by control diet for 102 weeks; group 7 (21 rats), control diet for two weeks followed by 5% sodium saccharin in the diet for 102 weeks; group 8 (23 rats), 0.2% FANFT in powdered diet for two weeks followed immediately by freeze-ulceration of the urinary bladder and 5% sodium saccharin in the diet for 102 weeks; group 9 (23 rats), 0.2% FANFT in the diet for two weeks followed by freeze-ulceration of the urinary bladder and control diet for 102 weeks; group 10 (23 rats), freeze-ulceration on day 0 followed by 104 weeks of 5% sodium saccharin in the diet; group 11 (26 rats), intraperitoneal injection of 100 mg/kg bw cyclophosphamide in distilled water on day 0 followed immediately by 0.2% FANFT in the diet for two weeks and then 102 weeks of 5% sodium saccharin in the diet; group 12 (26 rats), intraperitoneal injection of 100 mg/kg bw cyclophosphamide followed immediately by 0.2% FANFT in the diet for two weeks and then control diet for 102 weeks; group 13 (25 rats), intraperitoneal injection of 100 mg/kg bw cyclophosphamide followed by two weeks of control diet and then 5% sodium saccharin for 102 weeks; group 14 (26 rats), intraperitoneal injection of 100 mg/kg bw cyclophosphamide followed immediately by 104 weeks of control diet; group 15 (25 rats), intraperitoneal injection of 100 mg/kg bw cyclophosphamide followed immediately by 104 weeks of 5% sodium saccharin; group 16 (37 rats), 104 weeks of control diet (untreated control group); group 17 (21 rats), 5% sodium saccharin for 104 weeks. The experiment was terminated after 104 weeks. The survival rates of groups 12, 14 and 15 were significantly decreased, with 19, 16, 16, 20, 18, 16, 16, 19, 16, 16, 17, 0, 14, 4, 9, 28 and 14 rats alive at the end of the experiment in the various groups, respectively. The effective number of rats was considered to be the number alive after 76 weeks of the experiment, when the first bladder tumour was detected. The incidences of bladder carcinomas were 4/23 (17%), 0/22, 5/20 (25%), 0/23, 1/21 (5%), 0/19, 0/17, 8/22 (36%), 2/21 (10%), 2/21 (10%), 4/22 (18%), 0/9, 3/17 (18%), 0/7, 3/17 (18%), 0/32 and 0/20, respectively. The numbers of rats with urinary bladder papillomas were 1, 1, 2, 3, 2, 1 and 3, in groups 3, 8, 10, 11, 13, 14 and 15, respectively. Sodium saccharin enhanced the incidence of bladder tumours when administered after FANFT, cyclophosphamide or freeze-ulceration, but sodium saccharin alone administered at a concentration of 5% in the diet to rats for 102 or 104 weeks did not produce benign or malignant tumours of the urinary bladder (Cohen *et al.*, 1982).

3.4.6 N-*Nitrosobutyl*-N-*(4-hydroxybutyl)amine or* N-*nitrosodibutylamine*

Groups of 29–32 male and 29–32 female Fischer 344 rats, six weeks of age, were treated with 0.01% *N*-nitrosobutyl-*N*-4-(hydroxybutyl)amine (NBHBA) in the drinking-water for four weeks (groups 1–5) or received no treatment (groups 6–10), followed by 32 weeks of sodium saccharin in the diet (purity, > 99.5%, containing 7 ppm *ortho*-toluenesulfonamide) at concentrations of 5% (groups 1 and 6), 1% (groups 2 and 7), 0.2% (groups 3 and 8) or 0.04% (groups 4 and 9) or untreated diet (groups 5 and 10), respectively. All rats were killed at the end of 36 weeks. No bladder lesions were seen in the groups without pretreatment with NBHBA. In males, the incidences of papillomas were 6, 10, 8, 11 and 8, respectively, for groups 1–5. The incidences of papillary or nodular hyperplasia were 24, 19, 14, 12 and 11, respectively, which was significant ($p < 0.001$) only at the 5% dose when compared with NBHBA only. The number of hyperplastic lesions per 10 cm of basement membrane was also significantly increased at the 5% dose. Papillomas were seen in two females in group 2 and one in each of groups 1 and 3–5. The incidences of papillary or nodular hyperplasia were 23, 17, 14, 11 and 9 in groups 1–5, respectively; the increases were statistically significant only at 1 and 5%. The authors concluded that sodium saccharin caused dose-related promotion in both males and females, only for hyperplastic lesions and not for bladder papillomas (Nakanishi *et al.*, 1980a). [The Working Group noted the lack of effect on bladder tumours as an end-point.]

Male Wistar rats, eight weeks of age, were treated with 0.01% NBHBA in the drinking-water (groups 1–4) or with untreated drinking-water (groups 5–8) for four weeks and then received the following treatments for 32 weeks: 5% sodium saccharin (purity, > 99.5% with 7 ppm *ortho*-toluenesulfonamide) in the diet (groups 1 and 5); 0.1% caffeine in the drinking-water (groups 2 and 6); 5% sodium saccharin in the diet plus 0.1% caffeine in the drinking-water (groups 3 and 7); or untreated drinking-water and diet (groups 4 and 8). The authors stated that the water consumption was increased by approximately 50% in the groups treated with sodium saccharin when compared with other groups. No difference in growth or survival in the various groups was described. Rats that were not pretreated with NBHBA had no bladder tumours, but 5/26 rats treated with sodium saccharin (group 5) and 7/23 given sodium saccharin plus caffeine (group 7) had papillary or nodular hyperplasia compared with 0/12 in group 8. In group 1, 1/31 rats had a bladder carcinoma; and the incidences of bladder papillomas in groups 1–4 were 9/31 (29%), 6/28 (21%), 4/30 (13%) and 3/23 (13%), respectively; these were not statistically significantly different from each other. There were significant increases in the incidences and numbers of papillary/nodular hyperplasia in groups 1 and 3 compared with group 4. In a second experiment with 0.001% NBHBA, combinations of NBHBA, sodium saccharin and caffeine were administered simultaneously, with NBHBA and caffeine in the drinking-water and sodium saccharin in the diet. The treatments were as follows: group 1, NBHBA plus sodium saccharin plus caffeine; group 2, NBHBA plus sodium saccharin; group 3, NBHBA plus caffeine; group 4, NBHBA; group 5, sodium saccharin plus caffeine; group 6, sodium saccharin; group 7, caffeine; and group 8, no added chemical (untreated controls). The incidences of bladder papillomas were 9/32 (28%) and 10/24 (42%) in groups 1 and 2, respectively, compared with 0/22 in BBN controls, and the incidences of bladder carcinoma were 1/32 (3.1%), 2/24 (8.3%) and 0/22, respectively. No bladder tumours were induced in the other groups (Nakanishi *et al.*, 1980b). [The Working Group noted that the increased water consumption associated with sodium saccharin in the diet resulted in increased exposure of groups 1 and 2 to NBHBA, and this might have accounted for the increased incidences of tumours and other bladder proliferative lesions in these groups.]

Groups of 30 male Fischer 344 rats, six weeks of age, were treated with 0.01% NBHBA in the drinking-water for four weeks followed by either 5% sodium saccharin or 0.5% sodium saccharin in the diet for 34 weeks; a further group received NBHBA followed by basal diet, and additional groups received the same treatments after four weeks of untreated drinking-water. The body-weight gain of rats treated with 5% sodium saccharin with or without NBHBA was slightly decreased, but there was no apparent effect on survival. No bladder lesions were seen in rats that were not pretreated with

NBHBA. The incidences of bladder papillomas were 20% with NBHBA plus 5% sodium saccharin, 33% with NBHBA plus 0.5% sodium saccharin and 33% with NBHBA alone, and the incidences of papillary or nodular hyperplasia were 83%, 47% and 45%, respectively (Fukushima *et al.*, 1983b). [The Working Group noted the lack of effect on bladder tumour incidence and the relatively short duration of the experiment.]

Male Fischer 344 rats, six weeks old, were treated in two phases, the first phase consisting of administration of drinking-water with or without NBHBA for four weeks, followed by treatment with 5% sodium saccharin in the diet or untreated control diet for 32 weeks. The first group received 0.05% NBHBA followed by 5% sodium saccharin; group 2 received 0.05% NBHBA followed by untreated control diet; group 3 received 0.01% NBHBA followed by 5% sodium saccharin in the diet; group 4 received 0.01% NBHBA in the drinking-water followed by untreated control diet; and group 5 received untreated water followed by 5% sodium saccharin in the diet. No bladder tumours were observed in groups 3–5. Twenty of 25 rats in group 1 (80%) and 1/26 (3.8%) rats in group 2 developed bladder carcinomas. The number of papillary or nodular hyperplasias was increased in the group given 5% sodium saccharin after 0.05% NBHBA over that with the same dose of NBHBA alone (100% versus 46%); there were also significant increases in the incidences and numbers of hyperplasias in the rats pretreated with 0.01% NBHBA followed by sodium saccharin (83% versus 39%) (Ito *et al.*, 1983). [The Working Group noted the limited details reported for this experiment.]

Male Fischer 344 rats were treated as follows: group 1, 0.02% AAF in the diet for four weeks followed by 0.05% phenobarbital in the diet for 32 weeks; group 2, AAF followed by 5% sodium saccharin in the diet; group 3, AAF followed by untreated control diet; group 4, 0.01% NBHBA in the drinking-water for four weeks followed by 32 weeks of phenobarbital; group 5, NBHBA followed by 5% sodium saccharin; group 6, NBHBA followed by control diet; group 7, untreated water and diet followed by phenobarbital; group 8, untreated water and diet followed by 5% sodium saccharin in the diet; and group 9, untreated controls. No bladder papillomas were seen in groups 1–3 or 7–9. The incidences of bladder papillomas in groups 4–6 were similar: 9/30 (30%), 6/29 (21%) and 8/28 (29%), respectively. The incidences of papillary or nodular hyperplasia were 14 (47%), 24 (83%) and 11 (39%), respectively, in these groups; additionally, 4/29 (14%) rats in group 2 had papillary or nodular hyperplasia. Liver hyperplastic nodules were observed in 24/24, 27/29, 27/28 and 8/30 rats, respectively, in groups 1–4, with no hyperplastic nodules in groups 5–9. Five rats in group 1 had hepatocellular carcinoma, whereas none were seen in other groups. The authors concluded that phenobarbital enhances liver hyperplasia and sodium saccharin enhances bladder hyperplasia (Ito *et al.*, 1983). [The Working Group noted the lack of effect on bladder tumour incidences and the limited description of the details of this experiment.]

Male Fischer 344 rats, seven to eight weeks of age, received untreated water and control diet (group 1), control diet and 0.02% NDBA in the drinking-water (group 2), 5% sodium saccharin in the diet and untreated drinking-water (group 3) or 5% sodium saccharin in the diet and 0.02% NDBA in the drinking-water (group 4) for a total of 26 weeks with interim sacrifices at four and eight weeks. The end-points of the study were effects on γ-glutamyl transferase-positive foci, hyperplastic nodules and hepatocellular carcinomas in the liver. The number of foci at 26 weeks were 0.31 ± 0.31 (10 rats), 5.03 ± 1.06 (29 rats), 0.23 ± 0.23 (36 rats) and 31.3 ± 4.65 (21 rats), respectively. Similar trends were seen at four and eight weeks. The incidences of hyperplastic nodules were 0/11, 5/29 (17%), 0/36 and 17/21 (81%), respectively, and those of carcinomas were 0, 1 (3%), 0 and 17 (81%), respectively. A major confounding factor in the interpretation of these data is the marked increase in water consumption of rats given sodium saccharin. In group 4, this would have led to a marked increase in the consumption of NDBA, which was administered in the drinking-water, in comparison with group 2; however, the water consumption of these animals was not determined (Pereira *et al.*, 1983). [The Working Group noted the confounding issue of water consumption and therefore the dose of NDBA, suggesting that the effect on liver lesions might have been due to increased NDBA consumption rather than a direct effect of sodium saccharin.]

Groups of 25 male Fischer 344 rats, six weeks of age, were treated for four weeks with 0.01% NBHBA in the drinking-water followed by 32 weeks of 5% sodium saccharin in the diet or control diet for 32 weeks. A third group received no treatment for the first four weeks of the experiment followed by 32 weeks of 5% sodium saccharin in the diet. Rats treated with 5% sodium saccharin had a slight decrease in body-weight gain, but their survival was not affected. Papillomas were seen in five and six rats in groups 1 and 2, respectively, and none in group 3. The incidences of papillary or nodular hyperplasia were 23, 9 and 0 in groups 1–3, respectively (Hagiwara *et al.*, 1984). [The Working Group noted the lack of effect on bladder tumours but the increased incidence of nodular or papillary hyperplasia.]

Male Fischer 344 rats, six weeks old, were treated as follows: groups 1–4 were treated with 0.01% NBHBA in the drinking-water for four weeks; group 5 received no treatment during this period. Group 1 then received consecutive 10-week courses of 5% sodium saccharin, 2% DL-tryptophan and 5% sodium ascorbate in the diet, followed by two weeks of control diet; group 2 received consecutive 10-week courses of sodium saccharin and DL-tryptophan followed by basal diet; group 3 received one 10-week course of sodium saccharin followed by basal diet; and group 5 received consecutive 10-week courses of sodium saccharin, DL-tryptophan and sodium ascorbate followed by basal diet. All rats were killed at the end of 36 weeks. There was an increased incidence of bladder carcinomas, papillomas and papillary or nodular hyperplasia in group 1 but not in the other groups. No bladder lesions were seen in group 5. The incidences of carcinoma were 7/25 (28%), 2/24 (8.3%), 2/25 (8%), 0 and 0, respectively (Sakata *et al.*, 1984). [The Working Group noted the short period of administration of each chemical and the short duration of the experiment.]

Male Fischer 344 rats, six weeks of age, were pretreated with 0.05% NBHBA in the drinking-water for four weeks and then treated with chemicals in the diet for 32 weeks: group 1, untreated controls; group 2, 5% sodium saccharin in the diet; group 3, 5% sodium ascorbate in the diet; group 4, sodium saccharin plus sodium ascorbate in the diet; group 5, 5% ascorbic acid in the diet; and group 6, sodium saccharin plus ascorbic acid in the diet. All animals were killed at the end of 36 weeks. There was significant (> 10%) reduction in body-weight gain in all treated animals compared with controls. This was particularly marked in groups 4 and 6 in which the body-weight gain was decreased by approximately 20%. The incidences of bladder carcinomas were 0/15, 5/15 (33%), 11/16 (69%), 13/13 (100%), 2/16 (12%) and 1/16 (6.3%), respectively. The authors concluded that there was significant synergy between sodium saccharin and sodium ascorbate and that the significant inhibition seen with ascorbic acid might have been related to the decreased urinary pH (Fukushima *et al.*, 1990). [The Working Group noted the short period of administration and the small number of animals in each group.]

Male Fischer 344 rats, six weeks of age, were treated in two phases. The first phase lasted four weeks and consisted of treatment with either control drinking water (groups 1–4) or drinking-water containing 0.05% NBHBA (groups 5–8). The second phase consisted of 36 weeks of treatment with either control diet (groups 1 and 5), 5% sodium saccharin in the diet (groups 2 and 6), 5% sodium saccharin plus 0.1% nordihydroguaiaretic acid in the diet (groups 3 and 7) or 0.1% nordihydroguaiaretic acid in the diet (groups 4 and 8). The groups fed sodium saccharin plus nordihydroguaiaretic acid had significant growth retardation, but survival was not affected. No bladder hyperplastic lesions or tumours were seen in groups 1–4 (11 rats per group), which were not pretreated with NBHBA. In groups 5–8, the incidences of bladder carcinoma were 1/20 (5%), 2/23 (8.7%), 1/22 (4.5%) and 4/20 (20%), respectively; the incidences of papillomas were 2, 5, 0 and 3, respectively; and the incidences of papillary or nodular hyperplasia were 6, 19, 12 and 7, respectively. The authors concluded that nordihydroguaiaretic acid had anti-tumour promoting activity (Yu *et al.*, 1992). [The Working Group noted the inadequate number of animals, the short duration of the experiment and the lack of effect based on incidences of carcinoma.]

3.4.7 *Urethane*

In a bioassay to screen for lung adenomas, groups of 25 male A/St mice, eight weeks of age, were treated with one of four commercial saccharin preparations (Sweeta tablets, pharmaceutical powder, Sweet 10 liquid or Sweet-n-Low powder). The saccharin preparations were made up freshly each week in distilled water and administered at a dose of 1 g/kg bw daily by gavage on five days a week for a total of 17 weeks. Three groups of controls received distilled water. In the first series, no treatment other than saccharin or water was administered. In a second series, the mice also received an intraperitoneal injection of 0.1 mg/g bw urethane in 0.9% saline; the third group also received an intraperitoneal injection of 1 mg/g bw urethane. The urethane injections were given one week after initiation of saccharin administration. The incidences and numbers of adenomas per lung were determined; a few lungs from each group of mice were examined microscopically to confirm that the adenomas were being counted. The animals generally survived the treatment well, most of the deaths being due to trauma induced by gavage. The animals exposed to saccharin preparations gained somewhat less weight than the control animals during the course of this experiment, but their weight gain was substantial. The commercial saccharin preparations did not elicit a significant lung tumour response when given alone, with respect to either the incidence or number of lung tumours per mouse. At the low dose of urethane, the only sweetener that produced a lung tumour response greater than that in animals treated with urethane alone was Sweet-n-Low, which produced an approximately twofold increase in the number of lung tumours, although the incidence (47%) was the same as in the control group (52%) and was not statistically significant. At the high dose of urethane, all of the saccharin preparations significantly increased the number of lung tumours per mouse over that in animals treated with urethane alone: 2.13 ± 0.44, 4.36 ± 0.70, 5.95 ± 1.29, 6.08 ± 1.29 and 9.86 ± 3.65 in mice treated with 1 mg/g urethane plus either distilled water, Sweeta tablets, pharmaceutical powder, Sweet 10 liquid or Sweet-n-Low powder, respectively. The tumour incidences, however, were nearly the same and were not statistically different between the groups (Theiss *et al.*, 1980). [The Working Group noted the complex nature of the protocol, the lack of effect at the low dose of urethane and the lack of effect on incidence at the high dose of urethane and that there was no effect when the sweetener preparations were used without administration of urethane.]

3.4.8 N-*Methyl*-N′-*nitro*-N-*nitrosoguanidine*

Groups of 20 treated and 40 control male Wistar rats, seven weeks of age, were given 10 mg/L *N*-methyl-*N*′-nitro-*N*-nitrosoguanidine (MNNG) in the drinking-water and 10% sodium chloride in the diet for eight weeks (groups 1–5); groups 6–10 received neither MNNG nor sodium chloride during the first eight weeks. After these treatments, the rats in groups 1 and 6 were continued as the respective control groups without any further dietary supplementation for the remaining 32 weeks of the experiment (total experimental period of 40 weeks), animals in groups 2 and 7 were fed 10% sodium chloride in the diet, animals in groups 3 and 8 were fed 5% saccharin [form not specified] in the diet, groups 4 and 9 were fed 0.05% phenobarbital in the diet, and groups 5 and 10 received 1% aspirin in the diet. The growth of the animals was significantly retarded by the administration of MNNG plus sodium chloride; these animals showed a compensatory increase in growth rates once the treatments ended, although their weights at the end of the experiment were still lower than those in the groups not treated with MNNG. During the second phase of the experiment, the growth was similar, except for rats receiving the aspirin-supplemented diet, which showed a marked retardation of growth compared with the other groups. No gastric or duodenal tumours occurred in the rats that were not pretreated with MNNG plus sodium chloride. The incidences of gastric adenocarcinomas were 3/39 (7.7%), 4/20 (20%), 3/20 (15%), 1/19 (5.3%) and 0/20, respectively, for groups 1–5, and 3, 3, 1, 1 and 1 rats had duodenal adenocarcinomas, respectively. Only sodium chloride produced a significantly increased incidence in the total number of rats bearing tumours, including those of the stomach plus duodenum. In saccharin-treated rats, diffuse alterations in the fundic mucosa were observed, in which the thickness of the zone of proliferating cells was increased (Takahashi *et al.*, 1984).

3.4.9 *Betel nut*

Male and female C17 mice, 10–12 weeks of age, were either untreated (22 females and 12 males), received a diet containing 10% of a commercial preparation of saccharin-coated betel nut [no information on form or amount of saccharin] (18 females and 14 males), received 0.2 mL of a 0.1% solution of 1, 4-dinitrosopiperazine by oral intubation (14 females and 15 males) or received saccharin-coated betel nut powder in the diet plus 1,4-dinitrosopiperazine by gavage (12 females and 12 males). The mice were treated for 40 weeks and then allowed to live a normal life span on standard diet. There was no significant difference in mortality rate between the groups [overall survival was not indicated]. The incidences of squamous-cell carcinoma of the stomach were 0, 2, 7 and 6 in males and 0, 0, 4 and 3 in females. Reticular-cell neoplasms-type A of the uterus occurred in 2, 3, 5 and 3 female mice in groups 1–4, respectively (Pai *et al.*, 1981). [The Working Group noted the inadequate numbers of animals, the incomplete reporting of the experiment, the lack of information on exposure to saccharin, the lack of a group given saccharin only and the lack of information about the form of saccharin administered.]

3.4.10 *Freeze-ulceration*

Eight groups of 40 male Fischer rats, five weeks of age, were treated as follows: group 1, freeze-ulceration of the urinary bladder followed immediately by 5% sodium saccharin in powdered diet for 104 weeks; group 2, freeze-ulceration of the urinary bladder followed by two weeks of control diet and then 102 weeks of 5% sodium saccharin in the diet; group 3, freeze-ulceration of the urinary bladder followed by four weeks of control diet and then 100 weeks of 5% sodium saccharin in the diet; group 4, freeze-ulceration of the urinary bladder followed by six weeks of control diet and then 98 weeks of 5% sodium saccharin in the diet; group 5, freeze-ulceration of the urinary bladder followed by 18 weeks of control diet and then 86 weeks of 5% sodium saccharin in the diet; group 6, 104 weeks of 5% sodium saccharin in the diet; group 7, freeze-ulceration of the urinary bladder followed by 104 weeks of control diet; and group 8, 104 weeks of control diet (untreated control group). None of the treatments had a significant effect on survival or on body weight. The experiment was terminated after 104 weeks. The incidences of urothelial carcinomas were 11/36, 6/36, 12/40, 7/36, 9/39, 0/39, 1/39 and 0/39 in the eight groups, respectively. In addition, papillomas were found in two rats in group 2 and one rat in group 6. There were no significant differences in the incidences of bladder tumours between groups 1–5. Only one benign papilloma developed in the urinary bladder of rats fed 5% sodium saccharin alone throughout the experiment (group 6) (Hasegawa *et al.*, 1985).

Saccharin/cyclamate mixtures

Oral administration

Single-generation exposure

Rat: Two groups of 52 male and 52 female Sprague-Dawley rats aged 70–90 days, were given a 10:1 mixture of sodium cyclamate:sodium saccharin at a concentration of 2 or 5%

in the diet for up to 30 months. The cyclamate in the mixture contained less than 4 mg/kg cyclohexylamine, but no information on the purity of the saccharin was given. An untreated group of 52 male and 52 female rats served as controls. At 24 months, approximately 10% of the initial number of animals were still alive. The occurrence of bladder parasites (*Strongyloides capillaria*) was noted in 16% of animals. No bladder tumour was found. A similar frequency of benign neoplasms was seen in all groups, consisting of fibromas, fibroadenomas or adenomas of the mammary gland in females and thymomas in males (Schmähl, 1973).

In a study reported in an abstract, two groups of 54–56 Wistar rats [age unspecified] received 0 or 2.5 g/kg bw per day of a mixture of sodium cyclamate:sodium saccharin (10:1) [source and purity unspecified] in the diet for 28 months. Ten to 16 rats of each group were killed at 12 months, 11 at 24 months and all survivors at 28 months. No treated or control animals developed tumours of the urinary bladder (Furuya *et al.*, 1975). [The Working Group noted the incomplete reporting of the experiment.]

Groups of 35 male and 45 female weanling FDRL strain Wistar-derived rats were fed a 10:1 mixture of sodium cyclamate:saccharin [purity and method of manufacture unspecified] in the diet at concentrations providing doses of 0, 500, 1100 or 2500 mg/kg bw per day for two years. From week 79, the original groups were split, and 50% of the survivors in each group, except the untreated controls, received cyclohexylamine hydrochloride in the diet: at 25 mg/kg bw for the group receiving 500 mg/kg bw per day of the mixture, at 56 mg/kg bw for the group receiving 1100 mg/kg bw per day of the mixture and at 125 mg/kg bw for those receiving 2500 mg/kg bw per day of the mixture. The mortality rates were similar in control and test groups. Treatment-related pathological changes were seen only in the kidney and bladder. Pelvic hyperplasia was observed more often in the treated groups (8/80, 21/80 and 16/80, as compared with 3/80 in controls). Among animals surviving more than 49 weeks, 9/25 male and 3/35 female rats at 2500 mg/kg bw per day and 0/35 male and 0/45 female controls developed transitional-cell carcinomas of the urinary bladder. Of the treated rats with this tumour, three male and two female rats had received cyclohexylamine. Two of the bladder carcinoma-bearing animals had calculi, and 18 rats at 2500 mg/kg bw per day had non-malignant proliferative bladder lesions. Non-malignant proliferative lesions were found at the lower doses, but their incidence was not significantly higher than that in controls. Renal calcification was seen in 7/12 rats with bladder carcinomas; *Trichosomoides crassicauda* infection was present in one rat with bladder cancer and in four rats with non-neoplastic proliferative lesions at the highest dose, in four given 1120 mg/kg bw per day, in two given 500 mg/kg bw per day and in five control animals (Price *et al.*, 1970; Oser *et al.*, 1975).

Multigeneration exposure

Mouse: In a multigeneration study, a 10:1 mixture of sodium cyclamate:saccharin was fed at concentrations of 5 and 0.5% or 2 and 0.2%, respectively, in the diet continuously to Swiss mice over six generations. The saccharin contained 0.5% *ortho*-toluenesulfonamide; the cyclamate contained 2.1 mg/kg (ppm) cyclohexylamine. F_0 (parental), F_{3b} and F_{6a}

generations, consisting of 50 males and 50 females each, were used for the studies of carcinogenicity and were treated for 84 weeks. Pathological alterations and urinary bladder calculi occurred with similar frequencies in control and treated groups. Four neoplasms of the urinary bladder occurred: three anaplastic carcinomas (one in a female control of the F_0 generation and two in females of the F_0 and F_{6a} generations fed 2% cyclamate plus 0.2% saccharin) and one papilloma (in a male of the F_{6a} generation given 2% cyclamate plus 0.2% saccharin). The mean latent period was more than 80 weeks (Kroes *et al.*, 1977).

Rat: Four groups of 10 male and 20 female Sprague-Dawley rats were treated either with a cyclamate:saccharin (ratio 10:1) mixture at a total concentration of 5% or 2% of the diet, with a diet containing 20% sugar or with untreated diet for three months prior to mating. The F_0 females were continued on these diets throughout weaning of their offspring. Groups of 33–39 male and 34–39 female offspring (F_1 generation) were maintained on the respective diets for lifetime. Their body weights after one year were reduced when compared with controls. The average survival was 532, 480, 323 and 379 days for males and 530, 683, 450 and 464 days for females given 5% and 2% of the mixture or sugar and the control groups, respectively. A single bladder tumour (a papilloma) was found in one female rat given the 2% cyclamate:saccharin mixture, at 308 days of age. No other tumours of the urinary tract were noted, and there were no increased incidence of tumours at other sites. Calculi were observed in the bladder of two of the animals receiving the 5% mixture [sex not specified] and in the renal pelvis of eight of the rats at the high dose [sex not specified]. One rat [sex not specified] at 2% had a kidney stone, but no stones were seen in the sugar-treated animals or in the controls (Schmähl & Habs, 1984). [The Working Group noted the incomplete reporting of the experiment.]

***ortho*-Toluenesulfonamide**

Oral administration

Rat: In a two-generation study, groups of Charles River CD rats, 30 days of age, were fed daily doses of 0 (control), 2.5, 25 or 250 mg/kg bw *ortho*-toluenesulfonamide (purity, > 99.9%) or 250 mg/kg bw *ortho*-toluenesulfonamide plus 1% ammonium chloride in the drinking-water. Each group consisted of 50 males and 50 females, except for the group receiving ammonium chloride in the drinking-water, which comprised 40 males and 38 females. The F_0 animals were started on test at 32 days of age. After three months on test, the animals were mated on a one-to-one basis; all litters were culled randomly to eight pups (four males and four females) four days *post partum*. The pups were weaned onto their parents' diet, and 50 males and 50 females were selected randomly from each group to constitute the second generation (F_1). The two generations remained on test for 30 (F_1) and 32 (F_0) months. The animals were free of bladder parasites. Rats of both generations given 250 mg/kg bw *ortho*-toluenesulfonamide with or without ammonium chloride had lowered feed consumption. There were no treatment-related effects on longevity. The numbers of bladder tumours (all of which were benign) were: in F_0 males, one in a control and one each at 2.5 and 250 mg/kg bw *ortho*-toluenesulfonamide; F_0 females, one at 2.5 mg/kg bw; in F_1 females, two at 2.5 mg/kg bw (Arnold *et al.*, 1980).

Groups of 38 male and 38 female Sprague-Dawley rats, three months of age, were given daily doses of 0, 20 or 200 mg/kg bw *ortho*-toluenesulfonamide [source and purity unspecified] for life by adjusting the concentrations added to the diet. The average survival rates were 700 days for controls, 770 days at the low dose and 840 days at the high dose. The total incidences of malignant tumours were not different in treated groups compared with controls. Lymphosarcomas developed in 7/71 controls, 10/75 at the low dose and 10/76 at the high dose. In addition, 3/76 leukoses occurred at the high dose and 5/75 at the low dose, compared with 0/71 in controls. In rats at the high dose, 1/76 carcinoma and 4/76 papillomas of the bladder were found after 759–996 days [$p = 0.03$]; in those at the low dose, 3/75 papillomas of the bladder occurred after 539, 766 and 873 days. No bladder tumours occurred in 71 controls (Schmähl, 1978). [The Working Group noted that the presence or absence of bladder parasites was not recorded, and the sexes of animals with bladder tumours were not specified.]

Three groups of 63, 63 and 50 female Wistar rats [age unspecified] were given pure *ortho*-toluenesulfonamide at a concentration of 0 or 0.1% in the drinking-water or 79 mg/kg bw in the diet for two years. The survival rates were similar in all groups at 84 weeks. No difference in overall tumour incidence was observed between control and test groups. No bladder tumours were observed in any group, although mild diffuse urothelial hyperplasia was found in 1/50 rats fed *ortho*-toluenesulfonamide in the diet (Hooson *et al.*, 1980).

Administration with known carcinogens

Three groups of 63 female Wistar rats [age unspecified] were given a single intravesicular dose of 0.15 mL of a saturated solution of MNU in saline. Two weeks later, pure *ortho*-toluenesulfonamide was administered at a concentration of 0 or 0.08 mg/kg bw in the diet or 0.1% in the drinking-water for two years. The survival rates were similar in all groups at 84 weeks. No difference in overall tumour incidence was seen between control and test groups. Neoplasia and hyperplasia of the bladder occurred in 27% and 35%, respectively, of rats given MNU alone, but no statistically significant increase in bladder neoplasia or hyperplasia was observed in groups given MNU and *ortho*-toluenesulfonamide (Hooson *et al.*, 1980).

4. Other Data Relevant to an Evaluation of Carcinogenicity and its Mechanisms

4.1 Absorption, distribution, metabolism and excretion

4.1.1 *Humans*

Six women with an average oral daily intake of 100–300 mg saccharin [form not specified] had maximum plasma concentrations after 0.5–1 h and an elimination half-life of 7.5 h (Colburn *et al.*, 1981).

In three adult men given an intravenous bolus of 10 mg/kg bw sodium saccharin, the plasma concentration–time curve fitted a two-compartment open model with a terminal half-life of 70 min. There was no indication of metabolism, since the plasma clearance value was slightly less than that for renal clearance and saccharin was recovered in the urine quantitatively. Administration of probenecid decreased the elimination rate, suggesting renal tubular organic anion transport. After oral administration of 2 g sodium saccharin, 85% was adsorbed, as determined by recovery in the urine and by the concentration in plasma (Sweatman *et al.*, 1981).

Three groups of five men were given sodium saccharin in single oral doses of 50, 150 or 333 mg/60 kg bw. Peak plasma concentrations occurred between 30 and 60 min after dosing, and 60 and 76% was excreted unchanged in urine at 6 and 24 h, respectively (Pantarotto *et al.*, 1981).

Saccharin was detected in the sera and urine of six women aged 19–40 who had consumed saccharin in their diets during the last month of pregnancy, and was also found in the serum of the cord blood of the newborns, at a limit of detection of 20 ng/mL. The daily intake during the last month of pregnancy had been 25–100 mg (Cohen-Addad *et al.*, 1986).

After administration of 1-g doses of soluble (sodium) saccharin [form not specified] to three men, saccharin was excreted in the urine quantitatively unchanged by two of the subjects within 48 h. In a subsequent experiment involving six subjects, none excreted the dose quantitatively within 72 h, but no metabolism of saccharin was detected (McChesney & Goldberg, 1973).

Within 48 h, 92% of a dose of 500 mg [^{14}C]saccharin taken by six male volunteers was excreted in the urine and 5.8% in the faeces. Analysis of urine and faeces by high-performance liquid chromatography and thin-layer chromatography revealed only un-metabolized saccharin (Byard *et al.*, 1974).

One female and two male volunteers excreted 85–92% of a dose of 1g [3-^{14}C]-saccharin unchanged in the urine within 24 h, before or after taking 1 g saccharin daily for 21 days; no metabolites were found (Ball *et al.*, 1977).

4.1.2 *Experimental systems*

(*a*) *Saccharin*

[^{35}S]Sodium saccharin instilled into the bladder of male rats was absorbed into the plasma (Colburn, 1978).

[^{14}C]Saccharin administered by intravenous infusion to five rhesus monkeys at a dose of 4 μg/kg bw per min for 60 min during the last trimester of pregnancy crossed the placenta rapidly and was distributed in all fetal tissues except the central nervous system. During the infusion period, the fetal blood concentrations were approximately 30% those of the mothers. In contrast to the maternal organism, in which radiolabel disappeared quickly after infusion ended, the fetal compartment showed very slow clearance of saccharin and, 2 h after termination of the infusion, the fetal blood concentrations were higher than the maternal ones. The slow rate of fetal clearance suggests that considerable accumulation might result from repetitive maternal ingestion. No data were available on the penetration of saccharin into the embryonic compartment during organogenesis (Pitkin *et al.*, 1971a).

In male Sprague-Dawley rats fed 5% saccharin [about 2500 mg/kg bw per day] in the diet for 66 days, the plasma concentration showed a twofold diurnal variation. In three male rats given diets containing up to 10% saccharin [about 5000 mg/kg bw per day] in the diet for 22 days and one group of females exposed to 5% saccharin, the concentrations of saccharin were higher in the gut wall, kidneys and urinary bladder than in the plasma. There was evidence of decreased clearance at the highest doses. Probenecid was found to inhibit clearance (Sweatman & Renwick, 1980).

The tissue distribution of saccharin was investigated in two-generation feeding studies in Sprague-Dawley rats. After a single oral dose of 50 mg/kg bw [^{3}H]sodium saccharin dihydrate in late pregnancy, the concentrations of saccharin were lower in fetal than in maternal tissues after 6 and 12 h; however, concentrations were higher in fetal urinary bladder and liver after 24 and 48 h. Dams were exposed to 5% sodium saccharin [2500 mg/kg bw per day] in the diet beginning four weeks before mating and were either killed during late gestation or continued on treatment through the F_1 generation until 22 days of age. The concentration of saccharin in both maternal and fetal bladder walls showed wide interindividual variations, but the average concentration in fetal tissue was about twofold greater. The saccharin content of the stomachs of neonatal animals was very low (0.03%) and almost 200 times below the maternal dietary level. The tissue and urinary levels reflected these low dietary levels, but there was a large increase at 23 days, reflecting separation from the mother. In males, the urinary level increased over 10-fold from the neonatal period to 23 days of age, whereas the increase was somewhat less in females. During several time intervals up to 109 days of age, F_1 animals showed only equivocal evidence of accumulation of saccharin in the bladder when compared with other tissues (Sweatman & Renwick, 1982).

[^{35}S]Saccharin was observed to cross the placenta and enter the fetal circulation of Sprague-Dawley rats after treatment by gavage with 100 mg saccharin mixed with the radiolabelled compound (100 µCi, 266 mCi/mmol) on day 19 of gestation of animals that had been receiving 5% saccharin in the diet since gestation day 14. The concentrations in the fetal blood represented about 0.008% of the total dose up to 5 h after exposure. In contrast, the maternal blood levels during this time were 0.03–0.04% of the total dose (West, 1979).

The recovery of unmetabolized sodium saccharin was determined under conditions simulating one of the two-generation bioassays of carcinogenicity in which positive results were obtained (Arnold *et al.*, 1980). Male rats that had been exposed to a 5% acid saccharin diet [about 2500 mg/kg bw per day] *in utero* and maintained on this diet throughout the experiment were given 5% [^{3}H]sodium saccharin in the diet for 24 h when they weighed 290 g and were then returned to the unlabelled diet. Urine and faeces were collected at 24-h intervals and analysed. Almost all of the tritium was eliminated within 48 h, with 13–14% in the faeces and the remainder in the urine. Experiments with single low doses of [^{3}H]sodium saccharin and dosing after administration of 3-methylcholanthrene gave similar results. All of the urinary tritium was found in saccharin by thin-layer chromatography, with a limit of detection of 0.4% of the administered dose (Sweatman & Renwick, 1979).

The renal excretion of sodium saccharin infused into adult male and female Sprague-Dawley rats was found to exceed that of inulin at all plasma concentrations. Maximal tubular secretion was clearly demonstrable at a concentration of 14–20 mg/100 mL, and there was no evidence of tubular reabsorption. Clearance was inhibited when sodium saccharin and *para*-aminohippurate were infused simultaneously, indicating that excretion occurs via the carrier-mediated tubular organic anion transport system. No differences between male and female rats were found in secretory patterns or urinary saccharin levels (Bourgoignie *et al.*, 1980).

Purified [^{14}C]sodium saccharin was administered to six-month-old male and female Osborne-Mendel rats as a single oral dose of 5, 50 or 500 mg/kg bw. Between 0.03 and 0.55% of the radiolabelled sodium saccharin was metabolized to carbon dioxide. In groups of Charles River CD rats fed diets containing 0.01, 0.1 or 1% sodium saccharin for one year before administration of a radiolabelled dose of 5, 50 or 500 mg/kg bw per day, recovery of radiolabel in urine and faeces was 80–96% after seven days, which was slightly lower than the recovery (95–100%) from rats that had not been fed any saccharin before the test dose. Identification of metabolites in the urine showed that > 99% of the sodium saccharin remained as saccharin; two metabolites were reported: *ortho*-sulfamoylbenzoic acid and (probably) benzenesulfonamide. [The Working Group noted that the possibility could not be excluded that these represented contaminants of the batch of sodium saccharin administered.] The highest counts of radiolabel after administration of [^{14}C]saccharin were found in the kidney and urinary bladder, and the metabolic profiles in dogs, rabbits, guinea-pigs and hamsters were similar (Lethco & Wallace, 1975).

Two young male SIV50 Sprague-Dawley-derived rats were given single doses of 372 and 390 mg/kg bw [^{35}S]sodium saccharin by gavage and killed 50 h later. At least 99.6% of the radiolabel was found by thin-layer chromatography to correspond to unmetabolized saccharin. No binding of saccharin to DNA of liver or urinary bladder was found (Lutz & Schlatter, 1977).

Saccharin was not metabolized by liver microsomal preparations or by faecal homogenates taken from rats fed 1% hydrated sodium saccharin [approximately 0.2 g per day] in the diet for two years (Ball *et al.*, 1977). The accumulation of saccharin by rat renal cortical tissue incubated *in vitro* was dependent on oxygen and was reduced by metabolic inhibitors, suggesting that saccharin is eliminated by active tubular secretion (Goldstein *et al.*, 1978).

Saccharin was excreted rapidly and unchanged in the urine by rhesus monkeys (Pitkin *et al.*, 1971b). More than 90% of an administered dose was found within 24 h after dosing in the urine of guinea-pigs; about 70% was found in rat urine and the remainder in the faeces (Minegishi *et al.*, 1972). Although saccharin is rapidly excreted by rats, administration of multiple doses per day over several days resulted in accumulation in the bladder;

however, it was completely cleared within three days after removal of saccharin from the diet (Matthews *et al.*, 1973).

Another study showed that 90% of [^{14}C]sodium saccharin was excreted unchanged in the urine by rats and monkeys of each sex. Pretreatment with phenobarbital to induce mixed-function oxidase activity or prior intake of daily doses of sodium saccharin for over two years did not influence the metabolism of a single oral dose of [^{14}C]saccharin (Byard & Goldberg, 1973).

(*b*) *Impurities of saccharin*

The rates at which seven intragastrically administered impurities of saccharin (radio-labelled *ortho*-toluenesulfonamide, benz[*d*]isothiazoline-1,1-dioxide, 3-aminobenz[*d*]-isothiazole-1,1-dioxide, 5-chlorosaccharin, toluene-2- and -4-sulfonamides and 2- and 4-sulfamoylbenzoic acid) were eliminated in rats were similar. At doses ranging from 20 to 80 mg/kg bw, 80–95% of the impurities were recovered within 24 h in urine and faeces; urinary metabolites of these impurities were identified (Ball *et al.*, 1978; Renwick, 1978; Renwick & Williams, 1978; Renwick *et al.*, 1978).

In female Wistar rats given single oral doses of 20, 125 or 200 mg/kg bw [^{14}C]*ortho*-toluenesulfonamide, 79, 58 and 36% of the activity was recovered in 24-h urine samples; elimination at 24–48 h was 7, 14 and 33% of the dose, respectively. Within seven days, 4.5, 5.9 and 7% of the activity was recovered from the faeces. The main metabolites in the urine were 2-sulfamoylbenzyl alcohol and its sulfate or glucuronic acid conjugates (80%), *N*-acetyltoluene-2-sulfonamide (6%), saccharin (3%) and 2-sulfamoylbenzoic acid (2%) (Renwick *et al.*, 1978).

In a similar study, 50% of administered *ortho*- and *para*-toluenesulfonamides excreted in urine had been metabolized to *ortho*- and *para*-sulfamoylbenzoic acids, respectively (Minegishi *et al.*, 1972).

Low oral doses of 0.2–0.4 mg/kg bw [^{14}C]*ortho*-toluenesulfonamide were excreted more slowly in humans than in rats, an average of 56% of the activity being excreted in the urine within 24 h and almost 90% within 48 h. Less than 1% of the activity was found in faeces. The main urinary metabolites were 2-sulfamoylbenzoyl alcohol (unconjugated, 7%; conjugated with glucuronic acid, 11%; conjugated with sulfate, 20%), saccharin (35%) 2-sulfanoylbenzoic acid (4%) and *N*-acetyltoluene-2-sulfonamide (2%) (Renwick *et al.*, 1978).

4.1.3 *Comparison between humans and rodents*

A comparison of the rates of urinary excretion showed that the excretory and metabolic pattern of saccharin in humans is very similar to that observed in animals, most of the ingested saccharin being rapidly excreted in unchanged form (McChesney & Goldberg, 1973). These preliminary observations were confirmed in several subsequent experiments in humans, monkeys and rodents. The elimination half-life was longer in humans (70 min) than rats (30 min) (Sweatman & Renwick, 1980; Sweatman *et al.*, 1981). With one exception, all of the published studies indicate that saccharin is not metabolized. [The Working Group noted that in the one exception the possibility could not be excluded that the other urinary substances were contaminants in the batch of sodium saccharin administered.]

4.2 Toxic effects

4.2.1 *Humans*

Anecdotal evidence of effects in humans was related by Oser (1985) from a description of studies in about 12 male volunteers in the United States Department of Agriculture in the early part of this century, who were fed saccharin as a supplement to their diets for several weeks. The men experienced 'digestive disturbances' and, at even smaller doses, a 'renal effect'.

Idiosyncratic effects of saccharin on the liver were reported in a 70-year-old woman. Increased activities of alanine aminotransferase, aspartate aminotransferase, γ-glutamyl transferase and alkaline phosphatase were found after oral administration of three pharmaceutical drugs of which saccharin was the only common constituent. The drugs were lorazepam, dihydroergocristine and chlordemethyldiazepam. Exposure to saccharin alone reproduced the effects (Negro *et al.*, 1994).

As incorporation of sodium saccharin into the diet of experimental animals has been reported to have a rapid, pronounced effect on protein digestion in the intestine, which favours microbial metabolism of dietary tryptophan to indole, a urinary bladder co-carcinogen (Sims & Renwick, 1983), the metabolism of tryptophan was studied in 15 human subjects by analysing their daily urinary excretion of indican—a further metabolite of indole—before, during and after ingestion of sodium saccharin. The excretion of indican varied widely in both the control and the experimental groups and was not significantly affected by doses of 1 g sodium saccharin per day for one month (Roberts & Renwick, 1985).

4.2.2 *Experimental systems*

The LD_{50} values for sodium saccharin by oral administration are: mice, 18 g/kg bw; random-bred rats, 17 g/kg bw; Wistar rats, 14 g/kg bw (Taylor *et al.*, 1968); and hamster, 8.7 g/kg bw in males and 7.4 g/kg bw in females (Althoff *et al.*, 1975). The LD_{50} by intraperitoneal injection is 6.3 g/kg bw in mice and 7.1 g/kg bw in random-bred rats (Taylor *et al.*, 1968).

(*a*) *Cell proliferation*

In a two-generation study, the parents of the F_0 generation of Charles River CD rats were fed diets containing 0, 0.01, 0.1, 1, 5 or 7.5% sodium saccharin [0, 5, 50, 500, 2500 or 3750 mg/kg bw per day] from the weanling stage through mating and gestation to weaning of their litters. Of the F_1 generation, 48 animals per dose per sex were exposed to the same concentrations of sodium saccharin for life. The authors reported a statistically significant increase in urinary bladder hyperplasia only in female rats of the F_1 generation exposed to 7.5% sodium saccharin. The hyperplasia found was focal rather than diffuse and not morphologically precancerous. The incidence of hyperplasia in males was not statistically significantly increased, possibly because of a high incidence of hyperplasia in the male controls. A statistically significant increase in the incidence of urinary bladder neoplasms was found in males fed 7.5% sodium saccharin (Taylor *et al.*, 1980).

In a two-generation bioassay of sodium saccharin, 2500 F_1 male Charles River CD rats were divided into groups of 700 to 125 animals, the group at the lowest dose having the largest number. Dietary administration of 1, 3, 4, 5, 6.25 or 7.5% sodium saccharin [500, 1500, 2000, 2500, 3125 or 3750 mg/kg bw per day] was begun at six weeks for males and females of the F_0 generation; the F_1 generation was fed the same diet as the F_0 generation until the terminal kill at 30 months of age. The incidences of simple, papillary and nodular hyperplasia were analysed. Sodium saccharin increased the incidence of the combination of 'any hyperplasia' at 5, 6.25 and 7.5%, and the incidence in the last two groups achieved statistical significance (Schoenig *et al.*, 1985; re-examined by Squire, 1985).

No simple, papillary or nodular hyperplasia or papilloma was found among groups of 10-week-old male and female inbred Charles River Fischer 344 rats fed 0.04, 0.2, 1 or 5% sodium saccharin [20, 100, 500 or 2500 mg/kg bw per day] in a stock diet for 32 weeks (Nakanishi *et al.*, 1980a). In another experiment, two groups of 10-week-old male Wistar rats were exposed to 5% sodium saccharin in the diet for 36 weeks. In comparison with controls, which had no hyperplasia, sodium saccharin produced simple hyperplasia in 10/26 (38%) of one group and 11/21 (52%) of the other. The incidence of papillary or nodular hyperplasia was 5/26 (19%) and 9/21 (43%) in the two groups, respectively. The discrepancy between these results may be due to a strain difference in susceptibility (Nakanishi *et al.*, 1980b).

In a time-course study, six-week-old male Charles River Fischer 344 rats were exposed to 5% sodium saccharin [2500 mg/kg bw per day] in the diet for up to 18 weeks. Three animals per group were killed for histopathological analysis at 1, 3, 5, 7, 9, 12, 15 and 18 weeks, and DNA synthesis was measured at 1, 5, 9 and 18 weeks by [^{3}H]thymidine uptake and autoradiography. In exposed animals, vacuolar degeneration of the epithelial cells was found at three weeks, followed by simple hyperplasia at five weeks. By nine weeks, the degree of hyperplasia had increased, with a display of mitotic figures, hyperplastic foci and pleomorphic microvilli. Increased [^{3}H]thymidine uptake was seen in the exposed rats at all times, and the increase was five- to eightfold the rate seen in controls (Fukushima & Cohen, 1980).

In a study of dose–response, cell proliferation was measured by autoradiography and scanning electron microscopy in groups of three to four five-week-old male Fischer 344 rats after 10 weeks of exposure to 0.1, 0.5, 1, 2.5 or 5% sodium saccharin [50, 250, 500, 1250 or 2500 mg/kg bw/day] in the diet. A dose-related increase in [^{3}H]thymidine labelling index, hyperplasia and the presence of uniform and pleomorphic microvilli were found. At doses $\leq$ 1% sodium saccharin, there was no statistically significant increase in the incidence of hyperplasia or in the numbers of foci or cells exhibiting uniform and pleomorphic microvilli. At 0.1% sodium saccharin, there was no statistically significant change in the labelling index (Murasaki & Cohen, 1981). [The Working Group noted the small number of rats in each group and that subsequent studies showed labelling indices in occasional individual, untreated control rats that were similar to those seen in this study in rats treated with 1% sodium saccharin.]

Feeding of 7.5% sodium saccharin [3750 mg/kg bw per day] in the diets of male Sprague-Dawley rats from three weeks of age did not increase ^{3}H-thymidine incorporation in the DNA of urinary bladder epithelium at 1, 2, 3, 6, 10, 15, 20, 30 or 50 weeks after the beginning of exposure. Autoradiographic analysis of the thymidine labelling index at 1, 15 and 50 weeks also did not show statistically significant increases in sodium saccharin-exposed animals when compared with controls (Lawson & Hertzog, 1981).

The effects of 5% sodium saccharin [2500 mg/kg bw/day] in the diet for 20 weeks from six weeks of age were compared in male Fischer 344 rats, B6C3F1 mice, Syrian golden hamsters and Hartley guinea-pigs. Rats developed hyperplasia of the urinary bladder and significantly increased DNA synthesis at 20 weeks, as determined by [^{3}H]-thymidine autoradiography, but the other species did not have similar changes. These results indicated to the investigators that the urothelial-cell proliferative response to high doses of sodium saccharin was specific to the rat. In a comparative study with males of four strains of rats (ACI, Wistar, Fischer 344 and Sprague-Dawley), the ACI strain was reported to be the most susceptible to the effects on the urinary bladder of 5% sodium saccharin in the diet for 52 weeks (Fukushima *et al.*, 1983a).

In male Fischer 344 rats, the degree of hyperplasia and microvillus formation induced by freeze-ulceration in the bladder epithelium was similar during the subsequent two-week period whether or not 5% sodium saccharin was administered immediately after the procedure. The group receiving sodium saccharin only did not show hyperplastic changes in this time interval. Two weeks after freeze-ulceration, continuation or initiation of sodium saccharin exposure prolonged the duration of hyperplasia until termination of the experiment at eight weeks. The labelling index in the bladder epithelium of sodium saccharin-exposed groups with or without prior freeze-ulceration was increased above the control value in the last six weeks of the experiment. In another experiment, sodium saccharin given two or eight weeks after freeze-ulceration produced a similar increase in hyperplasia, microvillus formation and labelling index (Murasaki & Cohen, 1983b).

The effect of cation-associated saccharin was studied in five-week-old male Fischer 344 rats given 5% of the diet [2500 mg/kg bw per day] as sodium saccharin, acid saccharin, potassium saccharin or calcium saccharin for 10 weeks. Cell proliferation was measured by [^{3}H]thymidine incorporation, hyperplasia was determined by light microscopy and formation of microvilli by scanning electron microscopy. The labelling index was increased by approximately ninefold when compared with controls by sodium saccharin, threefold by potassium saccharin and twofold by calcium saccharin; there was no increase in labelling index with acid saccharin. Only the changes with the sodium and potassium salts reached statistical significance. Sodium saccharin also caused a statistically significant increase in the number of animals with simple hyperplasia when compared with controls. Although there was evidence of simple hyperplasia after treatment with potassium saccharin and calcium saccharin, these changes were not statistically significant. Pleomorphic microvilli were observed only in rats given sodium saccharin. Sodium saccharin in the diet increased the urinary excretion of sodium. The urinary concentration of saccharin was similar after administration of each of the four forms of saccharin (Hasegawa & Cohen, 1986).

When seven-week-old male Fischer rats were exposed to 5% sodium saccharin [2500 mg/kg bw per day] in the diet for 21 weeks, [^{3}H]thymidine labelling index and the ornithine decarboxylase activity in the bladder were about fivefold greater than in controls (Tatematsu *et al.*, 1986).

The proliferative effects of sodium saccharin were found to vary with diet in five-week-old male Fischer 344 and four-week-old Sprague-Dawley rats exposed to 5 or 7.5% [2500 and 3750 mg/kg bw per day] sodium saccharin. The diets containing sodium saccharin were continued for up to 10 weeks, at which time the animals were killed. The Fischer 344 rats showed statistically significant increases in the [^{3}H]thymidine labelling index with Prolab and NIH-07 diets at four weeks and with the Prolab diet at 10 weeks with 7.5% sodium saccharin. At the other times and doses, increased labelling indices were found, but they were not statistically significant, and no increase was seen in rats fed AIN-76A diet. The hyperplastic and epithelial changes in the groups on the three diets, monitored by scanning electron microscopy, were not remarkably different, except for an increase in the severity of changes with the Prolab diet and 7.5% sodium saccharin fed for 10 weeks. The animals fed AIN-76A diet had lower urinary volumes and higher concentrations of sodium saccharin and calcium, but lower levels of potassium than those on the Prolab and NIH-07 diets. The pH of the urine was also lower in this group (Garland *et al.*, 1989).

Weanling male Fischer 344 rats were fed 5% sodium saccharin [2500 mg/kg bw per day] in either a Wayne or an AIN-76A diet for 2, 4, 6, 10 and 16 weeks. Whereas the AIN-76A diet alone or with sodium saccharin resulted in a urinary pH of 5.5–6.5, the Wayne diet with sodium saccharin gave a urinary pH of 7.4. With both diets, sodium saccharin increased the [^{3}H]thymidine labelling index by about fivefold when measured at 2, 4, 6, 10 or 16 weeks. Addition of 2% sodium bicarbonate increased the labelling index for the group on the AIN-76A diet by six- to ninefold; sodium saccharin and sodium bicarbonate in the diet appeared to be additive (Debiec-Rychter & Wang, 1990).

In a dose–response experiment, sodium saccharin was administered in Prolab 3200 diet at concentrations of 0, 3, 5 or 7.5% [0, 1500, 2500 and 3750 mg/kg bw per day] to four-week-old male Fischer 344 rats, which were killed after 4, 7 and 10 weeks of exposure. [^{3}H]Thymidine was injected 1 h before killing, and hyperplasia was measured by light microscopy and scanning electron microscopy. No evidence of increased labelling index or hyperplasia was found with 3% sodium saccharin, but cell necrosis and exfoliation were evident after 10 weeks. A doubling of the labelling index was noted with exposure to 5% sodium saccharin at 10 weeks, with extensive cell damage. With 7.5% sodium saccharin, the labelling index was already increased by threefold after four weeks, with evidence of increasing hyperplasia over the 4- to 10-week period. In all three groups given sodium saccharin, there was an apparent progression of necrotic changes during treatment (Cohen *et al.*, 1990).

In two-generation studies, weanling male and female Sprague-Dawley and Fischer 344 F_0 rats were exposed to either 5% sodium saccharin or acid saccharin [2500 mg/kg bw per day] in Prolab 3200 diet for two weeks and then mated. Offspring were killed 1 h after injection of [^{3}H]thymidine *in utero*, during lactation or after weaning. In a study in which mostly male animals were evaluated, there was no effect of either sodium saccharin or acid saccharin through seven days of age; however, sodium saccharin increased the labelling indices above those of controls at 21, 63 and 91 days of age, while acid saccharin did not. In a study of both male and female Sprague-Dawley rats, increased bladder urothelial cell proliferation was found in animals of each sex at 21 but not at 7 days of age or on days 17 and 21 of gestation. There was also evidence of small foci of superficial necrosis and mild hyperplastic proliferation by 21 days of age in animals of each sex (Cohen *et al.*, 1995a).

The effects of exposure to concentrations of up to 6.84% sodium ascorbate [3400 mg/kg bw per day] as a single agent or 5 or 7.5% sodium saccharin [2500 and 3750 mg/kg bw per day] alone or combined with 1.23 or 1.85% ammonium chloride [620 and 920 mg/kg bw per day] in the diet on the urinary bladder of male Fischer 344 rats were measured on the basis of various histopathological and chemical parameters. Rats were placed on the experimental diets and mated, and the offspring were kept on the same diets as the F_0 generation. Female offspring were killed at 21 days of age and males at 16 weeks of age. One hour before death, the male F_1 rats were injected intraperitoneally with bromodeoxyuridine. Sodium saccharin but not sodium ascorbate increased the water consumption significantly. Groups of the F_1 generation at the high dose of sodium saccharin had to be terminated early because of toxic effects, and most of the other experimental groups showed some growth retardation. The urinary pH of rats at 5% sodium saccharin was decreased to less than 6.5 by co-administration of 1.23% ammonium chloride; it remained decreased but above 6.5 on day 37 of exposure to 5% sodium saccharin alone and was similar to that of controls by day 100. All of the groups given sodium ascorbate had urinary pH values significantly greater than those of controls. An amorphous precipitate containing calcium phosphate was present in the urine of male F_1 rats given sodium saccharin or higher doses of sodium ascorbate, but not in the controls, after the lowest dose of ascorbate or in rats given sodium saccharin plus ammonium chloride. The labelling index was increased and there was evidence of hyperplastic changes in the groups receiving 5% sodium saccharin alone or the highest dose of sodium ascorbate; the second highest dose of ascorbate induced evidence of hyperplasia, but the increase in labelling index was not statistically significant. No hyperplasia was observed in the group fed sodium saccharin plus ammonium chloride. In a small, one-generation study, hyperplasia was observed in male rats that had been kept on a diet containing 6.84% sodium ascorbate for 10 weeks but was completely inhibited in a group fed 2.78 or 3.7% ammonium chloride plus 6.84% sodium ascorbate. The caeca of rats given sodium saccharin with or without ammonium chloride were enlarged, but this effect was not seen with sodium ascorbate (Cohen *et al.*, 1995b).

Weanling male Fischer 344 male rats were exposed to 5% sodium saccharin [2500 mg/kg bw per day] in Prolab 3200 diet for up to 72 weeks, when their bladder epithelial cells were stained immunohistochemically for uroplakin expression and scored for hyperplastic changes. Simple hyperplastic lesions were induced by sodium saccharin and ascorbate, and the lesions showed identical uroplakin staining patterns (Ogawa *et al.*, 1996).

Twenty male and female monkeys (six African green, seven rhesus, six cynomolgus and one rhesus/cynomolgus hybrid) were exposed to 25 mg/kg bw sodium saccharin in the diet on five days per week from 24 h after birth up to 24 years of age. Eight monkeys died between 103 and 282 months of age, and the remainder were killed at between 207 and 283 months of age. At autopsy, none of the monkeys had any abnormalities of the urothelium, including the renal pelvis, ureter, urinary bladder and urethra. Of the monkeys that died, many had multiple abnormalities: two had septic hepatitis, five had lung infections and other abnormalities, one had chronic ulcers of the stomach and oesophagus, two had myocardial degeneration or fibrosis and one had chronic ileitis. The monkeys that were killed had abnormalities similar to those seen in 16 monkeys that served as controls, of which two died. There was no evidence of urothelial hyperplasia in either sodium saccharin-exposed animals or controls. No obvious differences in the chemical composition of the urine were seen in two cynomolgus and two rhesus monkeys of each sex given saccharin and in that of controls less than two years before they were killed. Examination of urine by scanning electron microscopy showed no increase in the frequency of microcrystalluria and no evidence of abnormal microcrystals, precipitate or calculi (Takayama *et al.*, 1998).

(*b*) *Physiological and biochemical changes in urine*

Sodium saccharin fed to weanling male Charles River rats at concentrations up to 7.5% [3750 mg/kg bw per day] for four weeks was found to increase the urine volume and decrease the urinary pH. It also increased faecal water content, faecal excretion of sodium and potassium and urinary excretion of calcium, magnesium and phosphorus (Anderson, 1979).

Administration to Wistar rats for two years of 2 g/kg bw per day sodium saccharin in the drinking-water or of 4 g/kg bw per day in the diet reduced the weight gain markedly; fluid intake was increased in the latter group and decreased in the former. The average urinary pH of males in the first group had risen to above 7.0 by 27 weeks, and some animals showed marked crystalluria. These pH changes could be reversed by the addition of ammonium chloride to the diet. The most important exposure-related findings were increased incidences of microcalculi and telangiectasia of the vasa recta in kidneys, of renal pelvic hyperplasia, of extramedullary haematopoiesis and of hepatic zonal necrosis. Hyperplasia of the bladder epithelium occurred earlier in animals of the second group (Chowaniec & Hicks, 1979).

Five-week-old male Fischer 344 rats were fed diets containing 5% sodium saccharin [2500 mg/kg bw/day] until week 104, beginning at week 0 or 4; further groups received

FANFT or L-tryptophan in the diet. The urine was analysed at weeks 1, 2, 4, 5, 6, 7, 8 and 12 and monthly thereafter. Exposure to sodium saccharin increased the water intake, which produced diarrhoea and increased the urinary volume. The concentration of sodium in the urine was not changed, and the only abnormality observed was slightly increased urinary pH during the first three months. There was no increase in crystal formation (Demers *et al.*, 1981).

Three groups of four-week-old male Crl:COBS[R]CD[R](SD)BR rats were exposed for 16 weeks to 5% sodium saccharin [2500 mg/kg bw per day] in the diet, 4% sodium saccharin [2000 mg/kg bw per day] in the drinking-water or control diet. Rats receiving saccharin in the diet had increased food and water consumption, urine elimination, precipitate and crystalline urinary sediment and some evidence of mild urothelial hyperplasia. Rats receiving saccharin in drinking-water showed increased urine osmolality (West & Jackson, 1981).

In a two-generation study, seven-month-old Charles River CD rats (F_0) and F_1 rats were exposed to 1, 3, 5 or 7.5% sodium saccharin in the diet [500, 1500, 2500 or 3750 mg/kg bw per day]. Controls were either unexposed or given 5% sodium hippurate, the latter to determine effects attributable to sodium. Sodium saccharin produced several physiological changes in the urine, including increased volume and sodium concentration, decreased osmolality and decreased potassium and zinc concentrations. Increases in bladder weight, hydration and the mineral content of the bladder tissue were also seen. Sodium hippurate caused similar changes, but they were less severe than those produced by sodium saccharin. Similar effects were found in an additional group of animals exposed to sodium saccharin from birth. In a group of animals exposed *in utero*, but not after birth, the measured parameters were similar to those in controls. Some differences in response to sodium saccharin were noted between males and females; for example, caecal weight was increased more in the females, but the mineral and sodium saccharin concentrations in the urine were higher in the males. In addition, at dietary concentrations of sodium saccharin ≥ 5%, the concentrations of sodium, potassium, magnesium and zinc were significantly increased in the bladders of males but not females. The pattern of and dietary concentrations at which these changes occurred suggested to the authors that changes in these mineral constituents in the urine and/or urine volume may play an important role in the etiology of bladder tumours in rats fed high dietary concentrations of sodium saccharin (Schoenig & Anderson, 1985).

Adult male Charles Rivers CD rats were fed either control or a diet containing 7.5% [3750 mg/kg bw/day] sodium saccharin for one month. Increased daily water intake, total urine volume, frequency of urination and average volume per urination were found (Renwick & Sims, 1983).

Histological changes in the urinary bladder related to cell proliferation and urinary chemistry were evaluated in male Fischer 344 rats in relation to dietary exposure to 5% sodium saccharin, acid saccharin, ascorbic acid or sodium ascorbate [2500 mg/kg bw per day]. Urinary pH, sodium, urinary bladder hyperplasia and scanning electron microscopic changes were measured at 8, 16 and 24 weeks. The histological changes seen by light microscopy were 'slight' or 'very slight' at the earlier times, and none were noted at 24 weeks. Scanning electron microscopy showed slight pleomorphic microvilli at 24 weeks in one of five animals given sodium saccharin and at eight weeks in one of five given sodium ascorbate. Short, uniform microvilli and ropy or leafy microridges were moderately prevalent with sodium saccharin or sodium ascorbate, whereas they were absent in the groups given saccharin or ascorbic acid. The urinary pH was increased by sodium saccharin and sodium ascorbate, was decreased by saccharin and was the same as that in controls with ascorbic acid. Urinary sodium excretion was increased by the sodium salts but not by the acidic forms (Fukushima *et al.*, 1986a).

Prolab 3200 or AIN-76A diets containing 5% sodium saccharin or calcium saccharin [2500 mg/kg bw per day] were administered to five-week-old male Fischer 344 rats for 10 weeks. Although the Prolab 3200 diet has a lower pH than the AIN-76 diet, the former contains larger amounts of sodium, calcium, potassium and most other ions than the latter. Exposure to either salt of saccharin resulted in a urinary pH above 6.5 with the Prolab diet and below 6.0 with the AIN-76A diet. The amount of sodium excreted in urine was lowest with the AIN-76A diet with or without calcium saccharin. With sodium saccharin administration, the sodium concentrations in urine were higher with the Prolab diet than with AIN-76A (Fisher *et al.*, 1989).

Changes in gastrointestinal and urinary tract physiology in young rats were investigated by a protocol simulating the two-generation bioassay of Schoenig *et al.* (1985; p. 548). Sodium saccharin was administered at 1, 3 or 7.5% [500, 1500 and 3750 mg/kg bw/day] in the diet, beginning with the F_0 generation; males and females in the F_1 generation were killed at approximately 30 days. Rats at 7.5% had decreased urinary pH, potassium and calcium and increased urinary volume, sodium, magnesium, phosphate and ammonia; animals at other doses were not examined for these parameters. In addition, rats fed 7.5% sodium saccharin had anaemia, a 50% increase in serum cholesterol concentration, a 10-fold increase in serum triglyceride concentration and decreased serum and hepatic concentrations of vitamins. These changes were not found at lower doses of sodium saccharin. In another experiment, newborn animals were dosed with sodium saccharin for 90 days, while others were given only control diet after 30 days on sodium saccharin. Some of the observed changes were found to be reversible; however, histopathological examination of the bladder showed no changes at 30 days and only slight changes at 90 days. The authors considered that the observed biochemical and physiological effects were not involved in bladder tumorigenesis. Many of the effects were found to be associated with anaemia due to iron deficiency, and some of them—but not the urinary or bladder effects—could be prevented by dietary iron and/or folate supplementation. This supplementation by itself increased the frequency of bladder hyperplasia (Garland *et al.*, 1991a,b, 1993).

In a study involving feeding of various sodium salts at doses equimolar to 7.5% sodium saccharin to male Fischer 344 rats for 10 weeks, urothelial-cell proliferation was studied by light microscopy (hyperplasia), by bromodeoxyuridine labelling and by scanning electron microscopy. The sodium salts of saccharin, ascorbate, glutamate, aspartate, citrate, erythorbate, bicarbonate and chloride caused various degrees of increase in urothelial proliferation and all resulted in formation of the calcium phosphate-containing urinary precipitate (amounts not quantified). A group of rats that received 1.85% ammonium chloride plus 7.5% sodium saccharin did not show increased proliferation or formation of the precipitate (Cohen *et al.*, 1995c).

(*c*) *Urinary precipitate formation and the role of urinary proteins*

In a two-generation lifetime feeding study, groups of 50 male and 50 female Sprague-Dawley rats were exposed to 5% [2500 mg/kg bw per day] sodium saccharin or to various doses of *ortho*-toluenesulfonamide in the diet, beginning when the F_0 generation was 32 days old. Rats were mated on day 90 of the study, and the F_0 generation and F_1 progeny were exposed to the same diets throughout life. The urine of older animals exposed to 5% sodium saccharin, especially the males, contained a flocculent-type precipitate, which dissolved in acetic acid. In 21-day-old pups and in 105-day-old male and female rats receiving *ortho*-toluenesulfonamide in another experiment reported by these investigators, a significant dose–response relationship was found for the incidence of bladder calculi, while sodium saccharin free of *ortho*-toluenesulfonamide did not have a similar effect (Arnold *et al.*, 1979, 1980).

Male Fischer 344 rats were fed 7.5% [3750 mg/kg bw/day] sodium saccharin in Prolab 3200 diet beginning at five weeks of age, and urine was collected on Millipore filters two and four weeks later. Whereas control rats had typical phosphate crystals, rats fed sodium saccharin had fewer crystals and approximately one-half contained silicate and were jagged in shape. These silicate crystals were found to result in occasional microabrasion of the urothelial surface. Gel filtration of urine with added radiolabelled sodium saccharin showed two fractions of saccharin-binding proteins: one corresponded to the size of α_{2u}-globulin, while the other corresponded to albumin. The authors postulated that saccharin–protein complexes form a precipitate with silicate in urine that has a pH greater than 6.5 (Cohen *et al.*, 1991b).

Support for the role of α_{2u}-globulin in sodium saccharin-induced cell hyperplasia and cell proliferation rates comes from studies with male Fischer 344 and NCI-Black-Reiter (NBR) rats. The latter strain does not produce the male-specific, low-molecular-mass urinary protein α_{2u}-globulin and does not undergo sodium saccharin-enhanced cell proliferation. Male NBR, Fischer 344 and castrated Fischer 344 rats were fed 7.5% sodium saccharin [3750 mg/kg bw per day] in Prolab 3200 diet for 10 weeks. Examination of the bladders by light microscopy revealed that 7/10 sodium saccharin-exposed Fischer 344 rats and 1/10 NBR rats had hyperplastic changes, but none were seen in the unexposed Fischer 344 rats; however, 4/10 castrated Fischer 344 rats also had hyperplastic bladders, although the α_{2u}-globulin urinary content was only 10% of that in normal Fischer 344 males. Examination of the bladder by scanning electron microscopy showed that the most severe changes occurred in castrated and normal sodium saccharin-exposed Fischer 344 rats, whereas the exposed NBR rats showed less severe changes. The increases in caecal weights showed a pattern similar to the changes observed by scanning electron miscroscopy. The urinary volume of NBR controls was threefold higher than that of Fischer 344 controls, and exposure to sodium saccharin increased the volume by three- to fourfold in NBR, Fischer 344 and castrated Fischer 344 rats (Garland *et al.*, 1994).

Six-week-old Fischer 344 and NBR rats were exposed to 5% sodium saccharin [2500 mg/kg bw per day], 5% sodium ascorbate or 3% uracil [1500 mg/kg bw per day] in the diet for eight weeks. Ascorbate produced simple hyperplasia in Fischer 344 rats but not in NBR rats, and uracil produced papillary hyperplasia in both strains. Scanning electron microscopy showed that uracil produced the most severe changes, and sodium saccharin and ascorbate produced some changes only in Fischer 344 rats. Large differences in the bromodeoxyuridine labelling index were found in Fischer 344 rats given sodium saccharin (20-fold) or ascorbate (36-fold) and in both strains exposed to uracil (over 50-fold). In Fischer 344 rats, the urinary pH and sodium concentration were increased by sodium saccharin and ascorbate, and the urine volume was decreased only by ascorbate. In ascorbate-treated NBR rats, a significant increase in urinary volume was observed (Uwagawa *et al.*, 1994).

Studies on the appearance of the crystalline and amorphous material in sodium saccharin-exposed male rats are described above (Cohen *et al.*, 1995b,c).

(*d*) *Studies primarily on gastrointestinal changes*

Dietary sodium saccharin was tested for its ability to alter caecal microflora in weanling male CD rats exposed to 7.5% sodium saccharin [3750 mg/kg bw/day] in the diet for 10 days. The weights of caecal tissue and its contents were higher than those of controls, which received 7.5% cellulose (Anderson & Kirkland, 1980).

Adult male Charles River (CD)-derived Sprague-Dawley rats (weighing about 300 g) were exposed to 0–10% sodium saccharin [0–5000 mg/kg bw per day], 2% tryptophan [1000 mg/kg bw per day] or 2% tryptophan plus 5% sodium saccharin [2500 mg/kg bw per day] in the diet for one to two months. The presence of sodium saccharin in the diet had a rapid, pronounced effect on the metabolism of dietary tryptophan. The excretion of indican, a metabolite of tryptophan, was increased 3.1-fold per 24 h in animals fed 10% sodium saccharin in the diet, and there was a linear relationship between the dietary concentration and indican excretion. High plasma concentrations of saccharin (200–300 μg/mL) reduced the renal clearance of both saccharin and indican; the authors suggested that this was due to saturation of renal tubular secretion. Indican concentrations in the urine, and the indole concentrations in the caecum were increased, possibly due to accumulation of protein and tryptophan in the caecum. Sodium saccharin produced a dose-related increase in both the weight of the caecal contents and the wall of the caecum. The effects of sodium saccharin and tryptophan were additive. These results are consistent with the concept that sodium saccharin has a major effect on protein digestion in the intestine, which favours increased microbial metabolism of dietary tryptophan to indole, a urinary bladder co-carcinogen (Sims & Renwick, 1983).

Indican and *para*-cresol excretion were found to be increased by three- to fourfold in male Charles River adult rats fed 7.5% sodium saccharin [3750 mg/kg bw per day] in the diet for 40 days, when compared with controls. As described above, indican is formed from indole, a microbial metabolite of tryptophan, whereas *para*-cresol is formed from tyrosine by the gut flora. The excretion of phenol, another microbial metabolite of tyrosine, was, however, abolished by the same regimen of sodium saccharin, indicating that there is an altered pattern of metabolism in addition to an increase in the amount of metabolites (Lawrie *et al.*, 1985).

Three-week-old male Sprague-Dawley rats were fed a diet containing 5% sodium saccharin [2500 mg/kg bw per day] for 4 or 20 weeks. Marked caecal enlargement and decreased β-glucuronidase, nitrate reductase and sulfatase activities were seen in the caecal content; however, there was no change in bacterial concentrations at either exposure interval. Incubation of the caecal contents from control rats with 75 mmol/L sodium saccharin *in vitro* produced similar enzyme inhibitions. The authors surmised that such inhibition may decrease the rate of formation of toxic bacterial products in the hindgut (Mallett *et al.*, 1985).

In a two-generation study, 7.5% [3750 mg/kg bw per day] sodium saccharin was fed in the diet to adult male and female Charles River (CD)-derived Sprague-Dawley rats from six weeks before mating. The pups of sodium saccharin-fed dams were found to be exposed to elevated levels of indican via the milk. Sodium saccharin-exposed pups were found to have increased caecal size and caecal protein, decreased caecal tryptophanase activity and increased urine volume and urinary indican excretion. Pups from dams fed sodium saccharin only from the time of parturition showed more variable responses than those from dams fed sodium saccharin from before conception; this was due to variations in tryptophanase activity. These changes were similar in males and females and were greatest during the first month after weaning (Sims & Renwick, 1985).

CD rat dams were fed increasing doses of sodium saccharin: 1% [500 mg/kg bw per day] beginning at parturition, 3% [1500 mg/kg bw] at day 8 and 5% [2500 mg/kg bw] at day 15. Pups were weaned at day 21 and continued on this diet. The pups of dams that had not received sodium saccharin were started on 5% sodium saccharin at weaning. When pups were exposed to sodium saccharin during nursing, no effect was seen on caecal or bladder mass at weaning but the caecal mass after weaning was almost doubled. The caecal mass of pups exposed from the time of weaning was intermediate between that of pups exposed from birth and that of controls. The changes in bladder mass followed a similar pattern but were not as extensive; the increased bladder mass correlated with increased urinary output (Anderson *et al.*, 1988a).

Although the studies described above suggest that gastrointestinal changes are implicated in the effects of sodium saccharin, the effects of saccharin on the caecal mass were not found to depend on the chemical form. There was no difference in the mass of the caecum plus contents or caecal tissue after 10 weeks of feeding male weanling CD rats 5% sodium saccharin [2500 mg/kg bw per day] or the molar equivalent of acid saccharin, potassium saccharin or calcium saccharin. Bladder hyperplasia was found only in rats given sodium or potassium saccharin, and increased relative bladder mass was found only with sodium saccharin. Sodium and potassium saccharin were also responsible for an increased relative urinary mass. The authors concluded that the caecal effects were due to the saccharin anion but that the urinary changes were dependent on the cation. Consequently, caecal mass changes do not appear to be involved in sodium saccharin-induced bladder tumours (Anderson *et al.*, 1988b).

The excretion of indican was found not to be responsible for the toxic effects on the bladder of dietary administration of 5% sodium saccharin. Male CD rats were exposed to 5% sodium saccharin [2500 mg/kg bw per day], 1.5% indole [750 mg/kg bw per day] or 5% sodium saccharin plus 1.5% indole added to diet for 10 weeks. Sodium saccharin and indole produced equivalent increases in bladder mass and epithelial hyperplasia; however, in rats exposed to sodium saccharin, the amount of indican excreted in the urine was less than one-tenth the amount produced after dietary exposure to indole. After exposure to indole and sodium saccharin together, the increase in bladder mass was additive, but there was no increase in hyperplasia over that observed with each compound alone (Anderson *et al.*, 1989).

(*e*) *Other mechanistic information*

In an assay to detect tumour promoters *in vitro*, sodium saccharin inhibited metabolic cooperation between Chinese hamster V79 cells in culture. A small number of *hprt*$^-$ (6-thioguanine resistant) cells were seeded in the presence of a large number of *hprt*$^+$ cells with 0–5 mg/L sodium saccharin in the culture medium. Sodium saccharin concentrations > 2 mg/L resulted in a dose-related increase in the recovery of 6-thioguanine-resistant cells (Trosko *et al.*, 1980).

Sodium saccharin inhibited binding of ^{125}I-labelled mouse epidermal growth factor to 18 cell lines, including HeLa (human carcinoma), MDCK (dog kidney), HTC (rat hepatoma), K22 (rat liver), HF (human foresekin), GM17 (human skin fibroblasts), XP (human xeroderma pigmentosum fibroblasts) and 3T3-L1 (mouse fibroblasts) (Lee, 1981).

Inhibition by sodium saccharin of urease and three proteases *in vitro* was not due to the sodium ion (Lok *et al.*, 1982).

Saccharin [type or source not specified] inhibited binding of epidermal growth factor to cultured rat pituitary tumour cells and enhanced prolactin production (Brennessel & Keyes, 1985).

In two initiation-promotion studies, inhibitors of lipid peroxidation were found to inhibit the tumour-promoting effects of sodium saccharin. Both aspirin and the antioxidant nordihydroguaiaretic acid inhibited bladder tumour formation when co-administered with sodium saccharin. These studies indicate that oxidative damage may play a role in the cytotoxic effects of sodium saccharin (Sakata *et al.*, 1986; Yu *et al.*, 1992).

In cultured bladders from young female Fischer 344 rats, 12 mmol/L sodium saccharin produced urothelial hyperplasia and dysplasia, as detected by histology. Sodium saccharin increased the number of foci of cell proliferation induced by MNU in explant bladder epithelium cultures of young female Fischer 344 rats. Only transient hyperplasia was found with sodium saccharin alone (Knowles & Jani, 1986; Nicholson & Jani, 1988).

Rat bladder explants were exposed continuously to sodium saccharin for up to 28 days. Hyperplastic effects and increased DNA synthesis were reported after exposure to 0.5% (Norman *et al.*, 1987), while explants treated with 0.1% resembled control cultures.

Saccharin [type not specified] was found to inhibit intercellular communication in a human urothelial cell-line (JTC-30), which was established from a well-differentiated transitional-cell carcinoma of the urinary bladder. Inhibition measured by dye transfer at 48 and 96 h occurred at a concentration of 3 mg/mL, which was relatively nontoxic. At lower concentrations, there was little or no effect, and higher concentrations were toxic (Morimoto, 1996).

The ionic structure of the saccharinate anion, as studied by two-dimensional nuclear magnetic resonance, was not altered by several ions at the wide ranges of concentrations found in urine after feeding of high doses of various salt forms of saccharin or its acid (Williamson *et al.*, 1987).

4.3 Reproductive and developmental effects

4.3.1 *Humans*

The teratogenic potential of saccharin in humans has been reviewed and determined to be minimal; however, the quality of the data considered in the analysis was poor to fair (Friedman & Polifka, 1994). No epidemiological studies of prenatal exposure to saccharin have been reported.

In a case–control study, the use of sugar substitutes was examined in 574 consecutive cases of spontaneous abortions and 320 age-matched controls from three Manhattan hospitals (United States) during 1974–77. Sugar substitutes (assumed to be saccharin) were used by 5.5% of the patients and 5.8% of the controls. There was no significant association between spontaneous abortion and the use of sugar substitutes (Kline *et al.*, 1977).

4.3.2 *Experimental systems*

Generally negative results were reported from a one-generation study in mice fed 1% sodium saccharin (Lorke & Machemer, 1975), a multigeneration study in Swiss mice given doses of 0.2 or 0.5% in the diet (Kroes *et al.*, 1977), in an abstract reporting a three-generation study in CD rats at 5 or 7% sodium saccharin in the diet (Taylor & Friedman, 1974), in studies for teratogenicity in hamsters and rats at 10 and 100 g per day calcium saccharin (Adkins *et al.*, 1972), in a study of exposure of rats before mating and during gestation to 0.4% sodium saccharin in the diet (Luckhaus & Machemer, 1978) and in an abstract of a study in which dogs received 0.5–1.5 g/kg bw of a 10:1 sodium cyclamate:sodium saccharin mixture during pregnancy while their offspring were kept on the same diet until one year of age (Fancher *et al.*, 1968). The finding that sodium saccharin was more toxic to fetal mice than to adults was not considered reliable (Tanaka, 1964, cited by Tanaka *et al.*, 1973). Morphological abnormalities of the eye and an increased mortality rate of offspring were reported after exposure of pregnant Wistar rats to 0.3 and 3% sodium saccharin in the diet (Lederer & Pottier-Arnould, 1973; Lederer, 1977), but these effects were attributed to impurities (primarily *ortho*-sulfobenzoic acid) arising from synthesis by the Remsen-Fahlberg method (IARC, 1980).

The studies on reproductive effects and teratogenesis were also reviewed by Arnold *et al.* (1983), who concluded that saccharin is not teratogenic to mice, rats or rabbits. The authors also reviewed the findings of a number of multigeneration studies that were designed primarily to examine effects on bladder tumour formation, i.e. those conducted by the Wisconsin Alumni Research Foundation (Tisdel *et al.*, 1974), the Food and Drug Administration (Taylor *et al.*, 1980), the Health Protection Branch (Arnold *et al.*, 1980) and several other modified multigeneration studies (one involving six generations; Kroes *et al.*, 1977). Significant effects on reproductive indices (primarily decrements in body weights) were observed in rats at dietary concentrations of 5–7.5%.

In another review of the teratogenic potential of saccharin in experimental systems (Friedman & Polifka, 1994), it was noted that the frequency of malformations was not increased in offspring of mice, rats or rabbits given up to 800, 1500 and 10 times the human maximum intake, respectively. They noted that a slightly increased incidence of bladder tumours was observed in rats in some studies in which perinatal exposure was to thousands of times the recommended daily intake of saccharin for humans; however, other studies did not show this effect.

Direct exposure of cultured rat embryos to 1 mmol/L saccharin on days 10.5–12.5 of gestation *in vitro* did not affect embryonic growth or morphology, even in the presence of a microsomal activating system (Kitchen & Ebron, 1983). Similar results were reported by Cicurel and Schmid (1988).

The concentration of sodium saccharin that inhibits proliferation of human embryonic palatal mesenchymal cells by 50% was reported to be 5350 μg/mL (26 mmol/L), whereas the authors considered a value < 1 mmol/L to be indicative of teratogenic potential in this assay (Pratt & Willis, 1985). A subsequent interlaboratory comparison of results showed no evidence for any teratogenic effect of saccharin in either an assay for growth of human embryonic palatal mesenchymal cells or an assay for inhibition of mouse ovarian tumour cell attachment (Steele *et al.*, 1988).

Exposure of developing *Drosophila* larva to saccharin caused a dose-related increase in the incidence of bent humeral bristles in adults, suggesting potential developmental toxicity in mammals (Lynch *et al.*, 1991).

Saccharin [form unspecified] was considered to be inactive in a screening test for teratogenicity in rat embryonic limb buds in culture. The median concentrations that affected chondrogenesis and cell proliferation were 2600 and 4100 μg/mL, respectively (Renault *et al.*, 1989). Saccharin at concentrations up to 500 μg/mL did not inhibit mouse embryonic stem cell differentiation (Newall & Beedles, 1996).

Acid saccharin was evaluated for effects on amphibian development in an assay for teratogenicity in frog embryos as part of an interlaboratory validation study. The mean median lethal concentration, the concentration that induced malformations in 50% of the surviving embryos and the teratogenic index resulting from those concentrations in four laboratories were 16 mg/mL, 16 mg/mL and 1 mg/mL, respectively. The authors concluded that saccharin had little, if any, potential developmental toxicity (Bantle *et al.*, 1994).

Saccharin [form unspecified] did not affect offspring viability, growth or morphology when administrated by oral gavage to ICR mice at a minimal maternally toxic dose in a short-term test for teratogenicity (Seidenberg *et al.*, 1986).

Pregnant ICR mice (10 controls and five in each treated group) received intraperitoneal injections of 0, 500, 1000 or 2000 mg/kg sodium saccharin on day 10 of gestation, by oral gavage at 0, 5, 10 or 25 mg/kg on days 5–15 of gestation, or via the drinking-water as a 0, 5, 10 or 20% solution on days 0–17 of gestation. Fetuses were examined on day 17 of gestation for viability, growth and gross external and internal malformations. Dams exposed to 25 mg/kg per day by gavage had a slightly elevated incidence of resorptions (5/52 implants versus 7/125 in controls), but this was not significant; the only defect noted in any fetus was an isolated case of cleft palate in this treatment group (Dropkin *et al.*, 1985).

In a protocol to assess reproductive toxicity during continuous breeding, CD-1 mice were exposed to 0, 1.25, 2.5 or 5% sodium saccharin in the drinking-water, equivalent to 0, 3.5, 5.9 and 8.1 g/kg per day. The water consumption of the group at the high dose was reduced by 10–20%, whereas it was increased by 20 and 40% at the intermediate and low doses, respectively. Mortality, attributed to dehydration, occurred at a significantly increased rate at the high dose, and the numbers of live pups per litter and pup weight adjusted for litter size were reduced in this group. Exposure to sodium saccharin was maintained for the last litters from both the control and the intermediate-dose groups, and these offspring were used to produce an F_1 generation. There were no treatment-related effects on reproductive function, despite increased fluid consumption (National Toxicology Program, 1997).

4.4 Genetic and related effects

The genetic toxicology of saccharin has been reviewed (Arnold *et al.*, 1983; Ashby, 1985; Arnold & Boyes, 1989). Additional information on the genetic and related effects of saccharin is available in a more recent review (Whysner & Williams, 1996).

4.4.1 *Humans*

No data were available to the Working Group.

4.4.2 *Experimental systems* (see Tables 3 and 4 for references)

Saccharin did not induce gene mutation in *Salmonella typhimurium* strains TA100, TA1535, TA1537, TA1538, TA98, TA92 or TA94 in the presence or absence of an exogenous metabolic activation system. It induced aneuploidy in *Saccharomyces cerevisiae* diploid strain D6 but did not induce mitotic recombination.

The results of an alkaline elution assay showed DNA single-strand breaks in rat hepatocytes. The frequency of chromosomal aberrations was not increased in Chinese hamster lung fibroblasts *in vitro*. Saccharin did not induce cell transformation in mouse C3H 10T1/2

Table 3. Genetic and related effects of saccharin

Test system	Result[a]		Dose[b] (LED or HID)	Reference
	Without exogenous metabolic system	With exogenous metabolic system		
Salmonella typhimurium TA100, TA98, TA1535, TA1538, reverse mutation	NT	–	2500 μg/plate	Ashby *et al.* (1978)
Salmonella typhimurium TA100, TA98, TA1535, TA1537, TA1538, reverse mutation	–	–	5000 μg/plate	Rao *et al.* (1979)
Salmonella typhimurium TA100, TA98, TA94, TA92, TA1535, TA1537, reverse mutation	–	–	10000 μg/plate	Ishidate *et al.* (1984)
Salmonella typhimurium TA100, TA98, TA1535, TA1537, reverse mutation	–	–	10000 μg/plate	Mortelmans *et al.* (1986)
Saccharomyces cerevisiae D6, homozygosis	–	NT	500[c]	Parry *et al.* (1981)
Saccharomyces cerevisiae D6, aneuploidy	+	NT	400[c]	Parry *et al.* (1981)
DNA single-strand breaks, rat hepatocytes *in vitro*	(+)	NT	549	Sina *et al.* (1983)
Chromosomal aberrations, Chinese hamster lung cells *in vitro*	–	NT	4000	Ashby & Ishidate (1986)
Cell transformation, C3H10T1/2 mouse cells	–	NT	100	Saxholm *et al.* (1979)
Cell transformation, RLV/Fischer rat embryo cells	–	NT	50[c]	Traul *et al.* (1981)
Sister chromatid exchange, human lymphocytes *in vitro*	–	–	100	Saxholm *et al.* (1979)
Sister chromatid exchange, human lymphocytes *in vitro*	–	NT	500	Brøgger *et al.* (1979)
Inhibition of gap-junctional intercellular communication, normal and *hprt*-deficient human fibroblasts *in vitro*	–	NT	10000	Mosser & Bols (1983)
Inhibition of gap-junctional intercellular communication, human urothelial carcinoma cells *in vitro*	+	NT	3000	Morimoto (1996)

Table 3 (contd)

Test system	Result[a]		Dose[b] (LED or HID)	Reference
	Without exogenous metabolic system	With exogenous metabolic system		
Inhibition of gap-junctional intercellular communication, Chinese hamster lung V79 cells *in vitro*	+	NT	2000	Umeda *et al.* (1980)
Inhibition of gap-junctional intercellular communication, Chinese hamster lung V79 cells *in vitro*	+	NT	3000	Trosko *et al.* (1980)

[a] +, positive; (+), weakly positive; –, negative; NT, not tested
[b] LED, lowest effective dose; HID, highest ineffective dose; unless otherwise stated, in-vitro tests, μg/mL
[c] Form of saccharin not specified

Table 4. Genetic and related effects of saccharin, sodium

Test system	Result[a]		Dose[b] (LED or HID)	Reference
	Without exogenous metabolic system	With exogenous metabolic system		
Prophage induction	NT	–	250 000[c]	Ho & Ho (1981)
Salmonella typhimurium TA100, TA98, reverse mutation	–	–	800 000 µg/plate[d]	Batzinger *et al.* (1977)
Salmonella typhimurium TA100, TA98, TA1535, TA1537, reverse mutation	–	–	5000 µg/plate	Stoltz *et al.* (1977)
Salmonella typhimurium TA100, TA98, TA1535, TA1538, reverse mutation	NT	–	2500 µg/plate	Ashby *et al.* (1978)
Salmonella typhimurium TA100, TA98, TA1535, TA1537, reverse mutation	–	–	1000 µg/plate	Pool (1978)
Salmonella typhimurium TA100, TA98, TA1535, TA1537, TA1538, reverse mutation	–	–	40 000 µg/plate	Eckhardt *et al.* (1980)
Salmonella typhimurium TA100, TA98, TA1535, TA1537, TA1538, reverse mutation	–	–	10 250 µg/plate	De Flora (1981)
Salmonella typhimurium TA100, TA98, TA1535, TA1537, reverse mutation	NT	–	2500 µg/plate	Herbold (1981)
Salmonella typhimurium TA100, reverse mutation	NT	–	10 000 µg/plate	Imamura *et al.* (1983)
Salmonella typhimurium TA100, TA98, TA94, TA92, TA1535, TA1537, reverse mutation	–	–	10 000 µg/plate	Ishidate *et al.* (1984)
Saccharomyces cerevisiae CM-1293, gene conversion	+	NT	2000	Moore & Schmick (1979)
Saccharomyces cerevisiae CM-1293, homozygosis	+	NT	2000	Moore & Schmick (1979)
Saccharomyces cerevisiae DIS 13, homozygosis	–	NT	18 300[c]	Persic (1986)
Saccharomyces cerevisiae CM-1293, reverse mutation	+	NT	2000	Moore & Schmick (1979)
Saccharomyces cerevisiae DIS 13, aneuploidy	+	–	1830[c]	Persic (1986)
Drosophila melanogaster, sex-linked recessive lethal mutations	+		1140 feed	Rao *et al.* (1971)

Table 4 (contd)

Test system	Result[a]		Dose[b] (LED or HID)	Reference
	Without exogenous metabolic system	With exogenous metabolic system		
Drosophila melanogaster, sex-linked recessive lethal mutations	?		1 µg/fly inj	Kramers (1977)
Drosophila melanogaster, sex-linked recessive lethal mutations	–		82 000 feed	Eckhardt *et al.* (1980)
Drosophila melanogaster, heritable translocations	–		8300 feed	Rao *et al.* (1971)
Unscheduled DNA synthesis, Fischer 344 rat primary hepatocytes *in vitro*	–	NT	10 250	Jeffrey & Williams (1999)
Unscheduled DNA synthesis, Sprague-Dawley rat primary hepatocytes *in vitro*	–	NT	10 250	Jeffrey & Williams (1999)
Gene mutation, mouse lymphoma L5178Y cells, *tk* locus	–	–	12 500[e]	Clive *et al.* (1979)
Sister chromatid exchange, Chinese hamster Don cells *in vitro*	+	NT	206	Abe & Sasaki (1977)
Sister chromatid exchange, Chinese hamster ovary cells *in vitro*	+	NT	5000	Wolff & Rodin (1978)
Sister chromatid exchange, Chinese hamster ovary cells *in vitro*	(+)	NT	100	Ray-Chaudhuri *et al.* (1982)
Chromosomal aberrations, Chinese hamster embryonic lung Cl-1-15 cells *in vitro*	+	NT	100	Kristoffersson (1972)
Chromosomal aberrations, Chinese hamster Don cells *in vitro*	+	NT	1030	Abe & Sasaki (1977)
Chromosomal aberrations, Chinese hamster lung cells *in vitro*	+	NT	8000	Ishidate & Odashima (1977)
Chromosomal aberrations, Chinese hamster ovary CHO-K1 cells *in vitro*	+	NT	20 000	Masubuchi *et al.* (1977)
Chromosomal aberrations, Chinese hamster lung cells *in vitro*	+	NT	4000	Ashby & Ishidate (1986)
Cell transformation, BALB/c3T3 mouse cells	–	NT	500	Sivak & Tu (1980)
Cell transformation, BALB/c3T3 mouse cells	–	NT	5000	Sakai & Sato (1989)
Cell transformation, C3H 10T1/2 mouse cells	–	NT	2000[c]	Mondal *et al.* (1978)
Cell transformation, Fischer 344 rat urothelial cells	–	NT	2200	Knowles & Jani (1986)
Cell transformation, rat bladder explant	–	NT	1230	Nicholson & Jani (1988)
Gene mutation, human embryo RSa cells, Na^+/K^+ ATPase *in vitro*	+	NT	15 000	Suzuki & Suzuki (1988)

Table 4 (contd)

Test system	Result[a]		Dose[b] (LED or HID)	Reference
	Without exogenous metabolic system	With exogenous metabolic system		
Gene mutation, human embryo RSa cells, K-*ras* *in vitro*	+	NT	15 000	Suzuki & Suzuki (1993)
Sister chromatid exchange, human lymphocytes *in vitro*	+	NT	1000	Wolff & Rodin (1978)
Sister chromatid exchange, human lymphocytes *in vitro*	–	NT	500	Brøgger *et al.* (1979)
Chromosomal aberrations, human lymphocytes *in vitro*	+	NT	2000	Chang & Stacey (1974)
Cell transformation, human neonatal foreskin fibroblasts	–	NT	50	Milo *et al.* (1988)
Body fluids, mouse urine, *Salmonella typhimurium*, reverse mutation	+		2500 po × 1[d]	Batzinger *et al.* (1977)
Body fluids, rat bile, *Salmonella typhimurium*, reverse mutation	–		100 iv × 1	Connor *et al.* (1979)
Host-mediated assay, *Salmonella typhimurium* TA100, TA98 in mouse peritoneal cavity	+		2500 po × 1[d]	Batzinger *et al.* (1977)
DNA single-strand breaks, CD1 mouse liver or renal DNA *in vivo*	+		50 ip	Cesarone *et al.* (1980)
DNA damage, Wistar rat bladder *in vivo*	–		800 iv × 1[c]	Miyata *et al.* (1980)
Somatic mutation, mice *in vivo*	–		1000 ip × 1	Fahrig (1982)
Somatic mutation, mice *in vivo*	+		750 po × 3	Mahon & Dawson (1982)
Sister chromatid exchange, Chinese hamster bone marrow cells *in vivo*	+		5000 po × 1	Renner (1979)
Sister chromatid exchange, ICR mouse embryo cells *in vivo*	–		2000 ip × 1	Dropkin *et al.* (1985)
Micronucleus formation, C57BL mouse erythrocytes *in vivo*	–		2000 ip × 1	Léonard & Léonard (1979)
Micronucleus formation, NMRI mouse bone marrow cells *in vivo*	–		1025 po/ip × 2	Eckhardt *et al.* (1980)
Chromosomal aberrations, Chinese hamster bone marrow cells *in vivo*	–		1500 po × 3	Van Went-de Vries & Kragten (1975)
Chromosomal aberrations, C57BL mouse bone marrow cells *in vivo*	–		4000 ip × 1	Léonard & Léonard (1979)
Chromosomal aberrations, ICR mouse bone marrow cells *in vivo*	+		1000 diet × 24 w[c]	Prasad & Rai (1987)
Chromosomal aberrations, C57BL mice, spermatogonia *in vivo*, spermatocytes observed	–		2000 ip × 1	Léonard & Léonard (1979)

Table 4 (contd)

Test system	Result[a]		Dose[b] (LED or HID)	Reference
	Without exogenous metabolic system	With exogenous metabolic system		
Chromosomal aberrations, C3H × 101 mice, spermatogonia *in vivo*, spermatocytes observed	–		500 po × 10	Pecevski *et al.* (1983)
Chromosomal aberrations, ICR mice, spermatogonia *in vivo*, spermatocytes observed	+		1000 diet × 24 w[c]	Prasad & Rai (1987)
Chromosomal aberrations, Chinese hamster spermatogonia *in vivo*, spermatogonia observed	–		5000 × 2 po	Machemer & Lorke (1975a)
Chromosomal aberrations, ICR mouse embryo cells *in vivo*	–		2000 × 1 ip	Dropkin *et al.* (1985)
Dominant lethal mutation, Swiss and C17 mice *in vivo*	+		240 × 1 sc	Tezabwala & Gothoskar (1977)
Dominant lethal mutation, CBA mice *in vivo*	+		340 drink 30 d	Rao & Qureshi (1972)
Dominant lethal mutation, NMRI/BOM mice *in vivo*	–		5000 × 5 po	Machemer & Lorke (1973)
Dominant lethal mutation, ICR mice *in vivo*	+		200 × 5 ip	Šrám & Zudová (1974)
Dominant lethal mutation, mice *in vivo*	–		2000 diet 10 w	Lorke & Machemer (1975)
Dominant lethal mutation, mice *in vivo*	–		10 000 × 1 po	Machemer & Lorke (1975b)
Dominant lethal mutation, C57BL mice *in vivo*	–		2000 ip × 1	Léonard & Léonard (1979)
Mouse (C3H x 101) heritable translocations *in vivo*	–		500 × 10 po	Pecevski *et al.* (1983)
Binding (covalent) to SD rat liver or bladder DNA *in vivo*	–		390 × 1 po[c]	Lutz & Schlatter (1977)

Table 4 (contd)

Test system	Result[a]		Dose[b] (LED or HID)	Reference
	Without exogenous metabolic system	With exogenous metabolic system		
Inhibition of gap-junctional intercellular communication, Chinese hamster V79 cells *in vitro*	–	NT	1000	Welsch & Stedman (1984)
Sperm morphology, CBA x BALB/c mice *in vivo*	–		500 × 5 ip	Topham (1980)

[a] +, positive; (+), weakly positive; –, negative; NT, not tested; ?, inconclusive

[b] LED, lowest effective dose; HID, highest ineffective dose; unless otherwise stated in-vitro tests, μg/mL; in-vivo tests, mg/kg bw per day; po, oral; iv, intravenous; ip, intraperitoneal; w, week; d, day

[c] Identification as sodium saccharin is not stated specifically in the reference but is based on solubility in water as identified by Whysner & Williams (1996).

[d] Purified sample

[e] HID is for purified sample; HID for unpurified sample, 19 000 μg/mL

cells, in baby hamster kidney cells or in virally enhanced RLV/Fischer rat embryo cells. It did not increase the frequency of sister chromatid exchange in human lymphocyte cultures. Gap-junctional intercellular communication was inhibited in Chinese hamster V79 lung fibroblasts and in a human urothelial carcinoma cell line, but intercellular communication in human fibroblasts was unaffected.

Sodium saccharin did not induce prophage and was not mutagenic to *S. typhimurium* strains TA100, TA1535, TA1537, TA1538, TA98, TA92 or TA94 in the presence or absence of an exogenous metabolic activation system. In one study, both a purified and an unpurified sample of sodium saccharin induced gene conversions, mitotic recombination and reverse mutation in *Saccharomyces cerevisiae*. It induced sex-linked recessive lethal mutations in *Drosophila melanogaster* treated by injection or feed in two of three studies, but it did not induce heritable translocations in one of the studies after injection of males with sodium saccharin.

Sodium saccharin did not induce unscheduled DNA synthesis or repair as evaluated by net nuclear grain counts in hepatocyte preparations from Fischer 344 and Sprague-Dawley rats. In a single study, neither a purified nor an unpurified sample of sodium saccharin induced gene mutation at the *tk* locus in mouse lymphoma L5178Y cells exposed to the test compounds for 4 h with or without exogenous metabolic activation. Sodium saccharin did increase the frequency of sister chromatid exchanges and chromosomal aberrations in Chinese hamster ovary, lung and Don cells, but did not induce cell transformation in rat bladder explants or urothelial cells, or in BALB/c3T3 mouse or baby hamster kidney cells treated *in vitro*. In a single study, sodium saccharin did not inhibit gap-junctional intercellular communication in Chinese hamster V79 cell cultures.

Sodium saccharin was mutagenic in RSa cells, a cell line derived from human embryos, inducing a dose-dependent increase in the number of ouabain-resistant mutants after a 24-h treatment. Point mutations in codon 12 of K-*ras* were also induced in the RSa cell line after six days of treatment with sodium saccharin. In one study, sister chromatid exchange frequencies were not increased in human lymphocytes obtained from one male donor and cultured with sodium saccharin for 24–48 h, but in a second study, sister chromatid exchanges were induced in lymphocytes that were cultured for 72 h in media containing sodium saccharin. In a single study, chromosomal aberrations were also induced in human lymphocytes cultured with sodium saccharin for 72 h. In another study, human neonatal foreskin fibroblast cultures were not transformed by treatment with sodium saccharin for 12 h.

In a single study, sodium saccharin did not bind covalently to DNA in liver or bladder of Sprague-Dawley rats treated once by gavage. In another study, measurements of DNA sedimentation patterns showed that sodium saccharin did not induce DNA damage in the bladder of Wistar rats after a single intravenous injection. Three of four sodium saccharin samples were mutagenic to *S. typhimurium* strains TA100 and TA98 in a host-mediated assay in which mice received a single oral treatment; only the highly purified sample gave negative results in this assay. Urine samples collected from mice over 24 h after treatment with the same four samples were also mutagenic to *S. typhimurium*. Bile from

Sprague-Dawley rats exposed to sodium saccharin by a single intravenous injection was not mutagenic to *S. typhimurium* in a single study.

Sodium saccharin induced single-strand breaks in liver and kidney DNA of CD1 mice treated by intraperitoneal injection in one study. It induced sister chromatid exchanges in the bone marrow of Chinese hamsters when cells were analysed 26 h after a single oral dose in one study, but not in a second study of ICR mouse embryo cells exposed *in utero* from a single intraperitoneal injection to pregnant dams on day 10 of gestation. Sodium saccharin did not induce micronuclei in C57BL mouse erythrocytes or NMRI mouse bone marrow, nor did it induce chromosomal aberrations in Chinese hamster or C57BL mouse bone marrow after treatment *in vivo*. A single intraperitoneal injection of sodium saccharin to mice did not induce somatic mutation; however, the compound induced somatic mutations when given daily for three days by stomach intubation.

Sodium saccharin induced dominant lethal mutations in mice in three of seven studies. Positive results were reported in CBA mice exposed to sodium saccharin in the drinking-water for 30 days, in ICR mice treated with five daily intraperitoneal injections and in Swiss and C17 mice treated with a single subcutaneous injection. Dominant lethal mutations were not induced in mice treated with two intraperitoneal injections, a single oral dose, five daily oral doses or fed a diet containing sodium saccharin for 10 weeks. The frequencies of chromosomal aberrations in the bone marrow and of spermatogonia of ICR mice were significantly increased after daily doses of sodium saccharin by gavage for 24 weeks. Chromosomal aberrations were not induced by sodium saccharin in ICR mouse embryos treated *in utero* by two intraperitoneal injections to pregnant dams on day 10 of gestation. Sodium saccharin did not induce chromosomal aberrations in spermatogonia of mice treated with a single intraperitoneal injection or with 10 daily oral doses or in spermatogonia of Chinese hamsters treated with two oral doses. In single studies, sodium saccharin did not induce heritable translocations or abnormal sperm morphology in mice given five daily intraperitoneal injections or 10 daily oral doses, respectively.

4.5 Mechanistic considerations

Sodium saccharin fed at high doses to rats increases the incidence of tumours of the urinary bladder if administered throughout the rats' lifetime, beginning before conception, at birth or at 30 days of age, and the effect is greater in male than in female rats. Bladder tumours are produced only sporadically in single rats when feeding is begun later, as in the usual one-generation bioassays. In addition, sodium saccharin increases the incidence of bladder tumours when administered to adult rats after pretreatment with a known genotoxic bladder carcinogen or after freeze-ulceration. As noted in section 3, no significant increase in the incidence of tumours in other organs is produced in rats, and no reproducibly increased incidence of tumours in any tissue, including the urinary bladder, was produced when sodium saccharin was administered to mice, hamsters, guinea-pigs or monkeys, although none of these species has been studied as extensively as the rat.

In all species including humans, about 80–95% of an orally administered dose of sodium saccharin is absorbed and rapidly eliminated in the urine, largely by renal tubular secretion. Studies of tissue distribution, including two-generation studies, provided no evidence of significant accumulation of saccharin in the bladder. Very small amounts of saccharin were found in the urine of male neonatal rats (up to 18 days of age), presumably from the small amounts of saccharin transferred to the pups during lactation, as evidenced by the low concentration in the stomach contents (Sweatman & Renwick, 1982).

Several mechanisms have been suggested to explain the effects of high dietary doses of sodium saccharin in rats. The possibility that an impurity might be responsible was evaluated extensively in bioassays with *ortho*-toluene sulfonamide, which gave either negative results or involved administration of doses far in excess of those that contaminate saccharin. In addition, *ortho*-toluene sulfonamide is not a contaminant of saccharin synthesized by the Maumee method. The biological responses in short-term studies and in two-stage carcinogenesis studies were similar with sodium saccharin synthesized by the Maumee and by the Remsen-Fahlberg methods. Furthermore, the contaminants are not electrophilic.

Saccharin exists in ionized form under physiological conditions. As the anion is a nucleophile (pKa of saccharin, 2.0), it would not form DNA adducts without prior metabolic alteration. As expected, no binding to DNA was detected after administration to rats *in vivo*. None of the studies in humans provided evidence for biotransformation of saccharin, and several studies in experimental animals showed no metabolism of sodium saccharin at a limit of detection of 0.4% of the administered dose. Trace amounts of metabolic products were found in one study, but the metabolites were not electrophiles; it is not possible to evaluate whether the investigators completely excluded contaminants in their purification process.

The dose-related caecal enlargement that is produced by sodium saccharin led Sims and Renwick (1983) to propose that sodium saccharin changes protein metabolism, leading to accumulation of tryptophan which is converted to indoles by the gastrointestinal microflora. Consequently, indole excretion may promote bladder tumours. Schoenig and Anderson (1985) found, however, that female rats fed sodium saccharin had larger caeca than males. Anderson *et al.* (1988b) found that the caecal enlargement was caused by the potassium, calcium and acid forms of saccharin. Therefore, the cation and sex specificity of sodium saccharin-induced cell proliferation and tumorigenicity cannot be explained by this hypothesis.

Another mechanistic hypothesis relates to sodium saccharin-induced increases in urine volume and sodium excretion. Anderson (1988) proposed that the high urine volume induced increases cell proliferation and bladder mass; however, this concept is unlikely to explain all of the sex-, age- and cation-specific results, and drugs that greatly enhance urine volume have not been associated with induction of bladder tumours.

The most plausible mechanism of the effects of high dietary doses of sodium saccharin in rats is the formation of a calcium phosphate-containing precipitate in the urine which is cytotoxic to the urothelium, resulting in mild regenerative hyperplasia which leads to tumour formation in a small percentage of rats.

Hyperplasia of the urothelium has been demonstrated in various long-term and short-term studies after dietary administration of high doses of sodium saccharin to rats. In a two-generation bioassay, hyperplasia of the bladder epithelium was found in conjunction with bladder tumour formation. At some doses at which tumours were found, a statistically significant increase in hyperplasia was found (Squire, 1985). In a species comparison, male Fischer 344 rats responded to 5% [2500 mg/kg bw per day] sodium saccharin with urothelial cell proliferation, whereas the male B6C3F$_1$ mice, Syrian hamsters and Hartley strain guinea-pigs did not (Fukushima *et al.*, 1983a).

Several other short-term studies have shown that exposure of male rats to sodium saccharin in the diet increases the frequency of cell proliferation in the bladder epithelium secondary to necrosis of superficial cells and exfoliation. The necrosis appears to be limited to the superficial cell layer, without ulceration and without inflammation. In investigations of the time-course of the effects of sodium saccharin on the bladder, vacuolar degeneration of epithelial cells has been demonstrated by light microscopy and superficial cell necrosis by scanning electron microscopy; these lesions are followed by hyperplasia and increased DNA labelling (tritiated thymidine or bromodeoxyuridine). In one study of male Fischer 344 rats, the rate of cell division after 10 weeks of treatment was found to be enhanced at dietary concentrations of 5 and 7.5% sodium saccharin [2500 and 3750 mg/kg bw per day] (Cohen *et al.*, 1990), even after four and seven weeks with 7.5% sodium saccharin, but no effect was found with 3% sodium saccharin [1500 mg/kg bw per day] in the diet. The sodium saccharin dose-related increases in cell proliferation correlated with evidence of cell damage, although cell damage without significant cell proliferation was found with 3% sodium saccharin at 10 weeks. This study indicates a close dose–response relationship between cell damage, cell proliferation, carcinogenesis in two-generation bioassays and tumour promotion. In a two-generation study of exposure to 5% sodium saccharin or acid saccharin [2500 mg/kg bw per day] in the diet, increased bladder epithelial cell proliferation was found only after administration of the sodium salt to males and females of the F$_1$ generation from 21 days of age.

A comparative study of various forms of saccharin in male rats demonstrated that cell proliferation was increased with sodium and potassium saccharin, but saccharin did not increase the labelling index (Hasegawa & Cohen, 1986); the results with calcium saccharin were equivocal and slight. The urinary concentration of saccharin was the same after administration of any of the four forms. Sodium bicarbonate also increased cell proliferation, and this effect appeared to be additive to that of sodium saccharin (Debiec-Rychter & Wang, 1990). Sodium chloride and sodium ascorbate both increased the thymidine labelling index by about fourfold, and in this experiment sodium saccharin increased the labelling index in bladder epithelium by about sevenfold over that in controls.

Diet has been shown to affect the ability of sodium saccharin to enhance bladder epithelial cell proliferation: animals fed AIN-76A diet (a semisynthetic diet with casein as the protein source, resulting in low urinary pH) did not show sodium saccharin-induced increases in cell proliferation, and diet-specific changes in urinary pH have been proposed to be an important factor (Garland *et al.*, 1989). Sodium ascorbate and sodium saccharin administered during one- and two-generation studies and in two-stage studies of carcinogenesis were found to have similar hyperplastic effects on the urinary bladder. The effects of saccharin and ascorbate were inhibited by co-administration of ammonium chloride, which acidified the urine (Ellwein & Cohen, 1990; Uwagawa *et al.*, 1994; Cohen *et al.*, 1995a, 1998; Cohen, 1999).

Sodium saccharin and sodium ascorbate are tumorigenic in male rats but usually only when administered in a two-generation protocol rather than in a standard two-year bioassay beginning at six to eight weeks of age (Ellwein & Cohen, 1990; Cohen *et al.*, 1998; Cohen, 1999). Several sodium salts administered at high doses in the diet have, however, produced bladder tumours in male rats after prior administration of a known genotoxic bladder carcinogen. These salts include sodium saccharin, sodium ascorbate, sodium aspartate, sodium citrate, sodium erythorbate, sodium succinate, sodium bicarbonate and sodium chloride. All these salts and sodium glutamate and sodium phosphate increased proliferation (hyperplasia) in the bladder in short-term studies in male rats when fed at doses comparable to 5 or 7.5% sodium saccharin (Ellwein & Cohen, 1990; Cohen *et al.*, 1995c; Cohen, 1999).

These data indicate that the sequence of events leading to the tumorigenicity of these chemicals is superficial cytotoxicity resulting in regenerative hyperplasia and ultimately in the production of bladder tumours. This effect appears to occur only in rats and more severely in males than in females. Administration from 30 days of age or earlier appears to be necessary to attain a significant incidence of bladder tumours in long-term bioassays.

The requirement for administration beginning early in life appears to be due to quantitative relationships with the total amount of urothelial cell proliferation occurring during the course of the experiment (Ellwein & Cohen, 1988). The urothelium proliferates rapidly during gestation, but the rate quickly decreases after birth, so that the tritiated thymidine labelling index (1-h pulse dose) is 0.1% or less by six weeks of age. Approximately one-third of the lifetime cell divisions of rat urothelium occur by six weeks of age. Feeding sodium saccharin in a two-generation protocol increased proliferation by 21 days of age, substantially increasing the number of cell divisions early in the life of the rat, which can then be sustained by continued administration of sodium saccharin. This process can be reproduced quantitatively by ulcerating the adult male rat bladder, allowing it to heal and then administering 5% sodium saccharin (Cohen *et al.*, 1982). The incidence of bladder tumours produced in this ulcer–saccharin protocol after two years is similar to that seen with high doses of sodium saccharin in two-generation studies in male rats.

Although several factors have been associated with the induction of urothelial toxicity, it appears to be due to the formation of a precipitate in the urine of rats after administration of high doses of sodium salts. This effect was first observed by Arnold *et al.* (1980) and subsequently by West and Jackson (1981) and Cohen *et al.* (1991). The effect has been observed in the urine of rats given high doses of sodium salts including those of saccharin, ascorbate, glutamate, aspartate, citrate, erythorbate, chloride and bicarbonate; in the urine of male rats more than in female rats (Arnold *et al.*, 1980); and not in mice or monkeys

(Takayama *et al.*, 1998; Cohen, 1999). In addition, co-administration of high doses of ammonium chloride with sodium saccharin or sodium ascorbate completely inhibits the appearance of the urinary precipitate (Cohen *et al.*, 1995a,c). Thus, there is a close correlation between the presence of this precipitate and the subsequent urothelial toxic and proliferative effects.

The major inorganic constituents of the precipitate appear to be calcium and phosphate, but there are significant amounts of a silicon-containing substance. In addition, the major organic components are mucopolysaccharides and urea, with small amounts of protein and saccharin (Cohen *et al.*, 1995b,c; Cohen, 1999). Calcium and phosphate in solution are essential ingredients for cell viability *in vitro* and *in vivo*, but calcium phosphate precipitate *in vitro* is cytotoxic to epithelial cells, including urothelial cells (Brash *et al.*, 1987; Cohen, 1999).

Several factors appear to be critical for the formation of the calcium phosphate-containing precipitate: the main ones are high concentrations of calcium, phosphate and protein, pH ≥ 6.5 and high osmolality (Table 5). These factors appear to be critical only in rats (Cohen, 1999). Adequate concentrations of calcium and phosphate are required for precipitation; the rat has approximately 10–20 times more urinary calcium than the mouse and an approximately two to four times higher phosphate concentration (Cohen, 1995). In addition, after being fed high doses of sodium saccharin, rats consume more water, with a consequently increased urinary volume and overall dilution of the urine; however, the urinary concentrations of calcium and phosphate do not decrease (Schoenig & Anderson, 1985).

Urinary precipitate formation is inhibited by a urinary pH below 6.5 (Cohen *et al.*, 1995b,c). After administration of high doses of sodium saccharin, the urinary pH may be similar to, lower than or higher than that of controls, but it remains above 6.5 (Ellwein & Cohen, 1990). If the compound is co-administered with ammonium chloride or if it is administered in AIN-76A semisynthetic diet, the urinary pH is below 6.0, no precipitate is found and there is no urothelial toxicity, regenerative hyperplasia or tumour formation. Thus, the parent acids, saccharin and ascorbic acid, do not cause these effects, since the urinary pH remains low after their administration. Sodium hippurate also does not produce these proliferative effects in rats, although the urinary pH remains below 6.3 after its administration (Fukushima *et al.*, 1983a; Schoenig *et al.*, 1985).

High urinary protein concentrations also appear to be necessary. Although the urinary concentration of protein is high in male and female rats, it is higher in males after sexual maturity because of the excretion of α_{2u}-globulin (Neuhaus & Flory, 1978; Hard, 1995). Studies of sodium saccharin- and sodium ascorbate-induced cell proliferation in NBR rats, which do not have very high urinary levels of the male rat-specific low-molecular-mass protein α_{2u}-globulin, have shown the importance of this protein (Garland *et al.*, 1994; Uwagawa *et al.*, 1994). Rats that do not produce this protein do not show the enhanced bladder epithelial cell proliferation caused by sodium saccharin or sodium ascorbate and behave similarly to females of other strains, such as Fischer 344. Male Fischer 344 rats given sodium saccharin in the diet had a statistically significantly greater

Table 5. Urinary concentrations of critical variables in various species and strains (control and treated) for the urothelial response to treatment with high doses of sodium saccharin in the diet

Variable	Species								
	Rat					Mouse[e]		Monkey[f]	Human
	Male[a]	Female[a]	Male[a,b]	Male[c]	Male[d]	Male	Female		
High protein[g]	++	+	++	+	±	++	+	–	–
High Ca^{++}, PO_4[g]	+	+	+	+	ND	–	–	+ or –	+ or –
pH ≥ 6.5[g]	+	+	–	+	+	+	+	+ or –	+ or –
High osmolality[g]	+	+	+	+	ND	+	+	–	–
Precipitate formation[h]	+	±	–	±	ND	–	–	–[i]	ND
Hyperplasia[h]	+	±	–	–	–	–	–	–[i]	ND
Tumorigenic effect[h]	+	±	–	ND	–	–	–	–[i]	

+, positive response; ±, equivocal response; –, negative response; + or –, both responses have been observed; ND, not determined; ++, higher protein concentrations in male rats and mice than in females

[a] Fischer 344 and Sprague-Dawley

[b] Rats given a treatment resulting in acidification of the urine, consisting of either acid saccharin, high doses of ammonium chloride with sodium saccharin or sodium saccharin in AIN-76A diet

[c] NBR rats deficient in α_{2u}-globulin

[d] Rats deficient in albumin

[e] Data on urinary parameters and hyperplasia for BALB/c and Swiss strains, data on tumorigenicity for BALB/c mice

[f] Cynomolgus, rhesus and African green

[g] Similar in control animals and in those treated with high doses of sodium saccharin

[h] Urinary precipitate formed in the urine and urothelial hyperplasia or tumours after administration of high doses of sodium saccharin in the diet; the tumorigenic effects include any found in one- or two-generation studies or the two-stage studies in different species

[i] Monkeys given sodium saccharin at a dose of 25 mg/kg bw per day for 18–23 years beginning at birth or within a few days of birth. The Working Group noted the relatively small dose of saccharin administered, the relatively small number of monkeys used and the multiplicity of species.

degree of hyperplasia and much higher cell proliferation rates than control Fischer 344 rats or NBR rats. Therefore, the difference in cell proliferation between these two strains of rats presumably correlates with the differences in urinary excretion of α_{2u}-globulin. Females were found to have no, or at most a very weak, tumorigenic response to sodium saccharin in two-generation studies (Tisdel *et al.*, 1974; Arnold *et al.*, 1980; Taylor *et al.*, 1980), and females do not excrete significant amounts of α_{2u}-globulin.

At three weeks of age, when proliferation increases after dietary administration of sodium saccharin, male and female rats have a similar urinary composition, with high protein concentrations due primarily to albumin. Albumin is present at higher concentrations in male and female rats than in humans and also appears to be effective in contributing to the proliferative effects caused by sodium saccharin. Feeding sodium saccharin to analbuminaemic rats does not produce a proliferative response in the urothelium (Homma *et al.*, 1991).

High osmolality also contributes to a greater likelihood of precipitation, and the osmolality of the urine of rats and mice is usually in the range of 1000–2000 mosm/kg or higher. In humans, urinary osmolality is usually < 300, and it has been calculated theoretically not to exceed 1000–1100. Rodents have a higher osmolality mainly because of their greater protein and urea concentrations.

The concentration of the administered anion does not appear to contribute much to formation of the precipitate. Although the urinary saccharin concentration after feeding at 5% of the diet is approximately 200 mmol/L, only small amounts are found in the precipitate. In addition, feeding sodium ascorbate at 5 or 7% in the diet produces the precipitate, but the urinary concentration of ascorbate is less than 20 mmol/L.

Thus, critical levels of multiple factors are required for the precipitate to form. The lower urinary protein concentrations in female rats appear to explain the differences in their response from that of male rats, and the lower urinary calcium and phosphate concentrations in mice appear to explain their lack of both precipitate formation and a urothelial proliferative response. Non-human primates and humans are not expected to develop the precipitate because they have lower urinary protein concentrations and osmolality.

Chemicals that induce urinary calculi, such as melamine and uric acid, produce urothelial toxicity, regenerative proliferation and tumours in rodent bladders. Calculi also appear slightly to increase the risk for bladder cancer in humans (Capen *et al.*, 1999). Since bladder tumours are induced only at doses that produce urinary calculi, this process represents a threshold phenomenon. The production of bladder tumours after the feeding of high doses of various sodium salts by a mechanism involving formation of a calcium phosphate-containing precipitate in the urine thus represents a process that is both species-specific (rat) and occurs only at high doses (threshold).

As described in Capen *et al.* (1999), calcium phosphate-containing precipitates in the urine of rats, such as those produced by the administration of high doses of some sodium salts, including sodium saccharin and sodium ascorbate, can result in the production of urinary bladder tumours. This sequence can be considered to be species- and dose-specific and is not known to occur in humans.

In making an overall evaluation of the carcinogenicity of saccharin and its salts to humans, it can be concluded that the production of bladder cancer in rats via a mechanism involving calcium phosphate-containing precipitates is not predictive of a carcinogenic hazard to humans, provided that the following criteria are met:

- the formation of the calcium phosphate-containing precipitate occurs under the conditions of the bioassay in which cancer is induced;
- prevention of formation of the urinary precipitate results in prevention of the proliferative effect in the bladder;
- the agent (and/or its metabolites) has no genotoxic activity *in vitro* or *in vivo*;
- the agent does not produce tumours at any other site in experimental animals; and
- there is evidence from studies in humans that precipitate formation or excess cancer risk does not occur in exposed populations.

Sodium saccharin produces urothelial bladder tumours in rats by a non-DNA-reactive mechanism. The calcium phosphate-containing precipitate occurs in the urine under the conditions of the bioassays. The proliferative effect of sodium saccharin and the formation of the precipitate are prevented by acidification of rat urine. In addition, urine acidification prevents the tumorigenic effect of sodium saccharin in two-stage bioassays. Sodium saccharin does not produce tumours at any other site in experimental animals. Epidemiological studies have not shown that the incidence of cancer is increased in saccharin-exposed populations.

5. Summary of Data Reported and Evaluation

5.1 Exposure data

Saccharin and its salts have been used as sweeteners for nearly a century. Saccharin (acid form), sodium saccharin and calcium saccharin are widely used as non-caloric table-top sweeteners, in beverages and foods, in personal care products and in a variety of non-food applications. The average daily dietary intake is generally less than 1 mg/kg bw.

5.2 Human carcinogenicity data

Case–control studies of the carcinogenicity of artificial sweeteners have been reported only for the urinary bladder or lower urinary tract. Most of the studies were published between 1975 and 1985, so that any association would be to sweeteners that were on the market over 25 years ago. The studies varied widely in the detail with which information on the source and nature of artificial sweeteners was identified, collected and presented. The terms used in the various studies include 'table-top', 'dietetic beverages', 'saccharin' and 'artificial sweeteners' with no further characterization; only the salts of saccharin are used in these ways. Eight of the studies considered were hospital-based, which raises uncertainty about the representativeness of the controls' consumption of artificial sweeteners in relation to the general population. The results of the population-based studies must also be viewed with caution, owing to the sizable proportion of non-respondents, which might reflect the occurrence of health-related conditions associated with the use of replacements for sugar.

A statistically significant relative risk in the order of 1.6 for the association between use of artificial sweeteners (and saccharin salts as such) and bladder cancer and a dose–response relationship between intake and odds ratio were found for men but not for women in an early study in Canada. In subsequent population-based studies, including a study of several thousand people in the United States, estimates for the entire population of each study did not confirm the existence of an assocation. In some studies, estimates of the strength of the association between consumption of sweeteners and bladder cancer differed between smokers and non-smokers, but the direction of the difference and its distribution between the sexes was inconsistent over the studies.

In spite of the fact that three studies showed high, statistically significant relative risks for small subsets of consumers of very large amounts of artificial sweeteners, the finding was limited to men in one study and to women in the other two. In addition, no consistent pattern of dose–response relationship between use of artificial sweeteners and cancers of the urinary bladder or lower urinary tract is apparent in the available literature.

5.3 Animal carcinogenicity data

Sodium saccharin was tested by oral administration in numerous experiments in rats and mice and in a few studies in hamsters, guinea-pigs and monkeys.

Sodium saccharin produced urinary bladder tumours in male rats in four two-generation studies, in one study in male rats in which administration commenced at birth and in one study commencing at 30 days of age. Sodium saccharin was not carcinogenic for the urinary bladder in several one-generation studies in male and female rats or in mice.

Saccharin (acid form) did not produce tumours in one study in male and female mice, in one study in male rats or in one study in female rats. Calcium saccharin did not produce tumours in one study in male rats.

A few studies with sodium saccharin in hamsters and guinea-pigs also showed no induction of bladder tumours but were considered inadequate. In one long-term (up to 23 years) study in monkeys in which oral administration of sodium saccharin was begun shortly after birth, no bladder tumours were observed, but a relatively low dose (25 mg/kg bw) and relatively few animals were used.

Sodium saccharin has been studied in numerous experiments in adult rats involving administration concurrently or, more frequently, sequentially with other chemicals or treatments. Enhanced bladder tumorigenesis has been observed after prior treatment with known urinary bladder carcinogens. In one study, saccharin (acid form) did not significantly enhance the incidence of bladder carcinogenesis, while calcium saccharin produced a marginal increase.

Thus, the only organ affected by sodium saccharin is the urinary bladder and only in rats exposed for periods including pre- and/or postnatal periods and/or when exposure was begun by 30 days of age.

5.4 Other relevant data

Studies in humans and rodents reveal that, after absorption, saccharin and sodium saccharin are excreted unchanged in the urine. Excretion occurs relatively rapidly with no evidence of accumulation. The strong nucleophilic character of the saccharin anion and the lack of metabolism are consistent with the lack of DNA reactivity. The urinary concentration of the saccharin anion is similar, regardless of the form administered.

Sodium saccharin has been shown to enhance urothelial cell proliferation in rats, primarily in males, resulting in hyperplasia. This regenerative cell proliferation follows urothelial cytotoxic effects. Administration of saccharin (acid form) does not produce these effects in rats. Sodium saccharin at doses that enhance cell proliferation in rats does not do so in other species, including mice, hamsters and guinea-pigs. Hyperplasia was not produced in non-human primates, although the dose used in this study was lower than that used in the studies in rodents.

The cytotoxicity has been shown to result from formation of a calcium phosphate-containing precipitate in rat urine after administration of high doses of sodium saccharin or a variety of other sodium salts. A combination of factors in urine composition appears to be critical for formation of the precipitate, including a pH of 6.5 or greater, high urinary concentrations of calcium phosphate and protein and high urinary osmolality. This combination of critical factors appears to be unique to the rat and is consistent with the species-specific urothelial proliferative and tumorigenic effects in rats.

Saccharin, generally as the sodium salt, has been tested for developmental and reproductive toxicity in mice, rats, hamsters and rabbits. The effects have generally been limited to reductions in body weights at high dietary concentrations. With the exception of a test in *Drosophila* larvae, no effects have been reported in a variety of short-term assays to screen for teratogenicity *in vivo* and *in vitro*.

Saccharin (acid form) was not genotoxic in human or rodent cells *in vitro*. It weakly induced DNA single-strand breaks in rat hepatocyte cultures. It induced aneuploidy in yeast but was not mutagenic to bacteria.

Sodium saccharin induced dominant lethality in three of seven studies in mice *in vivo*; it did not induce heritable translocations, chromosomal aberrations in spermatocytes or embryos or altered sperm morphology in rodents *in vivo*. Negative or conflicting results were obtained in most studies of chromosomal damage in bone marrow, somatic mutation and sister chromatid exchange in rodents *in vivo*. Sodium saccharin was mutagenic in host-mediated and body fluid assays and caused DNA single-strand breaks in hepatic and renal cells of mice; however, bile from rats exposed to sodium saccharin was not mutagenic. Sodium saccharin did not cause DNA damage and did not bind covalently to DNA of rat liver or bladder. It induced genotoxic effects in human and rodent cells and in *Drosophila* and yeast. It was not mutagenic to bacteria.

The positive results for genotoxicity found with sodium saccharin in mammalian cells *in vitro* have been hypothesized to result from increased osmolality (i.e. nonspecific ionic effects). This hypothesis would appear to explain some but not all of the findings of sister chromatid exchange, chromosomal aberrations and gene mutations *in vitro*. The few positive results seen in mice treated with sodium saccharin *in vivo* would not be readily explained by ionic influences.

Impurities in the test materials could explain the positive results obtained in some studies in mice treated with high doses of sodium saccharin. It is notable that no data are available on the genetic effects of saccharin or its salts in rats; however, the available evidence indicates no binding of sodium saccharin to DNA in rat bladder or liver. Overall, the results of tests for genotoxicity do not support a mechanism for the induction of urothelial-cell tumours in rats involving direct interaction of sodium saccharin with DNA.

5.5 Evaluation

There is *inadequate evidence* in humans for the carcinogenicity of saccharin salts used as sweeteners.

There is *sufficient evidence* in experimental animals for the carcinogenicity of sodium saccharin.

There is *inadequate evidence* in experimental animals for the carcinogenicity of saccharin (acid form) and calcium saccharin.

Overall evaluation

In making its evaluation, the Working Group concluded that sodium saccharin produces urothelial bladder tumours in rats by a non-DNA-reactive mechanism that involves the formation of a urinary calcium phosphate-containing precipitate, cytotoxicity and enhanced cell proliferation. This mechanism is not relevant to humans because of critical interspecies differences in urine composition.

Saccharin and its salts are *not classifiable as to their carcinogenicity to humans (Group 3).*

6. References

Abe, S. & Sasaki, M. (1977) Chromosome aberrations and sister chromatid exchanges in Chinese hamster cells exposed to various chemicals. *J. natl Cancer Inst.*, **58**, 1635–1641

Adkins, A., Hupp, E.W. & Gerdes, R.A. (1972) Biological activity of saccharins and cyclamates in golden hamsters (Abstract). *Texas J. Sci.*, **23**, 575

Akdas, A., Kirkali, Z. & Bili, N. (1990) Epidemiological case–control study on the etiology of bladder cancer in Turkey. *Eur. Urol.*, **17**, 23–26

Allen, M.J., Boyland, E., Dukes, C.E., Horning, E.S. & Watson, J.G. 1957) Cancer of the urinary bladder induced in mice with metabolites of aromatic amines and tryptophan. *Br. J. Cancer*, **11**, 212–231

Althoff, J., Cardesa, A., Pour, P. & Shubik, P. (1975) A chronic study of artificial sweeteners in Syrian golden hamsters. *Cancer Lett.*, **1**, 21–24

American Chemical Society (1998) *CAS Records*, Washington DC

Anderson, R.L. (1979) Response of male rats to sodium saccharin ingestion: Urine composition and mineral balance. *Food Cosmet. Toxicol.*, **17**, 195–200

Anderson, R.L. (1988) An hypothesis of the mechanism of urinary bladder tumorigenesis in rats ingesting sodium saccharin. *Food chem. Toxicol.*, **26**, 637–644

Anderson, R.L. & Kirkland, J.J. (1980) The effect of sodium saccharin in the diet on caecal microflora. *Food Cosmet. Toxicol.*, **18**, 353–355

Anderson, R.L., Lefever, F.R. & Maurer, J.K. (1988a) Comparison of the responses of male rats to dietary sodium saccharin exposure initiated during nursing with responses to exposure initiated at weaning. *Food chem. Toxicol.*, **26**, 899–907

Anderson, R.L., Lefever, F.R. & Maurer, J.K. (1988b) The effect of various saccharin forms on gastro-intestinal tract, urine and bladder of male rats. *Food chem. Toxicol.*, **26**, 665–669

Anderson, R.L., Lefever, F.R., Miller, N.S. & Maurer, J.K. (1989) Comparison of the bladder response to indole and sodium saccharin ingestion by male rats. *Food chem. Toxicol.*, **27**, 777–779

Anon. (1978) The food, drugs and chemical substances (food labelling, additives and standards) regulations, 1978. *Kenya Gazette*, **Suppl. 40**, special issue (Leg. Suppl. 27)

Anon. (1981) *Prevention of Food Adulteration Act 1954 (37 of 1954) and P.F.A. Rules, 1995, with Notifications and Commodity Index together with Comments as Amended up to 31 December 1980*, New Delhi, Army Educational Stores

Anon. (1983) *Tentative Safe Exposure Limits of Contaminants in Ambient Air of Residential Areas* (2947-83), Moscow, Ministry of Health Care of USSR

Anon. (1988) General statutory rules. *Gazette of India*, 1157 (E)

Association of Official Analytical Chemists International (1995) Food additives: Direct. In: Cunniff, P., ed., *Official Methods of Analysis of AOAC International*, 16th Ed., Arlington, VA, pp. 49–51

Arnold, D.L. & Boyes. B.G. (1989) The toxicological effects of saccharin in short-term genotoxicity assays. *Mutat. Res.*, **221**, 69–132

Arnold, D.L., Moodie, C.A., McGuire, P.F., Collins, B.T., Charbonneau, S.M. & Munro, I.C. (1979) The effect of *ortho* toluenesulfonamide and sodium saccharin on the urinary tract of neonatal rats. *Toxicol. appl. Pharmacol.*, **51,** 455–463

Arnold, D.L., Moodie, C.A., Grice, H.C., Charbonneau, S.M., Stavric, B., Collins, B.T., McGuire, P.F., Zawidzka, Z.Z. & Munro, I.C. (1980) Long-term toxicity of *ortho*-toluenesulfonamide and sodium saccharin in the rat. *Toxicol. appl. Pharmacol.*, **52**, 113–152

Arnold, D.L., Krewski, D. & Munro, I.C. (1983) Saccharin: A toxicological and historical perspective. *Toxicology*, **27**, 179–256

Ashby, J. (1985) The genotoxicity of sodium saccharin and sodium chloride in relation to their cancer-promoting properties. *Food chem. Toxicol.*, **23**, 507–519

Ashby, J. & Ishidate, M., Jr (1986) Clastogenicity in vitro of the Na, K, Ca and Mg salts of saccharin; and of magnesium chloride; consideration of significance. *Mutat. Res.*, **163**, 63–73

Ashby, J., Styles, J.A., Anderson, D. & Paton, D. (1978) Saccharin: An epigenetic carcinogen/ mutagen? *Food Cosmet. Toxicol.*, **16**, 95–103

Ball, L.M., Renwick, A.G. & Williams, R.T. (1977) The fate of [^{14}C]saccharin in man, rat and rabbit and of 2-sulphamoyl[^{14}C]benzoic acid in the rat. *Xenobiotica*, **7**, 189–203

Ball, L.M., Williams, R.T. & Renwick, A.G. (1978) The fate of saccharin impurities. The excretion and metabolism of ^{14}C toluene-4-sulphonamide and 4-sulphamoyl ^{14}C-benzoic acid in the rat. *Xenobiotica*, **8**, 183–190

Bantle, J.A., Burton, D.T., Dawson, D.A., Dumont, J.N., Finch, R.A., Fort, D.J., Linder, G., Rayburn, J.R., Buchwalter, D., Gaudet-Hull, A.M., Maurice, M.A. & Turley, S.D. (1994) Fetax interlaboratory validation study: Phase II testing. *Environ. Toxicol. Chem.*, **12**, 1629–1637

Bär, A. & Biermann, C. (1992) Intake of intense sweeteners in Germany. *Z. Ernährungswiss.*, **31**, 25–39

Batzinger, R.P., Ou, S.-Y.L. & Bueding, E. (1977) Saccharin and other sweeteners: Mutagenic properties. *Science*, **198**, 944–946

Bizzari, S.N., Leder, A.E. & Ishikawa, Y. (1996) High-intensity sweeteners. In: *Chemical Economics Handbook*, Menlo Park, CA, SRI International

Bourgoignie, J.J., Hwang, K.H., Pennell, J.P. & Bricker, N.S. (1980) Renal excretion of 2,3-dihydro-3-oxobenzisosulfonazole (saccharin). *Am. J. Physiol.,* **238,** F10–F15

Brash, D.E., Reddel, R.R., Quanrud, M., Yang, K., Farrell, M.P. & Harris, C.C. (1987) Strontium phosphate transfection of human cells in primary culture: Stable expression of the simian virus 40 large-T-antigen gene in primary human bronchial epithelial cells. *Mol. cell. Biol.*, **7**, 2031–2034

Brennessel, B.A. & Keyes, K.J. (1985) Saccharin induces morphological changes and enhances prolactin production of GH_4C_1 cells. *In Vitro cell. Dev. Biol.*, **21,** 402–408

British Pharmacopoeial Commission (1993) *British Pharmacopoeia 1993*, Vol. I, London, Her Majesty's Stationery Office, pp. 582–584

British Pharmacopoeial Commission (1995) *British Pharmacopoeia 1993*, Addendum 1995, London, Her Majesty's Stationery Office, pp. 1602–1603

Brøgger, A., Ardito, G. & Waksvik, H. (1979) No synergism between caffeine and saccharin in the induction of sister chromatid exchange in human lymphocytes. *Hereditas*, **91**, 135–138

Bryan, G.T., Erturk, E. & Yoshida, O. (1970) Production of urinary bladder carcinomas in mice by sodium saccharin. *Science*, **168**, 1238–1240

Budavari, S., ed. (1996) *The Merck Index*, 12th Ed., Whitehouse Station, NJ, Merck & Co., p. 1430

Byard, J.L. & Goldberg, L. (1973) The metabolism of saccharin in laboratory animals. *Food Cosmet. Toxicol.*, **11**, 391–402

Byard, J.L., McChesney, E.W., Goldberg, L. & Coulston, F. (1974) Excretion and metabolism with ^{14}C-labelled and unlabelled saccharin. *Food Cosmet. Toxicol.*, **12,** 175–184

Calorie Control Council (1996a) *Saccharin: A Scientific Review*, Atlanta, GA

Calorie Control Council (1996b) *Worldwide Status of Saccharin*, Atlanta, GA

Capen, C., Dybing, E., Rice, J. & Wilbourn, J., eds (1999) *Species Differences in Thyroid, Kidney and Urinary Bladder Carcinogenesis* (IARC Scientific Publications No. 147), Lyon, IARC

Cartwright, R.A., Adib, R., Glashan, R. & Gray, B.K. (1981) The epidemiology of bladder cancer in West Yorkshire. A preliminary report on non-occupational etiologies. *Carcinogenesis*, **2,** 343–347

Cesarone, C.F., Bolognesi, C. & Santi, L. (1980) [Study of the hepatic and renal toxicity induced by administration of sodium saccharin: Single-strand DNA breaks.] *Boll. Soc. Ital. Biol. sper.*, **56**, 2486–2491 (in Italian)

Chang, P. & Stacey, T. (1974) Sodium saccharin: Cytogenetic effect on human lymphocytes in vitro. *Proc. Pa. Acad. Sci.*, **48**, 50–51

Chemical Information Services (1995) *International Directory of Pharmaceutical Ingredients 1995/96 Edition*, Dallas, TX, pp. 860–867

Chowaniec, J. & Hicks, R.M. (1979) Response of the rat to saccharin with particular reference to the urinary bladder. *Br. J. Cancer*, **39**, 355–375

Cicurel, L. & Schmid, B.P. (1988) Post-implantation embryo culture: Validation with selected compounds for teratogenicity testing. *Xenobiotica*, **18**, 617–624

Clayson, D.B. (1974) Bladder carcinogenesis in rats and mice: Possibility of artifacts. *J. natl Cancer Inst.*, **52**, 1685–1689

Clive, D., Johnson, K.O., Spector, J.F.S., Batson, A.G. & Brown, M.M.M. (1979) Validation and characterization of the L5178Y/TK(+/–) mouse lymphoma mutagen assay system. *Mutat. Res.*, **59**, 61–108

Cohen, S.M. (1985) Promotion in urinary bladder carcinogenesis. *Environ. Health Perspectives*, **50**, 51–59

Cohen, S.M. (1995) Role of urinary physiology and chemistry in bladder carcinogenesis. *Food chem. Toxicol.*, **33**, 715–730

Cohen, S.M. (1999) Calcium phosphate-containing urinary precipitate in rat urinary bladder carcinogenesis. In: Capen, C., Dybing, E., Rice, J. & Wilbourn, J., eds, *Species Differences in Thyroid, Kidney and Urinary Bladder Carcinogenesis* (IARC Scientific Publications No. 147), Lyon, IARC, pp. 175–189

Cohen, S.M., Arai, M., Jacobs, J.B. & Friedell, G.H. (1979) Promoting effects of saccharin and DL-tryptophan in urinary bladder carcinogenesis. *Cancer Res.*, **39**, 1207–1217

Cohen, S.M., Murasaki, G., Fukushima, S. & Greenfield, R.E. (1982) Effect of regenerative hyperplasia on the urinary bladder: Carcinogenicity of sodium saccharin and *N*-[4-(5-nitro-2-furyl)-2-thiazolyl]formamide. *Cancer Res.*, **42**, 65–71

Cohen, S.M., Fisher, M.J., Sakata, T., Cano, M., Schoenig, G.P., Chappel, C.I. & Garland, E.M. (1990) Comparative analysis of the proliferative response of the rat urinary bladder to sodium saccharin by light and scanning electron microscopy and autoradiography. *Scanning Microsc.*, **4**, 135–142

Cohen, S.M., Ellwein, L.B., Okamura, T., Masui, T., Johansson, S.L., Smith, R.A., Wehner, J.M., Khachab, M., Chappel, C.I., Schonig, G.P., Emerson, J.L. & Garland, E.M. (1991a) Comparative bladder tumor promoting acrivity of sodium saccharin, sodium ascorbate, related acids, and calcium salts in rats. *Cancer Res.*, **51**, 1766–1777

Cohen, S.M., Cano, M., Earl, R.A., Carson, S.D. & Garland, E.M. (1991b) A proposed role for silicates and protein in the proliferative effects of saccharin on the male rat urothelium. *Carcinogenesis*, **12**, 1551–1555

Cohen, S.M., Cano, M., St John, M.K., Garland, E.M., Khachab, M. & Ellwein, L.B. (1995a) Effect of sodium saccharin on the neonatal rat bladder. *Scanning Microsc.*, **9**, 137–148

Cohen, S.M., Garland, E.M., Cano, M., St John, M.K., Khachab, M., Wehner, J.M. & Arnold, L.L. (1995b) Effects of sodium ascorbate, sodium saccharin and ammonium chloride on the male rat urinary bladder. *Carcinogenesis*, **16**, 2743–2750

Cohen, S.M., Cano, M., Garland, E.M., St John, M. & Arnold, L.L. (1995c) Urinary and urothelial effects of sodium salts in male rats. *Carcinogenesis*, **16**, 343–348

Cohen, S.M., Anderson, T.A., de Oliveira, L.M. & Arnold, L.L. (1998) Tumorigenicity of sodium ascorbate in male rats. *Cancer Res.*, **58**, 2557–2561

Cohen-Addad, N., Chatterjee, M., Bekersky, I. & Blumenthal, H.P. (1986) *In utero* exposure to saccharin: A threat? *Cancer Lett.*, **32**, 151–154

Colburn, W.A. (1978) Absorption of saccharin from rat urinary bladder. *J. pharm. Sci.*, **67**, 1493–1494

Colburn, W.A., Bekersky, I. & Blumenthal, H.P. (1981) Dietary saccharin kinetics. *Clin. Pharmacol. Ther.,* **30**, 558–563

Connor, T.H., Cantelli Forti, G., Sitra, P. & Legator, M.S. (1979) Bile as a source of mutagenic metabolites produced in vivo and detected by Salmonella typhimurium. *Environ. Mutag.*, **1**, 269–276

Coulston, F., McChesney, E.W. & Golberg, L. (1975) Long-term administration of artificial sweeteners to the rhesus monkey (*M. mulatta*). *Food Cosmet. Toxicol.*, **13**, 297–302

Council of Europe (1994) *European Pharmacopoeia*, 2nd Ed., Sainte-Ruffine, Maisonneuve, pp. 947-1–947-4

Council of Europe (1997) *European Pharmacopoeia*, 3rd Ed., Strasbourg

Debiec-Rychter, M. & Wang, C.Y. (1990) Induction of DNA synthesis by sodium phenobarbital, uracil and sodium saccharin in urinary bladder of the F344 rat. *Toxicol. appl. Pharmacol.*, **105**, 345–349

De Flora, S. (1981) Study of 106 organic and inorganic compounds in the *Salmonella*/microsome test. *Carcinogenesis*, **2**, 283–298

Demers, D.M., Fukushima, S. & Cohen, S.M. (1981) Effect of sodium saccharin and L-tryptophan on rat urine during bladder carcinogenesis. *Cancer Res.*, **41**, 108–112

DeSesso, I.M. (1989) Confounding factors in direct bladder exposure studies. *Comments Toxicol.*, **3**, 317–334

Dropkin, R.H., Salo, D.F., Tucci, S.M. & Kaye, G.I. (1985) Effects on mouse embryos of in utero exposure to saccharin: Teratogenic and chromosome effects. *Arch. Toxicol.*, **56**, 283–287

Eckhardt, K., King, M.-T., Gocke, E. & Wild, D. (1980) Mutagenicity study of Remsen-Fahlberg saccharin and contaminants. *Toxicol. Lett.*, **7**, 51–60

Ellwein, L.B. & Cohen, S.M. (1988) A cellular dynamics model of experimental bladder cancer: Analysis of the effect of sodium saccharin in the rat. *Risk Anal.*, **8**, 215–221

Ellwein, L.B. & Cohen, S.M. (1990) The health risks of saccharin revisited. *Crit. Rev. Toxicol.*, **20**, 311–326

Ershoff, B.H. & Bajwa, G.S. (1974) Inhibitory effect of sodium cyclamate and sodium saccharin on tumor induction by 2-acetylaminofluorene in rats. *Proc. Soc. exp. Biol. Med.*, **145**, 1293–1297

European Commission (1970) Council Directive of 23 November 1970 concerning additives in animal feeding stuffs (70/524/EEC). *Off. J. Eur. Com.*, **L270**, 1

European Commission (1978) Commission recommendation of 29 March 1978 to the Member States on the use of saccharin as a food ingredient and for sale as such in tablet form to the final consumer. *Off. J. Eur. Com.*, **L103**, 32

European Commission (1994a) European Parliament and Council Directive of 30 June 1994 on sweeteners for use in food stuffs (94/35/EC). *Off. J. Eur. Com.*, **L237**, 3

European Commission (1994b) Amendment to the Council Directive of 23 November 1970 concerning additives in animal feedingstuffs (70/524/EEC). *Off. J. Eur. Com.*, **L297**, 27

Fahrig, R. (1982) Effects in the mammalian spot test: Cyclamate versus saccharin. *Mutat. Res.*, **103**, 43–47

Fancher, O.E., Palazzolo, R.J., Blockus, L., Weinberg, M.S. & Calandra, J.C. (1968) Chronic studies with sodium saccharin and sodium cyclamate in dogs (Abstract No. 15). *Toxicol. appl. Pharmacol.*, **12**, 291

Fisher, M.J., Sakata, T., Tibbels, T.S., Smith, R.A., Patil, K., Khachab, M., Johansson, S.L. & Cohen, S.M. (1989) Effect of sodium saccharin and calcium saccharin on urinary parameters in rats fed Prolab 3200 or AIN-76 diet. *Food chem. Toxicol.*, **27**, 1–9

Fitzhugh, O.G., Nelson, A.A. & Frawley, J.P. (1951) A comparison of the chronic toxicities of synthetic sweetening agents. *J. Am. pharm. Assoc.*, **40**, 583–586

Food and Drug Administration (1998) Saccharin, ammonium saccharin, calcium saccharin, and sodium saccharin. *Code Fed. Regul.*, **Title 21**, Part 180.37, pp. 422–423

Frederick, C.B., Dooley, K.L., Kodell, R.L., Sheldon, W.G. & Kadlubar, F.F. (1989) The effect of lifetime sodium saccharin dosing on mice initiated with the carcinogen 2-acetylamino-fluorene. *Fundam. appl. Toxicol.*, **12**, 346–357

Friedman, J.M. & Polifka, J.E., eds (1994) *Teratogenic Effects of Drugs: A Resource for Clinicians: TERIS*, Baltimore, Johns Hopkins University Press, pp. 558–559

Fukushima, S. & Cohen, S.M. (1980) Saccharin-induced hyperplasia of the rat urinary bladder. *Cancer Res.*, **40**, 734–736

Fukushima, S., Friedell, G.H., Jacobs, J.B. & Cohen, S.M. (1981) Effect of L-tryptophan and sodium saccharin on urinary tract carcinogenesis initiated by *N*-[4-(5-nitro-2-furyl)-2-thiazolyl]formamide. *Cancer Res.*, **41**, 3100–3103

Fukushima, S., Arai, M., Nakanowatari, J., Hibino, T., Okuda, M. & Ito, N. (1983a) Differences in susceptibility to sodium saccharin among various strains of rats and other animal species. *Gann*, **74**, 8–20

Fukushima, S., Hagiwara, A., Ogiso, T., Shibata, M. & Ito, N. (1983b) Promoting effects of various chemicals in rat urinary bladder carcinogenesis initiated by *N*-nitroso-*n*-butyl(4-hydroxylbutyl)amine. *Food chem. Toxicol.*, **21**, 59–68

Fukushima, S., Shibata, M.-A., Kurata, Y., Tamano, S. & Masui, T. (1986a) Changes in the urine and scanning electron microscopically observed appearance of the rat bladder following treatment with tumor promoters. *Jpn. J. Cancer Res. (Gann)*, **77**, 1074–1082

Fukushima, S., Shibata, M.A., Khirai, T., Tamano, S. & Ito, N. (1986b) Roles of urinary sodium ion concentration and pH in promotion by ascorbic acid of urinary bladder carcinogenesis in rats. *Cancer Res.*, **46**, 1623–1626

Fukushima, S., Uwagawa, S., Shirai, T., Hasegawa, R. & Ogawa, K. (1990) Synergism by sodium L-ascorbate but inhibition by L-ascorbic acid for sodium saccharin promotion of rat two-stage bladder carcinogenesis. *Cancer Res.*, **50**, 4195–4198

Furuya, T., Kawamata, K., Kaneko, T., Uchida, O., Horiuchi, S. & Ikeda, Y. (1975) Long-term toxicity study of sodium cyclamate and saccharin sodium in rats (Abstract). *Jpn. J. Pharmacol.*, **25**, 55P–56P

Garland, E.M., Sakata, T., Fisher, M.J., Masui, T. & Cohen, S.M. (1989) Influences of diet and strain on the proliferative effect on the rat urinary bladder induced by sodium saccharin. *Cancer Res.*, **49**, 3789–3794

Garland, E.M., Kraft, P.L., Shapiro, R., Khachab, M., Patil, K., Ellwein, L.B. & Cohen, S.M. (1991a) Effects of *in utero* and postnatal sodium saccharin exposure on the nutritional status of the young rat. I. Effects at 30 days post-birth. *Food chem. Toxicol.*, **29**, 657–667

Garland, E.M., Shapiro, R., Kraft, P.L., Mattson, B.J., Parr, J.M. & Cohen, S.M. (1991b) Effects of *in utero* and postnatal sodium saccharin exposure on the nutritional status of the young rat. II. Dose response and reversibility. *Food chem. Toxicol.*, **29**, 669–679

Garland, E.M., Shapiro, R., Wehner, J.M., Johnson, L.S., Mattson, B.J., Khachab, M., Asamoto, M. & Cohen, S.M. (1993) Effects of dietary iron and folate supplementation on the physiological changes produced in weanling rats by sodium saccharin exposure. *Food chem. Toxicol.*, **31**, 689–699

Garland, E.M., St John, M., Asamoto, M., Eklund, S.H., Mattson, B.J., Johnson, L.S., Cano, M. & Cohen, S.M. (1994) A comparison of the effects of sodium saccharin in NBR rats and in intact and castrated male F344 rats. *Cancer Lett.*, **78**, 99–107

Gennaro, A.R. (1995) *The Science and Practice of Pharmacy*, 19th Ed., Vol. II, Easton, PA, Mack Publishing Co., pp. 1389–1390

Goldstein, R.S., Hook, J.B. & Bond, J.T. (1978) Renal tubular transport of saccharin. *J. Pharmacol. exp. Ther.*, **204**, 690–695

Green, U. & Rippel, W. (1979) Bladder calculi in rats treated with nitrosomethylurea and fed artificial sweeteners. *Exp. Pathol. Jena*, **17**, 561–564

Hagiwara, A., Fukushima, S., Kitaori, M., Shibata, M. & Ito, N. (1984) Effects of three sweeteners on rat urinary bladder carcinogenesis initiated by *N*-butyl-*N*-(4-hydroxybutyl)-nitrosamine. *Gann*, **75**, 763–768

Hard, G.C. (1995) Species comparison of the content and comparison of urinary proteins. *Food chem. Toxicol.*, **33**, 731–746

Hasegawa, R. & Cohen, S.M. (1986) The effect of different salts of saccharin on the rat urinary bladder. *Cancer Lett.*, **30**, 261–268

Hasegawa, R., Greenfield, R.E., Murasaki, G., Suzuki, T. & Cohen, S.M. (1985) Initiation of urinary bladder carcinogenesis in rats by freeze ulceration with sodium saccharin promotion. *Cancer Res.*, **45**, 1469–1473

Herbold, B.A. (1981) Studies to evaluate artificial sweeteners, especially Remsen–Fahlberg saccharin, and their possible impurities, for potential mutagenicity by the Salmonella/ mammalian liver microsome test. *Mutat. Res.*, **90**, 365–372

Her Majesty's Stationery Office (1983) *The Sweeteners in Food Regulations 1983* (Statutory Instruments 1211), London

Hibino, T., Hirasawa, Y. & Arai, M. (1985) Morphologic changes in the urinary bladder and stomach after long-term administration of sodium saccharin in F344 rats. *Cancer Lett.*, **29**, 255–263

Hicks, R.M., Chowaniec, J. & Wakefield, J.St J. (1978) Experimental induction of bladder tumors by a two-stage system. In: Slaga, T.J., Sivak, A. & Boutwell, R.K., eds, *Carcinogenesis*, Vol. 2, *Mechanisms of Tumor Promotion and Cocarcinogenesis*, New York, Raven Press, pp. 475–489

Ho, Y.L. & Ho, S.K. (1981) Screening of carcinogens with the prophage λcI*ts*857 induction test. *Cancer Res.*, **41**, 532–536

Homburger, F. (1978) Negative lifetime carcinogen studies in rats and mice fed 50,000 ppm saccharin. In: Galli, C.L., Paoletti, R. & Vettorazzi, G., eds, *Chemical Toxicology of Food*, Amsterdam, Elsevier/North-Holland Biomedical Press, pp. 359–373

Homma, Y., Kondo, Y., Kakizoe, T., Aso, T. & Nagase, S. (1991) Lack of bladder carcinogenicity of dietary sodium saccharin in analbuminaemic rats, which are highly susceptible to *N*-nitroso-*n*-butyl-(4-hydroxybutyl)amine. *Food chem. Toxicol.*, **29**, 373–376

Hooson, J., Hicks, R.M., Grasso, P. & Chowaniec, J. (1980) *ortho*-Toluene sulphonamide and saccharin in the promotion of bladder cancer in the rat. *Br. J. Cancer*, **42**, 129–147

Hoover, R.N. & Harge-Strasser, P.H. (1980) Artifical sweeteners and human bladder cancer: Preliminary results. *Lancet*, **i**, 837–840

Howe, G.R. & Burch, J.D. (1981) Artificial sweeteners in relation to the epidemiology of bladder cancer. *Nutr. Cancer*, **2**, 213–216

Howe, G.R., Burch, J.D., Miller, A.B., Morrison, B., Gordon, P., Weldon, L., Chambers, L.W., Fodor, G. & Winsor, G.M. (1977) Artificial sweeteners and human bladder cancer. *Lancet*, **ii**, 578–581

Howe, G.R., Burch, J.D., Miller, A.B., Cook, G.M., Esteve, J., Morrison, B., Gordon, P., Chambers, L.W., Fodor, G. & Winsor, G.M. (1980) Tobacco use, occupation, coffee, various nutrients and bladder cancer. *J. natl Cancer Inst.*, **64**, 701–713

Hulshof, K.F.A.M., Kistemaker, C., Bouman, M. & Löwik, M.R.H. (1995) *Use of Various Types of Sweeteners in Different Population Groups: 1992 Dutch National Food Consumption Survey (TNO Report V-95.301)*, Zeist, TNO Nutrition and Food Research Institute

IARC (1980) *IARC Monographs on the Evaluation of the Carcinogenic Risk of Chemicals to Humans*, Vol. 22, *Some Non-nutritive Sweetening Agents*, Lyon, pp. 111–170, 171–185

IARC (1987) *IARC Monographs on the Evaluation of Carcinogenic Risks to Humans,* Suppl. 7, *Overall Evaluations of Carcinogenicity: An Updating of* IARC Monographs *Volume 1 to 42*, Lyon, pp. 334–339

Imaida, K. & Wang, C.Y. (1986) Effect of sodium phenobarbital and sodium saccharin in AIN-76A diet on carcinogenesis initiated with *N*-[4-(5-nitro-2-furyl)-2-thiazolyl]formmide and *N,N*-dibutylnitrosamine in male F344 rats. *Cancer Res.*, **46**, 6160–6164

Imamura, A., Kurumi, Y., Danzuka, T., Kodama, M., Kawachi, T. & Nagao, M. (1983) Classification of compounds by cluster analysis of Ames test data. *Jpn. J. Cancer Res. (Gann)*, **74**, 196–204

International Sweeteners Association (1998) *Saccharin*, Brussels [http://www.isabru.org/]

Ishidate, M., Jr & Odashima, S. (1977) Chromosome tests with 134 compounds on Chinese hamster cells in vitro—A screening for chemical carcinogens. *Mutat. Res.*, **48**, 337–354

Ishidate, M., Jr, Sofuni, T., Yoshikawa, K., Hayashi, M., Nohmi, T., Sawada, M. & Matsuoka, A. (1984) Primary mutagenicity screening of food additives currently used in Japan. *Food chem. Toxicol.*, **22**, 623–636

Ito, N., Fuhushima, S., Shirai, T. & Nakanishi, K. (1983) Effects of promoters on *N*-butyl-*N*-(4-hydroxybutyl)nitrosamine-induced urinary bladder carcinogenesis in the rat. *Environ. Health Perspectives*, **50**, 61–69

Jeffrey, A.M. & Williams, G.M. (1999) Lack of DNA-damaging activity of five non-nutritive sweeteners in the rat hepatocyte/DNA repair assay. *Food chem. Toxicol.* (in press)

Jensen, O. & Kamby, C. (1982) Intra-uterine exposure to saccharine and risk of bladder cancer in man. *Int. J. Cancer*, **29**, 507–509

Johansson, S.L., Sakata, T., Hasegawa, R., Zenser, T.V., Davis, B.B. & Cohen, S.M. (1986) The effect of long-term administration of aspirin and sodium saccharin on the rat kidney. *Toxicol. appl. Pharmacol.*, **86**, 80–92

Jull, J.W. (1979) The effect of time on the incidence of carcinomas obtained by the implantation of paraffin wax pellets into mouse bladder. *Cancer Lett.*, **6**, 21–25

Kessler, I.I. (1976) Non-nutritive sweeteners and human bladder cancer: Preliminary findings. *J. Urol.*, **115**, 143–146

Kessler, I.I. & Clark, J.P. (1978) Saccharin, cyclamate and human bladder cancer. *J. Am. med. Assoc.*, **240**, 349–355

Kitchen, K.T. & Ebron, M.T. (1983) Studies of saccharin and cyclohexamine in a coupled microsomal activating/embryo culture system. *Food chem. Toxicol.*, **21**, 537–541

Kline, J., Stein, Z.A., Susser, M. & Warburton, D. (1977) Spontaneous abortion and the use of sugar substitutes (saccharin). *Am. J. Obstet. Gynecol.*, **130**, 708–711

Knowles, M.A. & Jani, H. (1986) Multistage transformation of cultured rat urothelium: The effects of *N*-methyl-*N*-nitrosourea, sodium saccharin, sodium cyclamate and 12-O-tetradecanoylphorbol-13-acetate. *Carcinogenesis*, **7**, 2059–2065

Kramers, P.G.N. (1977) Mutagenicity of saccharin in Drosophila: The possible role of contaminants. *Mutat. Res.*, **56**, 163–167

Kristoffersson, U. (1972) Effect of cyclamate and saccharin on the chromosomes of a Chinese hamster cell line. *Hereditas*, **70**, 271–282

Kroes, R., Peters, P.W.J., Berkvens, J.M., Verschuuren, H.G., De Vries, T. & Van Esch, G.J. (1977) Long term toxicity and reproduction study (including a teratogenicity study) with cyclamate, saccharin and cyclohexylamine. *Toxicology*, **8**, 285–300

Lawrie, C.A., Renwick, A.G. & Sims, J. (1985) The urinary excretion of bacterial amino-acid metabolites by rats fed saccharin in the diet. *Food chem. Toxicol.*, **23**, 445–450

Lawson, T.A. & Hertzog, P.J. (1981) The failure of chronically administered saccharin to stimulate bladder epithelial DNA synthesis in F_0 rats. *Cancer Lett.*, **11**, 221–224

Lederer, J. (1977) [Saccharin, its contaminants and their teratogenic effect.] *Louvain. méd.*, **96**, 495–501 (in French)

Lederer, J. & Pottier-Arnould, A.M. (1973) [Effect of saccharin on embryonal development in the pregnant rat.] *Diabète*, **21**, 13–16 (in French)

Lee, L.S. (1981) Saccharin and cyclamate inhibit binding of epidermal growth factor. *Proc. natl Acad. Sci. USA*, **78**, 1042–1046

Léonard, A. & Léonard, E.D. (1979) Mutagenicity test with saccharin in the male mouse. *J. Environ. Pathol. Toxicol.*, **2**, 1047–1053

Lessel, B. (1971) Carcinogenic and teratogenic aspects of saccharin. In: *SOS/70 Proceedings of the Third International Congress of Food Science and Technology, Washington DC, 1970*, Chicago, IL, Institute of Food Technologists, pp. 764–770

Lethco, E.J. & Wallace, W.C. (1975) The metabolism of saccharin in animals. *Toxicology*, **3**, 287–300

Lide, D.R., ed. (1997) *CRC Handbook of Chemistry and Physics*, 78th Ed., Boca Raton, FL, CRC Press, p. 3-66

Lok, E., Iverson, F. & Clayson, D.B. (1982) The inhibition of urease and proteases by sodium saccharin. *Cancer Lett.*, **16**, 163–169

Lorke, D. & Machemer, L. (1975) [Effect of several weeks' treatment of male and female mice with saccharin, cyclamate or cyclohexylamine sulfate on fertility and dominant lethal effects.] *Humangenetik*, **26**, 199–205 (in German)

Luckhaus, G. & Machemer, L. (1978) Histological examination of perinatal eye development in the rat after ingestion of sodium cyclamate and sodium saccharin during pregnancy. *Food Cosmet. Toxicol.*, **16**, 7–11

Lutz, W.K. & Schlatter, C. (1977) Saccharin does not bind to DNA of liver or bladder in the rat. *Chem.-biol. Interactions*, **19**, 253–257

Lynch, D.W., Schuler, R.L., Hood, R.D. & Davis, D.G. (1991) Evaluation of *Drosophila* for screening developmental toxicants: Test results with eighteen chemicals and presentation of a new *Drosophila* bioassay. *Teratog. Carcinog. Mutag.*, **11**, 147–173

Machemer, L. & Lorke, D. (1973) Dominant lethal test in the mouse for mutagenic effects of saccharin. *Humangenetik*, **19**, 193–198

Machemer, L. & Lorke, D. (1975a) Method for testing mutagenic effects of chemicals on spermatogonia of the Chinese hamster. *Arzneim.-Forsch.*, **25**, 1889–1896

Machemer, L. & Lorke, D. (1975b) Experiences with the dominant lethal test in female mice: Effects of alkylating agents and artificial sweeteners on pre-ovulatory oocyte stages. *Mutat. Res.*, **29**, 209–214

Mahon, G.A.T. & Dawson, G.W.P. (1982) Saccharin and the induction of presumed somatic mutations in the mouse. *Mutat. Res.*, **103**, 49–52

Mallett, A.K., Rowland, I.R. & Bearne, C.A. (1985) Modification of rat caecal microbial biotransformation activities by dietary saccharin. *Toxicology*, **36**, 253–262

Masubuchi, M., Nawai, S., Hiraga, K. & Hirokado, M. (1977) Lack of the cytogenetic effects of saccharin and its impurities on CHO-K1 cells. *Ann. Rep. Tokyo metr. Res. Lab. P.H.*, **28**, 159–161

Masui, T., Garland, E.M., Wang, C.Y. & Cohen, S.M. (1990) Effects of different types of diet and sodium saccharin on proliferation at the limiting ridge of the rat forestomach. *Food chem. Toxicol.*, **28**, 497–505

Matthews, H.B., Fields, M. & Fishbein, L. (1973) Saccharin: Distribution and excretion of a limited dose in the rat. *J. agric. Food Chem.*, **21**, 916–919

McChesney, E.W. & Goldberg, L. (1973) The excretion and metabolism of saccharin in man. I. Methods of investigation and preliminary results. *Food Cosmet. Toxicol.*, **11**, 403–414

McChesney, E.W., Coulston, F. & Benitz, K.-F. (1977) Six-year study of saccharin in rhesus monkeys (Abstract No. 79). *Toxicol appl. Pharmacol.*, **41**, 164

Milo, G.E., Oldham, J.W., Noyes, I., Lehman, T.A., Kumari, L., West, R.W. & Kadlubar, F.F. (1988) Cocarcinogenicity of saccharin and N-alkylnitrosoureas in cultured human diploid fibroblasts. *J. Toxicol. environ. Health*, **24**, 413–421

Minegishi, K.-I., Asahina, M. & Yamaha, T. (1972) The metabolism of saccharin and the related compounds in rats and guinea pigs. *Chem. Pharm. Bull.*, **20**, 1351–1356

Mitchell, M.L. & Pearson, R.L. (1991) Saccharin. In: O'Brien Nabors, L. & Gelardi, R.C., eds, *Alternative Sweeteners*, 2nd. Ed., New York, Marcel Dekker, pp. 127–156

Miyata, Y., Hagiwara, A., Nakatsuka, T., Murasaki, G., Arai, M. & Ito, N. (1980) Effects of caffeine and saccharin on DNA in the bladder epithelium of rats treated with n-butyl-n-(3-carboxypropyl)nitrosamine. *Chem.-biol. Interactions*, **29**, 291–302

Mohr, U., Green, U., Althoff, J. & Schneider, P. (1978) Syncarcinogenic action of saccharin and sodium-cyclamate in the induction of bladder tumours in MNU-pretreated rats. In: Guggenheim, B., ed., *Health and Sugar Substitutes*, Basel, Karger, pp. 64–69

Møller Jensen, O., Knudsen, J.R., Sorensen, R.L. & Clemmesen, J. (1983) Artifical sweeteners and absence of bladder cancer risk in Copenhagen. *Int. J. Cancer*, **32**, 577–582

Mommsen, S., Aagard, J. & Sell, A. (1983) A case–control study of female bladder cancer. *Eur. J. Cancer clin. Oncol.*, **19**, 725–729

Mondal, S., Brankow, D.W. & Heidelberger, C. (1978) Enhancement of oncogenesis in C3H/10T1/2 mouse embryo cell cultures by saccharin. *Science*, **201**, 1141–1142

Moore, C.W. & Schmick, A. (1979) Genetic effects of impure and pure saccharin in yeast. *Science*, **205**, 1007–1010

Morgan, R.W. & Jain, M.G. (1974) Bladder cancer: Smoking, beverages and artifical sweeteners. *Can. med. Assoc. J.*, **111**, 1067–1070

Morimoto, S. (1996) Alteration of intercellular communication in a human urothelial carcinoma cell-line by tumor-promoting agents. *Int. J. Urol.*, **3**, 212–217

Morrison, A.S. & Buring, J.E. (1980) Artifical sweeteners and cancer of the lower urinary tract. *New Engl. J. Med.*, **302**, 537–541

Morrison, A.S., Verhoek, W.G., Leck, I., Aoki, K., Ohno, Y. & Obata, K. (1982) Artificial sweeteners and bladder cancer in Manchester, UK, and Nagoya, Japan. *Br. J. Cancer*, **45**, 332–336

Mortelmans, K., Haworth, S., Lawlor, T., Speck, W., Tainer, B. & Zeiger, E. (1986) Salmonella mutagenicity tests: II. Results from the testing of 270 chemicals. *Environ. Mutag.*, **8** (Suppl. 7), 1–119

Mosser, D.D. & Bols, N.C. (1983) Effect of saccharin on metabolic cooperation between human fibroblasts. *Carcinogenesis*, **4**, 991–995

Munro, I.C., Moodie, C.A., Krewski, D. & Grice, H.C. (1975) A carcinogenicity study of commercial saccharin in the rat. *Toxicol. appl. Pharmacol.*, **32**, 513–526

Murasaki, G. & Cohen, S.M. (1981) Effect of dose of sodium saccharin on the induction of rat urinary bladder proliferation. *Cancer Res.*, **41,** 942–944

Murasaki, G. & Cohen, S.M. (1983a) Co-carcinogenicity of sodium saccharin and *N*-[4-(5-nitro-2-furyl)-2-thiazolyl]formamide for the urinary bladder. *Carcinogenesis*, **4**, 97–99

Murasaki, G. & Cohen, S.M. (1983b) Effect of sodium saccharin on urinary bladder epithelial regenerative hyperplasia following freeze ulceration. *Cancer Res.*, **43**, 182–187

Najem, G.R., Louria, D.B., Seebode, J.J., Third, I.S., Prusakowski, J.M., Ambrose, R.B. & Fernicola, A.R. (1982) Lifetime occupation, smoking, caffeine, saccharin, hair dyes and bladder carcinogenesis. *Int. J. Epidemiol.*, **11**, 212–217

Nakanishi, K., Hagiwara, A., Shibata, M., Imaida, K., Tatematsu, M. & Ito, N. (1980a) Dose response of saccharin in induction of urinary bladder hyperplasias in Fischer 344 rats pre-treated with *N*-butyl-*N*-(4-hydroxybutyl)nitrosamine. *J. natl Cancer Inst.*, **65**, 1005–1010

Nakanishi, K., Hirose, M., Ogiso, T., Hasegawa, R., Arai, M. & Ito, N. (1980b) Effects of sodium saccharin and caffeine on the urinary bladder of rats treated with *N*-butyl-*N*-(4-hydroxy-butyl)nitrosamine. *Gann*, **71**, 490–500

National Academy of Sciences (1996) *Food Chemicals Codex*, 4th Ed., Washington DC, National Academy Press, pp. 71–72, 343, 378–380

National Food Authority (1995) *Survey of Intense Sweetener Consumption in Australia. Final Report*, Canberra

National Institute for Occupational Safety and Health (1998) *National Occupational Exposure Survey (1981–83)*, Cincinnati, OH

National Research Council/National Academy of Sciences (1978) *Saccharin: Technical Assessment of Risks and Benefits*, Report No. 1, Committee for a Study on Saccharin and Food Safety Policy, Washington DC, Assembly of Life Sciences/Institute of Medicine

National Toxicology Program (1997) Sodium saccharin. *Environ. Health Perspectives*, **105** (Suppl. 1), 347–348

Negro, F., Mondardini, A. & Palmas, F. (1994) Hepatotoxicity of saccharin. *New Engl. J. Med.*, **331,** 134–135

Neuhaus, O.W. & Flory, W. (1978) Age-dependent changes in the excretion of urinary proteins by the rat. *Nephron*, **22**, 570–576

Newall, D.R. & Beedles, K.E. (1996) The stem-cell test: an *in vitro* assay for teratogenic potential. Results of a blind trial with 25 compounds. *Toxicol. In Vitro*, **10**, 229–240

Nicholson, L.J. & Jani, H. (1988) Effects of sodium cyclamate and sodium saccharin on focus induction in explant cultures of rat bladder. *Int. J. Cancer*, **42**, 295–298

Norman, J.T., Howlett, A.R., Spacey, G.D. & Hodges, G.M. (1987) Effects of treatment with *N*-methyl-*N*-nitrosourea, artificial sweeteners and cyclosphosphamide on adult rat urinary bladder *in vitro*. *Lab. Invest.*, **57**, 429–438

Ogawa, K., Sun, T.-T. & Cohen, S.M. (1996) Analysis of differentiation-associated proteins in rat bladder carcinogenesis. *Carcinogenesis,* **17**, 961–965

Okamura, T., Garland, E.M., Masui, T., Sakata, T., St John, M. & Cohen, S.M. (1991) Lack of bladder tumor promoting activity in rats fed sodium saccharin in AIN-76A diet. *Cancer Res.*, **51**, 1778–1782

Oser, B.L. (1985) Highlights in the history of saccharin toxicology. *Food chem. Toxicol.*, **23**, 535–542

Oser, B.L., Carson, S., Cox, G.E., Vogin, E.E. & Sternberg, S.S. (1975) Chronic toxicity study of cyclamate:saccharin (10:1) in rats. *Toxicology*, **4**, 315–330

Pai, S.R., Shirke, A.J. & Gothoskar, S.V. (1981) Long-term feeding study in C17 mice administered saccharin coated betel nut and 1,4-dinitrosopiperazine in combination. *Carcinogenesis*, **2**, 175–177

Pantarotto, C., Salmona, M. & Garattini, S. (1981) Plasma kinetics and urinary elimination of saccharin in man. *Toxicol. Lett.*, **9**, 367–371

Parry, J.M., Parry, E.M. & Barrett, J.C. (1981) Tumour promoters induce mitotic aneuploidy in yeast. *Nature*, **294**, 263–265

Pecevski, J., Vuksanovic, L., Savkovic, N., Alavantic, D. & Radivojevic, D. (1983) Effect of saccharin on the induction of chromosomal translocations in male mice and their F1 offspring. *Toxicol. Lett.*, **19**, 267–271

Penttilä, P.-L., Salminen, S. & Niemi, E. (1988) Estimates on the intake of food additives in Finland. *Z. Lebensm. Unters. Forsch.*, **186**, 11–15

Pereira, M.A., Herren, S.L. & Britt, A.L. (1983) Effect of dibutylnitrosamine and saccharin on glutamyl transpeptidase-positive foci and liver cancer. *Environ. Health Perspectives*, **50**, 169–176

Persic, L. (1986) Effect of saccharin on the meiotic division of *Saccharomyces cerevisiae. Mutat. Res.*, **174**, 195–197

Piper, J.M., Matanoski, G.M. & Tonascia, J. (1986) Bladder cancer in young women. *Am. J. Epidemiol.*, **123**, 1033–1042

Pitkin, R.M., Andersen, D.W., Reynolds, W.A. & Filer, L.J., Jr (1971b) Saccharin metabolism in *Macaca mulatta. Proc. Soc. exp. Biol. Med.*, **137**, 803–806

Pitkin, R.M., Reynolds, W.A., Filer, L.J., Jr & Kling, T.G. (1971a) Placental transmission and fetal distribution of saccharin. *Am. J. Obstet. Gynecol.*, **111**, 280–286

Pool, B. (1978) Non-mutagenicity of saccharin. *Toxicology*, **11**, 95–97

Prasad, O. & Rai, G. (1986) Induction of papillary adenocarcinoma of the thyroid in albino mice by saccharin feeding. *Indian J. exp. Biol.*, **24**, 197–199

Prasad, O. & Rai, G. (1987) Induction of chromosomal aberrations by prefeeding saccharin in albino mice. *Indian J. exp. Biol.*, **25**, 124–128

Pratt, R.M. & Willis, W.D. (1985) *In vitro* screening assay for teratogens using growth inhibition of human embryonic cells. *Proc. natl. Acad. Sci. USA*, **82**, 5791–5794

Price, J.M., Biava, C.G., Oser, B.L., Vogin, E.E., Steinfeld, J. & Ley H.L. (1970) Bladder tumors in rats fed cyclohexylamine or high doses of a mixture of cyclamate and sodium. *Science*, **167**, 1131–1132

Rao, M.S. & Qureshi, A.B. (1972) Induction of dominant lethals in mice by sodium saccharin. *Indian J. med. Res*, **60**, 599–603

Rao, M.S., Samuel, B.C. & Qureshi, A.B. (1971) Genetic effects of sodium saccharin in *Drosophila melanogaster. Indian J. Hered.*, **3**, 57–60

Rao, T.K., Stoltz, D.R. & Epler, J.L. (1979) Lack of enhancement of chemical mutagenesis by saccharin in the Salmonella assay. *Arch. Toxicol.*, **43**, 141–145

Ray-Chaudhuri, R., Currens, M. & Iype, P.T. (1982) Enhancement of sister-chromatid exchanges by tumour promoters. *Br. J. Cancer*, **45**, 769–777

Renault, J.-Y., Melcion, C. & Cordier, A. (1989) Limb bud cell culture for in vitro teratogen screening: Validation of an improved assessment method using 51 compounds. *Teratog. Carcinog. Mutag.*, **9**, 83–96

Renner, H.W. (1979) Possible mutagenic activity of saccharin. *Experientia*, **35**, 1364

Renwick, A.G. (1978) The fate of saccharin impurities: The metabolism and excretion of 3-amino-[3-^{14}C]benz[*d*]isothiazole-1,1-dioxide and 5-chlorosaccharin in the rat. *Xenobiotica*, **8**, 487–494

Renwick, A.G. (1995) Intense sweeteners intake surveys: Methods, results and comparisons. In: *Intake Studies—Lessons Learnt, ISA Symposium, Brussels, November 27, 1995*, Brussels, International Sweeteners Association, pp. 79–97

Renwick, A.G. & Sims, J. (1983) Distension of the urinary bladder in rats fed saccharin containing diet. *Cancer Lett.*, **18**, 63–68

Renwick, A.G. & Williams, R.T. (1978) The fate of saccharin impurities: The excretion and metabolism of [3-^{14}C]benz[*d*]-isothiazoline-1,1-dioxide (BIT) in man and rat. *Xenobiotica*, **8**, 475–486

Renwick, A.G., Ball, L.M., Corina, D.L. & Williams, R.T. (1978) The fate of saccharin impurities: The excretion and metabolism of toluene-2-sulphonamide in man and rat. *Xenobiotica*, **8**, 461–474

Reynolds, J.E.F., ed. (1998) *Martindale, The Extra Pharmacopoeia*, 31st Ed., London, The Pharmaceutical Press [MicroMedex CD-ROM]

Riggin, R.M., Kinzer, G.W., Margard, W.L., Mondron, P.J., Girod, F.T. & Birts, M.A. (1978) *Identification, Development of Methods for Analysis and Mutagenicity Testing of Impurities in Sodium Saccharin*, Columbus, OH, Battelle Columbus Laboratories

Risch, J.A., Burch, J.D., Miller, A.B., Hill, G.B., Steel, R. & Howe, G.R. (1988) Dietary factors and the incidence of cancer of the urinary bladder. *Am. J. Epidemiol.*, **127**, 1179–1191

Roberts, A. & Renwick, A.G. (1985) The effect of saccharin on the microbial metabolism of tryptophan in man. *Food chem. Toxicol.*, **23**, 451–455

Roe, F.J.C., Levy, L.S. & Carter, R.L. (1970) Feeding studies on sodium cyclamate, saccharin and sucrose for carcinogenic and tumour-promoting activity. *Food Cosmet. Toxicol.*, **8**, 135–145

von Rymon Lipinski, G.-W. (1995) Sweeteners. In: Elvers, B., Hawkins, S. & Russey, W., eds, *Ullmann's Encyclopedia of Chemical Technology*, 5th rev. Ed., Vol A26, New York, VCH Publishers, pp. 23–43

Sadtler Research Laboratories (1980) *1980 Cumulative Index*, Philadelphia, PA

Sakai, A. & Sato, M. (1989) Improvement of carcinogen identification in BALB/3T3 cell transformation by application of a 2-stage method. *Mutat. Res.*, **214**, 285–296

Sakata, T., Shirai, T., Fukushima, S., Hasegawa, R. & Ito, N. (1984) Summation and synergism in the promotion of urinary bladder carcinogenesis initiated by *N*-butyl-*N*-(4-hydroxybutyl)-nitrosamine in F344 rats. *Gann*, **75**, 950–956

Sakata, T., Hasegawa, R., Johansson, S.L., Zenser, T.V. & Cohen, S.M. (1986) Inhibition by aspirin of *N*-[4-(5-nitro-2-furyl)-2-thiazolyl]formamide initiation and sodium saccharin promotion of urinary bladder carcinogenesis in male F344 rats. *Cancer Res.*, **46**, 3903–3906

Salaman, M.H. & Roe, F.J.C. (1956) Further tests for tumour-inititating activity: N,N-Di-(2-chloroethyl)-*p*-aminophenylbutyric acid (CB1348) as an initiator of skin tumour formation in the mouse. *Br. J. Cancer*, **10**, 363–378

Saxholm, H.J.K., Iversen, O.H., Reith, A. & Broegger, A. (1979) Carcinogenesis testing of saccharin. No transformation or increased sister chromatid exchange observed in two mammalian cell systems. *Eur. J. Cancer*, **15**, 509–513

Schmähl, D. (1973) Lack of carcinogenic effect of cyclamate, cyclohexylamine and saccharin in rats. *Arzneimittelforschung*, **23**, 1466–1470 (in German)

Schmähl, D. (1978) Experiments on the carcinogenic effect of ortho-toluol-sulfonamid (OTS). *Cancer Res. clin. Oncol.*, **91**, 19–22

Schmähl, D. & Habs, M. (1980) Absence of a carcinogenic response to cyclamate and saccharin in Sprague-Dawley rats after transplacental application. *Arzneimittelforschung*, **30**, 1905–1906

Schmähl, D. & Habs, M. (1984) Investigations on the carcinogenicity of the artificial sweeteners sodium cyclamate and sodium saccharin in rats in a two-generation experiment. *Arzneimittelforschung*, **34**, 604–606

Schoenig, G.P. & Anderson, R.L. (1985) The effects of high dietary levels of sodium saccharin on mineral and water balance and related parameters in rats. *Food chem. Toxicol.*, **23**, 465–474

Schoenig, G.P., Goldenthal, E.I., Geil, R.G., Frith, C.H., Richter, W.R. & Carlborg, F.W. (1985) Evaluation of the dose response and *in utero* exposure to saccharin in the rat. *Food chem. Toxicol.*, **23**, 475–490

Seidenberg, J.M., Anderson, D.G. & Becker, R.A. (1986) Validation of an in vivo developmental toxicity screen in the mouse. *Teratog. Carcinog. Mutag.*, **6**, 361–374

Sieber, S.M. & Adamson, R.H. (1978) Long-term studies on the potential carcinogenicity of artificial sweeteners in non-human primates. In: Guggenheim, B., ed., *Health and Sugar Substitutes*, Basel, Karger, pp. 266–271

Silverman, D.T., Hoover, R.N. & Swanson, G.M. (1983) Artificial sweeteners and lower urinary tract cancer: Hospital vs. population controls. *Am. J. Epidemiol.*, **117**, 326–334

Simon, D., Yen, S. & Cole, P. (1975) Coffee drinking and cancer of the lower urinary tract. *J. natl Cancer Inst.*, **54**, 587–591

Sims, J. & Renwick, A.G. (1983) The effects of saccharin on the metabolism of dietary tryptophan to indole, a known cocarcinogen for the urinary bladder of the rat. *Toxicol. appl. Pharmacol.*, **67**, 132–151

Sims, J. & Renwick, A.G. (1985) The microbial metabolism of tryptophan in rats fed a diet containing 7.5% saccharin in a two-generation protocol. *Food chem. Toxicol.*, **23**, 437–444

Sina, J.F., Bean, C.L., Dysart, G.R., Taylor, V.I. & Bradley, M.O. (1983) Evaluation of the alkaline elution/rat hepatocyte assay as a predictor of carcinogenic/mutagenic potential. *Mutat. Res.*, **113**, 357–391

Sivak, A. & Tu, A.S. (1980) Cell culture tumor promotion experiments with saccharin, phorbol myristate acetate and several common food materials. *Cancer Lett.*, **10**, 27–32

Society of Japanese Pharmacopoeia (1996) *The Japanese Pharmacopoeia JP XIII*, 13th Ed., Tokyo, pp. 885–886

Squire, R.A. (1985) Histopathological evaluation of rat urinary bladders from the IRDC two-generation bioassay of sodium saccharin. *Food chem. Toxicol.*, **23**, 491–497

Šrám, R.J. & Zudová, Z. (1974) Mutagenicity studies of saccharin in mice. *Bull. environ. Contam. Toxicol.*, **12**, 186–192

Steele, V.E., Morrissey, R.E., Elmore, E.L., Gurganus-Rocha, D., Wilkinson, B.P., Curren, R.D., Schmetter, B.S., Louie, A.T., Lamb, J.C., IV & Yang, L.L. (1988) Evaluation of two *in vitro* assays to screen for potential developmental toxicants. *Fundam. appl. Toxicol.*, **11**, 673–684

Stoltz, D.R., Stavric, B., Klassen, R., Bendall, R.D. & Craig, J. (1977) The mutagenicity of saccharin impurities. I. Detection of mutagenic activity. *J. environ. Pathol. Toxicol.*, **1**, 139–146

Stoner, G.D., Shimkin, M.B., Kniazeff, A.J., Weisburger, J.H., Weisburger, E.K. & Gori, G.B. (1973) Test for carcinogenicity of food additives and chemotherapeutic agents by the pulmonary tumor response in strain A mice. *Cancer Res.*, **33**, 3069–3085

Sturgeon, S.R., Harge, P., Silverman, D.T., Kantor, A.F., Marston Linehan, W., Lynch, C. & Hoover, R.N. (1994) Associations between bladder cancer risk factors and tumor stage and grade at diagnosis. *Epidemiology*, **5**, 218–225

Suzuki, H. & Suzuki, N. (1988) Mutagenicity of saccharin in a human cell strain. *Mutat. Res.*, **209**, 13–16

Suzuki, H. & Suzuki, N. (1993) Detection of K-*ras* codon 12 mutation by polymerase chain reaction and differential dot-blot hybridization in sodium saccharin-treated human RSa cell. *Biochem. biophys. Res. Comm.*, **196**, 956–961

Sweatman, T.W. & Renwick, A.G. (1979) Saccharin metabolism and tumorigenicity. *Science*, **205**, 1019–1020

Sweatman, T.W. & Renwick, A.G. (1980) The tissue distribution and pharmacokinetics of saccharin in the rat. *Toxicol. appl. Pharmacol.*, **55**, 18–31

Sweatman, T.W. & Renwick, A.G. (1982) Tissue levels of saccharin in the rat during two-generation feeding studies. *Toxicol. appl. Pharmacol.*, **62**, 465–473

Sweatman, T.W., Renwick, A.G. & Burgess, C.D. (1981) The pharmacokinetics of saccharin in man. *Xenobiotica*, **11**, 531–540

Swiss Pharmaceutical Society (1998) *Index Nominum, International Drug Directory*, 16th Ed., Stuttgart, Medpharm Scientific Publishers [MicroMedex CD-ROM]

Takahashi, M., Kokubo, T., Furukawa, F., Kurokawa, Y. & Hayashi, Y. (1984) Effects of sodium chloride, saccharin, phenobarbital and aspirin on gastric carcinogenesis in rats after initiation with *N*-methyl-*N*′-nitro-*N*-nitrosoguanidine. *Gann*, **75**, 494–501

Takayama, S., Sieber, S.M., Adamson, R.H., Thorgeirrson, U.P., Dalgard, D.W., Arnold, L.L., Cano, M., Eklund, S. & Cohen, S.M. (1998) Long-term feeding of sodium saccharin to nonhuman primates: Implications for urinary tract cancer. *J. natl Cancer Inst.*, **90**, 19–25

Tanaka, S., Kawashima, K., Nakaura, S., Nagao, S., Kuwamura, T. & Omori, Y. (1973) Studies on the teratogenicity of food additives. 1. Effects of saccharin sodium on the development of rats and mice. *J. Food Hyg. Soc.*, **14**, 371–379

Tatematsu, M., Mera, Y., Kohda, K., Kawazoe, Y. & Ito, N. (1986) Ornithine decarboxylase activity and DNA synthesis in rats after long-term treatment with butylated hydroxyanisole, sodium saccharin or phenobarbital. *Cancer Lett.*, **33**, 119–124

Taylor, J.M. & Friedman, L. (1974) Combined chronic feeding and three-generation reproduction study of sodium saccharin in the rat (Abstract No. 200). *Toxicol. appl. Pharmacol.*, **29**, 154

Taylor, J.D., Richards, R.K. & Wiegand, R.G. (1968) Toxicological studies with sodium cyclamate and saccharin. *Food Cosmet. Toxicol.*, **6**, 313–327

Taylor, J.M., Weinberger, M.A. & Friedman, L. (1980) Chronic toxicity and carcinogenicity to the urinary bladder of sodium saccharin in the *in utero*-exposed rat. *Toxicol. appl. Pharmacol.*, **54**, 57–75

Tezabwala, B.U. & Gothoskar, S.V. (1977) Preliminary studies on mutagenicity of saccharin by induction of dominant lethals. *Indian J. Cancer*, **14**, 232–234

Theiss, J.C., Arnold, L.J. & Shimkin, M.B. (1980) Effect of commercial saccharin preparations on urethan-induced lung tumorigenesis in strain A mice. *Cancer Res.*, **40**, 4322–4324

Thorgeirsson, U.P., Dalgard, D.W., Reeves, J. & Adamson, R.H. (1994) Tumor incidence in a chemical carcinogenesis study of nonhuman primates. *Regul. Toxicol. Pharmacol.*, **19**, 130–151

Tisdel, M.O., Nees, P.O., Harris, D.L. & Derse, P.H. (1974) Long-term feeding of saccharin in rats. In: Inglett, G.E., ed., *Symposium: Sweeteners*, Westport, CT, Avi Publishing, pp. 145–158

Toledo, M.C.F. & Ioshi, S.H. (1995) Potential intake of intense sweeteners in Brazil. *Food Addit. Contam.*, **12**, 799–808

Topham, J.C. (1980) Do induced sperm-head abnormalities in mice specifically identify mammalian mutagens rather than carcinogens? *Mutat. Res.*, **74**, 379–387

Traul, K.A., Hink, R.J., Jr, Kachevsky, V. & Wolff, J.S., III (1981) Two-stage carcinogenesis in vitro: transformation of 3-methylcholanthrene-initiated Rauscher murine leukemia virus-infected rat embryo cells by diverse tumor promoters. *J. natl Cancer Inst.*, **66**, 171–175

Trosko, J.E., Dawson, B., Yotti, L.P. & Chang, C.C. (1980) Saccharin may act as a tumour promoter by inhibiting metabolic cooperation between cells. *Nature*, **285**, 109–110

Tsuda, H., Fukushima, S., Imaida, K., Kurata, Y. & Ito, N. (1983) Organ-specific promoting effect of phenobarbital and saccharin in induction of thyroid, liver, and urinary bladder tumors in rats after initiation with *N*-nitrosomethylurea. *Cancer Res.*, **43**, 3292–3296

Ulland, B., Weisburger, E.K. & Weisburger, J.H. (1973) Chronic toxicity and carcinogenicity of industrial chemicals and pesticides (Abstract No. 19). *Toxicol. appl. Pharmacol.*, **25**, 446

Umeda, M., Noda, K. & Ono, T. (1980) Inhibition of metabolic cooperation in Chinese hamster cells by various chemicals including tumor promoters. *Jpn. J. Cancer Res. (Gann)*, **71**, 614–620

United Nations Environment Programme (1998) *Recommendations and Legal Mechanisms. Saccharin*, Geneva (Internet 23 June 1998:http://irptc.unep.ch/irptc)

United States Pharmacopeial Convention (1994) *The 1995 US Pharmacopeia*, 23rd rev./*The National Formulary*, 18th rev., Rockville, MD, pp. 1392–1394, 2297–2298

Uwagawa, S., Saito, K., Okuno, Y., Kawasaki, H., Yoshitake, A., Yamada, H. & Fukushima, S. (1994) Lack of induction of epithelial cell proliferation by sodium saccharin and sodium L-ascorbate in the urinary bladder of NCI-Black-Reiter (NBR) male rats. *Toxicol. appl. Pharmacol.*, **127**, 182–186

Walker, A.M., Dreyer, N.A., Friedlander, E., Loughlin, J., Rothman, K.J. & Kohn, H.I. (1982) An independent analysis of the National Cancer Institute study on non-nutritive sweeteners and bladder cancer. *Am. J. public Health*, **72**, 376–381

Welsch, F. & Stedman, D.B. (1984) Inhibition of metabolic cooperation between Chinese hamster V79 cells by structurally diverse teratogens. *Teratog. Carcinog. Mutag.*, **4**, 285–301

West, R.W. (1979) The exposure of fetal and suckling rats to saccharin from dosed maternal animals. *Toxicology Lett.*, **4**, 127–133

West, R.W. & Jackson, C.D. (1981) Saccharin effects on the urinary physiology and urothelium of the rat when administered in diet or drinking water. *Toxicol. Lett.*, **7**, 409–416

West, R.W., Sheldon, W.G., Gaylor, D.W., Haskin, M.G., Delongchamp, R.R. & Kadlubar, F.F. (1986) The effects of saccharin on the development of neoplastic lesions initiated with *N*-methyl-*N*-nitrosourea in the rat urothelium. *Fundam. appl. Toxicol.*, **7**, 585–600

West, R.W., Sheldon, W.G., Gaylor, D.W., Allen, R.R. & Kadlubar, F.F. (1994) Study of sodium saccharin co-carcinogenicity in the rat. *Food chem. Toxicol.*, **32**, 207–213

WHO (1978) *Evaluation of Certain Food Additives* (WHO Technical Report Series 617), Geneva, pp. 24–26

WHO (1993a) *Evaluation of Certain Food Additives and Contaminants* (WHO Technical Report Series 837), Geneva, pp. 17–19, 46

WHO (1993b) *Guidelines for Drinking Water Quality*, 2nd Ed., Vol. 1, *Recommendations*, Geneva

Whysner, J. & Williams, G.M. (1996) Saccharin mechanistic data and risk assessment: Urine composition, enhanced cell proliferation, and tumor promotion. *Pharmacol. Ther.*, **71**, 225–252

Williamson, D.S., Nagel, D.L., Markin, R.S. & Cohen, S.M. (1987) Effect of pH and ions on the electronic structure of saccharin. *Food chem. Toxicol.*, **25**, 211–218

Wolff, S. & Rodin, B. (1978) Saccharin-induced sister chromatid exchanges in Chinese hamster and human cells. *Science*, **200**, 543–545

Wynder, E.L. & Goldsmith, R. (1977) The epidemiology of bladder cancer: A second look. *Cancer*, **40**, 1246–1268

Wynder, E.L. & Stellman, S.D. (1980) Artificial sweetener use and bladder cancer: A case–control study. *Science*, **207**, 1214–1216

Yu, A., Hashimura, T., Nishio, Y., Kanamaru, H., Fukuzawa, S. & Yoshida, O. (1992) Anti-promoting effect of nordihydroguaiaretic acid on *N*-butyl-*N*-(4-hydroxybutyl) nitrosamine and sodium saccharin-induced rat urinary bladder carcinogenesis. *Jpn. J. Cancer Res.*, **83**, 944–948

SIMAZINE

This substance was considered by a previous working group, in 1990 (IARC, 1991). Since that time, new data have become available, and these have been incorporated into the monograph and taken into consideration in the present evaluation.

1. Exposure Data

1.1 Chemical and physical data

1.1.1 *Nomenclature*

Chem. Abstr. Serv. Reg. No.: 122-34-9
Deleted CAS Reg. Nos: 11141-20-1; 12764-71-5; 39291-64-0; 119603-94-0
Chem. Abstr. Name: 6-Chloro-*N*,*N*′-diethyl-1,3,5-triazine-2,4-diamine
IUPAC Systematic Name: 2-Chloro-4,6-bis(ethylamino)-*s*-triazine
Synonyms: 2,4-Bis(ethylamino)-6-chloro-*s*-triazine; 4,6-bis(ethylamino)-2-chloro-triazine

1.1.2 *Structural and molecular formulae and relative molecular mass*

Cl, N, NH—C_2H_5, N, N, NH—C_2H_5

$C_7H_{12}ClN_5$ Relative molecular mass: 201.66

1.1.3 *Chemical and physical properties of the pure substance*

(*a*) *Description*: Crystals (Budavari, 1996)
(*b*) *Melting-point*: 226°C (Lide, 1997)
(*c*) *Density*: 1.302 g/cm³ at 20°C (Lide, 1997)
(*d*) *Solubility*: Practically insoluble in water; slightly soluble in dioxane (Budavari, 1996)
(*e*) *Volatility*: Vapour pressure: 8.1×10^{-7} Pa at 20°C (National Toxicology Program, 1991)
(*f*) *Octanol/water partition coefficient (P)*: log P, 2.18 (Hansch *et al.*, 1995)
(*g*) *Conversion factor*: mg/m³ = 8.25 × ppm

1.2 Production and use

Information available in 1995 indicated that simazine was produced in Brazil, Israel, Italy, Japan, Romania, the Russian Federation, South Africa, Switzerland and the United States (Chemical Information Services, 1995).

Simazine is used as a herbicide (Budavari, 1996). It is recommended for the control of broad-leaved and grass weeds in deep rooted crops, as a pre-emergence herbicide and as a soil sterilant. Simazine is used extensively on citrus and maize and, to a lesser extent, on other crops such as apples, grapes, peaches, nectarines, walnuts and almonds. In the United States, it has also been used to control algae in farm ponds, fish hatcheries and other surface waters (National Toxicology Program, 1991; National Library of Medicine, 1998a). [The Working Group estimated that the production of simazine was approximately 9700 tonnes in 1996 and 5900 tonnes in 1998.]

1.3 Occurrence

1.3.1 *Natural occurrence*

Simazine is not know to occur naturally.

1.3.2 *Occupational exposure*

According to the 1981–83 National Occupational Exposure Survey (National Institute for Occupational Safety and Health, 1998), approximately 360 chemical industry workers in the United States were potentially exposed to simazine. No data were available on the number of agricultural workers exposed. Occupational exposure may occur through dermal contact or inhalation during the manufacture, formulation or application of this herbicide.

1.3.3 *Environmental occurrence*

According to the Environmental Protection Agency Toxic Chemical Release Inventory for 1996, 2100 kg simazine were released into the air and 42 kg were discharged into water from manufacturing and processing facilities in the United States (National Library of Medicine, 1998b).

The worldwide use of simazine as a pre-emergent herbicide on a broad variety of crops and for weed control in industrial areas and effluents from manufacturing sites have resulted in its release into the environment in various waste streams.

Simazine and its degradation products have varying degrees of persistence in different soil types and seasons under aerobic and anaerobic conditions. The general mobility and stability of simazine are such that it has been detected at low concentrations in ambient rural and urban air, rainwater, surface and groundwater and, less frequently, in drinking-water. Simazine and its degradation products are detected less frequently than atrazine in ground- and surface waters and at lower concentrations (Environmental Protection Agency, 1988, 1990; Kolpin *et al.*, 1997; Tierney *et al.*, 1998; National Library of Medicine, 1998a). No residues of simazine (> 0.04 mg/kg) have been reported in surveys of various foods and feeds in the United States (Elkins *et al.*, 1998).

1.4 Regulations and guidelines

WHO (1993) has established an international drinking-water guideline for simazine of 2 mg/L.

2. Studies of Cancer in Humans

No data on simazine alone were available to the Working Group (see the monograph on atrazine).

3. Studies of Cancer in Experimental Animals

Previous evaluation

Simazine was tested for carcinogenicity in mice and rats by oral and subcutaneous administration and in mice by skin application. The studies were considered inadequate for an evaluation of carcinogenicity (IARC, 1991).

New studies

Oral administration

Mouse: Simazine was tested for carcinogenicity in a partly described study in CD-1 mice by administration in the diet at concentrations up to 400 mg/kg (ppm). Simazine did not increase the incidence of benign or malignant tumours (Hauswirth & Wetzel, 1998). [The Working Group considered this study to be inadequate for evaluation, since no data were available on the numbers of animals, numbers of dosed groups, study duration or observed tumour rates.]

Rat: Groups of 80–90 female Sprague Dawley rats [age unspecified] were fed diets containing 0, 10, 100 or 1000 mg/kg of diet (ppm) simazine (purity, 96.9% [impurities unspecified]) for 24 months. There was a significant ($p < 0.01$) decrease in the rate of survival at the intermediate and high doses. Significantly ($p < 0.01$) increased incidences of mammary gland fibroadenoma (control, 27/90, low dose, 28/80, intermediate dose, 19/80; high dose, 41/80) and mammary gland adenocarcinoma (16/90, 13/80, 20/80, 40/80) were observed at the high dose (Stevens *et al.*, 1994). In addition, the body-weight gain of animals at this dose was less than 30% that of controls (Hauswirth & Wetzel, 1998). The combined incidences of adenomas and carcinomas were 39/90 in controls, 33/88 at the low dose, 31/80 at the intermediate dose and 61/80 ($p < 0.01$) at the high dose. The incidence at the high dose was outside the range seen in historical controls (33–49%). There was also evidence of an earlier onset of mammary gland tumours at the high dose. The incidence of pituitary gland carcinoma was also significantly ($p < 0.05$) increased at the high dose (control, 1/90; low dose, 3/80; intermediate dose, 0/79; high dose, 6/80), but the rate of carcinoma at the high dose (8%) fell within the historical control range for the study laboratory (mean, 3%; range, 0–10%). Moreover, the incidence of pituitary gland adenoma and carcinoma (combined) was similar in all groups (74/90, 60/80, 63/79, 67/80) (Stevens *et al.*, 1994). In the same study [no detailed data reported], male Sprague Dawley rats receiving simazine did not show increased incidences of tumours (Hauswirth & Wetzel, 1998).

4. Other Data Relevant to an Evaluation of Carcinogenicity and its Mechanisms

4.1 Absorption, distribution, metabolism and excretion

4.1.1 *Humans*

No data were available to the Working Group.

4.1.2 *Experimental systems*

The primary route of metabolism for simazine in rats, rabbits and other species *in vivo* and *in vitro* is mono-N-dealkylation (Böhme & Bär, 1967; Adams *et al.*, 1990). Minor metabolites, other than some oxidation products of the alkyl side-chains, have not been identified. The chlorine group, which is linked directly to the aromatic ring, is a reactive site for the formation of glutathione conjugates, as in the case of atrazine (Timchalk *et al.*, 1990).

The metabolism of triazine herbicides (simazine and atrazine) has been evaluated *in vitro* with hepatic supernatant (10 000 × *g*) or microsomal systems from rats (Sprague-Dawley and Fischer 344), mice, goats, sheep, pigs, rabbits and chickens. All the species evaluated produced mono-deethylated metabolites of simazine and deisopropylated metabolites of atrazine. There was considerable variation among the species in the rate of metabolism and in the site-specificity of the reaction (Adams *et al.*, 1990).

4.2 Toxic effects

4.2.1 *Humans*

Simazine has been implicated as a cause of occupational contact dermatitis (Elizarov, 1972).

4.2.2 *Experimental systems*

Simazine toxicosis in sheep was reported to be associated with chronic ingestion of contaminated forage. Affected sheep had generalized muscular tremors that progressed to mild tetany, followed by collapse of the rear legs. Death occurred within two to three days after the onset of clinical signs. Histopathological evaluation revealed acute focal myocardial degeneration, focal non-suppurative encephalitis and hepatic congestion. Elevated simazine concentrations were found in affected tissues from the sheep that died (Allender & Glastonbury, 1992).

Sprague-Dawley rats were fed technical-grade simazine for two years at dietary concentrations of 0, 10, 100 or 1000 mg/kg of diet (ppm) with 40 rats of each sex in the control and high-dose groups and 30 rats of each sex at the low and intermediate doses. After approximately 52 weeks of treatment, 10 rats of each sex per group were killed, and an additional 10 rats of each sex from the control and high-dose groups were maintained on untreated diet for approximately 52 weeks, at which time all of the remaining animals were killed. After 104 weeks of treatment, all remaining animals were killed. The mean body weights and the mean body-weight gain of male and female rats at the high dose were significantly lower than those in the control group from day 7 of the study until the end. Females at the intermediate dose had significantly lower mean body weights than controls throughout the study and at termination (from National Toxicology Program Chemical Repository Database and USEPA Integrated Risk Information System, cited by Keith, 1997).

A number of haematological parameters appeared to be affected by treatment with simazine, mainly in females at the high dose. Significant differences between the controls and those at the high dose were as follows: the erythrocyte count was depressed at all sampling times; haemoglobin concentration and haematocrit were depressed when assayed on days 361, 537 and 725, while the mean corpuscular haemoglobin content was elevated on these days; the leukocyte count was elevated on days 174, 361, 537 and 725; the percentage of neutrophils was elevated on day 316; and the lymphocyte count was depressed on day 361. The mean corpuscular haemoglobin concentration of males at the high dose was significantly higher than that of controls on day 361, and the leukocyte count of males at the intermediate and high doses was significantly lower than that of controls on day 537. In summary, reductions in body-weight gain with accompanying haematological deficits appear to be the toxic end-points for simazine. These effects were seen in all studies that lasted at least one year, including a two-year feeding study in rats, a two-year feeding study in mice and a one-year feeding study in dogs (Keith, 1997).

In a one-year feeding study, dogs (four per sex per dose) were given simazine at dietary concentrations of 0, 20, 100 or 1250 mg/kg (ppm). Toxicity was manifested in males at the high dose by decrements in body-weight gain, variable but reversible decreases in erythrocyte counts, haemoglobin concentration and haematocrit and significant increases in platelet counts. Toxicity was manifested in females at the high dose by significantly larger decreases in body-weight gain and in females at the intermediate and high doses by decrements in erythrocyte counts, haemoglobin concentration and haematocrit. In males and females at the high dose, the absolute organ weights and the organ:brain weight and organ:body weight ratios were increased for the adrenal glands, kidney (males only) and liver and decreased for the spleen (males only) and thyroid/parathyroid (decreased in males, increased in females); however, the changes in organ weights were not accompanied by any histological findings (Keith, 1997).

Simazine did not induce luciferase activity *in vitro* in an oestrogen assay with a recombinant receptor–reporter gene construct integrated into HeLa cells (Balaguer *et al.*, 1996). Simazine also failed to induce oestrogen receptor-mediated responses *in vivo* in immature Sprague-Dawley rat uterus and *in vitro* in an oestrogen-responsive MCF-7 human breast cancer cell line and the oestrogen-dependent recombinant yeast strain PL3. Chloro-*s*-triazine also had no agonist activity and did not antagonize oestradiol-induced luciferase activity in MCF-7 cells transiently transfected with a Gal4-regulated luciferase reporter gene (17m5-G-Luc). These results taken together suggest that the oestrogenic and anti-oestrogenic effects of simazine are not mediated by the oestrogen receptor (Connor *et al.*, 1996).

It was reported in an abstract that the short-term effects of feeding female Sprague-Dawley rats with simazine at 100 or 1000 mg/kg bw of diet (ppm) included modification of the oestrus cycle with increased duration, a change in the uterotrophic response, alterations in the affinity of oestrogen and its receptors and changes in hormone concentrations in serum (Wetzel *et al.*, 1990).

4.3 Reproductive and developmental effects

4.3.1 *Humans*

No data were available to the Working Group.

4.3.2 *Experimental systems*

It was reported in an abstract that subcutaneous injection of simazine to neonatal rats on days 4–7 after birth prolonged the period of vaginal opening (Zeljenkova & Vargova, 1996).

Simazine altered the development of the gonads in birds (Didier & Lutz-Ostertag, 1972). In one study reported as an abstract, no developmental toxicity was seen in rats exposed by inhalation to concentrations up to 317 mg/m^3 on days 7–14 of gestation (Dilley *et al.*, 1977), while teratogenic effects were seen in rats in another study after exposure to a much lower concentration (0.2 mg/m^3) throughout pregnancy (Mirkova & Ivanov, 1981). [The Working Group noted that the effects in the latter study might have been due to an unspecified impurity.] Embryolethality and fetal growth retardation were seen in a study in which rats received oral doses > 312 mg/kg per day during organogenesis on days 6–15 of gestation (Chen *et al.*, 1981; see also IARC, 1991).

Simazine was a component of mixtures designed to mimic the contaminants of groundwater by agricultural practices that were evaluated for developmental and reproductive toxicity. The mixture contained several other pesticides, fertilizers and other organic substances commonly found in groundwater in the State of California (United States). The concentrations of simazine in drinking-water were 0, 0.3, 3 and 30 ng/mL, equivalent to 1, 10 and 100 times the median concentration of simazine in the groundwater. Swiss CD-1 mice were tested in a continuous breeding protocol, and a standard developmental toxicity study was conducted in which Sprague-Dawley rats were exposed on days 6–20 of gestation. In mice, no effects were noted on reproductive performance of F_0 or F_1 individuals or on spermatogenesis, epididymal sperm concentration, percentage of motile sperm, percentage of abnormal sperm or testicular tissues. In rats, no evidence of developmental toxicity was observed (Heindel *et al.*, 1994).

4.4 Genetic and related effects

4.4.1 *Humans*

No data were available to the Working Group.

4.4.2 *Experimental systems* (see Table 1 for references)

In single studies, simazine did not induce differential toxicity in *Bacillus subtilis* or *Salmonella* strains. It was inactive in the SOS DNA-repair assay in *Escherichia coli* and did not induce gene mutation in bacteriophage, bacteria or *Saccharomyces cerevisiae*, whereas mixed responses were obtained for mutation in plants. Simazine did not give rise to micronucleus formation in *Tradescantia*, but it induced chromosomal aberrations in various other plant species.

Mutations were induced at the *tk* locus in mouse lymphoma L5178Y cells, but DNA damage, as indicated by unscheduled DNA synthesis, was not induced in cultured human fibroblasts. Neither gene conversion nor mitotic recombination was induced in *S. cerevisiae*, nor aneuploidy in *Neurospora crassa*.

In single studies, simazine induced somatic mutation, sex-linked recessive lethal mutations, dominant lethal effects, but not aneuploidy, in *Drosophila melanogaster*.

Simazine did not induce sister chromatid exchange in cultured human lymphocytes or Chinese hamster cells, nor did it induce chromosomal aberrations in cultured Chinese hamster cells.

It did not induce micronucleus formation in bone-marrow cells of mice exposed *in vivo*.

4.5 Mechanistic considerations

Long-term feeding of 100 mg/kg of diet simazine per day for two years increased the incidence of mammary tumours in female Sprague-Dawley rats, but few data are available to establish a mechanism for that effect. Simazine administered at a high dose (300 mg/kg per day) for 14 days significantly prolonged the oestrous cycle in Sprague-Dawley rats (Wetzel *et al.*, 1990), suggesting that simazine may have a mechanism of action on the mammary gland similar to that of the structurally related atrazine (Stevens *et al.*, 1999).

5. Summary of Data Reported and Evaluation

5.1 Exposure data

Exposure to simazine occurs during its production, formulation and use as a herbicide. Simazine and its degradation products have been detected at low levels in ambient rural and urban air, rainwater, surface and groundwater and, less frequently, in drinking-water samples.

Table 1. Genetic and related effects of simazine

Test system	Results[a]		Dose[b] (LED or HID)	Reference
	Without exogenous metabolic system	With exogenous metabolic system		
Escherichia coli PQ37, SOS chromotest	NT	–	NR	Mersch-Sundermann *et al.* (1988)
Salmonella typhimurium TA1978/TA1538 and SL525/SL4700, differential toxicity	–	NT	2000 μg/disc	Environmental Protection Agency (1984)
Bacillus subtilis rec strains, differential toxicity	–	NT	1000 μg/disc	Kuroda *et al.* (1992)
Salmonella typhimurium TA100, TA98, TA1535, TA1537, TA1538, reverse mutation	NT	–	NR	Simmon *et al.* (1977)
Salmonella typhimurium TA100, TA98, reverse mutation	–	–	5000 μg/plate	Environmental Protection Agency (1984)
Salmonella typhimurium TA100, TA1535, TA1537, TA1538, reverse mutation	–	–	1000 μg/plate	Environmental Protection Agency (1977)
Salmonella typhimurium TA100, reverse mutation	NT	+[c]	NR	Means *et al.* (1988)
Salmonella typhimurium TA100, TA102, TA97, reverse mutation	–	–	1000 μg/plate	Mersch-Sundermann *et al.* (1988)
Salmonella typhimurium TA1530, TA1531, TA1532, TA1534, G46, reverse mutation (spot test)	–	NT	NR	Seiler (1973)
Salmonella typhimurium (eight unidentified strains), reverse mutation	–	NT	NR	Andersen *et al.* (1972)
Escherichia coli, forward mutation	–	NT	NR	Fahrig (1974)
Escherichia coli WP2 *uvr*, reverse mutation	–	–	1000 μg/plate	Environmental Protection Agency (1984)
Serratia marcescens, reverse mutation	–	NT	NR	Fahrig (1974)
Saccharomyces cerevisiae, gene conversion	–	NT	NR	Fahrig (1974)
Saccharomyces cerevisiae, gene conversion	–	NT	1000[d]	Siebert & Lemperle (1974)
Saccharomyces cerevisiae D3, homozygosis by recombination	–	–	50 000	Environmental Protection Agency (1977)

Table 1 (contd)

Test system	Results[a]		Dose[b] (LED or HID)	Reference
	Without exogenous metabolic system	With exogenous metabolic system		
Saccharomyces cerevisiae D7, mitotic recombination	–	–	25 000	Environmental Protection Agency (1984)
Saccharomyces cerevisiae D7, reverse mutation	–	–	25 000	Environmental Protection Agency (1984)
Saccharomyces cerevisiae D7, gene conversion	–	–	25 000	Environmental Protection Agency (1984)
Saccharomyces cerevisiae, reverse mutation	–	NT	5	Emnova *et al.* (1987)
Neurospara crassa, aneuploidy	–	NT	NR	Griffiths (1979)
Hordeum vulgare, mutation	+	NT	1000	Wuu & Grant (1966)
Hordeum vulgare, mutation	–	NT	200	Stroev (1968a)
Rizobium meliloti, mutation	–	NT	5000	Kaszubiak (1968)
Zea mays, chlorophyll mutation	+	NT	200	Morgun *et al.* (1982)
Zea mays, mutation	+	NT	NR	Plewa *et al.* (1984)
Fragaria ananassa, mutation	+	NT	2	Malone & Dix (1990)
Tradescantia paludosa, micronuclei	–	NT	200	Ma *et al.* (1984)
Hordeum vulgare, chromosomal aberrations	+	NT	500	Wuu & Grant (1966)
Hordeum vulgare, chromosomal aberrations	+	NT	500 spray	Wuu & Grant (1967a)
Hordeum vulgare, chromosomal aberrations	(+)	NT	500	Stroev (1968b)
Hordeum vulgare, chromosomal aberrations	(+)	NT	500[d]	Kahlon (1980)
Vicia faba, chromosomal aberrations	+	NT	200[d]	Wuu & Grant (1967b)
Vicia faba, chromosomal aberrations	+	NT	5	Hakeem & Shehab (1974)
Vicia faba, chromosomal aberrations	(+)	NT	1000	de Kergommeaux *et al.* (1983)
Allium cepa, chromosomal aberrations	+	NT	20	Chubutia & Ugulava (1973)

Table 1 (contd)

Test system	Results[a]		Dose[b] (LED or HID)	Reference
	Without exogenous metabolic system	With exogenous metabolic system		
Crepis capillaris, chromosomal aberrations	+	NT	1000	Voskanyan & Avakyan (1984)
Drosophila melanogaster, somatic mutation	+		2000 μg/g feed	Tripathy *et al.* (1995)
Drosophila melanogaster, sex-linked recessive lethal mutation	–		10 ng/fly inj	Benes & Šrám (1969)
Drosophila melanogaster, sex-linked recessive lethal mutation	+		6 ng/fly inj	Murnik & Nash (1977)
Drosophila melanogaster, sex-linked recessive lethal mutation	–		6000 μg/g feed	Murnik & Nash (1977)
Drosophila melanogaster, sex-linked recessive lethal mutation	+		2000 μg/g feed	Tripathy *et al.* (1995)
Drosophila melanogaster, dominant lethal mutation	+		6000 μg/g feed	Murnik & Nash (1977)
Drosophila melanogaster, aneuploidy	–		6000 μg/g feed	Murnik & Nash (1977)
Gene mutation, mouse lymphoma L5178Y cells *in vitro*, *tk* locus *in vitro*	–	(+)	300	Environmental Protection Agency (1984)
Sister chromatid exchange, Chinese hamster ovary cells *in vitro*	–	NT	1700	Environmental Protection Agency (1984)
Sister chromatid exchange, Chinese hamster lung V79 cells *in vitro*	–	NT	2	Kuroda *et al.* (1992)
Chromosomal aberrations, Chinese hamster ovary cells *in vitro*	–	NT	0.01	Biradar & Rayburn (1995)
Unscheduled DNA synthesis, human lung WI 38 fibroblasts *in vitro*	–	–	200	Environmental Protection Agency (1984)
Sister chromatid exchange, human lymphocytes *in vitro*	(+)	NT	NR	Ghiazza *et al.* (1984)

Table 1 (contd)

Test system	Results[a]		Dose[b] (LED or HID)	Reference
	Without exogenous metabolic system	With exogenous metabolic system		
Sister chromatid exchange, human lymphocytes *in vitro*	–	–	10	Dunkelberg *et al.* (1994)
Micronucleus formation, mouse bone-marrow and peripheral blood cells *in vivo*	–	NT	500 po × 2	Environmental Protection Agency (1984)

[a] +, positive; (+), weakly positive; –, negative; NT, not tested
[b] LED, lowest effective dose; HID, highest ineffective dose; unless otherwise stated, in-vitro test, µg/mL; in-vivo test, mg/kg bw per day; NR, not reported; inj, injection; po, oral
[c] Tested with extracts of simazine-treated *Zea mays*
[d] Commercial pesticide tested

5.2 Human carcinogenicity data

No data were available on simazine alone (see the monograph on atrazine).

5.3 Animal carcinogenicity data

Simazine was tested for carcinogenicity in one experiment by oral administration to Sprague-Dawley rats. It increased the incidences of benign and malignant mammary gland tumours in females.

5.4 Other relevant data

Simazine is metabolized by dealkylation. No interaction with an oestrogen receptor was seen *in vitro*. In Sprague-Dawley rats, simazine was not uterotrophic but prolonged the duration of the oestrus cycle. Long-term administration resulted in haematological effects in rats and dogs.

Simazine did not show developmental toxicity in one study by inhalation in rats, but it was embryolethal and decreased fetal body weights in a study in which it was administered orally.

No data were available on the genetic and related effects of simazine in humans. Simazine was not genotoxic to rodents *in vivo* or in cultured mammalian cells, yeast or bacteria. It induced genetic damage in *Drosophila* and in plants.

5.5 Evaluation

There is *inadequate evidence* in humans for the carcinogenicity of simazine.

There is *limited evidence* in experimental animals for the carcinogenicity of simazine.

Overall evaluation

Simazine is *not classifiable as to its carcinogenicity to humans (Group 3).*

6. References

Adams, N.H., Levi, P.E. & Hodgson, E. (1990) *In vitro* studies of the metabolism of atrazine, simazine, and terbutryn. *J. agric. Food Chem.*, **38**, 1411–1417

Allender, W.J. & Glastonbury, J.W. (1992) Simazine toxicosis in sheep. *Vet. hum. Toxicol.*, **34**, 422–423

Andersen, K.J., Leighty, E.G. & Takahashi, M.K. (1972) Evaluation of herbicides for possible mutagenic properties. *J. agric. Food Chem.*, **20**, 649–656

Balaguer, P., Joyeux, A., Denison, M.S., Vincent, R., Gillesby, B.E. & Zacharewski, T. (1996) Assessing the estrogenic and dioxin-like activities of chemicals and complex mixtures using *in vitro* recombinant receptor-reporter gene assays. *Can. J. Physiol. Pharmacol.*, **74**, 216–222

Benes, V. & Šrám, R. (1969) Mutagenic activity of some pesticides in *Drosophila melanogaster*. *Ind. Med.*, **38**, 442–444

Biradar, D.P. & Rayburn, A.L. (1995) Flow cytogenetic analysis of whole cell clastogenicity of herbicides found in groundwater. *Arch. environ. Contam. Toxicol.*, **28**, 13–17

Böhme, C. & Bär, F. (1967) [The metabolism of triazine herbicides in the animal organism.] *Food Cosmet. Toxicol.*, **5**, 23–28 (in German)

Budavari, S., ed. (1996) *The Merck Index*, 12th Ed., Whitehouse Station, NJ, Merck & Co., p. 1464

Chemical Information Services (1995) *Directory of World Chemical Producers 1995/96 Standard Edition*, Dallas, TX, p. 622

Chen, P.C., Chi, H.F. & Kan, S.Y. (1981) [Experimental studies on the toxicity and teratogenicity of simazine.] *Chin. J. prev. Med.*, **15**, 83–85 (in Chinese)

Chubutia, R.A. & Ugulava, N.A. (1973) [Cytogenetic effects of herbicides.] *Tr. Nauchno.-Issled. Inst. Zashch. Rast.*, **25**, 97–99 (in Georgian)

Connor, K., Howell, J., Chen, I., Liu, H., Berhane, K., Sciarretta, C., Safe, S. & Cachararewski T. (1996) Failure of chlor-s-triazine-derived compounds to induce estrogen receptor-mediated responses *in vivo* and *in vitro*. *Fundam. appl. Toxicol.*, **30**, 93–101

Didier, R. & Lutz-Ostertag, Y. (1972) [Action of simazine on the genital tract of chick and quail embryos *in vivo* and *in vitro*.] *C.R. Soc. Biol.*, **166**, 1691–1693 (in French)

Dilley, J.V., Chernoff, N., Kay, D., Winslow, N. & Newell, G.W. (1977) Inhalation teratology studies of five chemicals in rats (Abstract). *Toxicol. appl. Pharmacol.*, **41**, 196

Dunkelberg, H., Fuchs, J., Hengstler, J.G., Klein, E., Oesch, F. & Strüder, K. (1994) Genotoxic effects of the herbicides alachlor, atrazine, pendimethaline, and simazine in mammalian cells. *Bull. environ. Contam. Toxicol.*, **52**, 498–504

Elizarov, G.P. (1972) [Occupational skin diseases caused by simazine and propazine.] *Vestn. Derm. Venerol.*, **46**, 27–29 (in Russian)

Elkins, E.R., Lyon, R.S. & Jarman, R. (1998) Pesticide residues in processed foods: Not a food safety concern. In: Ballantine, L.G., McFarland, J.E. & Hackett, D.S., eds, *Triazine Herbicides: Risk Assessment* (ACS Symposium No. 683), Washington DC, American Chemical Society, pp. 116–122

Emnova, E.E., Merenіouk, G.V. & Turkan, L.G. (1987) [Genetic study of simazine-triazine herbicides on *Saccharomyces cerevisiae*.] *Tsitol. Genet.*, **21**, 127–130 (in Russian)

Environmental Protection Agency (1977) *Evaluation of Selected Pesticides as Chemical Mutagens.* In Vitro *and* In Vivo *Studies* (EPA-600/1-77-028), Washington DC

Environmental Protection Agency (1984) *In Vitro and In Vivo Mutagenicity Studies of Environmental Chemicals* (EPA-600/1-84-003; NTIS Report No. PB84-138973), Washington DC

Environmental Protection Agency (1988) *Health Advisories for 50 Pesticides: Simazine* (USNTIS, PB 88-245931), Washington DC, EPA Office of Drinking Water, pp. 765–788

Environmental Protection Agency (1990) *EPA National Pesticide Survey*, Washington DC, Office of Water—Office of Pesticides and Toxic Substances

Fahrig, R. (1974) Comparative mutagenicity studies with pesticides. In: Rosenfeld, C. & Davis, W., eds, *Environmental Pollution and Carcinogenic Risks* (IARC Scientific Publications No. 10), Lyon, IARC, pp. 161–181

Ghiazza, G., Zavarise, G., Lanero, M. & Feraro, G. (1984) [SCE (sister chromatid exchanges) induced in chromosomes of human lymphocytes by trifluralin, atrazine and simazine.] *Boll. Soc. It. Biol. Sper.*, **60**, 2149–2153 (in Italian)

Griffiths, A.J. (1979) Neurospora prototroph selection system for studying aneuploid production. *Environ. Health Perspectives*, **31**, 75–80

Hakeem, H. & Shehab, A. (1974) Cytological effects of simazine on *Vicia faba*. *Proc. Egypt. Acad. Sci.*, **25**, 61–66

Hansch, C., Leo, A. & Hoekman, D. (1995) *Exploring QSAR*, Washington DC, American Chemical Society, p. 34

Hauswirth, J.W. & Wetzel, L.T. (1998) Toxicity characteristics of the 2-chlorotriazines atrazine and simazine. In: Ballantine, L.G., McFarland, J.E. & Hackett, D.S., eds, *Triazine Herbicides: Risk Assessment* (ACS Symposium Series No. 683), Washington DC, American Chemical Society, pp. 370–383

Heindel, J.J., Chapin, R.E., Gulati, D.K., George, J.D., Price, C.J., Maa, M.C., Myers, C.B., Barnes, L.H., Fail, P.A., Grizzle, T.B., Schwetz, B.A. & Yang, R.S. (1994) Assessment of the reproductive and developmental toxicity of pesticide/fertilizer mixtures based on confirmed pesticide contamination in California and Iowa. *Fundam. appl. Toxicol.*, **22**, 605–621

IARC (1991) *IARC Monographs on the Evaluation of Carcinogenic Risks to Humans*, Vol. 53, *Occupational Exposures in Insecticide Application, and Some Pesticides*, Lyon, pp. 495–513

Kahlon, P.S. (1980) Seedling injury and chromosome aberrations induced by Bladex, Dowpon, Princep and Tenoran. *J. Tenn. Acad. Sci.*, **55**, 17–19

Kaszubiak, H. (1968) The effects of herbicides on *Rhizobium*. III. Influence of herbicides in mutation. *Acta microbiol. pol.*, **17**, 51–58

Keith, L.H. (1997) Simazine. In: *Environmental Endocrine Disruptors. A Handbook of Property Data*, New York, John Wiley & Sons, pp. 1033–1053

de Kergommeaux, D.J., Grant, W.F. & Sandhu, S.S. (1983) Clastogenic and physiological response of chromosomes to nine pesticides in the *Vicia faba* in vivo root tip assay system. *Mutat. Res.*, **24**, 69–84

Kolpin, D.W., Kalkhoff, S.J., Goolsby, D.A., Sneck-Fahrer, D.A. & Thurman, E.M. (1997) Occurrence of selected herbicides and herbicide degradation products in Iowa ground water, 1995. *Ground Water*, **35**, 679–688

Kuroda, K., Yamaguchi, Y. & Endo, G. (1992) Mitotic toxicity, sister chromatid exchange, and rec assay of pesticides. *Arch. environ. Contam. Toxicol.*, **23**, 13–18

Lide, D.R., ed. (1997) *CRC Handbook of Chemistry and Physics*, 78th Ed., Boca Raton, FL, CRC Press, p. 3-314

Ma, T.-H., Harris, M.M., Anderson, V.A., Ahmed, I., Mohammad, K., Bare, J.L. & Lin, G. (1984) Tradescantia-micronucleus (Trad-MCN) tests on 140 health-related agents. *Mutat. Res.*, **138**, 157–167

Malone, R.P. & Dix, P.J. (1990) Mutagenesis and triazine herbicide effects in strawberry shoot cultures. *J. exp. Bot.*, **41**, 463–469

Means, J.C., Plewa, M.J. & Gentile, J.M. (1988) Assessment of the mutagenicity of fractions from *s*-triazine-treated *Zea mays*. *Mutat. Res.*, **197**, 325–326

Mersch-Sundermann, V., Dickgiesser, N., Hablizel, U. & Gruber, B. (1988) [Examination of the mutagenicity of organic microcontaminations of the environment. I. Mutagenicity of selected herbicides and insecticides in the *Salmonella*-microsome test (Ames test) in relation to the pathogenic potency of contaminated ground- and drinking-water.] *Zbl. Bakt. Hyg. B.*, **186**, 247–260 (in German)

Mirkova, E. & Ivanov, I. (1981) [A propos of the embryotoxic effect of triazine herbicide Polyzin 50.] *Probl. Khig.*, **6**, 36–43 (in Russian)

Morgun, V.V., Logvinenko, V.F., Merezhinskii, Y.G., Lapina, T.V. & Frigorenko, N.V. (1982) [Cytogenetic and genetic activity of the herbicides atrazine, simazine, prometrin and linuron.] *Tsitol. Genet.*, **16**, 38–41 (in Russian)

Murnik, M.R. & Nash, C.L. (1977) Mutagenicity of the triazine herbicides atrazine, cyanazine and simazine in *Drosophila melanogaster*. *J. Toxicol. environ. Health*, **3**, 691–697

National Institute for Occupational Safety and Health (1998) *National Occupational Exposure Survey (1981–1983)*, Cincinnati, OH

National Library of Medicine (1998a) *Hazardous Substances Data Bank (HSDB)*, Bethesda, MD [Record No. 1765]

National Library of Medicine (1998b) *Toxic Chemical Release Inventory 1996* (TRI96), Bethesda, MD

National Toxicology Program (1991) *Simazine NTP Chemical Repository Data Sheet*, Research Triangle Park, NC

Oledzka-Slotwinska, H. (1974) The effect of simazine on the ultrastructure and activities of some hydrolases of the rat liver. *Ann. med. Sect. Pol. Acad. Sci.*, **19**, 141–142

Plewa, M.J., Wagner, E.D., Gentile, G.J. & Gentile, J.M. (1984) An evaluation of the genotoxic properties of herbicides following plant and animal activation. *Mutat. Res.*, **136**, 233–245

Seiler, J.P. (1973) A survey on the mutagenicity of various pesticides. *Experientia*, **29**, 622–623

Siebert, D. & Lemperle, E. (1974) Genetic effects of herbicides: Induction of mitotic gene conversion in *Saccharomyces cerevisiae*. *Mutat. Res.*, **22**, 111–120

Simmon, V.F., Kauhanen, K. & Tardiff, R.G. (1977) Mutagenic activity of chemicals identified in drinking water. In: Scott, D., Bridges, B.A. & Sobels, F.H., eds, *Progress in Genetic Toxicology*, Amsterdam, North Holland Biomedical Press, pp. 249–258

Stevens, J.T., Breckenridge, C.B., Wetzel, L.T., Gillis, J.H., Luempert, L.G., III & Eldridge, J.C. (1994) Hypothesis for mammary tumorigenesis in Sprague-Dawley rats exposed to certain triazine herbicides. *J. Toxicol. environ. Health*, **43**, 139–154

Stevens, J.T., Breckenridge, C.B., Wetzel, L., Thakur, A.K., Liu, C., Werner, C., Luempert, L.G., III & Eldridge, J.C. (1999) A risk characterization for atrazine: Oncogenicity profile. *J. Toxicol. environ. Health*, **56**, 69–109

Stroev, V.S. (1968a) [The mutagenic effect of herbicides on barley.] *Genetika*, **4**, 164–167 (in Russian)

Stroev, V.S. (1968b) [Cytogenetic activity of the herbicides simazine and maleic acid hydrazide.] *Genetika*, 4, 130–134 (in Russian)

Tierney, D.P., Clarkson, J.R., Christensen, B.R., Golden, K.A. & Hines, N.A. (1998) Exposure to the herbicides atrazine and simazine in drinking-water. In: Ballantine, L.G., McFarland, J.E. & Hackett, D.S., eds, *Triazine Herbicides: Risk Assessment* (ACS Symposium Series No. 683), Washington DC, American Chemical Society, pp. 252–265

Timchalk, C., Dryzga, M.D., Langvardt, P.W., Kastl, P.E. & Osborne, D.W. (1990) Determination of the effect of tridiphane on the pharmacokinetics of [^{14}C]-atrazine following oral administration to male Fischer 344 rats. *Toxicology*, **61**, 27–40

Tripathy, N.K., Routray, P.K., Sahu, G.P. & Kumar, A.A. (1995) Simazine: Genotoxicity studies in Drosophila melanogaster. *Biol. Zent. Bl.*, **114**, 378–384

Voskanyan, A.Z. & Avakyan, V.A. (1984) [Cytogenetic effect of simazine and linuron herbicides on the chromosomes of *Crepis capillaris*.] *Biol. Zhuv. Armenii*, **9**, 741–744 (in Russian)

Wetzel, L.T., Breckenridge, C.B., Eldridge, J.C., Tisdel, M.O. & Stevens, J.T. (1990) Possible mechanism of mammary tumor formation in Sprague-Dawley rats following the administration of chloro-triazine herbicides (Abstract). *J. Am. Coll. Toxicol.*, **9**, 650

WHO (1993) *Guidelines for Drinking Water Quality*, 2nd Ed., Vol. 1, *Recommendations*, Geneva, pp. 90–91

Wuu, K.D. & Grant, W.F. (1966) Morphological and somatic chromosomal aberrations induced by pesticides in barley (*Hordeum vulgare*). *Can. J. Genet. Cytol.*, **8**, 481–501

Wuu, K.D. & Grant, W.F. (1967a) Chromosomal aberrations induced by pesticides in meiotic cells of barley. *Cytologia*, **32**, 31–41

Wuu, K.D. & Grant, W.F. (1967b) Chromosomal aberrations in somatic cells of *Vicia faba* by pesticides. *Nucleus*, **10**, 37–46

Zeljenkova, D. & Vargova, M. (1996) Possible estrogenic effects of some herbicides (Abstract). *Teratology*, **53**, 39A

SUMMARY OF FINAL EVALUATIONS

Agent	Degree of evidence of carcinogenicity		Overall evaluation of carcinogenicity to humans
	Human	Animal	
Allyl isothiocyanate	I	L	3
ortho-Anisidine	I	S	2B
Atrazine	I	S	3[a]
Butyl benzyl phthalate	I	L	3
Chloroform	I	S	2B
Chlorothalonil	I	S	2B
Cyclamates	I	I	3
Dichlorobenzenes			
ortho-Dichlorobenzene	I	ESL	3
meta-Dichlorobenzene	I	I	3
para-Dichlorobenzene	I	S	2B[a]
Hexachlorobutadiene	I	L	3
Hexachloroethane	I	S	2B
d-Limonene	I	S	3[a]
Melamine	I	S	3[a]
Methyl *tert*-butyl ether	I	L	3
Nitrilotriacetic acid and its salts	I	S	2B
Paracetamol	I	I	3
ortho-Phenylphenol and its sodium salt			
ortho-Phenylphenol	I	L	3
Sodium *ortho*-phenylphenate	I	S	2B
Potassium bromate	I	S	2B
Quercetin	I	L	3
Saccharin and its salts	I		3[a]
Sodium saccharin		S	
Saccharin (acid form) and calcium saccharin		I	
Simazine	I	L	3

I, inadequate evidence; L, limited evidence; S, sufficient evidence; ESL, evidence suggesting lack of carcinogenicity; group 1, carcinogenic to humans; group 2B, possibly carcinogenic to humans; group 3, not classifiable as to its carcinogenicity to humans; for definitions of criteria for degrees of evidence and groups, see preamble, pp. 23–27.

[a] Mechanistic data were taken into account in making the overall evaluation.

CUMULATIVE CROSS INDEX TO *IARC MONOGRAPHS ON THE EVALUATION OF CARCINOGENIC RISKS TO HUMANS*

The volume, page and year of publication are given. References to corrigenda are given in parentheses.

B

C

D

G

K

L

M

N

O

Q

R

S

T

List of IARC Monographs on the Evaluation of Carcinogenic Risks to Humans*

Volume 1
Some Inorganic Substances, Chlorinated Hydrocarbons, Aromatic Amines, *N*-Nitroso Compounds, and Natural Products
1972; 184 pages (out-of-print)

Volume 2
Some Inorganic and Organometallic Compounds
1973; 181 pages (out-of-print)

Volume 3
Certain Polycyclic Aromatic Hydrocarbons and Heterocyclic Compounds
1973; 271 pages (out-of-print)

Volume 4
Some Aromatic Amines, Hydrazine and Related Substances, *N*-Nitroso Compounds and Miscellaneous Alkylating Agents
1974; 286 pages (out-of-print)

Volume 5
Some Organochlorine Pesticides
1974; 241 pages (out-of-print)

Volume 6
Sex Hormones
1974; 243 pages (out-of-print)

Volume 7
Some Anti-Thyroid and Related Substances, Nitrofurans and Industrial Chemicals
1974; 326 pages (out-of-print)

Volume 8
Some Aromatic Azo Compounds
1975; 357 pages

Volume 9
Some Aziridines, *N*-, *S*- and *O*-Mustards and Selenium
1975; 268 pages

Volume 10
Some Naturally Occurring Substances
1976; 353 pages (out-of-print)

Volume 11
Cadmium, Nickel, Some Epoxides, Miscellaneous Industrial Chemicals and General Considerations on Volatile Anaesthetics
1976; 306 pages (out-of-print)

Volume 12
Some Carbamates, Thiocarbamates and Carbazides
1976; 282 pages (out-of-print)

Volume 13
Some Miscellaneous Pharmaceutical Substances
1977; 255 pages

Volume 14
Asbestos
1977; 106 pages (out-of-print)

Volume 15
Some Fumigants, the Herbicides 2,4-D and 2,4,5-T, Chlorinated Dibenzodioxins and Miscellaneous Industrial Chemicals
1977; 354 pages (out-of-print)

Volume 16
Some Aromatic Amines and Related Nitro Compounds—Hair Dyes, Colouring Agents and Miscellaneous Industrial Chemicals
1978; 400 pages

Volume 17
Some *N*-Nitroso Compounds
1978; 365 pages

Volume 18
Polychlorinated Biphenyls and Polybrominated Biphenyls
1978; 140 pages (out-of-print)

Volume 19
Some Monomers, Plastics and Synthetic Elastomers, and Acrolein
1979; 513 pages (out-of-print)

Volume 20
Some Halogenated Hydrocarbons
1979; 609 pages (out-of-print)

Volume 21
Sex Hormones (II)
1979; 583 pages

Volume 22
Some Non-Nutritive Sweetening Agents
1980; 208 pages

Volume 23
Some Metals and Metallic Compounds
1980; 438 pages (out-of-print)

Volume 24
Some Pharmaceutical Drugs
1980; 337 pages

Volume 25
Wood, Leather and Some Associated Industries
1981; 412 pages

Volume 26
Some Antineoplastic and Immunosuppressive Agents
1981; 411 pages

Volume 27
Some Aromatic Amines, Anthraquinones and Nitroso Compounds, and Inorganic Fluorides Used in Drinking-water and Dental Preparations
1982; 341 pages

Volume 28
The Rubber Industry
1982; 486 pages

Volume 29
Some Industrial Chemicals and Dyestuffs
1982; 416 pages

Volume 30
Miscellaneous Pesticides
1983; 424 pages

---

*Certain older volumes, marked out-of-print, are still available directly from IARCPress. Further, high-quality photocopies of all out-of-print volumes may be purchased from University Microfilms International, 300 North Zeeb Road, Ann Arbor, MI 48106-1346, USA (Tel.: 313-761-4700, 800-521-0600).

Volume 31
Some Food Additives, Feed Additives and Naturally Occurring Substances
1983; 314 pages (out-of-print)

Volume 32
Polynuclear Aromatic Compounds, Part 1: Chemical, Environmental and Experimental Data
1983; 477 pages (out-of-print)

Volume 33
Polynuclear Aromatic Compounds, Part 2: Carbon Blacks, Mineral Oils and Some Nitroarenes
1984; 245 pages (out-of-print)

Volume 34
Polynuclear Aromatic Compounds, Part 3: Industrial Exposures in Aluminium Production, Coal Gasification, Coke Production, and Iron and Steel Founding
1984; 219 pages

Volume 35
Polynuclear Aromatic Compounds, Part 4: Bitumens, Coal-tars and Derived Products, Shale-oils and Soots
1985; 271 pages

Volume 36
Allyl Compounds, Aldehydes, Epoxides and Peroxides
1985; 369 pages

Volume 37
Tobacco Habits Other than Smoking; Betel-Quid and Areca-Nut Chewing; and Some Related Nitrosamines
1985; 291 pages

Volume 38
Tobacco Smoking
1986; 421 pages

Volume 39
Some Chemicals Used in Plastics and Elastomers
1986; 403 pages

Volume 40
Some Naturally Occurring and Synthetic Food Components, Furocoumarins and Ultraviolet Radiation
1986; 444 pages

Volume 41
Some Halogenated Hydrocarbons and Pesticide Exposures
1986; 434 pages

Volume 42
Silica and Some Silicates
1987; 289 pages

Volume 43
Man-Made Mineral Fibres and Radon
1988; 300 pages

Volume 44
Alcohol Drinking
1988; 416 pages

Volume 45
Occupational Exposures in Petroleum Refining; Crude Oil and Major Petroleum Fuels
1989; 322 pages

Volume 46
Diesel and Gasoline Engine Exhausts and Some Nitroarenes
1989; 458 pages

Volume 47
Some Organic Solvents, Resin Monomers and Related Compounds, Pigments and Occupational Exposures in Paint Manufacture and Painting
1989; 535 pages

Volume 48
Some Flame Retardants and Textile Chemicals, and Exposures in the Textile Manufacturing Industry
1990; 345 pages

Volume 49
Chromium, Nickel and Welding
1990; 677 pages

Volume 50
Pharmaceutical Drugs
1990; 415 pages

Volume 51
Coffee, Tea, Mate, Methyl-xanthines and Methylglyoxal
1991; 513 pages

Volume 52
Chlorinated Drinking-water; Chlorination By-products; Some Other Halogenated Compounds; Cobalt and Cobalt Compounds
1991; 544 pages

Volume 53
Occupational Exposures in Insecticide Application, and Some Pesticides
1991; 612 pages

Volume 54
Occupational Exposures to Mists and Vapours from Strong Inorganic Acids; and Other Industrial Chemicals
1992; 336 pages

Volume 55
Solar and Ultraviolet Radiation
1992; 316 pages

Volume 56
Some Naturally Occurring Substances: Food Items and Constituents, Heterocyclic Aromatic Amines and Mycotoxins
1993; 599 pages

Volume 57
Occupational Exposures of Hairdressers and Barbers and Personal Use of Hair Colourants; Some Hair Dyes, Cosmetic Colourants, Industrial Dyestuffs and Aromatic Amines
1993; 428 pages

Volume 58
Beryllium, Cadmium, Mercury, and Exposures in the Glass Manufacturing Industry
1993; 444 pages

Volume 59
Hepatitis Viruses
1994; 286 pages

Volume 60
Some Industrial Chemicals
1994; 560 pages

Volume 61
Schistosomes, Liver Flukes and *Helicobacter pylori*
1994; 270 pages

Volume 62
Wood Dust and Formaldehyde
1995; 405 pages

Volume 63
Dry Cleaning, Some Chlorinated Solvents and Other Industrial Chemicals
1995; 551 pages

Volume 64
Human Papillomaviruses
1995; 409 pages

Volume 65
Printing Processes and Printing Inks, Carbon Black and Some Nitro Compounds
1996; 578 pages

Volume 66
Some Pharmaceutical Drugs
1996; 514 pages

Volume 67
Human Immunodeficiency Viruses and Human T-Cell Lymphotropic Viruses
1996; 424 pages

Volume 68
Silica, Some Silicates, Coal Dust and *para*-Aramid Fibrils
1997; 506 pages

Volume 69
Polychlorinated Dibenzo-*para*-Dioxins and Polychlorinated Dibenzofurans
1997; 666 pages

Volume 70
Epstein-Barr Virus and Kaposi's Sarcoma Herpesvirus/Human Herpesvirus 8
1997; 524 pages

Volume 71
Re-evaluation of Some Organic Chemicals, Hydrazine and Hydrogen Peroxide
1999; 1586 pages

Volume 72
Hormonal Contraception and Post-menopausal Hormonal Therapy
1999; 660 pages

Volume 73
Some Chemicals that Cause Tumours of the Kidney or Urinary Bladder in Rodents and Some Other Substances
1999; 674 pages

Volume 74
Surgical Implants, Prosthetic Devices and Foreign Bodies
1999 (in preparation)

Supplement No. 1
Chemicals and Industrial Processes Associated with Cancer in Humans (*IARC Monographs*, Volumes 1 to 20)
1979; 71 pages (out-of-print)

Supplement No. 2
Long-term and Short-term Screening Assays for Carcinogens: A Critical Appraisal
1980; 426 pages (out-of-print)

Supplement No. 3
Cross Index of Synonyms and Trade Names in Volumes 1 to 26 of the *IARC Monographs*
1982; 199 pages (out-of-print)

Supplement No. 4
Chemicals, Industrial Processes and Industries Associated with Cancer in Humans (*IARC Monographs*, Volumes 1 to 29)
1982; 292 pages (out-of-print)

Supplement No. 5
Cross Index of Synonyms and Trade Names in Volumes 1 to 36 of the *IARC Monographs*
1985; 259 pages (out-of-print)

Supplement No. 6
Genetic and Related Effects: An Updating of Selected *IARC Monographs* from Volumes 1 to 42
1987; 729 pages

Supplement No. 7
Overall Evaluations of Carcinogenicity: An Updating of *IARC Monographs* Volumes 1–42
1987; 440 pages

Supplement No. 8
Cross Index of Synonyms and Trade Names in Volumes 1 to 46 of the *IARC Monographs*
1990; 346 pages (out-of-print)

All IARC publications are available directly from IARCPress, 150 Cours Albert Thomas, F-69372 Lyon cedex 08, France (Fax: +33 4 72 73 83 02; E-mail: press@iarc.fr).

IARC Monographs and Technical Reports are also available from the World Health Organization Distribution and Sales, CH-1211 Geneva 27 (Fax: +41 22 791 4857) and from WHO Sales Agents worldwide.

IARC Scientific Publications, IARC Handbooks and IARC CancerBases are also available from Oxford University Press, Walton Street, Oxford, UK OX2 6DP (Fax: +44 1865 267782).

www.ingramcontent.com/pod-product-compliance
Lightning Source LLC
Chambersburg PA
CBHW081238220326
41597CB00023BA/4029

* 9 7 8 9 2 8 3 2 1 2 7 3 7 *